Community-based Nursing Practice:

Learning Through Students' Stories

D1476406

Community-based Nursing Practice:

Learning Through Students' Stories

By

Jeanne M. Sorrell, RN, PhD

Professor

College of Nursing and Health Science

George Mason University

Fairfax, Virginia

and

Georgine M. Redmond, RN, EdD

Associate Professor

College of Nursing and Health Science

George Mason University

Fairfax, Virginia

F. A. DAVIS COMPANY • Philadelphia

F. A. Davis Company
1915 Arch Street
Philadelphia, PA 19103
www.fadavis.com

Printed in the United States of America

Last digit indicates print number: 10 9 8 7 6 5 4 3 2 1

Acquisitions Editor: Joanne Patzek DaCunha, RN, MSN
Developmental Editor: Ron Watson
Production Editor: Bette Haitsch
Designer: Melissa Walters
Cover Designer: Louis J. Forgione

As new scientific information becomes available through basic and clinical research, recommended treatments and drug ther-apies undergo changes. The author(s) and publisher have done everything possible to make this book accurate, up to date, and in accord with accepted standards at the time of publication. The authors, editors, and publisher are not responsible for errors or omissions or for consequences from application of the book, and make no warranty, expressed or implied, in regard to the contents of the book. Any practice described in this book should be applied by the reader in accordance with professional stan-dards of care used in regard to the unique circumstances that may apply in each situation. The reader is advised always to check product information (package inserts) for changes and new information regarding dose and contraindications before ad-ministering any drug. Caution is especially urged when using new or infrequently ordered drugs.

Library of Congress Cataloging-in-Publication Data
 Community-based nursing practice : learning through students' stories / [edited by]
Jeanne Sorrell and Georgine Redmond.
      p. cm.
  Includes bibliographical references and index.
  ISBN 0-8036-0607-9
  1. Community health nursing—United States. 2. Community health nursing—Canada. I.
 Title: Community based nursing practice. II. Sorrell, Jeanne Merkle. III. Redmond,
 Georgine.

RT98 .C627 2001
610.73′43′0973—dc21

                                                              2001028654

DEDICATION

We dedicate this book to our husbands, Greg Sorrell and Bob Redmond, whose lives have overlapped ours so meaningfully in the process of completing the circle of this book.

And to our students, for sharing their stories
That speak to the essence of nursing in community-based practice.

Jeanne Sorrell and Georgine Redmond

Growing, we move through worlds of differences,
The cycles and circles of a life,
Fulfilled by overlapping with the lives of others.

Mary Catherine Bateson, in *Full Circles, Overlapping Lives*

PREFACE

For those of you who read this book either willingly or unwillingly (assigned reading!), it is important to know that this book did not grow out of an esoteric exercise in some ivory tower. This book, rather, is the outgrowth of our dedicated faculty members faced with the challenge of making a major curriculum shift to respond to real-world needs and a real-world change in the delivery of health care in our society.

The decade of the 1990s brought major changes in the delivery of health care, unraveling health-care expectations, and even entitlements. Those changes mandated a transformation in the education of health-care providers. The status quo is always easier to maintain; change is always threatening. The College of Nursing and Health Science faculty at George Mason University did not take these challenges lightly.

Although care in the community has always been part of nursing education, the shift to a community-based curriculum illustrated by this book was a quantum change. Not only did this shift involve knowledge, skill, and expertise, but it also struck at the very fabric of what many believed to be the basic foundations of nursing education. The move to a community-based curriculum involved a change in the culture of our college and in our beliefs about how and where students learn to become professional nurses.

This book will bring you many insights, whether read cover to cover or in selected sections. Each chapter represents an actual part of a curriculum that serves more than 500 students each year at George Mason University. Each chapter was written by a faculty member who was actively engaged in developing the curriculum, courses, and student experiences detailed in this book.

The book is designed for students in both associate degree and baccalaureate nursing programs and provides information that is unique to community-based practice, specifically in the United States and Canada. It is meant to supplement, rather than replace, population-based community health texts. Stories from students and faculty are integrated throughout the text to engage you in learning practical information that you will need in your practice.

The first section of the text provides basic information to help you differentiate between community health and community-based nursing in both the United States and Canada, to understand concepts related to primary health care, and to gain a beginning understanding of various approaches to community-based nursing with diverse groups of clients. The second section of the text focuses on selected primary-care skills that you will need in your work with clients in the community, such as skills in teaching, communication, and working with families and other groups. The final section of the text features application of community-based concepts in specific community sites, such as an elementary school, a campus community, and a faith community.

I would like to think that as you read and learn important concepts in this text, you can identify with the stories that our students and faculty have shared with you.

Rita M. Carty
Dean, College of Nursing and Health Science
George Mason University

ACKNOWLEDGMENTS

We gratefully acknowledge the many persons who have contributed to the completion of this book. We cannot possibly list all of these special individuals, but would like to specifically acknowledge the following:

Dean Rita M. Carty for her vision and support of the many phases of the project;

Our research assistants, Shelly Kollar, Judith A. Rogers, Pamela R. Cangelosi, and Nancy Sloan for their resourcefulness and attention to detail;

Nasim Khawaja and Luanne Pearce for their careful typing of the manuscripts and willingness to work without watching the clock;

Laura Sikes for her persistence in seeking out the right picture;

Our talented editor, Joanne DaCunha, for her unflagging enthusiasm for the project;

Noelle Barrick, Production Editor, for her patience and attention to detail;

And, finally, our colleagues and friends, who never seemed to doubt that our efforts would arrive at a successful ending.

Jeanne Sorrell and Georgine Redmond

Acknowledgments for Student Stories and Photos

We would like to acknowledge the following students, including those who wish to remain anonymous, for their contributions.

Students from George Mason University

Daniell Aldrich	Janet Garcia	Leslie Jo Mitchell
Kathy Alexander	Elaine Grazziano	Mariam Mokhtarzada
Rosalyn J. Alvarez	Michael Holland	Felicia Parkman
Ramona Beal	Heidi Hoff Johnson	Nicole Price
Christi Bradley	Joan Johnson	Deborah Quinn
Christine Brocious-Zaccaria	Georgiana Junor	Brenda Reed
Jennifer Marie Brothers	Prudence Karangera	Lori Sandstrom
Michelle Cantey	Jonathan Laryea	Florie A. Spellerberg
Sherlyn Carter	Jennifer Lawrence	Richard Tatic
Linda Torres Catzoela	Anne Lohr	Huyen Thai
Karen Emily Downey	Tammy McBride	Laura Tissinger
Susan Fentress	Kim McCartney	Kelly Ann Williams
Karen Fish	Shawn A. McManamey	

Students from the University of Windsor

Carolyn Ballantine
Miranda Burgess
Anu Chopra

Bean Duguay
Laura Sollazzo

Additional Ackowledgments
Shelley Kollar
Rose Powell
Shelley Kollar
Christine Sorrell

CONTRIBUTORS

Pamela A. Avent, MSN, RN
Assistant Professor
Northern Virginia Community College
Annandale, Virginia

Christine T. Blasser, MSN, RN
Instructor
College of Nursing and Health Science
George Mason University
Fairfax, Virginia

M. Lucille Boland, MSN, RN
Assistant Professor
College of Nursing and Health Science
George Mason University
Fairfax, Virginia

Rosemarie C. Brenkus, MEd, RN
Assistant Dean for Student Academic Affairs
College of Nursing and Health Science
George Mason University
Fairfax, Virginia

Ann H. Cary, PhD, MPH, RN, A-CCC
Director, Institute for Research, Education,
and Consultation
American Nurses Credentialing Center
Washington, D.C.

Margaret J. Cofer, PhD, RN
Adjunct Faculty
College of Nursing and Health Science
George Mason University
Fairfax, Virginia

Charlene Yvonne Douglas, PhD, RN
Associate Professor
College of Nursing and Health Science
George Mason University
Fairfax, Virginia

Susan W. Durham, MPH, RN
Instructor
College of Nursing and Health Science
George Mason University
Fairfax, Virginia

Joyce A. Hahn, MSN, RN
Clinical Practice Coordinator
INOVA Health System
Fairfax, Virginia

Janet Fraser Hale, PhD, RN
Professor
Graduate School of Nursing
University of Massachusetts
Worcester, Massachusetts

Marie Kodadek, PhD, RN
Assistant Professor
College of Nursing and Health Science
George Mason University
Fairfax, Virginia

Joanne Langan, PhD, RN
Adjunct Assistant Professor
School of Nursing
St. Louis University
St. Louis, Missouri

Christena Langley, PhD, RN
Assistant Professor and Assistant Dean,
Undergraduate Programs
College of Nursing and Health Science
George Mason University
Fairfax, Virginia

Maureen Kirkpartick McLaughlin, MS, RN
Child Care Health Consultant
Doctoral Student
College of Nursing and Health Science
George Mason University
Fairfax, Virginia

Janet Schwab Merritt, MSN, RN
Instructor
College of Nursing and Health Science
George Mason University
Fairfax, Virginia

Margaret M. Moss, MSN, RN
Instructor
College of Nursing and Health Science
George Mason University
Fairfax, Virginia

Mary Narayan, RN, MSN, RC, CS, CTN
Education Coordinator
INOVA VNA Home Health
Alexandria, Virginia

Mary Anne Noble, DNSc, RN
Associate Professor
College of Nursing and Health Science
George Mason University
Fairfax, Virginia

Loretta Brush Normile, PhD, RN
Assistant Professor
College of Nursing and Health Science
George Mason University
Fairfax, Virginia

Georgine M. Redmond, RN, EdD
Former Associate Dean, Undergraduate
Programs
Associate Professor
College of Nursing and Health Science
George Mason University
Fairfax, Virginia

E. Francine Roberts, PhD, RN
Assistant Professor
College of Nursing and Health Science
George Mason University
Fairfax, Virginia

Mary Cipriano Silva, PhD, RN, FAAN
Professor
College of Nursing and Health Science
George Mason University
Fairfax, Virginia

Jeanne M. Sorrell, PhD, RN
Coordinator, PhD in Nursing Program
Professor
College of Nursing and Health Science
George Mason University
Fairfax, Virginia

Lynnette Leeseberg Stamler, PhD, RN
Associate Professor and Director
Collaborative BScN Program
Nipissing University
North Bay, Ontario, Canada

REVIEWERS

Ida Androwich, RN, PhD, FAAN
Associate Professor
BSN, MSN, & PhD Programs
Loyola University of Chicago
Maywood, Illinois

Carol Alvates Brooks, RN, DNSc
Associate Professor
BSN, MSN, & Post-Master's Programs
Syracuse University
Syracuse, New York

Rosemary Kohl, RN, MSN
Clinical Nurse Specialist, Medical Care Program
BSN and Inservice Education
London Health Sciences Centre
London, Ontario, Canada

Patricia A. Gonser, RN, PhD
Associate Professor
MSN Program
University of Southern Mississippi
Meridian, Mississippi

John R. Lowe, RN, PhD
Assistant Professor
BSN & MSN Programs
Florida International University
Fort Lauderdale, Florida

M. Peggy MacLeod, RN, MN
Associate Professor
BSN Program
College of Nursing
University of Saskatchewan
Saskatoon, Saskatchewan, Canada

Sheila Favro Marks, RN, MS
Chair, Department of Nursing
RN-BSN Program
Florida Southern College
Lakeland, Florida

Eleanor McClelland, RN, MPH, PhD
Associate Professor
BSN, MSN, and Continuing Education
Programs
The University of Iowa
College of Nursing
Iowa City, Iowa

Nancy J. Michela, RN, C, MS
Associate Professor
BSN Program
Russell Sage College
Troy, New York

Anne K. Moshtael, RN, BSN
Nursing Instructor
LPN Program
Macon Technical Institute
Macon, Georgia

Linda Pearce, RN, C, MEd, CDE, CPNA
Consultant
Clinical Practice
Brandon, Mississippi

Patricia Schafer, RN, PhD
Associate Professor
BSN, Diploma, MSN Programs
Carlow College
Pittsburgh, Pennsylvania

Julie A. Slack, RN, BSN, MSN(c)
Instructor of Nursing
Dixie College
LPN program
St. George, Utah

Patricia Torsella, RN, DNSc
Associate Professor
BSN & MSN Programs
Bloomsburg University
Bloomsburg, Pennsylvania

Carol Zeller, RN, MSN
Nursing Instructor
ADN Program
College of Marin
Kentfield, California

Contents

Section 1
General Concepts of Community-based Practice

Section 2
Applying Primary-care Skills for Community-based Practice

General Concepts of Community-based Practice

CHAPTER 1

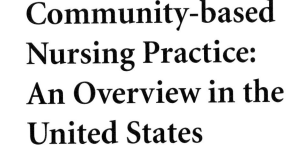

Community-based Nursing Practice: An Overview in the United States

Christena Langley

LEARNING OBJECTIVES

1) Outline the historical development of community-based nursing care.

2) Differentiate community-based nursing practice from nursing in acute and public health settings.

3) Explore the concepts of community, and community, neighborhood, and home assessment.

4) Describe nursing roles in community-based health care.

5) Discuss community-based nursing care across the life span with individuals, families, and groups.

6) Examine changes in nursing practice resulting from community-based practice research.

COMMUNITY-BASED NURSING: A STUDENT'S PERSPECTIVE

I really love the hospital setting, and I just couldn't imagine anything as interesting . . . or anywhere else that I could make as much difference in the life of my client. Community nursing is such a different arena than acute care. It takes a big attitude

shift . . . community nursing involves long-term interventions that must be followed over time, and many times the results of the nurse's actions may not be seen. . . . I think this field requires a lot of patience and aggressiveness to ensure that clients are well cared for. . . .

I was especially nervous about home visiting. Having never done home visits in any clinical situation, I was anxious about going into the home of someone I'd never met and "interfering" with their life. Why would this person want to listen to a complete stranger, let alone a student, talk about how they should change their health patterns?

The first home visit client assigned to me was a 3-month-old infant, born 2 months prematurely. I was to deal with developmental delays and teach the parents how to encourage the growth and development of their infant. But in addition, the family was of another culture (I was worried about language barriers) and the mother had had a positive Purified Protein Derivative (PPD) and had just started isoniazid (INH) therapy when her pregnancy ended. Not exactly the "simple newborn" I had expected!

I was grateful that I was able to make the first visit with an experienced nurse. She helped locate the family's home and began to develop a trusting relationship. It helped me to see her interact with the baby and his mother. My client's mother was anxious about being a good parent, but also lonely and concerned because she had no transportation and felt housebound during the day. She was an extremely involved parent with many questions that she wanted answered.

One important thing that I learned through this experience is the value of really knowing my material. Many times I had to do research to find answers to questions. Nurses working in the community are resources to their clients, and it is important to be well versed in their problem areas or know where to get the answers to their questions. I found networking was very important. Other students in my clinical group were also visiting families with preterm infants and we were able to collaborate in finding valuable resources . . . and in teaching ourselves to be more able caregivers.

My obstetrics textbook and other textbooks were good for information, but those sources helped me more than they helped my client. The public library was a great resource. I used "normal people" books about preterm infants, infant nutrition, and play and sleep patterns to show my client's mother important and easy concepts. She appreciated everything I taught her about "adjusted developmental patterns" because of her great concern that her baby was behind already. We talked a lot about nutrition and play patterns to increase his motor development.

I was very excited when I was able to participate in a physical therapy session with the infant and his therapist. The therapist reinforced everything I had been talking about with my client! I was so proud that the baby wasn't as far behind as his gestational age.

As the semester is ending, I look back and laugh that I was so scared to go on that first solo home visit. Clients that we home visit are incredibly grateful that we are taking the time to come and see them and share our resources. With this particular family, I know I made a difference not only in the baby's life but also with the mom by supporting her with her INH medication and teaching her about tuberculosis (TB). To show her appreciation, she has made many interesting foods for me. She always tells me how much the baby enjoys my visits, and I know she does, too.

Students often begin their experiences in community-based nursing with some of the same feelings of apprehension expressed in the preceding student's story. They wonder why they are placed in nontraditional settings outside the hospital environment when there are so many procedures and technologies that they want to learn and practice before they graduate from nursing school and seek out their first jobs. They often ask, "Why do I have to do this, when what I really want to know is how to care for postoperative open-heart surgery patients, how to assist in labor and delivery, how to care for patients in isolation, and how to treat trauma victims? Someday I want to be a nurse practitioner and work in an Emergency Department or a Medical ICU. That's where nursing is really exciting! How is this community-based rotation ever going to help me reach my goals?"

Once nursing students become actively involved in nursing care in the community, they begin to make the connections that our student telling the story made: They begin to see health and health care from the client's perspective, and they experience the continuum of health care through acute, community-based, and public health settings, which is critical to their professional development.

This textbook is intended to assist students in making that transition in thinking from acute care nursing to community-based health care that not only includes the client's use of acute care facilities, but also encompasses the client's health needs throughout the life span. This first chapter introduces some of the philosophical underpinnings of community-based health care and provides an overview of the roles of nursing in this dynamic field.

A BRIEF HISTORICAL PERSPECTIVE

Nursing in the United States began as "community-based" nursing. Self-trained women cared for the sick and dying, assisted women in laboring and delivering infants, and provided education to those without access to information about protecting the health of their families. The first hospitals were built during the late 1700s with the goal of preventing the spread of infectious diseases. Unfortunately, they were usually places of last resort for the poor or homeless who had no other resources available to them during bouts of serious illness. For the most part, across all socioeconomic classes, people were cared for in their homes by family members whenever possible. Physicians and nurses continued to be self-educated and trained through apprenticeships rather than through formal education programs.

In England in the late 1850s, Florence Nightingale published her work "Notes on Nursing: What It Is and What It Is Not," which for the first time made the distinction between "health nursing" and "sick nursing" (Buchholtz & Klainberg, 1998). Nightingale defined health nursing as assisting healthy persons outside of hospitals to remain free of disease, whereas sick nursing entailed helping those suffering from disease to regain their health. A few years later in the United States, Clara Barton worked with other untrained but dedicated women to provide nursing care to the Civil War-wounded in their communities—the battlefields. With minimal supplies and equipment, these nurses worked to protect their patients from the communicable diseases that were rampant and to treat their battle wounds.

In 1893, Lillian Wald, a trained nurse from a privileged background, made her first home visit in New York City in response to a request from a small child for help with her mother who, as it turned out, was hemorrhaging in her bed following childbirth. Wald resolved to help people in their homes. She began a district nursing service in New York City. She and other nurses lived in the neighborhood and let their neighbors know that they were there to help.

Through her outspoken activism, Wald served as an agent of change and brought national attention to the existence of grave health and social problems in the homes, schools, and work settings of urban families. She had a vision of nurses in the community linking families' social, economic, and health needs with the services that they needed to acquire or maintain health. She also envisioned the "health nursing" described by Florence Nightingale as being concerned with the health of the public rather than individuals or families.

At the turn of the century (1895–1910) 90 percent of health care occurred in the home. Now, 100 years later, health care is returning to home and other noninstitutional settings. A rapid expansion of health-care services developed between the 1940s and the 1980s with a burgeoning of medical technologies and pharmaceutical innovations that took more and more health care into hospital environments. In addition, the passage of Medicare and Medicaid during the 1960s contributed to increased health-care spending and the expansion of home-care services for the care of the homebound ill. Voluntary visiting nurses and official public health agencies expanded their home visiting programs as a result.

The 1960s marked the beginning emergence of "community nursing," as society became more concerned with social inequities. Community-based mental health programs came into being. The Economic Opportunity Act provided funding from the federal level for Head Start and neighborhood health centers. As understanding of the preventable aspects of several chronic diseases grew, an increasing number of clinical nurses moved out of hospitals to work in programs designed for the early detection and treatment of major health problems such as cardiovascular disease, diabetes, and cancer. The focus of care across all of these programs was the individual and family.

Through the late 1980s and early 1990s, other shifts in health care occurred. As public concern grew regarding quality, accessibility, and affordability of health care, the

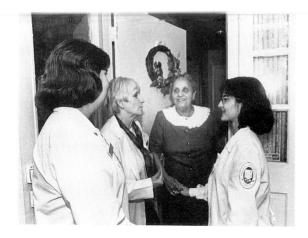

health-care system evolved into a managed-care system more attentive to health promotion and disease prevention activities, and treatment shifted from acute settings to ambulatory settings and a team approach to health-care delivery.

WHAT LIES AHEAD?

Now in a new century, health-care delivery will continue to change, bringing new opportunities to nurses ready to accept the challenges. As primary and preventive care continue in importance, our client populations will include both healthy and ill consumers. Preventive health care serves people of all ages and at all levels of health. Improving access to health care means bringing health services to people where they live, work, play, or worship through primary-care networks that support a continuum of care, including acute, community, and home-based health services.

Because managed care networks include acute care, ambulatory care, long-term care, and home-based services within one system of client services, nurses will be faced with the challenge of maintaining multiple skills in multiple settings (O'Neill & Pennington, 1996). Case management, health-promotion and disease-prevention skills, and principles of epidemiology, as well as excellent physical assessment skills, will be crucial elements of the repertoire of the 21st-century nurse. Critical thinking and excellent therapeutic communication skills will be

essentials for professional nurses working in multiple settings with diverse client populations. Nurses prepared during their basic nursing education for responsibilities across the continuum of care will have an advantageous beginning for their careers.

THE CONTINUUM OF CARE

Because community-based nursing care is part of the continuum of health-care services, it is important to understand the similarities and differences among services offered by acute care centers, community-based organizations, and public health agencies. In addition, there has been international discussion of the significance of primary health care for the world's population. Nursing students need to understand the differences between the concepts of primary health care and primary care (Barnes et al., 1995). **Primary care** is the first contact in a given episode of illness that leads to a decision regarding the course of action needed to resolve the problem (Starfield 1992). Much of primary care is aimed at promotion of health, early diagnosis of disease, and prevention of illness for individuals and families. Clients of primary-care providers have direct access to the appropriate source of care for maintenance of health over time. Family practice physicians and nurse practitioners are the major providers of primary care in the United States. In contrast, **primary health care** refers to the international consensus reached during the World Health Assembly meeting in 1979 outlining essential health services for all people throughout the world. Population-focused health-care providers are responsible for ensuring that all members of communities receive these essential services. Table 1–1 examines several aspects of community-based nursing as compared to acute care and population-focused nursing as outlined in the nursing literature (Baldwin et al., 1998; Barnes et al., 1995; Clarke & Cody, 1994; Deal, 1994; Rothman, 1990; Zotti et al., 1996).

When thinking about this continuum of care, it is important to understand that the categories of acute care, community-based care, and population-focused care are not mutually exclusive. Health-care professionals working in acute care are mindful of the collectivity of their clients as well as their individual needs. When an acute-care nurse begins to see a number of clients admitted to

Table 1-1

Comparison of Acute, Community-based, and Population-focused Care

	ACUTE-CARE NURSING	COMMUNITY-BASED NURSING	POPULATION-FOCUSED NURSING
What is the goal of intervention?	Immediate treatment of an individual with an existing condition or problem.	Managing acute or chronic conditions while promoting self-care among individuals and their families.	Health promotion and disease prevention among aggregates and populations through the core functions of assessment, policy development, and assurance (may sometimes involve providing care to high-risk individuals; i.e., those with communicable diseases).
What is the underlying philosophy?	*Episodic Care*—treatment of individuals for an acute episode of an illness, for the sequelae of an accident or trauma, or during recovery from surgery. Concerned with individual autonomy.	*Direct Primary Care*—may be preventive, curative, or rehabilitative. Care of individuals, families, and groups with the goal of contributing to the health of the larger population. Uses the Human Ecological Model—understanding the client within his/her social networks. Supports and promotes individual and family autonomy.	*Primary Health Care for Communities*—(as defined by the World Health Organization in 1978 at Alma Ata USSR). Calls for the universal distribution of these essential services: 1. Education for the identification and prevention/control of prevailing health problems 2. Proper food supplies and nutrition 3. Adequate supply of safe water and basic sanitation 4. Maternal and child health services including family planning 5. Immunization against the major infectious diseases, prevention and control of locally endemic diseases 6. Appropriate treatment of common diseases using appropriate technology 7. Promotion of mental health 8. Provision of essential drugs (All eight are considered valid for all countries, but are applied differently throughout the world.) Individual's rights may be sacrificed for the greater good of the larger community.
Who is the client?	Ill individuals within families and/or social systems.	Individuals and their families at various points on the wellness-illness continuum. Family members and significant others are included in decisions and in designing and evaluating services.	Aggregate groups and communities through population-based community outreach and education.

Table 1–1

Comparison of Acute, Community-based, and Population-focused Care—cont'd

	ACUTE-CARE NURSING	**COMMUNITY-BASED NURSING**	**POPULATION-FOCUSED NURSING**
Where is the client located?	Inpatient and outpatient units of hospitals and long-term care facilities where personnel are specialized and use complex and sophisticated equipment and materials for diagnostic and treatment purposed. May involve emergency or intensive care.	In home, neighborhood, and community environments. Homes, schools, occupational settings, churches, recreational facilities, specialty ambulatory care clinics, or managed care organizations. The nurse assists clients and their significant others in moving through networks of care. For example, a client receiving instructions for foot care from a nurse in a community-based Diabetes Clinic may enter the hospital for surgery, be discharged to home care provided by the community-based clinic nurse, and be seen at the hospital outpatient clinic for surgical follow-up.	Public Health Departments serving the population of a defined geographical area (i.e., census tracts, zip codes, state, region of a country, or an entire country).
How is the client located?	Individuals seek out services or are brought to services as the result of emergency situations.	Through referral and case finding as well as clients who seek services.	Referral and case finding. Through consultation with other providers for the good of the larger population.
What type of service is offered?	Direct care of clients.	A mixture of direct and indirect services.	Predominantly indirect services.
What level of prevention dominates?	Secondary and tertiary.	Primary, secondary, and tertiary.	Predominately primary with some secondary.
What are the diagnostic tools used?	History taking and physical assessment X-ray examination Laboratory testing (Done with individual clients)	Same as in acute care, plus, home and neighborhood assessment Family assessment Cultural assessment	Epidemiological techniques such as community assessment, diagnosis, planning, and evaluation Tracking disease patterns Collecting morbidity and mortality data Investigating infectious disease outbreaks

the medical unit of a community hospital with the same antibiotic-resistant infectious disease, the nurse analyzes and reports this data to the appropriate resource person for follow-up. Excellent care that improves the health of individuals and families will also improve the health of the population in general. In turn, nurses working in population-focused public health departments are ever mindful of the health needs of individuals and families without access to services. Box 1–1 applies "continuum of care."

Table 1–1

Comparison of Acute, Community-based, and Population-focused Care—cont'd

	ACUTE-CARE NURSING	COMMUNITY-BASED NURSING	POPULATION-FOCUSED NURSING
What are the primary tools for intervention?	Medications, surgery, radiation therapy	Patient counseling and education	Community education Immunizations Sanitation inspection and licensure of food supplies and water systems Tracing exposures to communicable disease ("contact tracing")
What are the secondary tools for intervention?	Counseling and education of clients	Case management	Case management (for medically indigent populations such as children, HIV-infected individuals, TB, and STD clients) Health education Consultation and collaboration with community members

---

Box 1–1   Student Learning Activity

Continuum of Care

Elizabeth Moore is a student nurse visiting Mrs. Kelly, 74, who lives alone in a high-rise apartment. Mrs. Kelly suffers from diabetes and is insulin dependent. While performing the assessment, Elizabeth discovers a large area of ulceration on Mrs. Kelly's left foot. The wound is open and has a foul smell and exudate. Elizabeth finds that Mrs. Kelly has a low-grade fever. She contacts Mrs. Kelly's physician, who makes arrangements for hospitalization. How does this case example reflect your understanding of the continuum of care?

COMMUNITY ASSESSMENT

Regardless of the setting in which they work, nurses need to understand the concepts of community and community assessment. For the nurse working in an acute-care facility, the community may be the geographic area surrounding the hospital.

Although it may seem to have no significance to the nursing care provided in the hospital, the surrounding community is the source of patients and staff members. The resources within that community may very well provide crucial follow-up services to clients after discharge from the hospital.

Often **community** is defined simply as a group, population, or cluster of people with at least one common characteristic, such as geographic location, occupation, ethnicity, or health concern (Anderson & McFarlane, 1996). In community-based nursing, the community is the unit of service. For example, if you are working in a prenatal clinic, all of the pregnant women in your area are your clients and represent the community that you serve. If the clinic also offers pregnancy testing and family planning services, your clients may include all women of childbearing age in your catchment area. In community-based settings, the

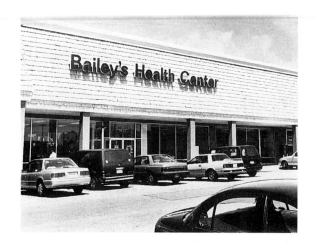

providers of care are concerned not only with the clients who present themselves for services, but also with the larger population of potential or at-risk clients.

How do nurses working in community-based settings know their community? A crucial piece of community-based nursing is ongoing community assessment, a term that is often used to encompass the whole of the nursing process as applied to the community (Arnold, 1998). Community assessment is, therefore, the process of systematically determining the

community's health status, identifying real or potential health concerns, developing plans of intervention, initiating activities to implement the plan, and evaluating the outcomes of the interventions for evidence of success.

Part of the challenge for nursing students assigned for a brief period of time to a community-based clinical rotation is becoming adequately acquainted with the community to feel competent in providing nursing care. Anderson and McFarlane (1996) have outlined the critical components of community assessment. These are the population or people (the core of the community), the surrounding physical environment, and the subsystems within the community. These subsystems are the interdependent service systems that are available to the residents of the community. Table 1–2 outlines the aspects of these components of community assessment that are most valuable to community-based health care providers.

Community assessment is accomplished through a variety of sources of information. The nurse can use observation by walking, driving a car, or riding the bus through the community. This is called conducting a "windshield survey." Just as head-to-toe inspection of a client presenting in acute care provides an impression of that client and

Table 1–2

Components of Community Assessment

POPULATION	PHYSICAL ENVIRONMENT	SUBSYSTEMS
Demographics: Age distribution, marital status, ethnicity, employment, and income levels	Climate Terrain Flora and fauna	Recreation Safety and transportation
Vital Statistics: Birth and death rates	Natural and political boundaries Housing	Communication Education
Morbidity Data: Rates of diseases within the community	Locations of businesses Air and water quality	Health and social services Economics
Values, Beliefs, and Religious Practices	Parks Traffic patterns	Politics Government

his or her health state, this inspection of the community provides a cursory first impression and assists in getting acquainted with the overall topography of the community as well as the locations of community services. This process often eases students' minds about the safety of the neighborhood as well.

Other sources of data include the local Chamber of Commerce, the Internet, and library reference rooms for census and other statistical data. Key informants in the various agencies of local government are also helpful in gathering information about the community and its health needs.

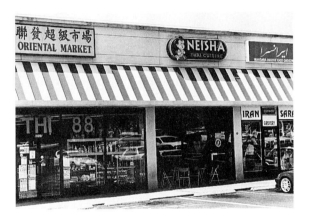

It is important for the community-based nurse to be mindful of the environmental hazards that have been associated with health problems. The *Healthy People 2010 Objectives: Draft for Public Comment* (United States Department of Health and Human Services, 1998) includes 34 priority areas in environmental health. These objectives cover a broad range of exposure media including air, water, and soil and target a number of pollutants such as radon, toxic chemicals, industrial waste, and lead. Several of the objectives relate to healthy homes and healthy communities.As nurses travel through communities, they need to be aware of evidence of these types of health risks. Community-based nurses often work closely with public health sanitarians to ensure the safety of their communities.

Here is one student's description of her first experience with community assessment:

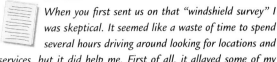

When you first sent us on that "windshield survey" I was skeptical. It seemed like a waste of time to spend several hours driving around looking for locations and services, but it did help me. First of all, it allayed some of my fears. This was a new geographic area to me—I've never been a city person and I was worried about safety.

It was comforting to see mothers walking with their babies in strollers, older people out walking their dogs, and businessmen and women going out to lunch in groups. There is a lot of traffic and everything's very congested. A lot of the businesses and houses look very old and are very close together. But it wasn't as scary as I had imagined. I also found that later in the semester when I went to make home visits I remembered streets we had used during the windshield survey—I think that saved me time and kept me from getting lost frequently.

When we reported our findings on resources and services in this community, as well as the morbidity and mortality data, I found myself making mental comparisons to the county where I live. This helped me figure out ideas for my health education project that might or might not be useful for this population.

Community Assessment in Daily Practice

The nurses in a tuberculosis treatment and prevention clinic were concerned that in the past year they had seen six clients newly diagnosed with active TB whose addresses were within a few blocks of each other. None of the three nurses was familiar with the neighborhood, so they decided to conduct a windshield survey of the area. They discovered a small cluster of older garden apartments with a number of extended families living together. Through home visits to one or two of their clients, they learned that the people living in these apartments socialized together, shared food, and often baby-sat for each other's children. Through their visits and interviews, they were able to establish opportunities to offer TB screening and education to the residents regarding health practices to prevent the spread of communicable diseases, including tuberculosis. If they had not stepped out of the clinic to see where their clients lived, they would not have identified the need for these important nursing services. Box 1–2 allows you to complete a community assessment.

Box 1–2   Student Learning Activity

Community Assessment

Take 2 weeks to conduct a community assessment. Begin by walking or driving through your locality and observing the following:

Who do you see on the streets?

_____

_____

_____

How congested are the streets? Is public transportation available?

_____

_____

_____

_____

_____

What types of housing are available? (apartments, town homes, single-family dwellings, farms, trailers, etc.)

_____

_____

_____

_____

_____

Where are the parks, schools, community centers, and shopping centers?

_____

_____

_____

Describe what is most striking about the community.

Now locate some information about the population. Use census data to determine:

Age distribution: Employment status:

Ethnicity: Income levels:

How does the data for your community compare with the rest of your state?

_____

_____

_____

How does your community compare with the nation?

_____

_____

What are the leading causes of illness and death in your community?

_____

_____

Where do the people in your community go for health care?

_____

_____

What other information would you like to have about the community?

_____

_____

Neighborhood and Home Assessment

One of the most important methods of interventions by community-based nurses is home visitation. As more health-care services become available through ambulatory and outpatient facilities and hospital stays are shortened, clients have required more nursing services, both direct and indirect, in their homes. Visiting clients in their homes provides an environment conducive to accomplishing health education and care coordination goals by involving the whole family and facilitating the development of self-care among family members (Deal, 1994; Olds & Kitzman, 1990). In addition, direct observation of family interactions as well as their living conditions support tailored nursing interventions that are realistic and useful. Therefore, it is extremely important that the community-based nurse become skilled in home and neighborhood assessment as well as assessment of the broader community. Addressing areas of concern, especially safety issues, is an important part of the nurse's role in community-based practice.

As community-based nurses travel to the homes of their clients, they are actively involved in the daily assessment of the neighborhoods in which their clients reside. Some important aspects of the neighborhood to consider are:
- Convenience of drug stores, grocery stores, schools, and parks
- Location of fire, police, and rescue services
- Lighting of streets at night
- Condition of streets, pavement, sidewalks, and curbs
- Presence of crosswalks
- Evidence of stray animals

Within the clients' home, it is important to notice:
- Evidence of unsafe debris in the yard or in the hallways of apartments
- Overall size and spatial arrangements of rooms
- Adequacy of heating and ventilation systems
- Safety of floors, windows, stairwells, elevators, electrical wiring and appliances, pipes, and radiators
- Availability of electricity, lighting fixtures, hot and cold running water, and telephone services
- Safekeeping of medications, firearms, and kitchen knives
- Presence of working smoke detectors and fire extinguishers
- Adequacy of bathroom and kitchen facilities
- Safe handling of pets

Although community-based nurses are not directly responsible for ensuring the safety of their clients' homes and neighborhoods, they are part of the team of health workers collaborating to improve the health of clients in all settings. Community-based nurses are also in a position to take advantage of the "teaching moments" in relation to home and neighborhood issues as they work with clients. Box 1–3 will help you to think about teaching moments.

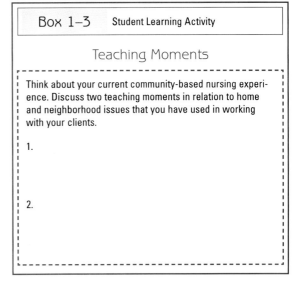

Box 1–3   Student Learning Activity

Teaching Moments

Think about your current community-based nursing experience. Discuss two teaching moments in relation to home and neighborhood issues that you have used in working with your clients.

1.

2.

NURSING ROLES IN COMMUNITY-BASED PRACTICE

Nurses working in community-based nursing share the same roles as their colleagues working in acute-care or population-focused nursing. They are providers of care, members of their profession, and coordinators of care; however, in community-based practice, the nursing roles of coordinator of care and member of the profession may predominate over the direct provision of care. Table 1–3 provides examples of activities of community-based nurses within each of these roles. What other activities can you think of that would be appropriate for a community-based nurse in your setting?

Table 1–3

Examples of the Roles of Community-based Nurses

PROVIDER OF CARE	MEMBER OF THE PROFESSION	COORDINATOR OF CARE
Primary Prevention—Teaching and counseling clients across the life span.	Collaborating with other professionals in interdisciplinary teams.	Facilitating clients' transitions between hospital and long-term care or home, so that care is continuous and distributed over time.
Secondary Prevention—Screening activities and follow-up advice in prenatal, child health, occupational, spiritual, and recreational settings. Community-based nurse-midwives deliver babies in birthing centers.	Collaborating with and supervising a large corp of allied health providers, such as home-health aides, companions, translators, lay visitors (for example, directly-observed therapy with TB clients).	Assisting clients to locate resources and coordinate services. Working with parents and school staff on behalf of children.
Tertiary Prevention—Home visits and educational programs to improve living with chronic illnesses.	Interacting with community groups and volunteers as participants in program planning, execution, and evaluation.	Case management in managed care settings. Interpreting care options and services to clients.

A STUDENT DESCRIBES HER ROLES IN COMMUNITY-BASED NURSING PRACTICE

One of the main nursing interventions in the community is the home visit. Families often present with various problems that need to be addressed by a multitude of sources. Your job as a home-health nurse in the community is to be aware of the surrounding environment, including resources for the whole family. You may have to refer a young grandchild to an immunization clinic or a teenager to a maternity clinic while visiting an elderly client . . . you need to know where thrift shops and used furniture stores are, as well as drugstores that deliver. You might have to locate Meals-on-Wheels or Respite Care.

Collaboration is also a big part of home-health service. It is important for the nurse to be involved with the other team members who visit—the social worker, the occupational therapist, the physical therapist, the home-health aide, or the companion service. Each of these people has a piece of the family's story. The clients depend on the nurse to teach them how to use resources, practice health-promoting behaviors, and act independently in their health care.

As you build your experiences in community-based settings, you will develop your skills in case management, patient education, collaborative practice, and advocacy for individuals and families. You will also gain an increasing understanding of health and illness conditions in clients of all ages and multiple cultures. Often, nursing experiences in community-based settings bring together the pieces of knowledge that students have gathered in more acute settings into a wholeness of information about their clients. Rather than being a less challenging area that depends little on scientific information, community-based nursing actually demands a synthesized understanding of nursing science, pathophysiology, epidemiology, and family and group dynamics. All of the relevant material can be shared with clients in layperson's terms so that they can understand and use the information to enhance their self-care practices. As generalists, community-based nurses must be well versed to answer questions that frequently arise spontaneously. They must also recognize when they cannot answer a question and need to consult additional sources. The next section of this chapter presents stories written by nursing students to portray their experiences in community-based nursing practice.

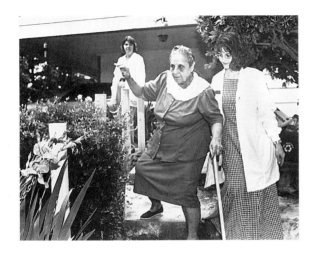

that the baby was born with seizures of unknown origin, and that they were in need of county services. I accompanied my nurse mentor on the first visit. This very experienced nurse brought formula, diapers, and me.

The first visit was to get acquainted and to determine the needs of mother and baby. We discovered that they needed a lot! The mother was still covered by her parents' insurance, but the baby was not. The baby had spent several days in the neonatal intensive care unit (NICU) and was now being maintained on phenobarbital, but would require regular appointments with the neurologists and rehabilitation therapy for hypertonia. There would be medications and many tests to determine the cause of the seizures as well as to monitor his progress.

I began meeting weekly with baby and mother. She was a senior in high school and a nondriver. Together, we arranged for the baby to receive Medicaid and Women, Infants, and Children (WIC) services; to be seen by the neurologist, pediatrician, and rehab; for mom to have a postpartum checkup and investigate family planning options. The mother also needed education on everything from recognizing seizure activity in an infant to medication administration, formula preparation, and bathing techniques.

As I spent time with this family, I was able to garner their trust. I showed them the way to much needed help and to independence with their health care. I felt so exhilarated because I was able to assist this family with problems that were staggering for them.

This experience changed my outlook on community-based nursing because I had no idea that it could be so personal and gratifying. It made me consider that in hospital nursing, when patients leave we really lose track of them. We treat them for one tiny moment in their lives, and then, they're gone.

Community-based Nursing Practice throughout the Life Span of Clients

One of the most enjoyable aspects of community-based nursing practice is the variety of clients encountered. Unlike acute-care facilities where clients are assigned rooms based on their conditions, gender, and often age, clients in the community present in a more randomized fashion. Community-based nurses often describe themselves as "generalists," or nurses who know "a little bit about a lot," as opposed to nurses working in acute care who often know a specialized area in great depth. Opportunities abound in the community to work with clients across the life span.

MAKING A DIFFERENCE AT THE BEGINNING OF A LIFE

When I began this clinical, I thought I knew what to expect. I was going to participate in ambulatory-care clinics for immunizations, cancer screening, well-baby checkups . . . that sort of thing. What took me by surprise was the opportunity to be a case manager. . . .

The first week of clinical I was assigned a client to home visit throughout the semester. She was an 18-year-old Hispanic woman who had just delivered her first baby. The only information that I had was that she was 42 weeks pregnant at delivery,

HELPING JUAN

My clinical assignment in community-based nursing was in an elementary school with a very diverse population. When I first visited my assigned class of kindergartners, I did not even notice Juan. At first glance, he appeared to be a rather typical, happy, healthy 5-year-old boy. But Juan had a secret that only a few people in the school knew. He was diagnosed with epilepsy when he was a year old and even with multiple medications and careful monitoring of dosages, he continued to have tonic/clonic seizures on a regular basis.

As I began working with his teacher and his mother, I was struck by something—this is still a "secret" disease. It's something we still whisper about. Although his mother agreed that the other children and teachers needed to be taught about the disease, she did not want Juan to be labeled. His teacher feared that he would have a seizure in class and the other children would be terrified by the experience. She also questioned her own ability to handle the situation if it arose in the classroom. She had never seen a seizure and knew little about it. She had been given a simple one-page instruction sheet from the physician about what to do during a seizure. She had no information about how to handle his classmates or their questions about a seizure episode. I was worried . . . Juan had had two seizures at home during the preceding weekend.

I started by trying to devise a teaching plan for the class. Where to start? What to cover? How could I teach 5-year-olds without frightening them? How much information is appropriate? How could I do this without upsetting Juan and his mother?

My answers came when I phoned the Epilepsy Foundation. They immediately sent an information packet for the teacher and provided me with facts about programs they already have in place for children in schools. I quickly realized that reinventing the wheel was not necessary. Many of the volunteers at the Epilepsy Foundation are epileptic themselves and understand the feelings and frustrations associated with misinformation and myths. Now I understood my job: connecting the school community with the foundation and other community resources. By having the experts come to teach, I benefited by learning about the disease and how to pass the knowledge to others.

Even though Juan has a serious health condition, he is lucky in a sense. His school and neighborhood are offering help. Although epilepsy is not a communicable disease, it still affects the family, the school, and the broader community. By educating everyone about epilepsy, the whole community will benefit. The laws about disabilities have changed and have opened opportunities for many people, but laws do not always change attitudes. Only education and awareness can do that.

WHEN YOU LEAST EXPECT IT!

I had a very interesting experience today. I went out with the Environmental Sanitarian to do restaurant inspec-

tions. I know that safe water and safe food are very important to health, but I have to admit, I was not at all sure what I would learn or how this related to my nursing education! It was great! First of all, I did learn about food handling and how important that is for the community's health, but I had a "nursing experience" within the experience. At one of our stops, one of the kitchen workers started sweating profusely even though it wasn't hot in the kitchen. She was shaky and looked awful—pale and clammy skin. I asked her whether she was feeling okay and she explained that she had recently been diagnosed with diabetes. She had taken her "pill" that morning but had not eaten anything because she never likes eating breakfast. After I got her juice and a snack, we talked for quite awhile about diet and medication and the importance of balance with diabetes. I surprised myself and her with what I knew. So I guess the teaching really is everywhere.

CULTURE

My client was a 37-year-old woman from Sudan who speaks a fair amount of English. She has two teenage sons that were born in the United States. Her social support network is not extensive, but she does have several neighbors (from her country) and relatives in the area. She does not work outside the home nor does she have government assistance.

The focus of our home visits was prevention of complications from a mitral valve prolapse repair as well as treatment for some gynecological abnormalities. Adherence to her medication regimen and keeping appointments with physicians has been inconsistent. My initial goal was to understand her reasons for her inconsistent self-care. After some rapport building, I learned that her husband is a very controlling man who does not always allow her to go to the doctor for scheduled appointments and who sometimes refuses to pick up her cardiac medications even when she has run out. She also shared with me some of her spiritual background and culture that is so important to her.

Her most recent missed appointment was for a cryoscopy that was scheduled as follow-up to several abnormal pap smears. My client and I discussed the procedure and its importance. After a 20-minute conversation, she asked, "Why do I need to do this?"

Very puzzled by this question, considering I had just explained it several times, I paid special attention to her body lan-

guage and facial expression during her question. She seemed to be shocked or surprised rather than inquisitive because of a lack of knowledge. I decided to use "therapeutic silence" and let her elaborate.

After a few minutes, she exclaimed, "But I only have one husband; how can this be possible?" A lightbulb came on for me. She went on to tell me in broken English that her husband was sure that the only way to have "such problems" was to have had multiple sexual partners. Now understanding her concerns and her husband's reasoning, I was able to assure her that there were other possible reasons. When she persisted in her skepticism, another lightbulb appeared for me. I said, "Perhaps Allah has given this to you, and we do not know why." This explanation was acceptable to her. She acknowledged that this was possible, that "Allah has his ways," and she was satisfied with this. She agreed to return to the clinic at the next available appointment time.

AN EPISODE WITH THE ELDERLY

When I went on my home visit to see Mrs. C., her husband asked me to check his blood pressure. He has been on medication for hypertension for several years. When I checked his pressure, it was quite high—180/120. He said he was still taking his daily medication, so I asked him to show me his pills. He brought the container to me and when we opened it I noticed that the pills were all cut in half. He explained that his wife thought that "her pressure was too high, too," and they were sharing his prescription. He could not afford to refill his prescription early, and they still had not been to her doctor about her blood pressure. They thought that if they each took some medicine, they would both improve their blood pressures a little bit and that would be good. I spent a long time explaining the importance of the right dose of medicine for each of them and the dangers of taking a medication for hypertension that had not been prescribed. I was really glad that I had asked to see that medicine container!

As you read these stories, what struck you about the roles the nursing students played? What particular skills did they demonstrate that enabled them to be successful in their endeavors with their clients? How would you have approached these clients?

COMMUNITY-BASED PRACTICE RESEARCH

As health-care services move from acute-care facilities into community-based settings, health-care research will also focus more extensively on the efficacy of services provided in the community. Two longitudinal studies published in recent years represent the significance of community-based practice research in the delivery of nursing care. Both studies have been accomplished through several years of work and have caused changes to be made in the delivery of community-based nursing care. This is typical of research dealing with preventive strategies. Unlike pharmaceutical and technological modalities that can produce change in the short term, preventive practices take a longer time frame to prove effective and are often confounded by other variables. In addition, both studies represent the human ecological model of intervention with clients through multiple approaches by an interdisciplinary team. In both studies, the approach to clients included social, economic, behavioral, and psychological approaches.

The first study evolved from a community assessment done by nurses (Mahon, et al., 1991). The results of their assessment indicated that only 60 percent of the pregnant women in their community received early prenatal care. Low-birth-weight infants, infant mortality, and pregnancy complications were more prevalent than in the surrounding population.

The nurses formed a network with women in the community and initiated de Madres a Madres, a volunteer-based primary health-care program to circulate information on prenatal care to neighborhood women (Fehir, 1996). The project eventually received funding from both the March of Dimes and W. K. Kellogg Foundation.

Community partnerships were forged with the general public, businesses, volunteer community members, and community-based nurses to increase outreach to Hispanic women to begin early prenatal care (Fehir, 1996; Mahon et al., 1991). Volunteer mothers from within the community learned to provide social support and guidance regarding community resources through the efforts of the community-based nurses. During the first year of

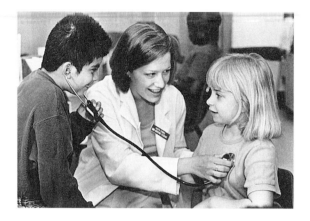

the program, these volunteers contacted over 2000 at-risk women. After five years, no low-birth-weight baby has been born to a woman working with a de Madres a Madres volunteer, and the infant mortality rate for the neighborhood has fallen from 16.5 to 11.4 (Fehir, 1996).

The second study was conducted over a 15-year period to examine the long-term effects of prenatal and early childhood home visitation by nurses on the life course of young mothers and their children (Olds et al., 1997). Child abuse and neglect were also studied within this population in comparison with the community at large. Data were compiled through self-reporting by the participants and a review of state records. The results revealed that teen mothers who received home visitation by nurses during the prenatal and early childhood period with their first infants had fewer subsequent pregnancies, less use of welfare, and fewer reported cases of child abuse and neglect.

As health-care services based in the community continue to grow in number, multidisciplinary research will need to increase in frequency. Linkages between health promotion strategies, the mix of team members, and health outcomes need to be examined closely. As you pursue clinical rotations in community-based settings, use the Internet and other library services to access research studies reporting on nursing activities in the community setting. Consider forming a journal club with some of your classmates to share information and discuss some of the research and its application to your clinical activities.

References

Anderson, E., & McFarlane, J. (1996). Community as partner: Theory and practice in nursing (2nd ed.). Philadelphia: Lippincott-Raven.

Arnold, J. (1998). Community assessment and diagnosis. In M. Klainberg, S. Holzemer, M. Leonard, & J. Arnold (Eds.), Community health nursing: An alliance for health. (pp. 139-172). New York: McGraw-Hill Nursing Core Series.

Baldwin, J. H., Conger, C., Abegglen, J. C., & and Hill, E. M. (1998). Population-focused and community-based nursing: Moving toward clarification of the concepts. Public Health Nursing, 15(1), 12-18.

Barnes, D., Eribes, C., Juarbe, T., Nelson, M., Proctor, S., Sawyer, L., Shaul, M., & Meleis, A. I. (1995). Primary health care and primary care: A confusion of philosophies. Nursing Outlook, 43(1), 7-16.

Buchholtz, S., & Klainberg, M. (1998). An historical perspective of community health nursing. In M. Klainberg, S. Holzemer, M. Leonard, & J. Arnold (Eds.), Community health nursing: An alliance for health. (pp. 23-36). New York: McGraw-Hill Nursing Core Series.

Clarke, P. N., & Cody, W. K. (1994). Nursing theory-based practice in the home and community: The crux of professional nursing education. Advances in Nursing Science, 7(2), 41-53.

Deal, L. W. (1994). The effectiveness of community health nursing interventions: A literature review. Public Health Nursing, 11, 315-325.

Fehir, J. (1996). De madres a madres: Community empowerment and health through collaboration partnerships and coalitions. In E. T. Anderson, & J. McFarlane (Eds.), Community as partner: Theory and practice in nursing (2nd ed.). Philadelphia: J. B. Lippincott.

Mahon, J., McFarlane, J., & Golden, K. (1991). De madres a madres: A community partnership for health. Public Health Nursing, 8, 15-19.

Olds, D. L., & Kitzman, H. (1990). Can home visitation improve the health of women and children at environmental risk? Pediatrics, 86, 108-116.

Olds, D. L., Eckenrode, J., Henderson, C. R., Kitzman, H., Powers, J., Cole, R., Sidora, K., Morris, P., Pettitt, L. M., & Luckey, D. (1997). Long term effects of home visitation on maternal life course and child abuse and neglect. Journal of the American Medical Association, 278, 637-643.

O'Neil, E. S., & Pennington, E. A. (1996). Preparing acute care nurses for community-based care. Nursing & Health Care: Perspectives on Community, 17(2), 62-65.

Rothman, N. L. (1990). Towards description: Public health nursing and community health nursing are different. Nursing & Health Care, 11, 481-483.

Starfield, B. (1992). Primary care: Concept, evaluation, and policy. New York: Oxford University Press.

United States Department of Health and Human Services. (1998). Healthy people 2010: Draft for public comment. Washington DC: Authors.

Zotti, M. E., Brown, P., & Stotts, R. C. (1996). Community-based nursing versus community health nursing: What does it all mean? Nursing Outlook, 44, 211-217.

CHAPTER 2

Community-based Primary Health Care and the Public Health Perspective

Janet Fraser Hale

LEARNING OBJECTIVES

1) Delineate the global and national historical development and rationale for population-based primary-care initiatives.

2) Define community-oriented primary health care.

3) Describe nurses' unique contributions to their role and function in community-based primary health care.

4) Apply an interdisciplinary model of primary care as a means of community assessment, intervention, and evaluation.

OVERVIEW OF HEALTH CARE IN THE UNITED STATES

From the end of World War II until the late 1970s, the method of health care delivery in the United States was relatively stable. Typically, health care was delivered and managed by doctors and nurses in small, locally based, usually nonprofit organizations. Care for most people was provided through a relatively unrestricted fee-for-serve insurance system generously financed to provide high levels of intervention with the most up-to-date technological supports. Unfortunately, this level, quality, and method of care delivery came at a high price. Now, as we enter the new millennium, we must accept that our health-care system is the most expensive in the world, although our morbidity and mortality statistics are not exemplary compared to many other developed countries.

Consequently, since the early 1980s, public and private initiatives have begun to emerge to control costs, leading to a redesign of how health care is delivered and financed in the United States. In 1993, the Clinton administration initiated dramatic health-care reform efforts to stop the continued exponential escalation of health-care costs in this country and to increase access to care for vulnerable populations. Although the efforts to enact comprehensive legislative reforms were not successful, they did force the country to focus on the issues of access, consumer satisfaction, quality, and cost of care, particularly for our medically underserved populations who either have no health insurance or who have health insurance, but no access to adequate health care.

This forced change in how we think about and view health care has resulted in a paradigm shift in health care and health professions education as follows:

- Managed care pressures providers to restrain costs and control health-care use.
- "For-profit" corporations have dramatically influenced the way hospitals and physician practices operate.
- Health care has moved from hospital-based, highly technological health care to community-based primary care (i.e., the current health-care system is moving health care out of the hospital).
- Our health-care system has moved from a system that encourages specialty practice to a system that recognizes the value and need for primary-care generalist professionals.
- We recognize the need to move from a primary focus on illness care to an emphasis on disease prevention and health promotion.
- Focus has moved from a primary concern for the individual who is identified as "sick" to the impact of that illness on the family (however, they may choose to define family) within the context of their community, as well as on the identified patient.
- Focus has moved from the "sick patient" to the concept of population-based behaviors and care recognizing and addressing the primary causes of morbidity and mortality within a given population.
- Focus has moved from a single organization or institution model to an integrated network or health systems model.
- Focus has moved from an illness/critical events management model to a health/life processes management model.
- Focus has moved from a privatized fee-for-service model to a capitated cost-managed model.

These concerns also initiated the effort for professional schools to realign their training and education to be consistent with the changing needs of the health-care delivery system. The Pew Health Professions Commission's 1998 report stresses the following:

- The health professions workforce should reflect the diversity of the nation's population.
- Health-care provider education should move from hospital focus to ambulatory care.
- Interdisciplinary competence should be required in all health professions educational programs.
- Health professions students and graduates should be encouraged to participate in public service.

For nursing education, the 1998 Pew report specifically suggests:

- The introduction of students to the importance of healthy lifestyles early in their program, emphasizing their responsibility for promoting health by serving as role models and resources for health information.
- Teaching principles of prevention, health promotion, risk reduction, and behavior change.
- Provision of community-based learning experiences in health promotion and self-management of health for defined groups, such as schoolchildren, employees, and church and civic groups.
- Provision of learning experiences that help students understand the link between prevention and the cost of health care.
- Focus more on ambulatory, long-term care, and community-based settings.

Nurses have historically had a valued impact on communities. Community/public health experiences have always been a part of baccalaureate education. As more and more health care is moving from hospitals to communities, nursing education at all levels (including graduate level) is incorporating more community-based care as a key component of the curriculum. Between 1980 and 1996, registered nurse (RN) employment increased 137 percent in ambulatory care, 116 percent in public and community health, and 64 percent in long-term care. Nursing education reform has been relatively slow to reflect these changes in RN practice (Pew, 1998, p. 63).

Here is a student's description of her early experiences with a health department:

My first experience with a health department was back in rural West Virginia when I was a very little girl. The health department was where we went for

our immunizations. It was at the health department that I first learned I was about to become a teenage pregnancy statistic during my senior year in high school. Everybody I knew went to the health department for shots, WIC, and birth control, and it seemed to me for most all health matters. Very rarely did people go to a regular doctor, only when they were really ill.

I was looking forward to my rotation in the health department. I am working in the very same place (albeit a different building) that I brought my daughter for her shots so she could go to preschool 22 years earlier. At the time, I was so ignorant about the importance of shots. I remember the Public Health Nurse (PHN) berating me because my child was so delinquent in her immunizations. The nurse wasn't trying to make me feel bad; I now realize that she was trying to educate me. I find it ironic that life has taken me full circle and now I'm the person talking to parents about the importance of getting those immunizations.

Therefore, in addition to needing knowledge to provide episodic and direct primary care, nurses need a population-wide perspective of public health care. They must have a basic knowledge of clinical epidemiology, biostatistics, behavioral and political sciences, and how these concepts apply to the communities or defined populations with whom nurses share responsibilities for health outcomes. Population-based services should include identifying, tracking, and serving members with unmet needs and allocating resources appropriately and efficiently to maximize the targeted community's health.

This concept of shared responsibility among the health-care disciplines requires the coordinated efforts of practitioners from many disciplines to work together in a focused manner to provide the best outcomes for the sickest patients and to manage the health care of defined communities. This type of comprehensive care of individuals, families, and groups requires a wide range of knowledge and skills in a variety of delivery settings. Nurses and other health-care disciplines need to work interdependently to carry out roles and responsibilities and to convey mutual respect, trust, support, and appreciation of each discipline's unique contributions to health care. To achieve this, nursing education needs to incorporate planned community-based, interdisciplinary experiences in the curriculum through courses, seminars, clinical experiences, and research projects (Pew 1998, p. 39).

Nurses must learn as students to actively build interdisciplinary bridges and also to develop a better understanding of what each health profession brings to the service setting. The shift to community-based health care requires that nursing students be educated to provide care to individuals, families, and groups in settings that are located within the community (Korniewicz & Palmer, 1997). This means that health-care services must be provided where the people are, in the neighborhood where they live, in the schools they attend, and in their workplace approaches (Korniewicz & Palmer, 1997). Box 2–1 allows you to think further about the interdisciplinary team.

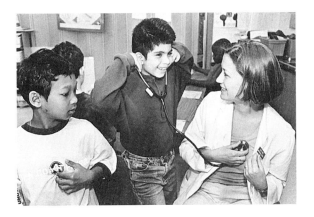

Box 2-1	Student Learning Activity

Interdisciplinary Team

Think about the families with whom you have worked this semester in your community-based sites. List members of the interdisciplinary team who were essential to providing quality health care for your families.

This chapter provides the historical background on global and national community-based care. Chapter 2 is a foundation for other chapters in the book in that it offers working definitions and explanations of some of the more common terms (many with overlapping definitions) and concepts of care that describe community-based health care efforts. This chapter also offers opportunities to see how nurses fit in as members of interdisciplinary, collaborative teams working in communities. Finally, the chapter presents an example of one model to identify and address the health-care needs of a community.

How did we arrive at this point of health care delivery in the United States?

To answer that question, it is probably best to start by asking: How does the global world of health care contribute to U.S. community-based primary health care?

THE EVOLUTION OF GLOBAL PRIMARY HEALTH CARE

In the 1960s and early 1970s, it was believed that if there could be development in "third-world" countries, then the achievement of health goals worldwide would naturally follow. Large investments through international loans were made to stimulate development in these countries. However, as the world economy subsequently began to lag, it was apparent that there was little improvement in health status. In fact, health improvement was even farther behind than originally imagined. Consequently, countries facing the burden of payment of these large loans began to put less funding toward health efforts. The World Health Organization (WHO) took the lead by looking at countries in which there had been at least some health improvement and then evaluated the data for identified commonalities. This effort resulted in the World Health Assembly (WHA), which met in Geneva in 1977 (World Health Assembly, 1977) and developed the goal of Health for All in the Year 2000 (HFA, 2000). This initiative then led to the planning of the historic Alma-Ata (Russia) Conference on Primary Health Care (PHC) by the WHA and the United Nations Children's Fund (UNICEF) in 1978. Attendance at Alma-Ata included representatives from 134 governments and delegates from 67 United Nations organizations and other specialized and nongovernmental agencies. Globally, the Declaration of Alma-Ata established Primary

Health Care as the strategy for achieving the objective of Health for All in the Year 2000 (Collado, 1992).

The Alma-Ata conference defined health as a state of complete physical, mental, and social well-being, and not merely the absence of disease or infirmity, emphasizing that health is a fundamental human right that should be a worldwide social goal. The conference attendees recognized the gross inequality in health status by comparing individuals from developed versus developing countries. They recognized that economic and social development is required to attain health for all and to reduce the health status gap between developed and developing nations. Likewise, they recognized promotion and protection of health as necessary to sustain economic and social development. The Alma-Ata attendees believed populations have the right and duty to participate as individuals and as a collective group in the planning and implementation of their own care. And, finally, the attendees supported the HFA/2000 goal that all people should have a high level of health by 2000 (WHO, 1978). Box 2–2 allows you to apply the Alma-Ata definition.

Box 2-2	Student Learning Activity

Alma-Ata Definition

Using the Alma-Ata definition of health, briefly discuss the health status of a family whom you have met in your community-based practice.

To achieve the goal of HFA/2000, the Alma-Ata attendees recognized primary health care as the key. They explained primary health care as the first level of contact with a national health system and the importance of bringing that level of care to where the people live and work. The attendees believed:

- Primary health care should address the main health problems of a community.
- Solutions to community health problems should include health promotion and disease prevention, as well as curative and rehabilitative services.
- Primary health care includes education about the predominant health problems and methods of preventing and controlling them including:
  - Food availability and nutrition management
  - Adequate pure water and basic sanitation
  - Maternal and child health care
  - Family planning and immunizations
  - Disease and injury management

These educational efforts are all areas in which community-based nurses and nursing students can have an impact. This is discussed in Chapter 1, which compares acute-care nursing with community-based nursing and public health nursing. The Alma-Ata attendees recommended maximum individual and community self-reliance with their collective participation in the management of primary health care. They invited all countries to cooperate to ensure primary health care for all people because the quality of health in one country directly affects every other country (WHO, 1978).

Furthermore, the Alma-Ata attendees believed that primary health care would be a practical way to make health care universally accessible to individuals and families in communities in an acceptable and affordable way, which ensured their participation to reach healthy outcomes. Participants recognized that health is not achieved by the health-care system alone, but rather must be attained through economic development, antipoverty measures, food production, water, sanitation, housing, environmental protection, and education (WHO, 1978, p. 38–40).

Primary health care guarantees a minimum level of basic, essential health care for all people. Four assumptions support this philosophy (Zotti, Brown, & Stotts, 1996, pp. 211–217):

- Health is a political and social right. Equity is fundamental, and universal coverage is the norm, with care provided according to need.
- The community as a whole, rather than the individual, is the client, and the community determines its greatest priority and allocates resources based on priorities. Thus the overall public good is promoted, but needs of individuals may go unmet.
- Because conditions in many sectors of communities affect health, multisectoral cooperation is necessary to promote, maintain, and improve the health of the community.
- The philosophy of primary health care can be applied to any country or community on the globe.

How Has Nursing Fit into Global Primary Health Care?

Historically, nursing's social commitment to justice and equity support the concepts of PHC. An overview of the evolution of community-based nursing in the United States is specifically addressed in Chapter 1. Nursing has always had an integral part to play in primary health care by combining preventive and curative aspects of health care along with community advocacy. Since the 1977 World Health Assembly (WHA), nursing and midwifery have been identified as a valuable human resource for PHC; subsequently, governments and organizations were encouraged to review the roles and functions of nursing and midwifery in meeting the HFA/2000 goal through primary health care (World Health Assembly, 1983, 1992).

In 1987, the WHO developed the structure for the selection of World Health Organization Collaborating Centres for Nursing and Midwifery Development to be awarded to selected schools or colleges of nursing around the world to work collaboratively between and among themselves in terms of research, policy, and legislation to further the goal for HFA/2000. As of 2001, there were 32 World Health Organization Collaborating Centres for Nursing and Midwifery designated worldwide that have formed the Global Network of World Health Organization Collaborating Centres for Nursing and Midwifery Development. Network members are committed to strengthening and promoting nursing leadership toward the realization of health for all through primary health care. This is achieved through a process of collaboration, coordination, and mobilization of resources in the area of nursing and midwifery, education, research, and practice.

U.S. Efforts in Primary Health Care

In the early 1960s, the lack of allocation of resources to primary care settings was recognized. A study by White and associates (1961) noted that during a one-month period, in a population of 1,000 individuals, 750 experienced some aspect of illness or injury, 250 consulted a physician, and 9 were hospitalized. Only one of these hospitalizations was in a university medical center. The authors questioned why the United States financially supports and trains health-care providers in academic health science centers when the experience of physicians and patients with diseases is overwhelmingly in the community. More than three decades ago, these authors proposed that the training and education process should reflect this reality and that greater numbers of primary-care physicians needed to be developed.

Consequently, the United States was left with three major concerns: (1) a lack of adequate numbers of health-care providers of the types needed, (2) many geographical areas of the United States had inadequate or in some cases no local health-care providers, and (3) a need for a fiscal way of looking at promoting health and disease management through community-based population medicine practices. Later in the 1960s, in response to this concern, general practice evolved into family practice and was formalized with postgraduate training and a specialty family practice board examination. The American Academy of Family Practice assumed a leadership role for this primary-care specialty. Subsequently, the Health Professions Educational Assistance Act in 1972 and 1976 provided federal support for the training of family practitioners, general internists, and general pediatricians. In addition, to try to help decrease the deficit of primary-care providers, these acts provided for the training of the two new primary-care disciplines of nurse practitioners (NPs) and physicians assistants (PAs). Private foundations also provided funding to support the education of primary-care-oriented professions. However, despite the realization of the value and importance of primary care, the preponderance of educational support for graduate medical education as well as physician reimbursement continued to favor training for medical specialists. In the early 1980s, more than two-thirds of American physicians were still engaged in specialty practice. In 1990, only 14.6 percent of graduating medical students indicated that they intended to pursue careers in primary care. These were not adequate numbers for primary care, and the need for a change in the way the United States looked at health care became more obvious—setting the stage for the health-care reform initiatives of 1993.

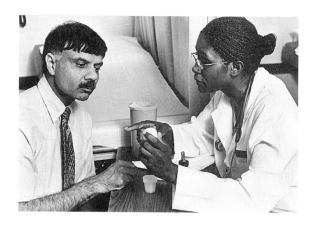

As a WHO member, the United States enthusiastically subscribed to the concept of primary health care as a mechanism for achieving the goal of Health for All by the year 2000. The U.S. focus has been on disease prevention and health promotion as formally depicted by the *Healthy People* initiatives—the prevention agenda for the nation, which targets increasing years of healthy life for Americans and reducing the health disparities among Americans. The *Healthy People* initiative has become the nation's road map to good health. The first set of national health targets was published in 1979 in *Healthy People: The Surgeon General's Report on Health Promotion and Disease Prevention*. The second set of national health targets was published in 1991 in *Healthy People 2000: National Health Promotion and Disease Prevention Objectives* by the Public Health Service. This publication identified our nation's top causes of morbidity and mortality. Measurable objectives (319 objectives organized into 22 priority areas) were set, and the percentage of reduction was set as the goal was determined. The national targets have served as the basis for monitoring and tracking health status, health risks, and use of preventive services. Many states and localities have used the same process to guide local public health policy and program development. The year 2000 objectives focused on three major goals: (1) increasing the life span for healthy Americans, (2) reducing the disparities in health among Americans and decreasing the race-based disparity in life expectancy, and (3) the provision of access to preventive services for all Americans. A third set of national health targets was published in 2000 in "Healthy People 2010: Understanding and Improving Health." This publication was designed to achieve two overarching goals: (1) Increase quality and years of healthy life, and (2) Eliminate health disparities.

Success is measured by positive changes in health status or reductions in risk factors, as well as improved provision of certain services. Specifically, the areas of health promotion, health protection, preventive service priorities, and system improvement priorities were clarified (Healthy People 2000, 1991):

- *Health promotion*: Nutrition; physical activity and fitness; reduction of consumption of tobacco, alcohol, and other drugs; family planning; reduction of violent and abusive behavior; mental health; and educational and community-based programs (Healthy People 2000, 1991). Individual decisions about sexual behavior, tobacco use, alcohol consumption, diet, and exercise create most of the disease burden experienced by the nation, but at the same time a significant number of health-care consumers are becoming more interested in—and more knowledgeable about—health maintenance and promotion as evidenced by the significant increase in behaviors seeking alternative and complementary health care (Pew, 1998).
- *Health protection*: Environmental health, occupational safety and health, accidental unintentional injuries, food and drug safety, and oral health.
- *Preventive services priorities*: Maternal and infant health, immunizations and infectious diseases, human immune virus infection, sexually transmitted diseases, heart disease and stroke, cancer, diabetes, and other chronic disabling conditions, as well as mental and behavioral disorders.
- *System improvement priorities*: Health education and preventive services and surveillance and data systems.

THE EARLY YEARS OF THE NEW MILLENNIUM—THROUGH 2010

To push health-care objectives forward into the 21st century, the United States Department of Health and Human Services has developed objectives for the year 2010. Nurses (through representatives from the American Nurses Association, the American Association of Colleges of Nursing, the Association of Pediatric Oncology Nurses, and the Association of Women's Health, Obstetric, and Neonatal Nurses) were part of the consortium developing these 300 objectives. Major changes from the 2000 objectives include a broadened disease prevention base, improved surveillance and data systems, a heightened awareness and demand for preventive health services and quality of care, and a focus on eliminating health disparities among all Americans including racial and ethnic groups, age groups, economic groups, disability groups, gender groups, and geographic locations. Progress toward the goals will be measured, initially, in 2005. The national efforts "beg" for outcomes that improve the health and quality of life of the American public.

HOW DO WE KNOW IF WHAT WE DO MAKES A DIFFERENCE? OUTCOMES!

How do we know if what we do makes a difference? That's what the health planners and the funders of health care want to know. To truly understand if your community-based nursing intervention has worked—that is, if the intervention has been successful in changing behavior and then actually impacting on the *Healthy People Objectives*—you must have measurable objectives. Did our actions make a difference? The answer is between preintervention and postintervention. Has the unhealthy behavior changed to healthier behavior? Ultimately, has the changed behavior resulted in better individual, family, or population health? For example: A decrease in the number of strokes and heart attacks in an "at risk" group in your community would be a good goal. A short-term outcome would be that these "at risk" individuals would attend a class or health fair that your nursing student group has planned. An intermediate outcome might be that as a result of having attended your class, the targeted family or group attitudes changed favorably toward positive health behavior. A long-term outcome would be a decrease in cardiovascular disease (stroke or MI) 10, 20, or 30 years after they implement behavior changes that decrease fat intake, decrease measured cholesterol, increase exercise, and manage stress. Box 2–3 will help you focus on setting health goals for a family.

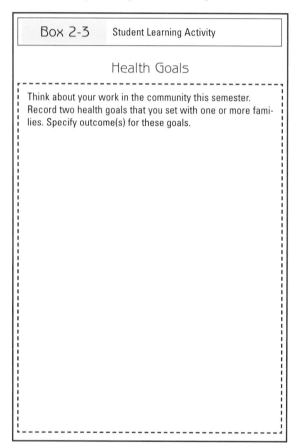

Box 2-3	Student Learning Activity

Health Goals

Think about your work in the community this semester. Record two health goals that you set with one or more families. Specify outcome(s) for these goals.

KEY CONCEPTS ESSENTIAL FOR UNDERSTANDING COMMUNITY-BASED PRIMARY HEALTH CARE

For clarification and a common understanding of the terms used throughout this book, we look at some of the most frequently used explanations for terms and concepts.

Public Health

A good place to start is with the concept of public health, because this is probably how nurses first began their education and practice outside of the hospital setting. The mission of public health is to "fulfill society's interest in assuring conditions in which people can be healthy." Unlike clinical disciplines, public health focuses on whole communities and large populations of people, rather than the health of any single individual. The core essential services of public health follow (IOM, 1996, pp. 75–76).

- Monitoring health status to identify community health problems
- Diagnosing and investigating health problems and health hazards in the community
- Informing, educating, and empowering people about health issues
- Mobilizing community partnerships to identify and solve health problems
- Developing policies that support individual and community health efforts
- Enforcing laws and regulations that protect health and ensure safety
- Linking people to needed personal health services and ensuring the provision of health care when otherwise unavailable
- Ensuring a competent public health and personal health-care workforce
- Evaluating the effectiveness, accessibility, and quality of personal and population-based health services
- Research innovative solutions to health problems

Primary Care

Historically, primary care was considered a physician-patient dyad and the first contact with the health-care system. In 1994, the Institute of Medicine began to reconceptualize primary care, and ultimately in 1996 the Institute of Medicine updated its definition of primary care in a useful and inclusive manner:

Primary care is the provision of *integrated, accessible, health-care services* by *clinicians* who are *accountable* for addressing a large *majority of personal health-care needs*, developing a *sustained partnership* with *patients,* and practicing in the **context of family and community** (IOM, 1996, p. 31).

Further clarification of the terms used to explain this definition of primary care is as follows (IOM, 1996, pp. 32–33):

- *Integrated* is intended to encompass the provision of comprehensive, coordinated, and continuous services that provide a seamless process of care. Integration combines events and information about events occurring in disparate settings, levels of care and over time, preferably throughout the life span.
- *Comprehensive* care addresses any health problem at any given stage of a patient's life cycle.
- *Coordination* ensures the provision of a combination of health services and information that meets a patient's needs. It also refers to the connection between, or the rational ordering of, those services, including the resources of the community.
- *Continuity* is a characteristic that refers to care over time by a single individual or team of health-care professionals ("clinician continuity") and to effective and timely communication of health information such as events, risks, advice, and patient preferences ("record continuity").
- *Accessible* refers to the ease with which a patient can initiate an interaction for any health problem with a clinician (e.g., by phone or at a treatment location) and includes efforts to eliminate barriers such as those posed by geography, administrative hurdles, financing, culture, and language.

Box 2–4 helps you to think about barriers to health care in your community.

```
┌─────────────────────────────────────────────────────┐
│  ┌──────────────────────────────────────────────┐   │
│  │  Box 2-4     Student Learning Activity        │   │
│  └──────────────────────────────────────────────┘   │
│                                                       │
│           Barriers to Health Care                     │
│                                                       │
│  Access to health care is a major problem in poor and under-│
│  served communities. Reflect on the experience you are hav- │
│  ing in the community this semester. Identify three barriers to │
│  health care for your families and discuss how you overcame │
│  them.                                                │
│                                                       │
└─────────────────────────────────────────────────────┘
```

- *Health care services* refers to an array of services that are performed by health-care professionals or under their direction, for the purpose of promoting, maintaining, or restoring health. The term refers to all settings of care (such as hospitals, nursing homes, clinicians' offices, intermediate care facilitates, schools, and homes).
- *Clinician* means an individual who uses a recognized scientific base and has the authority to direct the delivery of personal health services to patients.
- *Accountable* applies to primary-care clinicians and the systems in which they operate. These clinicians and systems are responsible to their patients and communities for addressing a large majority of personal health needs through a sustained partnership with a patient in the context of a family and community and for quality of care, patient satisfaction, efficient use of resources, and ethical behavior.
- *Majority of personal health-care needs* refers to the essential characteristic of primary-care clinicians: that they receive all problems that patients bring—unrestricted by problem or organ system—and have the appropriate training to diagnose and manage a large majority of those problems and to involve other health-care practitioners for further evaluation or treatment when appropriate. *Personal health-care needs* include physical, mental, emotional, and social concerns that involve the functioning of an individual.
- *Sustained partnership* refers to the relationship established between the patient and clinician with the mutual expectation of continuation over time. It is predicated on the development of mutual trust, respect, and responsibility.
- *Patient* means an individual who interacts with a clinician either because of illness or for health promotion and disease prevention.
- *Context of family and community* refers to an understanding of the patient's living conditions, family dynamics, and cultural background.
- *Community* refers to the population served, whether patients or not. A community can be a geographically or geopolitically defined population such as a town or country; or it can be neighbors who share values, experiences, language, religion, culture, or ethnic heritage.

As discussed in Chapter 1, our communities are more likely to be a specific group (e.g., infants, mothers, school-age children, elderly) or it may be a group of people congregated at a particular site, such as a church, school, jail, neighborhood, or workplace (Rhyne, Bogue, Kukulka, & Fulmer, 1998). It might be a group of individuals or neighbors who share common values or attributes such as

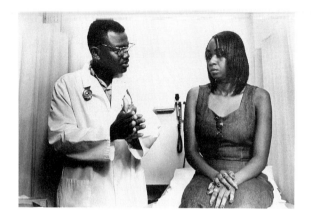

lifestyle, culture, experiences, language, ethnic heritage, or religion (e.g., a monastery or an Amish community) (NINR, 1993).

Primary Health Care

Primary health care is considered essential health care that is made universally accessible to individuals and families in the community…through their full participation and at a cost that the community and country can afford (WHO, 1978, p. 3). More recently the NINR Panel agreed that "primary health care focuses on promotion of health and prevention of disease across the continuum of care" with a focus of concern on the health of the community (NINR, 1993, p. 2). According to the NINR definition, primary health care not only includes the concepts of primary care and community-oriented primary care, but also brings in public health delivery along with epidemiological principles. Community residents and health-care professionals are partners in the goal of improved health. In addition, primary health care includes the components of self-care and self-management, with community populations empowered to use their knowledge, attitudes, and skills to improve their own health as well as that of the community (NINR, 1993).

Epidemiology

Epidemiology is an important concept in community-oriented primary health care. It is the study of the occur-rence, distribution, and cause of disease in humankind. For example, an emergency room might have a sudden influx of patients complaining of nausea and vomiting; the commonality tracked might be that all of the individuals had eaten the same meal at the same restaurant the evening prior to the onset of similar symptoms. Further investigation of the food served reveals bacterial contamination with *E. coli* or salmonella from unsanitary food handling.

The medical knowledge of morbidity and mortality statistics, population risk factors, and diseases comes from large epidemiological studies published in medical and public health journals and in the news media. These studies span 5 to 10 years and longer. Vast quantities of these up-to-date national statistics are widely available on the Internet through the Centers for Disease Control (CDC) and the Department of Health and Human Services (DHHS). Locally, the information can be obtained from state and county government agencies.

OTHER PERTINENT TERMS

Case Management

Case management typically focuses on coordination, cost containment, quality of care, and collaboration on individual cases, such as patients with complex health issues who frequently require costly hospitalizations.

For example, individuals with severe cardiovascular disease who have congestive heart failure and are known to be at risk for frequent costly hospitalizations might be closely monitored and frequently assessed by a nurse case manager for signs of decompensation, sequelae, or the onset of new problems that if left unattended would result ultimately in hospitalization. Early interventions, which can often be managed successfully at home or on an outpatient basis, preclude these problems from becoming disabling or severe enough to warrant hospitalization.

Nurse case managers plan health-care services and integrate them across the health-care delivery continuum—an important concept in the emerging health care delivery systems (O'Neil & Coffman, 1998).

In the preceding example, if early interventions did not prevent hospitalization, the case manager would continue to monitor and work with the patient and staff of the hospital to increase the likelihood of an earlier discharge, with patient and family teaching, arrangements for home care, and daily follow-up at home as needed.

Continuum of Care

Continuum of care begins with health promotion and disease prevention and works through acute care, transitional care, and long-term services for individuals, families, and communities (NINR, 1993). It subsumes monitoring, tracking, and managing of an individual throughout the continuum and gives one person (i.e., one health-care provider known most recently as the primary-care provider) total oversight for the outcome of the movement of the patient through the "system." In other words, this concept includes care at all levels of prevention: primary, secondary, and tertiary (NINR, 1993). How this applies specifically to nurses is discussed in Chapter 1. Box 2–5 gives you an opportunity to think about continuity of care in your community.

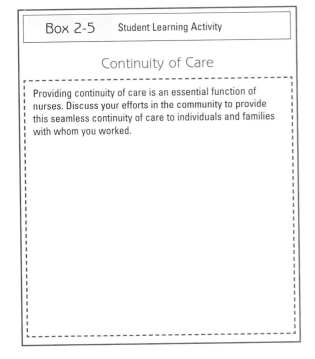

Box 2-5 Student Learning Activity

Continuity of Care

Providing continuity of care is an essential function of nurses. Discuss your efforts in the community to provide this seamless continuity of care to individuals and families with whom you worked.

Health Maintenance Organizations

Health maintenance organizations (HMOs) provide medical care (often preventive as well as for illness) to members for a fixed monthly fee by contracting with hospitals, physicians, and other health-care professionals and facilities (Knight, 1998). HMOs are economically motivated to respond to the health needs of their populations and offer opportunities and incentives (Nevin & Gohel, 1996).

Integrated Delivery Systems

Integrated delivery systems provide a full array of services from a variety of levels of facilities for a given price to a defined population in settings that are most appropriate to patients' needs. This definition ensures that primary care cannot be defined or assessed in isolation from the overall system of which it is a part (IOM, 1996).

Managed Care

Managed care refers to health plans that have a selective list of providers, both health professionals and hospitals, and that include mechanisms for influencing the nature, quantity, and site of services delivered (IOM, 1996). Managed care attempts to create an organized system in which health care that is medically necessary is promptly delivered by the appropriately trained and educated provider, in appropriate locations and level of facilities, under practice guidelines that will most likely result in the most favorable outcome for the patient (Knight, 1998).

Managed care plans usually include the following (Knight, 1997):

- Arrangements with physicians, hospitals, and other health-care professionals to provide a defined set of health-care services to subscribers of their plan
- Criteria and processes for selecting and monitoring providers
- A mechanism to gather, monitor, and measure data on health services use, physician referral patterns, and other quality and performance measures
- Incentives or requirements for subscribers to use providers and services associated with the plan
- Incentives for providers to encourage the appropriate use of health-care resources

NEWER TERMS ENTERING THE HEALTH-CARE VERNACULAR

Care Management

Care management expands on case management to focus on disease or need management of large numbers of individuals experiencing the same need or concern, such as hypertension, hyperlipidemia, cardiovascular disease, and diabetes. Care management assumes a team approach that includes clinical pathways, disease management programs, and benchmarking data and analyses. It may require the collection and synthesis of data from each of the team members—physicians, nurses, ancillary providers, managed care organizations, and the patients who are targeted as members of the population of concern. Nurses are leaders of these teams, and student nurses should look to this as a viable nursing role for them in health-care delivery and management in integrated health-care systems (O'Neil & Coffman, 1998).

Population Health Management

Population health management suggests the assumption of accountability for and the management of an entire community of people, regardless of system membership or insurance status. It requires management of medical care as well as health promotion and disease prevention efforts (O'Neil & Coffman, 1998). Population health management offers opportunities and incentives within the HMO and managed care systems.

What is the result of combining all of the above and looking at the concepts of primary care, primary health care, managed care (to a degree), and community partnerships? Perhaps it can best be described as community-based primary health care, although this is not yet a commonly used term.

Community-based Primary Health Care

Community-based primary health care focuses on communities and populations and incorporates coordination, interaction, and partnerships with institutions providing acute and chronic health care, as well as community members, providers, and insurers (NINR, 1993) with an overall health promotion, risk screening, and disease prevention focus. To access and identify the needs of the population or targeted community, nurses need to look at a community from the bottom up rather than from the top down. That is to say, when first entering a community as a health-care worker, it is best to ensure that the community members (along with the identified community leaders and administrators) participate on an ongoing basis in all discussions and decisions affecting the programs and planning for the desired outcomes for the community. From the beginning, involve those whose needs you are trying to meet and those for whom the outcomes are identified. A key question to ask the community members as well as the leaders is, "What do they perceive to be their problems? What are their needs?" This is vital if you want to make a real, measurable impact on the health status of a population. You need to find out what they, the community members, believe are their health problems or the social problems that contribute to their health problems, and you need to know what outcomes they would like to see result from interventions.

Nurses need community members to be involved in helping to plan the intervention as well as to ensure that it will be a program in which community members will participate. Interventions must be planned in conjunction with the values and beliefs of the culture of the population to be served. Just as a nurse does a comprehensive health history and physical examination of a patient, the nurse who is working on population-based efforts needs to do a comprehensive assessment and examination of the community that is the focus of "treatment" attention and efforts. Furthermore, just as the hospital-based nurse involves the patient in the assessment and plan, so does the community-based nurse involve those individuals or groups who will be making (or not) the requisite behavior change in the assessment and plan to provide greater assurance that they "buy into" and believe in the changes and programs that are planned. Many times, nurses and other health-care professionals perceive themselves as the authorities who know what the patient or community's problems are; they tend to go into the relationship with predetermined solutions. There are a number of frameworks to assess a community, all of which resemble the nursing process to a certain degree. The Community-Oriented Primary Care model embodies community-based primary health care and is described in the following section.

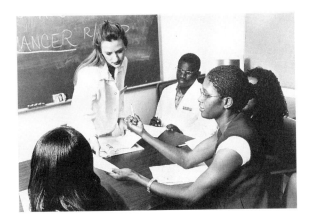

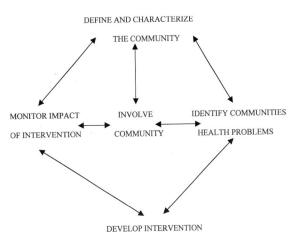

FIGURE 2–1

Community-oriented Primary Care Model

From Rhyne, R., Bogue R., Kukulka, G., & Fulmer, H. (1998). Community-oriented primary care: Health care for the 21st century. Washington, DC: American Public Health Association, p. 12.

COMMUNITY-ORIENTED PRIMARY CARE

Community-oriented Primary Care (COPC) is a community-responsive model of health-care delivery that integrates public health with primary care. For over 20 years, COPC has been discussed as a viable mechanism for dealing with current health problems through a coordinated effort to combine elements of primary care with community-based medicine in an innovative and creative way to improve health outcomes of an identified community. The thought is that when a model of health care allocates more resources into community care, it will ultimately save money, increase access, and result in better health outcomes. COPC was introduced in the United States in the early 1980s. The philosophical constructs have been in place in publicly funded clinics for many years and have been documented as being a component of the curricula of a selected number of universities and medical education programs since 1993 (Nevin & Gohel, 1996).

An operational definition of COPC requires three criteria: (1) a primary-care practice, (2) an involved and definable community, and (3) a set of activities that systematically address the major health issues of the community (IOM, 1984). Simply put, COPC is a systematic process for identifying and addressing the health problems of a defined population. Rhyne and associates note nothing special about the name of COPC; it could just as easily be called community-responsive health care or community-based primary care. They note that it is

the process and the inclusion of the community as partner at every step that is the vital component (1998).

The COPC model offers providers a unified approach and process for identifying and responding to the health-care problems of a specific community. The model for COPC is seen as circular, and theoretically you can enter the model at any of the steps:

1. Define the community.
2. Systematically identify and prioritize the major health problems of the defined community.
3. Design interventions that will modify or improve the health problems.
4. Evaluate the impact of these programs on targeted health problems (IOM, 1984; Mullan & Kalter, 1988).
5. Involve the community at every step (Rhyne et al., 1998). See Figure 2–1.

Applying the COPC Framework

To define and characterize the community, the nurse collects objective data from sources such as census data, geographical maps representing the area, vital statistics, and local surveys from a variety of sources including public libraries, insurance companies, and local government agencies. Community assessment includes "windshield surveys of the area at various times of the day and days of the week (e.g., morning, evening, night during a weekday, and a weekend day). The nurse also notes the businesses, schools, and community resources that are (or are not) available to community members. Always be sure to include the community members and leaders in your survey and assess their perceptions of the problems. Sometimes the interests of the community members do not coincide with the perceptions of need as determined by health-care professionals. Negotiation and compromise are essential for any program to be successful. Politically, it may be much more important to address a perceived need of the community to gain its trust before pursuing a problem supported only by objective data.

Try to identify the health problems and then prioritize them when working on the second step of the model. Partnering with community members and community leaders again is very important.

When problem solving, deciding on, and planning the interventions, the partnership with community members and leaders continues to be vital, as noted in Figure 2–1. Health planners must always take into consideration the "culture," both obvious and subtle, of those with whom they work.

Evaluation consists of ongoing monitoring and feedback regarding the outcomes of the intervention. Evaluation is essential to further define the community, identify new health problems or reprioritize those already identified, redesign the interventions, or perhaps contribute to the development of new programs. The process is valuable in that it seeks measurable outcomes, which are becoming increasingly important in the managed care environment.

Here is another student's description of her first day in the community. It exemplifies a cursory look with the COPC process and the importance of involving the target group or community of people throughout the process. It also demonstrates the import of full recognition of their culture; the array of multiple, competing needs; and again, the importance of involving community members in all phases of COPC.

At my clinical site, one of the rotations we had to do was to spend three hours in the lobby, without a name tag, talking to the people who came to the clinic. I'm

sure a lot of people would think that this was a waste of our time. It was to give us the opportunity to sit and observe so that for a few moments we could put ourselves in the shoes of the clients we serve. We were to see what it is they see when they come to the clinic: How are they treated, how do they think they are being treated, what are some of the reasons they are at the health department. While I was in the lobby, I noticed how the faces of the people who are at the clinic have changed since the days I came to the health department. There are a lot of different languages spoken now. With the different languages come cultural barriers that the public health nurse (PHN) must break through. It is difficult enough getting health information to a client when you are speaking the same language; it is twice as hard to educate a client who speaks a language you barely recognize.

While sitting in the lobby, I spoke with a woman who brought her daughter and her daughter's five children to the health department so she could add her 2-month-old baby to the Women, Infants, and Children (WIC) program. This lady asked me to make a call for her because neither she nor her daughter had the 35 cents required for the pay phone. She needed me to call someone to come and give her some money so that she could put enough gas in the car to get home. Only a few dollars stood between this family and peace of mind, far less than the money I would probably spend for lunch that day, yet I couldn't help them, not financially at least. It was hard for me not to just hand them the money. I know that my job as a PHN is not to give a handout but to help them learn to help themselves.

I struggled to make some sense about what my role would be this semester. For the longest time I couldn't see that anything I did would make a difference to anyone. I soon realized that the changes I make would not be to any other person; the changes would have to be in me. I am not to judge people; I know that I won't always understand these clients and I won't always like them. I need to look beyond anything that I may see as a fault and help the clients with their needs.

Community-based registered nurses are ideally suited to serve as the liaison between the health-care team and the community leaders and volunteers working together to combine health promotion, disease prevention, and the curative and restorative components of health care (NINR, Chapter 1). The nurse is responsible for considering all cultural aspects that could influence a group's health and program preferences and build them into intervention efforts. Nurses are generally educated to use more preventive and health-promoting interventions, to counsel and communicate with patients more frequently, and to take advantage of health education, community resources, and behavioral interventions to manage disease and disability. These are precisely the skills required by a health-care system that values continuous and comprehensive engagement with patients to preserve their health.

Health-care professionals wishing to have COPC as a lived experience must be willing and able to think outside the walls of their offices and treatment rooms. They need to look at the community in which they work and those they serve and apply the additional knowledge and skills of epidemiology, defining the community, collaborating with community members and leaders within the framework of the economic, political, legal, and administrative climate. The complexity and enormity of this task points to the need for the expertise of multiple health-care professionals in partnership with the community to accomplish the desired health outcomes.

Primary-care Research in Public Health

A number of recent research studies provide valuable information about primary-care research in public health. Bates and Wolinsky (1998) investigated the personal, financial, and structural barriers to immunization of socioeconomically disadvantaged urban children in the first two years of life. Mothers were recruited from the postpartum unit of a large municipal teaching hospital. Mothers who had healthy term newborns were interviewed 24 to 72 hours postpartum regarding personal and financial barriers to immunization. They were also asked where they intended to take their newborns for well-child care. Researchers found that family environment, history of prenatal care use, and financial barriers were important factors related to whether or not the children received immunizations. In addition, the researchers found that mothers who had less continuity with physicians were less likely to have their children fully vaccinated, although this finding was not statistically significant. An important conclusion of the study was that mothers may need a more realistic expectation of the health benefits of vaccination to prevent them from being disillusioned if their children should get sick.

Another research study focused on the benefits and barriers to well-child care. To address the concern that many children do not receive regular well-child care, Earle and Burman (1998) conducted a qualitative study to explore how mothers in a rural state perceived well-child care, its benefits, and the barriers to obtaining this service. The study was guided with a framework adapted from the Health Belief Model. Twenty-one women in two counties of Wyoming were interviewed about their knowledge and beliefs related to well-child care and the care their own children had received. The researchers found that most of the mothers valued well-child care in areas of maternal reassurance, information, identification of problems, developmental testing, preventive care, and health maintenance. They perceived that barriers such as financial limitations and inconvenience discouraged use of well-child care. The researchers noted the need for primary-care providers to promote the use of well-child care through educating consumers on the purposes, benefits, and schedule for preventive care, as well as providing cues for encouraging consumers to make and keep appointments.

A third study looked at the global distribution of physicians and nurses and the influence of the gross national product (GNP) per capita on this distribution. Wharrad and Robinson (1999) used a database compiled from various United Nations (UN) sources for 147 countries. The researchers concluded that 70 percent of the distribution of nurses globally could be explained by the distribution of physicians. The GNP appeared to have a substantial influence on these distributions. Only a minority of the world's very poorest countries substituted higher numbers of nurses for lower numbers of physicians. One conclusion, however, was that the potential inaccuracies of the presently available UN global data sets raise questions about how seriously findings from the research should be taken.

CONCLUSION

In summary, as nurses, we are being challenged to be actively involved in the development and implementation of cost-effective, high-quality, innovative systems of care that are available to all individuals. To accomplish this, nursing students and faculty are shifting the education and training grounds to the community to practice nursing. We are realigning our practices and our accountability away from institutions and out into the community (NLN, 1993). Nursing students need to master assessment skills that not only address the needs of individuals and families, but also the homes, work environments, and communities where they live.

Although the U.S. health-care system is in constant flux as it tries to envision and formulate its future, nurses, as the largest single discipline of all the health professions, are perfectly postured to take the lead in the efforts to manage the health of individuals, families, and groups within the context of the community. The enormity and magnitude of community health problems create unlimited opportunities for role expansion, and they create new positions for nurses and the nursing profession (O'Neil & Coffman, 1998). Nurses can be the leaders in promoting health for all in the new millennium!

Active Learning Strategies

1. Discuss with a classmate the national and global historical development for population-based primary health care. How does this development relate to community-based primary health care today?

2. Discuss with your clinical group the World Health Organization's goal of "Health for All" as it relates to the immigrant populations with whom you work. In what ways is their health care consistent with what you would expect in a developed country? Inconsistent?

3. Define a community of interest. To identify the needs of this community, involve several community members in your assessment. Identify at least five members and discuss how you will go about seeking their involvement.

4. Discuss with one of the nurses in your clinical experience how the COPC model could be used to assess health-care problems in your community.

References

Bates, A. S., & Wolinsky, F. D. (1998). Personal, financial, and structural barriers to immunization in socioeconomically disadvantaged urban children. Pediatrics, 101(4), 591–596.

Collado, C. B. (1992). Primary health care: A continuing challenge. Nursing & Health Care 13(8), 408–413.

Earle, L. P., & Burman, M. E. (1998). Benefits and barriers to well-child care: Perceptions of mothers in a rural state. Public Health Nursing, 15(3), 180–187.

Healthy People 2000 (1991). National health promotion and disease prevention objectives. Washington, DC: United States Department of Health and Human Services.

Healthy People 2010 (2000). Understanding and improving health. Washington, DC: United States Department of Health and Human Services.

Institute of Medicine. (1978). A manpower policy for primary health care: Report of a study. Washington, DC: National Academy Press.

Institute of Medicine. (1984). Community-oriented primary care: A practical assessment. Washington, DC: National Academy Press.

Institute of Medicine. (1996). Primary care: America's health in a new era. Washington, DC: National Academy Press.

Knight, W. (1997). Managed care contracting: A guide for health care professionals. Gaithersburg, MD: Aspen Publishers, pp. 2–3.

Knight, W. (1998). Managed care: What it is and how it works. Gaithersburg, MD: Aspen Publishers.

Korniewicz, D. M., & Palmer, M. H. (1997). The preferable future for nursing. Nursing Outlook, 45 (3), 108–113.

Mullan, F., & Kalter, H. D. (1988). Population-based and community-oriented approaches to preventive healthcare. American Journal of Preventive Medicine, 4(suppl 4), 141–154.

National League for Nursing. (1993). A vision for nursing education. New York: Author.

National Nursing Research Agenda (NINR). (1993). Developing knowledge for practice: Challenges and opportunities. In Community-based care: Concepts and definitions. National Institute of Nursing Research. www.nih.gov/ninr/vol7.

Nevin, J. E., & Gohel, M. M. (1996, March). Community-oriented primary care. Models of Ambulatory Care, 23(1), 1–15.

O'Neil, E., & Coffman, J. (Eds.). (1998). Strategies for the future of nursing: Changing roles, responsibilities, and employment patterns of registered nurses. The University of California, San Francisco: The Center for the Health Professions.

Pew Health Professions Commission. (1998). Recreating health professional practice for a new century. Fourth Report of the Pew Health Professions Commission. San Francisco: Author.

Rhyne, R., Bogue R., Kukulka, G., & Fulmer, H. (1998). Community-oriented primary care: Health care for the 21st century. Washington, DC: American Public Health Association.

Wharrad, H., & Robinson, J. (1999). The global distribution of physicians and nurses. Journal of Advanced Nursing, 30(1), 109–120.

White, K., Williams, T., & Greenberg, B. (1961). The ecology of medical care. New England Journal of Medicine 265, 885–893.

World Health Assembly. (1977, May 19). Resolution 30.48. The role of nursing/midwifery in the strategy of Health for All. Geneva: Author.

World Health Assembly. (1983, May 13). Resolution 36.11. The role of nursing/midwifery in the strategy of Health for All. Geneva: Author.

World Health Assembly. (1992, May 11). Resolution 45.5. Strengthening of nursing and midwifery in support of strategies for Health for All. Geneva: Author.

World Health Organization (1978). Primary Health Care: Report of the International Conference on Primary Health Care. Alma-Ata, USSR. Geneva: Author.

World Health Organization. (1988). From Alma-Ata to the year 2000: A midpoint perspective. Geneva (Switzerland): Author.

Zotti, M. E., Brown, P., & Stotts, R. C. (1996). Community-based nursing versus community health nursing: What does it all mean? Nursing Outlook, 44.

Community-based Practice: An Overview in Canada

Lynette Leeseberg Stamler

LEARNING OBJECTIVES

1) Acquire factual information about the historical evolution of a single-payer health-care system.

2) Compare and contrast the single-payer system with other health-care plans.

3) Examine the role of community nursing in a single-payer system.

As a nursing student, I was assigned a prenatal client to follow for a semester. She was 17 years old and experiencing her third pregnancy. I was 19 and just starting my maternity experience, concurrent with my community experience. I felt intimidated by my lack of knowledge. For instance, when I asked her if she had any questions about labor and delivery, she told me she had watched the first birth with a mirror. She did seem interested in having a tour of the hospital she was to deliver at for this pregnancy and was also interested in birth control. I was able to arrange a tour and also was able to correct some misconceptions about birth control, both for my client and her mother. She and her mother both favored tubal ligation. Upon further questioning, it was evident that they thought this procedure could easily be reversed at a later date, when my client was more mature and ready for more children. She was active in her 10th grade class and frequently just didn't show for appointments we had made. I finished the semester feeling that I had somehow failed her. Imagine my surprise when I got a phone call during finals week from my client. She had just delivered a healthy baby and she wanted to share that with me! I guess I made a difference after all!

Author

This story may not sound much different from that of a U.S. student. The system of financing and delivery of health care developed in Canada, however, is much different in many ways than in the United States. Although the actual nursing tasks of hospital and community care for the patient with appendicitis or AIDS may look very similar in each of the two countries, payment for such care and the context and accessibility of community care may look quite dissimilar. To understand the similarities and differences in community-based practice between the two countries, students must first explore the historical roots of health care in Canada, as well as the social context that nurtured those roots.

In this chapter we explore the history of health care in Canada and its influence on health-care system realities today. The current picture of health care in general and community-based care will be discussed. Nursing education for community-based care will also be addressed.

CANADA'S HEALTH-CARE SYSTEM—AN HISTORICAL VIEW

There are several intertwined factors that have strongly influenced the development of the health-care system in both the United States and Canada. These include religious and family beginnings, immigration history, and legislation. The majority of Canada's first settlers were from England and France. Although nurses were known in both English and French settlements, it was nuns from France who were instrumental in providing nursing care. Priests from France were a common sight in early Canada, but they were unable to take sick persons into their homes; thus the nuns were a socially acceptable source of assistance. As immigration moved westward, the nuns moved as well, ensuring that nursing care was available. These women worked both with the immigrants and the aboriginal peoples—who viewed these early efforts as a charm against disease. The most famous of these groups of nuns were the Grey Nuns, sometimes referred to as the first visiting nurses in Canada (Kerr, 1996a, 1996b). Most cities in Canada still have at least one hospital that was founded by one of the religious orders.

In addition, women who were family members of health-care workers also were active in nursing in early Canada. For instance, Marie Rollet Hebert, wife of Louis Hebert, a surgeon-apothecary, partnered with him by

nursing his patients. She was also noted for her work with aboriginal peoples (Kerr, 1996a). The Canadian immigration patterns differed somewhat from those of the United States. Many immigrants to the United States were disaffected or dissatisfied individuals or families fleeing from something such as persecution or a lack of opportunity in their own countries. These people tended to be rugged individualists, and frequent stories are told of families moving westward when the eastern part of the United States became "too crowded." Canada also had immigrants who fit this picture, including some Loyalists who fled the Revolutionary War in the United States, but Canada also advertised throughout Europe for people to settle in the new land. Thus, whole families or groups of families would often come and form a settlement together. The success of the whole community, as opposed to the United States's rugged individualists, became a desired goal. This desire is demonstrated by the fact that as early as 1665 Dr. Etienne Bouchard offered prepaid health coverage to 26 families in Montreal. This met two aims. First, it helped ensure that physicians would remain in the area because they had a livelihood. Second, it helped to ensure health care whenever needed, regardless of ability to pay (Health and Welfare Canada, 1974).

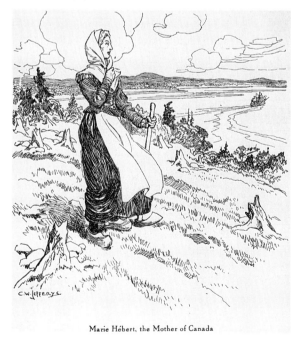

Marie Hébert, the Mother of Canada

Legislation was another instrumental factor in the development of the Canadian health-care system. In 1867, the British North America (BNA) Act was passed in Britain creating the Dominion of Canada. The Dominion became a part of the British Commonwealth, linking Canada with other countries and cultures in a common bond. Although there were battles in Canada's history to decide the dominance of English over French or white over aboriginal, Canada was created by evolution rather than revolution. There was little mention of health in the BNA Act, but it did allot management of quarantine and marine hospitals as the responsibility of the federal government. Any other public health initiative was to be the purview of the provincial governments (Baumgart, 1992). However, the federal government retained the majority of the resources (Armstrong & Armstrong, 1994). This basic allocation of responsibilities and resources played a very important role in future initiatives.

Although Canada had the responsibility of passing its own legislation, it turned to Britain for the basis of many of its laws. For instance, most of the original provincial public health acts were patterned on the British Public Health Act of 1875 (Du Gas, Esson, & Ronaldson, 1999). The British Act included such community problems as safe drinking water and assistance for the poor. Ontario was the first province to pass such an act in 1884; other provinces followed as they joined confederation. All the provincial acts had the creation of both a board of health and sanitation regulations in common (Baumgart, 1992). In 1910, the Flexner report on medical education in the United States and Canada reinforced the need for rigorous scientific inquiry as the basis for medical care. Nurses were striving to demonstrate an equally rigorous scientific basis for nursing care, beginning with Nightingale's "Notes on Nursing." However, the absence of a similar report in nursing, which resulted in the closing of nursing schools that did not meet medical schools' standards, contributed to an ongoing public and professional perception that medicine and curative activities were more important than promotion of healthy living or ongoing maintenance of chronic health problems (Rafael, 1999).

Just as the presence of disease was once considered a personal fault of the afflicted individual, asking for or receiving assistance of any kind has frequently been perceived as a personal failure. Those who were rich could afford to pay for whatever health care they required, whereas the very poor, albeit reluctantly, were forced to accept charity. The middle class, who had a small amount

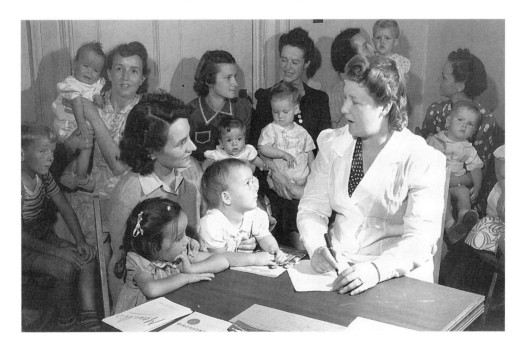

of money, sometimes had the greatest difficulty. In addition, the rural areas had the greatest problem with attracting and keeping medical practitioners. Thus, it is not surprising that the initial legislation that eventually led to Canada's health insurance system arose out of the province of Saskatchewan, a primarily agrarian province where the principle crop is wheat. In 1916, Saskatchewan passed the Union Hospital Act and the Rural Municipality Act. In each act, municipalities were allowed to band together, one to pay for physicians and the other to raise taxes for the purpose of building hospitals. The basic goal of these acts was to improve the health care of the population through the provision of practitioners and hospitals, and the acts did have the desired effect. Other provinces followed suit, although on a lesser scale. During the Great Depression of the 1930s, employment fell, and both physicians and hospitals found themselves almost unable to carry on as a result of lack of payment. In addition, the general health of the population was decreasing, in part because of the widespread poverty. Canada's federal government attempted to intervene in 1935 with the proposed Employment and Social Insurance Act, an act that would have established a federal health and welfare program. However, the provinces held fast to their rights under the BNA Act, and in 1937 the Supreme Court of Canada upheld the provincial rights to govern health care (Baumgart, 1992).

Saskatchewan once again was the leader. In 1944, Tommy (T. C.) Douglas won the provincial election and led the first Socialist government in Canada. Mr. Douglas had immigrated to Canada as a child and soon after was diagnosed with osteomyelitis. Because his family could not afford immediate care, he almost lost his leg. It was a lesson that he never forgot. Mr. Douglas, originally a minister, had been in politics since the 1930s, and among other things, helped to organize a local labor party. This group joined with others to become the Cooperative Commonwealth Federation, Canada's first national socialist party. Goals of the new party included universal hospital care, unemployment insurance, and a universal pension (Wong, 1998). So it was not surprising that in 1947, under Douglas's leadership, Saskatchewan passed the first universal hospital program, which ensured hospital care all for residents regardless of ability to pay. British Columbia was the next province to pass such a plan, and

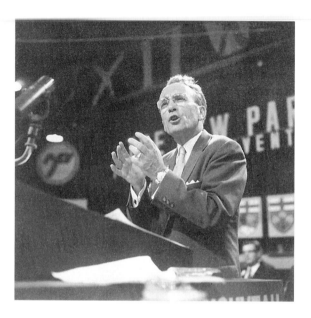

other provinces followed. Although the provinces held the final say in health care, the federal government was able to pass the National Health Grant Program in 1948. This program allowed the federal government to give monies to the provinces for the purpose of strengthening public health services, especially for specific diseases, such as tuberculosis, and for building additional hospitals.

In the next several years, the provinces realized that the cost of health care was quickly becoming a burden and began lobbying the federal government for additional funds. In response, the federal government proposed the National Hospital and Diagnostic Services Act, passed in 1957. Under this act, the federal and provincial governments shared the costs of hospital insurance. By 1961, 99 percent of Canadian residents were able to have standard benefits. These included basic acute and chronic hospital care, diagnostic services, and some outpatient services (Baumgart, 1992; Du Gas, Esson, & Ronaldson, 1999).

Saskatchewan once again was the leader for the next step. Still under the leadership of T. C. Douglas, now considered the father of Medicare in Canada, the province introduced a government-sponsored medical insurance plan in 1962 to cover physician expenses. Although the general public was overjoyed, the medical profession was very unhappy, and even went on strike to protest the legislation. When the physicians realized that the public as well as the government was against them, they signed an agreement with the province. Under this agreement, physicians would accept the medical insurance payments, but retained the right to bill patients more than the suggested government fee. This practice became known as "extra billing" and influenced future legislation. In the next few years, each province proposed some form of medical insurance, but no plan covered all residents. The federal government sponsored the Hall Commission in 1964. This was a very comprehensive study of health care in Canada and examined all options for health-care delivery. As a result of the commission's recommendations, the Medical Care Bill was passed in 1966 and implemented in 1968 (Baumgart, 1992; Du Gas, Esson, & Ronaldson, 1999).

In keeping with the BNA Act, each province had to decide to participate in the federal program. In addition, each province had to promise to abide by the principles of the Medical Care Bill. The first principle of the Medical Care Bill was that each plan had to be comprehensive and cover all physician and treatment services whenever there was a demonstrated medical need. Next, each plan had to be accessible regardless of income and universal in that each had to cover 95 percent of the eligible population. In addition, each plan had to be portable; individuals could move between provinces without losing their benefits. Finally, each plan had to be nonprofit and publicly administered. In return, the federal government promised to provide 5 percent of the funding for each of the provincial plans (Baumgart, 1992). Thus, Canada's health-care system became a group of provincial health plans with common principles. However, the federal government had not anticipated how quickly the costs of health care would escalate, and, in 1977, it moved to a block funding formula. Under this legislation, home-care, nursing home, and ambulatory services were included.

During the 1970s, a federal discussion paper, *A New Perspective on the Health of Canadians,* was released by the Minister of Health and Welfare, Marc Lalonde (Lalonde, 1974). In this paper, determinants of health were identified and strategies for reducing illness and improving health were noted. The report was also the first time that the government had put forward the notion that more physicians and medical care would not necessarily ensure greater health, but that improved environments and

changing individual health behaviors were more significant (O'Neill & Pederson, 1994). Beginning with the Lalonde Report, Canada has been a leader in health promotion efforts. The struggle between the illness care view and the health promotion view has continued since the 1970s. In some cases, it has been perceived as a struggle between medicine and nursing, or between acute care and community.

Provinces and service providers were always searching for a way to increase funding for the costs of health care. User fees and extra billing were being considered as a primary source of extra funds, a potential violation of the principle of accessibility. In 1982, the Medical Care Bill was opened, and much debate ensued. This debate was of great importance to nurses because, among the other items, was the identification of point of entry into the health-care system. At the time of the Medical Care Bill, the physician was the primary point of entry. The Canadian Nurses Association (CNA) advocated multiple entry points, including nursing. Moreover, the CNA wanted nursing care to be placed on the list of insured services and suggested that more community services be included. The federal Minister of Health at the time, Monique Begin, was adamant that the principles of the Medical Care Bill be reiterated within the new health act, which the CNA also supported. The CNA decided to focus its energies on the key statement "physicians and other health-care providers" to identify providers who could bill the health plans under the act. Following significant grassroots and sophisticated lobbying efforts, nurses under the leadership of the CNA were successful in ensuring the statement was included (Adaskin, 1988). Thus they paved the way for nurses to be named as health-care providers within the provincial acts, a precursor to the full use of advanced practice nurses in community and acute care.

When the Canada Health Act was finally passed in 1984, not only was the statement of health-care providers included, but provisions were also in place providing retribution for provinces that violated the principles of the act. This was especially applicable to the concept of extra billing, and the act provided that the federal government could withhold funds equal to the estimate of the extra billing. By 1987, all the provinces had agreed to the provisions of the Canada Health Act (Baumgart, 1992).

Provinces must still provide the federal government documentation of compliance with the provisions and principles of the Canada Health Act to qualify for federal health funding.

CANADA'S HEALTH-CARE SYSTEM: CURRENT CONCERNS AND ISSUES

The author remembers one of her community clients:

 It was our custom to phone clients before making the first visit. This particular client was a retired teacher, who had had childhood polio and walked with the aid of a leg brace. However, she was very independent and had managed her own care up to this point. She had recently broken her elbow and was unable to bathe herself, hence the referral to visiting nursing. The big news of the day was the signing of the repatriation agreement with Britain, which would make Canada an independent country, rather than part of Britain. The signing ceremony was to be that morning, and although my new client was very anxious for me to come, she was adamant that my visit not interfere with her viewing this historic occasion on television. I grew to love this independent and intelligent woman and found that what she most missed was the ability to have a "real" bath or shower, instead of a sponge bath. However, the bathtub in her condominium was too low for her to maneuver her brace on to her leg and then rise to a standing position. In consultation with the community occupational and physiotherapists, a rope ladder was fixed to the wall behind her bathroom door. Using this, she could slide from the bath board, and rise and pivot on her sound leg to the raised toilet seat on her toilet. From this vantage point, she could easily put on her brace, and continue her independent movement. What began as an acute difficulty became the solution to a lifelong dream.

Author

Currently, each province and territory has a health plan. Each has a hospital plan as well as a medical plan, and some have additional services, such as dental plans for children or plans for prescription drugs. Only two provinces levy premiums; for others all costs are covered by the tax base, federally and provincially. All include

some form of health plan for home care, and some also cover other practitioners, such as physiotherapists (outside hospital care), podiatrists, and chiropractors. Coverage for any item must be initiated by medical need, usually decided by the practitioner at point of entry. The physician is the primary point of entry. He or she works on a fee-for-service basis and bills the provincial plan for all services. Individuals are free to choose their physician, although the choice of a specialist may be limited to those who have privileges in the same hospitals as the family physician. This is, however, for convenience, rather than legislation or regulation.

Many employers also offer additional health insurance, which typically covers things such as dental care, vision care, chiropractic, mental health (e.g., psychologists), and alternative therapy services, drug plans, ambulance services, private duty nursing, and private rooms during hospital stays. Each plan may place annual caps on insured services. Although the federal government is considering the initiation of additional services such as universal child care, the provinces remain adamant that under the BNA Act, the federal government should give them the money, and they should decide on specific purchasing options. Money for health care and other services such as postsecondary education, social assistance, and other social services is transferred to the provinces under the Canada Health and Social Transfer block fund. This means that the provinces may spend the money according to their own priorities, within the principles of the Canada Health Act. Another condition is that there can be no minimum residency period to qualify for social assistance (Finance Canada, 1999).Health care does remain a provincial mandate. There are some health areas, however, that remain under federal jurisdiction. Table 3–1 provides an outline of the various branches of Health Canada and the mandates of each branch. The federal branches work with the regional and provincial counterparts to provide national consistency in these areas.

As in many countries that have single-payer systems (and some who do not), Canadians are concerned with the cost of their health-care system. According to Health Canada, Canada currently spends approximately $2,694 (Cdn) or $1,785 (US) per capita on health. This represents 9.3 percent of the gross domestic product, with the

Table 3-1

Areas of Health Care under Federal Jurisdiction

GOVERNMENT AGENCY	MANDATE
Population and Public Health Branch	-Centre for Surveillance Coordination: includes risk and intervention assessment -Centre for Healthy Human Development: includes the Canadian Health Network (health promotion on the Internet) -Centre for Chronic Disease Prevention and Control: includes addiction -Centre for Infectious Disease Prevention and Control: includes human immunodeficiency virus/acquired immunodeficiency syndrome (HIV/AIDS)- Emergency Response -Center for Emergency Preparedness and Response: includes global and domestic public health threats. -National Microbiology Laboratory: includes national reference centers.
Health Products and Food Branch	-Promotes informed use of drugs, food and natural health products -Promotes good nutrition nationally -Maximizes safety of products in the marketplace and health system
Healthy Environments and Consumer Safety Branch	-Promotes safe environments, with an emphasis on work and occupational health -Works to reduce environmental health risks Edit ok: -Promotes reduction of use of tobacco and alcohol and other controlled substances -Regulates safety of industrial and consumer products
First Nations and Inuit Health Branch	-Assists these communities in addressing health inequalities and disease threats -Ensures access to and availability of health services -Assists in moving control of health care to the aboriginal communities
Health Policy and Communications Branch	-Administration of the Canada Health Act -Works with intergovernmental and international affairs -Sets nursing policy -Works with public communication and relations -Creates linkages with regional programs -Works with policy and planning
Information Analysis and Connectivity Branch	-Creation of knowledge and information through analysis and research -Dissemination of that knowledge
Corporate Services Branch	-Financial planning and administration -Coordinates human resources -Regulates occupational health and safety

Other Health Canada Agencies
Science Advisory Board
Canadian Institutes of Health Research
Hazardous Materials Information Review Commission
Patented Medicine Prices Review Board

Source: www.hc-scgc.ca/english/about.htm

Health Expenditures in Canada - 1998

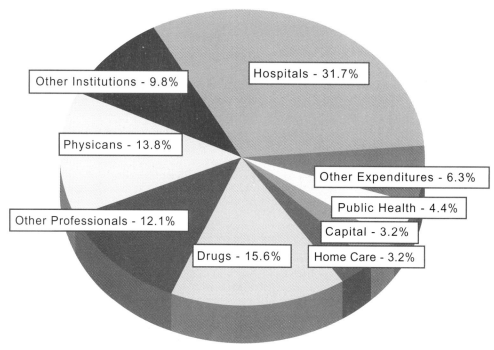

Other Institutions - 9.8%

Hospitals - 31.7%

Physicans - 13.8%

Other Expenditures - 6.3%

Public Health - 4.4%

Other Professionals - 12.1%

Capital - 3.2%

Drugs - 15.6%

Home Care - 3.2%

Figure 3–1
Health Expenditures in Canada—1998

provinces spending almost one-third of their budgets on health care (Health Canada, 1999). Of that, only 4 percent is spent on home care (Health Canada, 1999*).*

Home care, as defined by Health Canada, refers to support services in addition to health care that is delivered to an individual at home. Support services can include homemaker services, meal services, therapy services, and nursing services, including the assessment and delivery of nursing care. In most provinces, these services are directed by a government or related agency (e.g., Workers' Compensation) that contracts with trained personnel (usually nurses or social workers) to assess the situation and decide on the services needed. The actual nursing services are either provided by a government agency or contracted out, often on a fee-per-visit basis (Health Canada, 1999). An ongoing debate has focused on the definitions/distinctions of community-health nursing and public-health nursing. Table 1-1 in Chapter 1 identifies the differences between acute-care

nursing, community-based nursing, and public-health nursing. In Canada, the distinctions between community-based nursing and public-health nursing have not always been so clear. The Canadian Public Health Association (CPHA) (1990) published a document that defined the roles and activities of community-health nurses and public-health nurses. They noted that in some areas of Canada, the term *community-health nurse* was a more generic term, of which public-health nursing was a part. Home nursing or home-care nursing was then described as another part. They noted that the focus of community-health and public-health nursing is "health promotion, illness and injury prevention, health maintenance and community development regardless of the settings in which the nurses work" (p. 3). Similarly, King, Harrison, and Reutter (1995) viewed community-health nursing as the more inclusive term and stated that it included "public health nursing, home care nursing, community mental health nursing, and occupational health nursing" (p. 410). Kerr and MacPhail (1996), in describing the history of community-health nursing in Canada, include both public-health nursing and home-visit nursing. Because many of the community-health textbooks used in Canadian nursing schools are still U.S. based, the discussion over definitions continues. Generally, however, community nursing in Canada refers to *both* the last two columns in Table 1-1 in Chapter 1, with the "Community-based Nursing" column renamed "Home-care Nursing." The rest of the information in that table is applicable to community nursing in Canada. Later in this chapter, we will explore home-care nursing in greater detail.

When the history of health care in Canada is read, it is easy to realize how Canadians were socialized into illness care rather than health care. Because illness was such a catastrophic event, both personally and economically, it was what the early legislators focused on. The message to Canadians was clear—one had to be "sick" to benefit from the health-care system. Over the last decade, *health-care reform* has been a common term. Health-care reform was initiated in an effort to contain hospital costs. However, it has become evident that prevention is a better way to both contain costs and improve the health of Canadians. Box 3–1 gives you practice in accessing information electronically.

| Box 3-1 | Student Learning Activity |

Using the Web

Access the Health Canada Website *(www.hc-sc.gc.ca)*. Click on "Public Health." Scroll down until you see the "Electronic Magazine" on the left-hand side. Read the October 1998 issue on Child and Family violence. Describe here how you, as a community nurse, could use the information in the electronic magazine, and how you would promote this method of accessing information.

The Alma-Ata Conference defined primary care as "essential health care made universally accessible to individuals and families, through their full participation, and at a cost the community and country can afford" (WHO, 1978). The principles of primary health care include: "accessibility of services, increased emphasis on prevention and promotion, lay participation, intersectoral cooperation, and appropriate technology" (Reutter & Harrison, 1996, p. 46). Primary health care became and continues to be the philosophy behind community-health nursing in Canada (CPHA, 1990; Kerr & MacPhail, 1996). The Epp Report (Epp, 1986) clearly set out strategies to promote better health. The strategies are noted in Figure 3–2. Some may be implemented on an individual/family basis, whereas others involve whole communities or populations. The strategies are consistent with the definition of primary health care and have distinct implications for education, practice, and research within community-health nursing.

As each of the provinces and territories grappled with health-care reform, some commonalities in their efforts emerged. The most striking of these is the "strong movement to home- and community-based care" and a "reduction in hospital beds." In addition, "more effective utilization of health personnel" and the reduction of "inequities existing between regions within a province as well as between specific groups within the population" are considered important goals (Du Gas, Esson, & Ronaldson, 1999, p. 46). These goals are consistent with the principles of primary health care and strongly influence the role and scope of community-based nursing.

In 1994, a national health forum was begun to examine health care in Canada. The report was entitled Canada Health Action: Building on the Legacy (National Forum on Health, 1997). The main recommendations from this report include the following. First, there is a need for restructuring the system. Specifically, the report suggested that Canada should fund the care rather than the provider. There was a concern that under the current fee-for-service agreements, the temptation was to increase the provider's client case load to maximize income. The report also suggested including all home care and drugs under the umbrella of the health-care system. This would be a national effort—to standardize care across the country. Second, some additional programs were suggested. One was an integrated

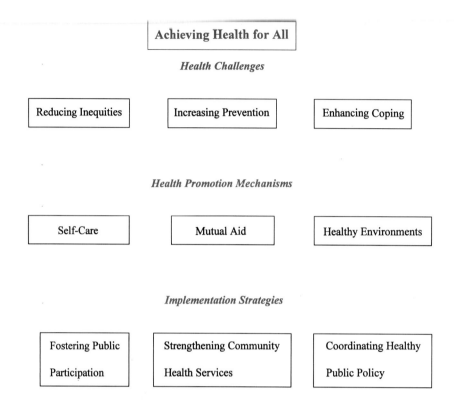

Figure 3–2
Health Promotion Framework

Source: Adapted from Epp. J. (1986). Achieving health for all: A framework for health promotion. Ottawa: Minister of Supply and Services Canada.

child and family strategy and another was an aboriginal health institute. These would address the health concerns of some specific populations who had perhaps been traditionally underserved. In addition, the report noted that an evidence-based system was very important. A nationwide population health information system was proposed, so that treatments and strategies could be compared across the country for efficacy. As always, the issue was that the federal government may propose programs, but the provinces have the last say in how health dollars will be spent. An additional topic for discussion is the inclusion of home care under the umbrella of the Canada Health Act. This was proposed as an amendment, to avoid opening the entire act. This meant that home care would need to meet the principles of the Canada Health Act, including accessibility and universality. If home care were a mandated health activity within the act, provinces would have to demonstrate that they were meeting that mandate, although the methods used could vary from province to province.

Home-care Nursing in Canada

A nurse remembers her first home visit:

It was my first day in the district as a visiting nurse with the Victorian Order of Nurses (VON). I was assigned to go with another nurse on her visits, and the

next day I would be on my own. Although I had been a nurse for several years, this was my first community job. The day progressed as planned, and I admired the nurse's skill in knowing her clients and functioning as an informal teacher with each conversation. That afternoon one of our visits was with an elderly couple. The wife was wheelchair bound, with some cognitive deficits. The husband had an ostomy, and the nurse was going to check on his skin and see how he was managing. After some conversation, we followed the husband into the small bedroom. Pulling up his shirt, we found that the ostomy pouch was filled with herniated bowel, which thankfully was still moist and pink. We both tried hard to remain calm, mostly me. The nurse asked him when he had first noticed this problem, and if he had called anyone about it. He replied, "It only happened this morning, and since I knew you were coming, I knew that you would know what to do." I will never forget the trust on his face.

Author

Canada has had a long history of home and community nursing. By the end of the 19th century, the new country was growing rapidly, and health-care needs were escalating beyond what the health-care providers could deliver. In 1897, Countess Ishbel Aberdeen, wife of the Governor-General of Canada, proposed a system of home helpers. These women were qualified nurses, with additional preparation in home nursing. The group was modeled after the Jubilee Institute of District Nurses in Britain. The project was a memorial for the 60th anniversary of the crowning of Queen Victoria. Although the medical profession was not in favor of the project, mostly because of concerns about lost midwifery income, this woman of influence prevailed. Dr. Alfred Worchester, founder of the Waltham Training School for District Nurses in Massachusetts, assisted Countess Aberdeen in her lobbying efforts. In December 1897, Queen Victoria granted a royal charter to the Victorian Order of Nurses (VON) (Du Gas, Esson, & Ronaldson, 1999; VON, 2000).

At first, there were only a few branches. They were governed by local boards as well as by a national director. During the Gold Rush of 1898, four VON nurses traveled to the Yukon, ensuring a greater national awareness of the services offered. In 1898, a cottage hospital was opened in Regina, Saskatchewan, to provide health services to early settlers. Forty-three more hospitals were opened over the

next several years, with the last being handed over to local boards in 1924. Over time, VON branches could be found in most major cities across the country, with services delivered to several rural areas as well (Du Gas, Esson, & Ronaldson, 1999; VON, 2000).

Services offered are decided on locally, but generally include prenatal and postnatal care, infectious disease care, and services to the elderly and the poor. All services are offered on a nonprofit basis, with payments based on ability to pay. Fiscal deficiencies are offset by monies from charitable organizations such as United Way and its precursors. Eventually the VON greatly expanded its services to include, for example, Meals on Wheels and foot care clinics. As each provincial health plan was established and refined, the VON has become the preferred provider from whom the government purchases home-care visits. Nurses, in consultation with government health agencies and other community agencies, assess clients' needs and make recommendations for amount and type of care. These recommendations are rarely overturned, and most VONs work quite independently with their clients within the organization. Another group with long roots in Canada's district nursing history is Saint Elizabeth Health Care. Begun in 1908 as Saint Elizabeth Visiting Nurses, this group was established in Toronto and contributed to health-care efforts in the area of maternity and child care. Although not as well known nationally as the VON, Saint Elizabeth's has become another recognized not-for-profit agency for home-health care. Over the last few decades, Saint Elizabeth's has expanded the number of locations with offices and services (Saint Elizabeth Health Care, 2000).

Currently, referrals for home nursing are made from many sources. One source is hospitals, where special nurses coordinate the plans for discharge with the home-care needs. Another is the physician, who may call the agency about a patient with a concern or a learning need. The client or primary caregiver may be the person who initiates the referral, whereas in some cases it may be through word of mouth. For instance, the caretaker of an apartment building may know of a tenant with a health concern. When the caretaker sees the nurse visiting another client in the same building, he or she may make a verbal referral, on which the nurse follows up through the office. All referrals must have the permission of the physician as the entry point into the system. Within health plan guidelines, and guided by medical need, the plan of nursing care is then established, implemented, and evaluated over time.

Another group that functions in the community, although not necessarily in home nursing, is the primary-care nurse practitioner. Nurse practitioners have been in Canada for over two decades. Originally, the role of the nurse practitioner was to provide primary health care in places where there was an undersupply of physicians, such as in the North. A variety of university programs prepared nurses for this role. Many of the programs, however, ceased to function in the early 1980s. In Ontario, in the mid 1990s, a province-wide collaborative university program to prepare nurses for the primary-care nurse practitioner role was begun. It was envisioned that these nurses would function in a variety of primary-care settings. In 1998, the Expanded Services for Patients Act was passed in Ontario, giving nurse practitioners the legal authority to independently practice those skills covered under the act (Nurse Practitioner Association of Ontario, 2000).

With concerns about health-care costs and reform, home care was also examined. Some provinces chose to effectively take over the care networks and organizations established by the VON and other providers and rehired many of the nurses to staff a government organization to deliver home care as required. Other provinces, such as Ontario, chose to use a government agency (Community Care Access Centres [CCAC]) to oversee the delivery of home health care, while opening up the competition between providers. For many cities and citizens, this meant great change. The VON had both a long history and a virtual monopoly in the area of not-for-profit home nursing in many geographic centers. Thus when other companies began moving in and acquiring the right to provide home care under the provincial health acts, items such as cost and quality of care became important issues. Agencies were now required to respond to requests for proposals on how they might deliver home care for a given population during a given length of time. This process has raised many concerns. One concern is the process of choosing providers. How will the decision be made, and will cost rather than quality of care be the deciding factor in the

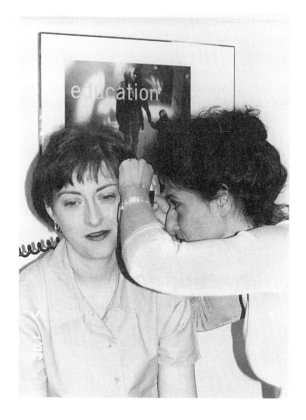

granting of contracts? How would quality of care be measured for such a proposal? Another concern is the quality of work life for the nurses. If cost becomes the deciding factor, will salaries be cut in an effort to cut costs? What kind of mentorship, supervision, and continuing education will be available for home-care nurses? Will home-care agencies be staffed with mostly new graduates looking for part-time or entry-level work, and then quickly moving on to a higher-paying job? What will this do to continuity and quality of care in the community? How will patient outcomes be measured, and who will be authorized to make the comparisons? A third issue becomes the entry of for-profit agencies into the health-care system. Does this violate the accessibility, universality, and public administration principles of the Canada Health Act?

Currently, none of the provincial and territorial health acts permit nurses to bill the system. Ontario is considering legislation that would permit advanced practice nurses such as primary-care nurse practitioners to function as entry points into the system. Ontario and Quebec have begun to create community health centers. These centers are sometimes part of the overall health-care system or targeted to underserved or priority population areas. Because all multidisciplinary staff (including physicians) are salaried and the funding is to the center, primary-care nurse practitioners can work to the full scope of their practice without worrying about billing the provincial health systems. However, community nurse-run clinics are still a dream in Canada. As nurses, we would like to believe that nurse-run clinics and care would focus more on health promotion than strictly illness care, thus saving time, money, and efforts in the long run through prevention of disease, disability, and complications. Although there is some compelling evidence of the efficacy of home nursing and discharge nursing in preventing future hospitalizations and reducing costs (Arnold et al., 1995; Brooten, 1995), other research continues to point

to the physician as the preferred source of some health information and advice (May, Kiefe, Funkhouser, & Fouad, 1999; Metsch et al., 1998).

Education for Community-based Nursing in Canada

In Canada, there are currently two educational paths to becoming a registered nurse. When students attend a nursing program in a community college, they receive a diploma in nursing. A university graduate in nursing receives a baccalaureate degree. Traditionally, community nursing has been more of a focus in university nursing education than in community college nursing education. As in the United States, there has been a professional impetus to move to the baccalaureate degree as the entry to practice nursing. Although some provinces have already moved in that direction, others have been slower to do so. Some university programs offered a diploma in public-health nursing, but have discontinued it in favor

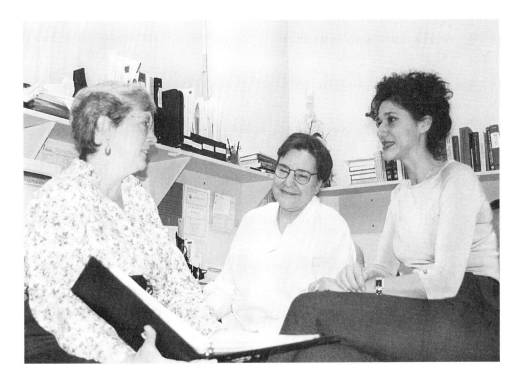

of post-registered nurse (RN) baccalaureate programs. Under many of the provincial health acts, a community nurse is defined as a nurse with a baccalaureate degree and preparation in community nursing. Thus, although agencies can hire diploma-prepared RNs, as well as licensed (or registered) practical nurses to deliver care to patients in their homes, technically it is the degree-prepared nurse who completes the initial nursing assessment and plan of care. Nurses who are eligible for the Extended Class RN designation (nurse practitioners) in Ontario have advanced education in addition to the baccalaureate degree. There is not yet a requirement for a master's degree for the RN (EC) designation, but that may well be the case in the future.

Any educational divisions in community nursing have tended to focus on the client. For instance, if the client is an individual, family, or aggregate, the education focuses on home-care nursing. If the client is the community, the focus is on public-health nursing. In most baccalaureate programs in Canada, students have an opportunity to participate in clinical practice in both areas. In home-care nursing, clinical practice may include well-family health education, health teaching to community groups or classes in schools, or participating in a community prenatal program. In public-health nursing, clinical practice can include delivering sex education in university dormitories, assisting the cancer society with an educational program, or working with a seniors' group. The focus of the clinical experience determines whether the student completes an assessment, intervention, and evaluation of a family or a community.

Culture has also become an important part of community nursing. The "melting pot" notion was never part of Canada's past. In fact, Canada's history and legislation has ensured that multiculturalism is an important part of the social context of Canada. Early nurses recognized the great influence of cultural beliefs on the health behaviors of their clients. Although that recognition may have been misplaced at times in history, there is a greater reawakening of the need for nursing education to incorporate the study of culture into all phases of nursing. However, the use of culturally congruent care is even more important in community nursing, as discussed in Chapter 6 of this book. Box 3–2 helps you compare your community's health care needs with those of Canadian communities.

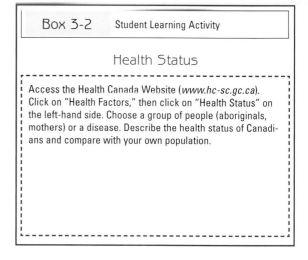

Box 3-2   Student Learning Activity

Health Status

Access the Health Canada Website (*www.hc-sc.gc.ca*). Click on "Health Factors," then click on "Health Status" on the left-hand side. Choose a group of people (aboriginals, mothers) or a disease. Describe the health status of Canadians and compare with your own population.

In Ontario, the College of Nurses of Ontario (CNO) is the body that registers nurses. The College has recently identified a list of competencies for the new registered nurse graduate, to take effect January 1, 2005 (CNO, 1999). This document provided the greatest impetus toward the baccalaureate as entry to practice in that province. Within the list of competencies are items such as "forms partnerships with clients to achieve mutually agreed health outcomes with individuals, families, populations and communities (both stable and unstable)" (p. 15). In addition, the registered nurse is expected to promote clients' rights and responsibilities, advocate for clients, and attend to health-service needs availability. A thorough grounding in the principles of community nursing is necessary to achieve success in the competencies.

Students' Perceptions of Health Care in Canada

In the process of compiling information for this book, students in nursing programs at the University of Windsor and George Mason University participated in an online international discussion about nursing student experiences in their communities. The University of Windsor is in Windsor, Ontario, the only place in Canada that is south of the Canada/U.S. border. The university is medium-sized, with both a generic and post-RN baccalaureate program. George Mason University has approximately 1,000 nursing students at various levels. It also has a generic and post-RN baccalaureate program. George Mason is located in Northern Virginia, near Washington, D.C., and has a culturally diverse student body. Students from the two universities dialogued about how they perceived community-based nursing practice in their countries.

One student in Canada wrote:

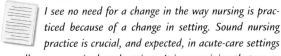 *I think [community-based nursing experiences have] broadened the view of some nurses. I have found being with people in the hospital and being with them in their homes to be two different experiences. By incorporating this rotation into our education, we have been given a broad view of what nursing is. At the same time, I think how we practice has changed and will continue to change as long as we increase health promotion across all social classes in our communities and as long as people are sent home from the hospital much sooner than they ought to be. This extends to working with people that we students haven't worked with before, in situations that we may have never encountered; for example, in homes where there is no soap or cleaning agent. How we practice changes dramatically, though our foundations don't change . . . I think it's a good thing, maybe hard, but a good thing.*

An American student continued:

I see no need for a change in the way nursing is practiced because of a change in setting. Sound nursing practice is crucial, and expected, in acute-care settings as well as community-based settings. It is my opinion that we as nurses ought to operate from a principle of "how" we practice, not "where" we practice. With this in mind, it is my belief that by incorporating community-based nursing into our education we will be prepared to practice and deliver quality nursing skills and interventions no matter what setting we may find ourselves operating in. I see this as adding positively to our nursing education.

Another student from Canada summarized her thoughts about her community-based student experiences:

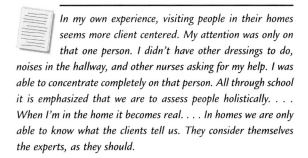 *In my own experience, visiting people in their homes seems more client centered. My attention was only on that one person. I didn't have other dressings to do, noises in the hallway, and other nurses asking for my help. I was able to concentrate completely on that person. All through school it is emphasized that we are to assess people holistically. . . . When I'm in the home it becomes real. . . . In homes we are only able to know what the clients tell us. They consider themselves the experts, as they should.*

Students' comments online suggested that there were many similarities in both nursing education and community-based health care in the two countries. They enjoyed the opportunity to learn from each other and to discuss various experiences they had with their clients. Further excerpts from this dialogue are included in other chapters in this text.

Research in Canadian Community Nursing

Canada has greater land mass than the United States, but only one tenth of the population, with correspondingly fewer nurse researchers. In addition, the single-payer system of health care may have lessened the impetus to move quickly to provide evidence of the fiscal and health efficacy of community-nursing interventions. Whatever the reason, Canadian nurse researchers have not been prolific in publishing research based on community-nursing care. However, Canada was a leader in research examining the role of the nurse practitioner in group practice. In this section, we examine that early literature as well as some published and in-progress research regarding community-nursing care.

In July 1971, the members of a suburban medical practice began to systematically collect data on the effectiveness of nurse practitioners contrasted with physicians in primary care (Spitzer et al., 1974). The methodology was a randomized controlled trial, with data collected over one year. The data collected included mortality experience, physical functional capacity, social function, emotional function, and quality of care. In addition, satisfaction of both the patients and the health-care professionals was tested. Finally, the cost-effectiveness of the whole project was examined. The nurses involved were nurses who had previously practiced with these physicians and completed a training program jointly delivered by the nursing and medical schools. The patients were randomized by families, and the two groups were found to be similar in physical function, activities of daily living (ADL) abilities, freedom from bed disability, and baseline health status. The results indicated that in all areas examined, there was no statistically significant difference between the outcomes of the patients cared for by physicians and nurse practitioners. A serendipitous finding was that the physicians believed that their work had become more efficient because of the increased communication with other care providers, especially the nurse practitioners. It was found that the method of practice was fiscally responsible in terms of societal cost; however, because of the inability to charge the provincial health system for the nurse practitioners' work, the physicians, in fact, lost income.

More recently, a group of nursing researchers (Ciliska et al., 1996) undertook a systematic overview of the effectiveness of home visiting as demonstrated in the literature. They examined literature from 1979 through 1993, both electronically and by hand. From a possible 6000 titles, only 77 studies were found that evaluated an intervention or program within the scope of public-health nursing in Canada, used a control or comparison group, and provided client-focused or cost outcomes. Of these, 19.2 percent were Canadian, and 46.6 percent were produced in the U.S. The authors found that home visiting increased the effectiveness of other interventions, but that effectiveness varied with the intensity of the home-visiting intervention. In other words, a small-intensity visiting intervention (e.g., few visits, lack of focus) might not make a measurable difference, whereas a well-designed program that was intensive and targeted to a high-risk population was found to be not only effective in terms of health of the client, but also in terms of cost to society.

A strong research project is based on an articulated theoretical background or framework and uses clear measurements of relevant concepts. In community-based nursing, one such concept is quality of life. In an effort to provide a well-defined starting point, Harrison, Juniper, and Mitchell-DiCenso (1996) examined the concept of quality of life, as well as the proliferation of research instruments that purport to measure this concept. They articulated a view that differentiated what contributes to quality of life from what quality of life actually is. In addition, they offered an operational definition as well as a discussion of important issues in measuring quality of life. These studies provided a foundation for other nurse researchers to build on to design research studies that are methodologically strong. This research also has produced results that other nurses can depend on, moving nursing knowledge forward and providing evidence to support nursing care.

Community-based nursing research in Canada is moving forward. As nursing care moves back to the community and fiscal and political influences are more strongly felt, it is becoming incumbent on nursing to demonstrate the effectiveness of our care. Currently, structured collaborative practice between nurse practitioners and family physicians is being examined, and many of the agencies delivering nursing care in the community are participating in research that looks at effectiveness of and satisfaction with nursing interventions.

CONCLUSION

There are many issues that need to be addressed in community nursing, whether in Canada or elsewhere. The single-payer system may be advantageous in some ways, but no system is perfect and all have drawbacks. The nursing care that is rendered to clients in the community will use the same nursing theories, the same communication skills, and many of the same nursing therapeutics regardless of the system. However, the community nurse needs to be aware of the legislative and societal context of both the clients and the community. It is only with that knowledge that she or he can assist the client to take full advantage of all the services possible and contribute to the client's independence and well-being.

A final story illustrates one difference between home visits in Canada and the United States:

Many of my VON patients really liked to have someone visit, and near the end of the visit would frequently ask me to stay for tea. Having tea meant that first the

kettle had to boil, the tea was steeped, and then I had to wait while it cooled long enough that I didn't burn my tongue! Having tea with a client was very pleasant, and acceptance of this gift was a part of establishing and continuing my therapeutic relationship with clients in the community. However, having tea with several clients in one day can wreak havoc with the nursing schedule. I soon learned that tea with my regular clients had to be on a sort of rotating schedule, so that none felt slighted, and I got my work done. Finally, I persuaded all of them (over time) that the only way I liked tea was to have it with ice cubes, which also saved time.

Author

Active Learning Strategies

1. Meet with two or three other students. Using the information in this chapter as well as what you have learned on the Internet, draft a list of benefits and drawbacks of a single-payer health system.

2. Examine the box of federal health programs in Table 3–1. Do you agree that these activities are better managed by a federal rather than a provincial body? Why or why not?

3. When examining the Health Promotion Framework, notice that the first row of boxes are the health challenges. Looking at your own population, are these also your health challenges? Suggest some ways that nursing could meet these challenges in your area.

4. You are the Minister of Health in a Canadian province. You want to increase home-health services, while ensuring that quality care is given. How might you go about allocating the additional funds?

References

Adaskin, E. J. (1988). Organized political action: Lobbying by nurses' associations. In A. J. Baumgart & J. Larsen (Eds.), Canadian nursing faces the future (pp. 475–488). St. Louis, MO: Mosby.

Armstrong, P., & Armstrong, H. (1994). Health care in Canada. In P. Armstrong, H. Armstrong, J. Choiniere, G. Feldberg, & J. White (Eds.), Take care: Warning signals for Canada's health system. Toronto, ON: Garamond Press.

Arnold, L., Gennaro, S., Kirby, A., Atendido, M., Laverty, M., & Brooten, D. (1995). The perinatal evaluation center: A nurse practitioner service delivery model. Journal of Perinatal and Neonatal Nursing, 9(1), 45–51.

Baumgart, A. J. (1992). Evolution of the Canadian health care system. In A. J. Baumgart & J. Larsen (Eds.), Canadian nursing faces the future (2nd ed.) (pp. 23–44). St. Louis, MO: Mosby.

Brooten, D. (1995). Perinatal care across the continuum: Early discharge and nursing home follow-up. Journal of Perinatal and Neonatal Nursing, 9(1), 38–44.

Canadian Public Health Association. (1990). Community health-public health nursing in Canada: Preparation and practice. Ottawa, ON: Author.

Ciliska, D., Hayward, S., Thomas, H., Mitchell, A., Dobbins, M., Underwood, J., Rafael, A., & Martin, E. (1996). A systematic overview of the effectiveness of home visiting as a delivery strategy for public health nursing interventions. Canadian Journal of Public Health, 87(3), 193–198.

College of Nurses of Ontario. (1999). Entry to practice competencies for Ontario registered nurses as of January 1, 2005. Toronto, ON: Author.

Du Gas, B. W., Esson, L., & Ronaldson, S. E. (1999). Health care in Canada. In Nursing foundations: A Canadian perspective (2nd ed.) (pp. 33–52). Scarborough, ON: Prentice Hall Canada.

Epp, J. (1986). Achieving health for all: A framework for health promotion. Ottawa: Minister of Supply and Services Canada.

Finance Canada. (1999). Online. Available: www.fin.gc.ca/fedprove/chse.html.

Harrison, M. B., Juniper, E. F., & Mitchell-DiCenso, A. (1996). Quality of life as an outcome measure in nursing research—"May you have a long and healthy life." Canadian Journal of Nursing Research, 28(3), 49–68.

Health and Welfare Canada. (1974). Social security in Canada. Ottawa: Information Canada.

Health Canada. (1999). Online. Available: www.hc-sc.gc.ca.

Kerr, J. R. (1996a). Early nursing in Canada, 1600–1760: A legacy for the future. In J. R. Kerr & J. MacPhail (Eds.), Canadian nursing: Issues and perspectives (3rd ed.) (pp. 3–10). St. Louis, MO: Mosby-Year Book.

Kerr, J. R. (1996b). Nursing in Canada from 1760 to the present: The transition to modern nursing. In J. R. Kerr & J. MacPhail (Eds.), Canadian nursing: Issues and perspectives (3rd ed.) (pp. 11–22). St. Louis, MO: Mosby-Year Book.

Kerr, J. R., & MacPhail, J. (1996). An introduction to issues in community health nursing in Canada. St. Louis, MO: Mosby-Year Book.

King, M., Harrison, M. J., & Reutter, L. I. (1995). Public health nursing or community health nursing: What's in a name? In M. J. Stewart (Ed.), Community nursing: Promoting Canadians' health. Toronto, ON: W. B. Saunders Canada.

Lalonde, M. (1974). A new perspective on the health of Canadians. Ottawa: Health and Welfare Canada.

May, D. S., Kiefe, C. I., Funkhouser, E., & Fouad, M. N. (1999). Compliance with mammography guidelines: Physician recommendation and patient adherence. Preventive Medicine, 28(4), 386–94.

Metsch, L. R., McCoy, C. B., McCoy, H. V., Pereyra, M., Trapido, E., & Miles, C. (1998). The role of the physician as an information source on mammography. Cancer Practice: A Multidisciplinary Journal of Cancer Care, 6(4), 229–36.

National Forum on Health. (1997). Canada health action: Building on the legacy. Vol. 1. Ottawa, ON: Minister of Public Works and Government Services.

Nurse Practitioner Association of Ontario. (2000). About PHC and AC NPs. Online: www.npao.org/phcac.html.

O'Neill, M., & Pederson, A. (1994). Two analytic paths for understanding Canadian developments in health promotion. In A. Pederson, M. O'Neill, & I. Rootman (Eds.), Health promotion in Canada: Provincial, national & international perspectives. Toronto, ON: W. B. Saunders Canada.

Rafael, A. R. F. (1999). The politics of health promotion: Influences on public health promotion nursing practice in Ontario, Canada from Nightingale to the nineties. Advances in Nursing Science, 22(1), 23–39.

Reutter, L., & Harrison, M. J. (1996). Primary health care and the health of families. In J. R. Kerr & J. MacPhail (Eds.), An introduction to issues in community health nursing. St. Louis, MO: Mosby-Year Book.

Saint Elizabeth Health Care. (2000). Online. Available: www.saintelizabeth.com/index1.htm.

Spitzer, W. O., Sackett, D. L., Sibley, J. C., Roberts, R. S., Gent, M., Kergin, D. J., Hackett, B. C., & Olynich, A. (1974). The Burlington randomized trial of the nurse practitioner. New England Journal of Medicine, 290, 251–256.

Victorian Order of Nurses. (2000). Online. Available: www.von.ca/english/front.htm.

Wong, K. (1998). Tommy Douglas: A remarkable Canadian. Online. Available: www.sfn.saskatoon.sk.ca/business/cupe1975/burs5.html

World Health Organization. (1978). Primary health care: Report of the international conference on primary health care. Alma-Ata, USSR, Geneva: Author.

Storytelling as a Nursing Intervention in Community-based Nursing Practice

Jeanne Merkle Sorrell

LEARNING OBJECTIVES

1) Describe the use of storytelling as a nursing intervention.

2) Explore important aspects of listening to stories.

3) Discuss strategies for using storytelling as a therapeutic nursing intervention for clients in community-based nursing practice.

4) Identify research that has focused on storytelling as a therapeutic intervention.

5) Write a story that illustrates a "lived experience" of a health-care system encounter in the community.

Mrs. Cahill, an 83-year-old woman with kidney failure, told the following story:

I would go to the dialysis center three times a week. Sometimes when I was there, my legs started jumping so bad. It was awful. I couldn't sit still. The nurses sometimes would get angry and scold me because they were afraid the needle would come out of my arm, because I was moving so much in my chair, but I couldn't help it. Sometimes the doctor would come by and ask me this question or that. He told the nurses that my jumping legs were leg cramps from changes in my calcium and told them to give me some calcium, but it never helped. I tried to tell the doctor and the nurses that I had restless legs and that was what was wrong, but they didn't seem to listen. They told me to try to sleep, and then the dialysis would be over faster. I tried to sleep in the chair because I was so tired, but usually my jumping legs woke me up. It seemed like everyone else at dialysis could sleep, but not me. It was so discouraging. Sometimes I just cried.

Mrs. Cahill suffered for years from a chronic condition called restless legs syndrome (RLS), a condition in which a person experiences a creepy, crawling feeling deep within the legs that creates an almost irresistible urge to stand up and walk or at least move the legs. This condition seems to be especially common in individuals who are undergoing dialysis. The involuntary leg movements often occur just prior to or during sleep, and they wake the person. Unfortunately, many health-care professionals are unfamiliar with this syndrome and tend to dismiss it as unimportant. The causes of RLS are not completely understood, but the condition differs from the common leg cramps that dialysis patients often experience, and it can be very debilitating. Because the involuntarily leg movements can occur hundreds of time during the night when the person is trying to sleep, it is considered a serious sleep disorder. Individuals with RLS are often extremely sleep deprived. For Mrs. Cahill, the RLS symptoms were much more frustrating than having to undergo dialysis treatment three times each week. Physicians, nurses, and social workers who interacted with her, however, never seemed to realize this. They thought her depression and exhaustion were caused by her kidney failure and long-term dialysis. They spent hours studying detailed reports of lab values and nutritional intake, but no one bothered to listen to her story. Yet it was through her *story* that health-care professionals could begin to understand the unique interaction between the various pathophysiological processes that she was experiencing and how these chronic conditions affected her "lived experience" of adapting to her illness.

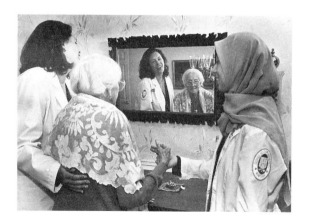

STORYTELLING AS A NURSING INTERVENTION

What do we mean by storytelling? Storytelling is an individual's account of an event that creates a memorable picture in the mind of the listener. Stories are told for many reasons, including entertainment, passing on traditions, or relieving tensions. The use of storytelling in this text is designed to help nurses think about how stories can aid understanding of the unique needs of clients in community-based nursing practice and also how to better understand themselves.

Most communication with clients in community-based practice are storylike, or narrative, in structure. They are intertwined with events in the clients' lives, which are part of their evolving stories (Eide, 1996). Listening to clients' stories can help the nurse to understand clients' illness experiences through their own eyes, as well as provide the clients an important form of self-understanding.

Think about what it would be like if three of your friends suddenly learned that they had a serious chronic illness. What would you need to know as you interacted with them and their families and tried to help them adjust to the illness? Certainly, you would want a scientific understanding of the illness, including the causes, various approaches to treatment, and ways to halt the progress of the disease. You would want to know the side effects and adverse reactions of any medications prescribed and what the overall prognosis for remission or cure would be. Do you think, however, that each of your three friends would react to the diagnosis and treatment of the disease in the same way? They would probably differ considerably in their responses, depending on many factors, such as the current state of their overall health, personality traits, and extent of support from their family. Listening to an individual's story of an illness can help you to understand that person's unique perspective.

The following story, written by a nursing student, helps us to understand the impact that a serious illness had on her.

MY DECISION

In April of 1995, I suffered a serious illness that led to my decision to become a nurse. My husband took me to the emergency room on a Sunday because I was vomit-

ing blood and bleeding rectally after a week of abdominal pain. Extensive testing went on for several days without revealing anything definitive. By Thursday, a team of six doctors decided they had no choice other than to perform exploratory surgery the next day. That evening, my condition continued to deteriorate. During the surgery on Friday morning, the surgeon found all but the last foot of my small intestine infarcted, because of a clot, with most of it black and dead. He removed about 70 percent of it, keeping that last foot and the first four feet, which looked gray and "dusky." The surgeon did not close the incision, but put in a zipper so he could monitor what remained of my small intestine to see if it would survive. I was put in the intensive care unit on a respirator and kept completely sedated.

On Saturday, the surgeon reexamined me and called my family together. He said they had a "very difficult decision to make." It looked like the dusky part of the small intestine was dying, and that he had to take me back to surgery and possibly remove that part. He told them that if he didn't, I would die. But even if he did, the mortality rate was very high. Even if successful, I would never be able to eat again and would have to be fed intravenously (IV) for the rest of my life. My family told him, "Do what you have to do to give her a chance to live."

The surgeon took me back into surgery for the second time, and an hour later walked into the waiting room with the first report of good news. Although it still looked bad, ultrasound revealed some traces of blood flow to the tissue, which meant there was a chance for recovery of the remaining intestine. So he zipped me up again, and I returned to ICU.

Over the next two days, I showed great improvement. When the surgeon looked at my intestine again, he liked what he saw so much that he called to my mom, who was standing outside the room, to come in and look! Some color had returned to the tissue, some peristalsis was occurring, and healing was definitely in progress. With that news, he removed the sedatives and kept me on IV pain medications, and I began to wake up. I pulled out the respirator myself, quite unexpectedly, while still sedated. The next day, I was awake and talking. However, I was so weak that I could barely move my arms and legs and couldn't even squeeze the clip that held the call light to my pillow. The last thing I remembered was the Sunday night that I came into the emergency room, some 10 days earlier.

The following day, the surgeon again took me back to surgery, took out the zipper, and sewed me up. I remember waking up in the recovery room, crying because I was in pain and apologizing to the nurse for being in pain and crying. She kept telling me it was okay to cry, that it wasn't my fault that I was in pain, and she gave me something for the pain. The next day, I left the ICU and returned to a regular hospital room—14 days after I entered the hospital.

I spent two more weeks in the hospital recovering. Of course, I remember this time the best. During those two weeks I watched and visited with the nurses. I was very impressed with their knowledge, professionalism, and caring attitudes. I don't remember all their names, but I definitely remember the people. They were wonderful.

I remember my first night on the floor after being in ICU. I was brought to the floor with three IV poles (morphine pump, antibiotics, heparin, and total parenteral nutrition [TPN]) and a pole for my gastric feeding tube. I had two subclavian catheters because the vessels in my arms couldn't handle the IVs any longer. I couldn't remember the previous two weeks, and some of the medications I was on were giving me bizarre dreams. I was a mess physically and emotionally. I was afraid to be alone, but because I was in a semiprivate room, my husband couldn't stay with me. When I finally felt ready to try to go to sleep, I couldn't figure out how to turn off my overhead light and called the nurse. She came in to find me frustrated and crying. I can't remember exactly what she said, but I do remember that she calmed me down, fixed my light switch so I could reach it, and told me she was here if I needed her again. She didn't make fun of me for crying or tell me I was weak and a nuisance; she was kind and understanding.

Even the most basic things like washing my hair meant so much to me. I had been in the hospital about three weeks with only bed baths, and my hair felt terrible. One morning my nurse came in and asked if I would like her to wash my hair. She even took the time to massage my head while she washed and then helped me dry it. Just that simple act of washing my hair made me feel more like myself again and helped as much as anything in my recovery.

What impressed me most about my nurses was the care they gave me, not how well they gave injections or performed various procedures. It is this aspect of nursing that I want to remember as I perform my duties as a nurse. I never want to forget what it was like to be a patient on the receiving end of nursing care.

We each respond to a common set of conditions in a unique way. It is important to understand individual variances in clients to identify the therapeutic interventions most likely to help an individual to cope with an illness. Encouraging clients to tell you stories of their illness is one important strategy to understand how intervention can minimize disability imposed by the illness and foster renewed health.

Storytelling is an art that has its roots in long-ago traditions of many cultures. Throughout history, stories have been used to pass on important concepts from the past to new generations. Included in these concepts are those related to the maintenance of mental, physical, and spiritual health. With the amazing increase in scientific knowledge in the past century, we have come to rely mainly on scientific information for knowledge about clients and health conditions. The nonscientific knowledge gained from stories has, at times, seemed unimportant.

When first assigned to the clinical area, nurses probably encourage rich autobiographical stories from their clients. With increased client loads, however, many nurses eventually resort to more concise, dry, and structured client reports. It appears that the higher one climbs on the educational ladder in health care, the less time there is for relaxed, storytelling reflection (Coles, 1989).

Stories help create a shared world between nurses, clients, and clients' families. Often, stories can create an immediate bond between storyteller and listener. The Russian novelist Tolstoy said that storytellers should always strive to love the ones listening to their stories and to transmit that love to the audience through stories (Eide, 1996). Nurses may not always meet this standard of storytelling, but it is important to strive for it. Have you ever heard a nurse tell a story about a particular patient who no one wants to visit because he or she isn't compliant with treatments and is unappreciative of anything the nurses do? Often, these types of stories create negative mental pictures for the listener, who then forms a preconceived unfavorable impression of the client. What would happen if, instead, the nurse told a story about how she or he came to realize *why* this particular patient was acting in a combative manner—for example, that he was terrified of being left alone and falling in his home?

This would, no doubt, create an immediate bond of empathy with listeners and motivate the nurses to identify resources to support the client and minimize his fears.

The following story shows how one student came to understand herself and her client better through writing her story about "A Crabbity Old Woman."

MY VERY OWN CRABBITY OLD WOMAN

On the first day of junior clinical blitz, my instructor, Ms. Moss, gave each nursing student a poem entitled "Crabbity Old Woman." The poem contained the reflections of an elderly woman living in a nursing home and how she felt about the treatment she received from others. The old woman felt others judged her quickly and harshly, never taking the time to know her as a person. The poem also drove home the point that all people deserve respect, kindness, and understanding from others. I did not realize that, in just a few short weeks, I would meet my very own Crabbity Old Woman.

I always thought I would enjoy working with older people and was really looking forward to beginning my long-term care clinical. The first week went off without a hitch; the residents I was assigned to were delightful and I was having a great time. Then my second week began.

During preconference I was assigned to work with Emily, a resident who was described as "challenging." No problem, I thought, as I made my way to Emily's room. We'll get along just fine. A nurse's aide stood in the hallway, across from Emily's door. "Have fun," she said as I entered the room. I soon understood what she meant.

Emily was indeed a challenge! She was 78 years old and had a serious heart condition. Even though she could be extremely forgetful, she was a woman who knew exactly what she wanted. During her shower she barked orders constantly; the water was either too hot or too cold, her feet weren't properly dried, we didn't have an extra towel, and so forth. When the shower was over, it was time to tidy her room. She critically analyzed my bed-making skills and then announced, "You'll need to leave now." With a wave of her hand, I was dismissed from the room. Several of the nursing staff laughed. They told me not to take it personally; according to them, Emily was mean to everybody.

I continued to work with Emily. Each day, as she barked or-ders, I would cheerfully comply. And each day, she would tell me just a little bit more about herself. Did I want to listen to her "jazzed-up" heart? She had an amazingly irregular beat! Did I like chiffon cake? She made the best one! She told me stories about her life: where she had grown up, what her fa-vorite things were, and how, most of all, she hated being in the nursing home.

On my last clinical day, Emily invited me to sit down on the bed that I had so carefully made. Not being one to mince words, she said, "Kelly, you're my kind of girl. You'll make a wonderful nurse." And then she leaned over and quickly kissed my cheek. With a wave of her hand, she said, "You'll need to go now, I wouldn't want them to know I really am nice."

As I left Emily's room for the final time, it occurred to me that I had indeed met my very own Crabbity Old Woman. Though Emily was indeed a challenge to work with, she will forever re-mind me to treat all of my patients with the kindness, respect, and understanding they so deserve.

LEARNING TO LISTEN

Coles (1989) reminds us that our clients bring us their stories. They hope they tell them in a way that will help us understand their lived experiences. It is important that we *listen* to these stories. In our fast-paced and techno-logically sophisticated society, we may not want to take time to listen, a condition that Fiumara (1990) refers to as "benumbment." In the midst of the constant noise of our modern world, we need to create sufficient silence to hear ourselves and to hear others.

Many of us, as we rush from one task to another, speak to others without really listening. To listen, we need to be *open*—open to concerns that our clients may want to share with us. These concerns may not be elicited from the struc-tured interview tools often used by nurses and may only be heard through carefully listening to the client's story. Can you think of times when you did not listen carefully to someone who wanted to tell you his or her story? What kinds of distractions seemed to detract from your ability to listen? Write in Box 4–1 the factors that you think discour-age nurses from being open to listening to their clients.

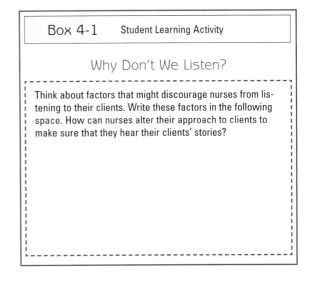

Box 4-1   Student Learning Activity

Why Don't We Listen?

Think about factors that might discourage nurses from lis-tening to their clients. Write these factors in the following space. How can nurses alter their approach to clients to make sure that they hear their clients' stories?

Stories require a special method of listening: It is impor-tant to note the manner in which the story is presented, the development of a plot in the story, the characters who are described and the emphasis given to one or another, and the degree of enthusiasm and coherence of the accounting of the story (Coles, 1989). Does your client have difficulty thinking of a story? Does he or she seem to forget parts and repeat them? Is there anger expressed in the story? Does the story pour out along with tears? Does telling the story seem to have a cathartic effect? All of these aspects are important in listening to stories as you try to understand the lived ex-perience of the client.

The following story, written by a junior-level baccalaure-ate student, describes what she learned from her client about the importance of listening. Does her story help you think about the importance of listening in a new way? Why?

LISTENING

It was near the end of our clinical rotation. As excited as I had been for it to start, I was ready now for it to end. I was tired and I wanted a break. I had made my decision that I wanted to work in the neonatal intensive care unit (NICU) or in pediatrics. To be blunt, I'm not that interested in work-ing with sick, older people. Then I met her. She was a 98-year-old who was recovering from pneumonia and a urinary tract infection (UTI). I thought it was going to be like any other day, but this day was better. I greeted her and explained who I was. As soon as I entered the room, her face lit up. She was just happy to see somebody. I told her I was her student nurse for the day and that I would let her rest a bit more before I did her assessment. She told me that would be fine, because she didn't get that much sleep the previous night. I asked her why, and she explained that someone had given her two shots, she didn't know why, and they wouldn't explain anything to her. At first I thought she may have been experiencing some dementia, and I called to find out what really happened. I found out that they had drawn blood from her and had to stick her twice. I explained this to her and did her assessment. She was grateful for my explanation and added that she tried to ask them what it was for, but no one would discuss it with her. She stated that she was scared and couldn't get back to sleep. She told me she rang her call bell a number of times, but no one came to her. All she wanted was for someone to comfort her for a few minutes, and no one tried. I told her how long I would be there and that if she called me I would come. I took care of her that day by doing her assessments, giving her a bed bath, massaging her back and feet with lotion, helping to feed her, and answering all of her call lights. At one point her daughter wanted to go eat lunch. I told her to go and that I would sit with her mother until she came back with her lunch. Those 15 minutes were the most enjoyable time spent during my clinical rotation. I listened to her talk about her husband, children, grandchildren, and how she had lived here all her life. Her daughter came back and thanked me. I told her it was my pleasure and part of what I'm supposed to do. She stated that none of the other nurses would have done that. It was at that time I realized I don't ever want to become like one of the "other nurses." I don't want to stop caring about people in general, whether they are young or old. No matter how many patients I may have each day, I won't ever stop listening to them. Listening to our patients is one of our most important responsibilities as nurses.

STRATEGIES FOR USING STORYTELLING AS A THERAPEUTIC NURSING INTERVENTION

The interaction between nurse and client is an important factor in using storytelling as a nursing intervention.

As a client tells his or her story, the nurse may engage in a dialogue related to the story, creating a mutual understanding through the telling and listening of the story. Because all stories create a relationship between the teller and the listener, there is a need for openness and involvement. This open and accepting environment is created through various therapeutic communication approaches. Nonverbal behaviors, as well as verbal comments, should suggest interest in the client's story—listen actively, nod encouragingly, be comfortable with silence. Prompt the client occasionally with phrases such as, "How did that make you feel?" or "Can you tell me more about that?" The interest and acceptance that is communicated will help clients to continue the dialogue.

Increasingly, health professionals are using stories as therapeutic interventions with different client populations. This section provides four examples of strategies for the use of stories as nursing interventions for clients in community-based settings—assessment of health needs, reminiscence therapy, narrative reframing, and nurses as storytellers.

Assessment of Health Needs

Assessment of a client's condition often results in scientific information in numerical form. Assessment of a client's condition through stories, however, is also important. The essence of the story, or narrative, is a detailed description of an experience, not a measurement of variables related to cause and effect.

Stories may be able to cross individual, cultural, and educational differences more powerfully than other types of information. Stories can integrate facts, emotions, thoughts, physical and mental sensations, intuition, and imagination in a way that is unique to the individual storyteller. Think about a client who is at home recovering from a heart attack. To care for this client, a nurse will need both scientific data and stories. In Box 4–2, write three types of data you think are important related to both scientific data and stories for this client.

Coles (1989) noted that clients often come to us with preconceived ideas of what they think we want to know, and they do their best to relate those facts to us. They are used to answering many "yes/no" questions on forms in their physicians' offices, with the result that they think they

---

Box 4-2   Student Learning Activity

Data Using Numbers and Stories

When caring for a client recovering from a heart attack at home, you want to think about all the important data for planning the client's care. Write at least three types of data that you think are important related to both numbers and the client's stories. An example for each type of data is provided to get you started. Examples of questions in Box 4–3 may be helpful.

Numerical Data   Data from Stories

Blood pressure   Story of how he rests and sleeps at home

1.

2.

3.

Box 4-3   Student Learning Activity

Using a Story Format for Assessing Health Status

When you meet with clients in your community-based practice, you can learn a great deal about their health needs by encouraging them to tell you stories about their lives. Sharing stories establishes an atmosphere of interest and trust. As the story unfolds, it may provide clues to your client's health needs, which you can then explore further. Try comments and questions such as the following:

I see that you live alone in your apartment. What is it like to live by yourself?

I understand that you've lived with arthritis for a long time now. How has this changed your life?

I'd love to hear you tell about how you have kept yourself so healthy to live to age 92. What kinds of things do you do that you think are important?

What additional questions might help gather important health information for your own clients through stories? Write at least two of your ideas in the following space:

1.

2.

---

know what they should stress when presenting their history to health-care professionals. They are unaccustomed to telling stories to illustrate their health history and needs. Stories can be used, however, as a valuable nursing intervention for gathering important client information and, in the process, strengthening communication between nurse and client (Banks-Wallace, 1999). Stories have the capacity to bring ideas and facts together in a sharpened focus, helping the nurse to picture a client's situation from his or her perspective (Emden, 1998). As a result, important information can be gained for structuring a plan of care.

Think of what it would be like for an elderly woman who lives alone in her apartment, with little contact with the outside world. She goes to her church on a Friday to get her blood pressure checked at the annual Health Fair. If you were the nurse at that Health Fair, you could use this as a valuable opportunity to engage her in telling the story of what her life is like. In this way, you could learn important information about her needs. Box 4–3 contains examples of questions you might ask to elicit this type of information. Write in the box at least two more examples from your own ideas.

Storytelling as a means of assessing health needs can be very helpful in work with clients of diverse cultures (Evans & Severtsen, 2001). Clients' stories are never just their stories—they connect the listener with larger cultural narratives of shared meanings (Emden, 1998). Canales (1997) notes that health care professionals often construct the identity of ethnic minority women from stereotypes and myths evoked by their appearance. As a result, ethnic minority women may experience a feeling of double jeopardy by enduring the consequences of living in a society that devalues both women and members of specific racial or ethnic groups. Although Canales focused primarily on Hispanic women, these concerns related to stereotyping on the part of health-care professionals can apply to many other client minority groups. Through listening to personal stories of interaction with the health-care system as members of ethnic minorities, nurses can better understand the unique health-care needs of these individuals.

Reminiscence Therapy

One strategy for the use of stories as a nursing intervention is through reminiscence therapy. This approach to storytelling has been used effectively with a variety of client populations, including elderly clients with confusion and dementia. Sometimes it is combined with other interventions, such as tai chi (Gibb, Morris, & Gleisberg, 1997). Reminiscence therapy can be enjoyable and empowering for clients. It appears that reminiscing about one's life through stories can be a beneficial coping strategy—it helps to process information, feelings, and thoughts into a broader life perspective and enriches the identification of self. Reminiscence activities as described in Box 4–4 can enhance empathy between you and your future clients.

Research suggests that as we age, we have cognitive and spiritual goals to achieve, and that even people with moderate dementia still want to progress toward these goals (Gibb et al., 1997). Persons with Alzheimer's disease and other dementias often experience devastating losses and multiple transitions in the progression of the disease. These individuals need nursing interventions that help to preserve integrity, generate self-esteem, and enhance

---

Box 4-4	Student Learning Activity

A Reminiscing Activity

Reminiscence activities can encourage important connections between you and another person. Try engaging a classmate that you do not know well in reminiscing about some part of her or his life. Or try this activity with a senior citizen in your neighborhood. Some examples of "leads" are presented to help you get started. Once the person is engaged in telling the story, you will probably not have to "prompt" very often—just sit back and listen!

Some suggestions for leads for stories of reminiscence:

I can't believe that Thanksgiving is going to be here in a few weeks. I always enjoy that holiday. Do you have memories of a special holiday celebration?

You've lived in this house for a long time. Does it bring back any special memories for you?

Doesn't it seem like we've been in school forever? What were your early experiences in elementary school like? Can you think of special memories of those school times?

I noticed that you almost always are working on some needlework project. How did you get started with this hobby?

After listening carefully to the person reminisce about a memory, think about the story. What did you learn about the person from this experience? Do you see her or him any differently after this activity? What strategies did you use to help the person tell the story? Write your ideas in the following space:

well-being. One advantage of reminiscence as an intervention for persons with Alzheimer's disease is that it focuses on remote memory, making short-term memory less important. Interestingly, even the pseudoreminiscences, or confabulation, common to persons with dementia, seem to have a positive effect. Even though these storytellers may confuse past and present, truth and fantasy, the stories do have identifiable themes and appear to serve as a helpful means for social interaction and for reconstructing an identity (Crisp, 1995).

One creative way to enhance reminiscence for persons with dementia is to involve family members in preparing a scrapbook or videotape that tells an autobiographical story through pictures and information about important events in the person's life. Early research suggests that when the scrapbook or videotape is presented to the person with dementia, wandering, fidgeting, irritable behaviors, and aggressive outbursts may decrease, and attention span increases as the individual becomes involved in "reliving" his or her story. Often, children and other family members feel awkward and confused about how to interact with persons who have dementia and thus may avoid visiting them. The use of creative autobiographies such as the scrapbooks and videotapes can fa-cilitate enjoyable interactions between family members and the person with dementia.

Reminiscence therapy can be done as a one-to-one intervention or with small groups. When visiting clients at home, nurses may want to engage clients in recounting stories about certain aspects of their life. Of course, nurses do not function as mental health specialists attempting to diagnose a mental health problem. Rather, they intervene as nurses focused on a method to enhance their clients' enjoyment and sense of well-being. Family photographs displayed in the home may offer clues to what to use as prompts for initiation of storytelling. Observe clients' demeanor as they tell the story: Do they become animated and tell the story with obvious joy? Or does the reminiscing lead to sadness? It is important to validate clients' feelings related to this activity.

Small groups may be set up in the community through various organizations in which participants, in conjunction with a facilitator, share in reminiscence therapy. Acting as a facilitator in this type of group requires expert skills in group communication and a sensitivity to knowing when a reminiscing activity may be distressing a person. If possible, try to observe reminiscence therapy in a group setting so that you can see the powerful potential of this intervention.

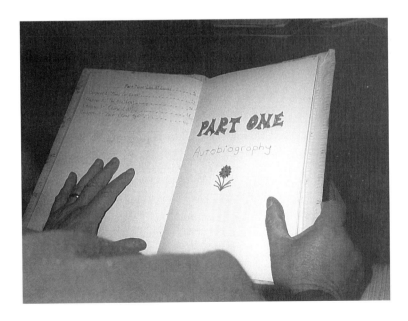

Narrative Reframing

Narrative reframing is a storytelling approach that nurses can use to help clients reassess and restructure their life experiences. Think about your early childhood and later years and how your family's and friends' beliefs and attitudes may have affected your view of different experiences in your life. Did these experiences encourage you to feel that you had control over events in your life? Did they help you feel that you could accomplish almost anything you wanted? Or did you grow up feeling that you were at the mercy of "fate" and could do little to change your life? The way we learn to view experiences in our lives affects how we relate to these experiences. Some people see the "glass as half empty." Others may see the same "glass as half full." Through listening to how clients tell stories of experiences in their lives, you can help them to reframe these stories into a more optimistic outlook and empowering approach.

Clark and Standard (1997) describe the use of this technique for reducing the sense of caregiver burden for individuals caring for dependent family members at home. They describe how a daughter, Karen, who was caring for her "disabled" and "complaining" mother, was feeling "anxious" and "depressed" (words in quotations were Karen's terms as described in the article). Karen was encouraged to *story* her *experience* of caring for her mother, rather than focusing on identification of specific activities that were making her anxious. Karen's story helped the health professional better understand the context of the problem. In turn, the health professional prompted Karen to identify times when her mother was *not* disabled (Karen's main frustration with her mother's disability was related to her incontinence) and when she was *not* complaining (her mother's complaints seemed to occur primarily when she was getting up in the morning or going to bed). Karen was helped to think about *exceptions* to the problems of disability and complaining—problems that seemed to have jeopardized the close relationship she always had with her mother. She learned to *restory* various contexts in the experience of caring for her mother and to focus on the courage, rather than the inadequacy, of her contributions as caregiver. Through

restorying negative aspects of her experiences, Karen was able to transform her feelings of depression and burden into a healthy acceptance of her contributions as a skillful and loving daughter and caregiver. You can use this restorying approach for both caregivers and clients for whom you are caring.

You may also want to consider narrative reframing to explore ethical issues with clients. Ethical principles, as discussed in Chapter 7, provide important guidelines for interacting with clients. It is also important to hear clients' stories of ethical dilemmas. For example, how does the concept of autonomy relate to a client with increasing dementia, whose "self" is increasingly fragmented? Post (1995) suggests that for clients with dementia, we may need to move beyond a standard approach to the use of ethical principles, and involve clients and caregivers in a dialogue that develops understanding of their lived experience with dementia. For the client with increasing cognitive loss from Alzheimer's disease, this may help the family caregiver find a balance between autonomy and a paternalism that will protect the safety of the client.

As nurses listen to their clients' and caregivers' stories, they are drawn into a dialogue in which they can help clients and caregivers restory their ethical concerns. For example, one caregiver, when talking to a nurse about her husband's Alzheimer's disease, wondered aloud about how to balance teachings from her Catholic upbringing about the sanctity of life with the need for advanced directives to protect her husband. As she talked about her concerns, she realized that she was not clear on current teachings of the Catholic Church and thus had been avoiding outlining advanced directives. She then decided to seek out a priest to clarify her concerns. The priest helped her to write a set of advanced directives with which she was comfortable. Using stories in this way helps elicit ethical concerns from clients, guides clients in reframing their concerns, and sheds light on feasible approaches for addressing these concerns. Has any client in your community-based nursing experience expressed an ethical concern to you? In Box 4–5, write down one of these concerns and an opening prompt that you could use to help the client restory the concern.

Box 4-5	Student Learning Activity

Using Stories to Elicit Ethical Concerns

Clients you encounter in your community-based experiences may be concerned about ethical issues related to themselves or their family members. Often, they do not have ready access to a nurse who can help sort out some of these concerns. Through encouraging your clients to "story" their concerns about an ethical issue, you can guide them in thinking through the issue and reframing their concerns. They may then be able to address the ethical concern more directly.

In the following space, write an ethical concern that you sense one of your clients has experienced. Then write an opening prompt that you can use to help the client restory the concern.

Nurses as Storytellers

In addition to encouraging clients to tell nurses their stories, Lawlis (1995) points out that nurses should also learn to *tell* stories to clients as an integral part of the health-care delivery process. To do this, nurses must develop storytelling skills. Lawlis points out that combining storytelling with therapies such as relaxation and imaging can help clients internalize these techniques as needed in future situations. For example, he describes his efforts to teach relaxation therapy to a 6-year-old boy, Timmy, who was being prepared for a repeat spinal tap. The child was so anxious and fearful that as soon as he faced the upcoming procedure, he seemed to forget all that he had been taught about relaxation techniques. When Lawlis created and told Timmy a story about how a "boy very much like him" became a hero in his village by showing others how to deal with pain through relaxation techniques, Timmy seemed to gain a new understanding of what had been taught him about relaxation strategies, and he withstood the spinal tap procedure well. Using stories in this way helps to provide a coping technique in a generalized context of the client's experience, not in a situation-specific event. This encourages clients to integrate the coping technique into their life experiences. Lawlis also suggests that training parents as storytellers helps them to develop an effective coaching approach to help their child deal with illness.

Lawlis (1995) identifies the important features in this type of storytelling. As the storyteller, the nurse's relaxation and ability to involve the client in the story are more important than the content of the story. As the client concentrates on the story and begins to relax, the story serves as an excellent vehicle for education, because the problem can be examined from a distance, encouraging the client to judge his or her own crisis from the safe viewpoint of a character in the story. Use of story imagery can provide the client with a different perspective for viewing and understanding a disease and the methods to manage it. Finally, participation of the listener (i.e. the client) is important in this therapeutic approach to storytelling; the storyteller may want to ask the client to continue the story at some point or to resolve the problem basic to the story. Lawlis (1995) notes that the purpose of this type of storytelling is to involve the client as an active participant in the healing process.

Nurses have not traditionally used stories in this way, but further exploration of this technique as a nursing intervention could create important possibilities for new approaches to caring for clients in the community. Think about a client you met in your community-based nursing experiences who was experiencing chronic pain. In Box 4–6, write down images that you could include in a story to help the client visualize that the pain is decreasing.

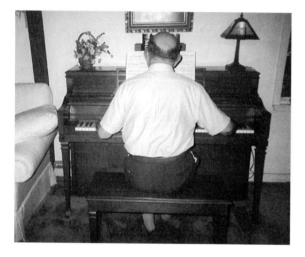

Box 4-6   Student Learning Activity

Images in Storytelling

Many people who experience chronic pain find that the use of imagery helps them learn to live with the pain. Sometimes telling a client a story that uses imagery can help him or her understand how to use this technique. For example, a pianist who lives with chronic back pain, yet sits at the piano for hours each day, may benefit from a story about how musical notes form a beautiful harmony to surround the painful area and protect it. As the pianist sits and plays, he can imagine that the music he creates is also helping to protect his body from pain.

Think about a client you met in your community-based nursing experiences who was experiencing chronic pain. In the following space, write images that you could include in a story to help the client visualize that his pain is decreasing.

This section has presented only four examples of ways to use stories as nursing interventions. There are many more. For example, start a support group for diabetic teenagers to provide a forum for them to share their stories. Structure a storytelling time for children in a preschool to talk about their concerns about going to a health-care provider's office. Meet with members of a parish to hear their stories about how they maintain their health. Use stories as catalysts for individuals to identify their personal preferences related to advanced directives (Kirkpatrick, et al., 1997). What other strategies can you think of for using stories as a nursing intervention? Write at least three ideas in Box 4–7.

Box 4-7   Student Learning Activity

Strategies for Using Stories as a Nursing Intervention

Think about ways you can use stories as you work with your clients in community-based experiences. What strategies can you think of for using stories as a nursing intervention? Write at least three ideas.

1.

2.

3.

RESEARCH IN THE USE OF STORIES AS THERAPEUTIC INTERVENTION

A variety of research studies have focused on the use of stories as therapeutic intervention for clients in the community. This section presents four examples of research from different countries.

Researchers (Good, et al., 1994) conducted interviews with a sample of persons in Turkey who were diagnosed with epilepsy or seizure disorders. Analysis of interview transcripts revealed that participants' life stories of illness had an overall narrative structure and that this structure was composed of a set of shorter, identifiable stories. Specific types of information were present in the stories that appeared to allow participants and their families to justify continued care seeking and to maintain hope for positive, even "miraculous" outcomes. The researchers concluded that the stories represented possibilities for healing.

Another research study (Steffen, 1997) focused on social and process aspects of personal narratives told at Alcoholics Anonymous (AA) groups in Denmark from 1990 to 1993. Analysis of the stories suggests that the ongoing telling of personal narratives in AA groups takes place in a continuum between autobiography and myth. It appears that individual and collective experiences are merged into a shared therapeutic process.

A third research study (Draucker, 1998) explored storytelling as an intervention with women in the United States who had multiple experiences of sexual violence and abuse within the context of their intimate relationships. Narrative therapists elicited discussion of moments of strength, autonomy, and emotional vitality that were embedded in life stories otherwise saturated with suffering and oppression. Results of this research study suggest that narrative therapy may be a useful intervention for opening up possibilities for these women to construct new life narratives.

An interesting study carried out by Chelf, Deshler, Hillman, and Durazo-Arvizu (2000) explored attitudes and beliefs about storytelling as a strategy for coping with cancer among participants who attended a cancer-related storytelling workshop. Participants included persons with a diagnosis of cancer, their loved ones, and members of the public. Findings showed that 97 percent of the respondents agreed that storytelling was a helpful way to cope with cancer. Eighty-five percent of the respondents stated that hearing others' stories of living with cancer gave them hope. The authors suggested further research to demonstrate the benefits of storytelling as a strategy for coping with cancer.

WRITING YOUR STORY

It is important to be able to express clients' stories in writing, so that other health-care professionals can read them and arrive at new understandings of the clients' lived experiences with illness. As nurses, it is also important for us to write our own lived experience stories. Gordon (1997) suggests that nurses need to realize the value that stories can play in understanding the tapestry of care that enfolds the essence of nursing. Stories can be used to stimulate discussions among nursing students at various levels and between novice and expert nurses (Benner, 1984; Vezeau, 1993). We come to know essential content of nursing knowledge through the lived

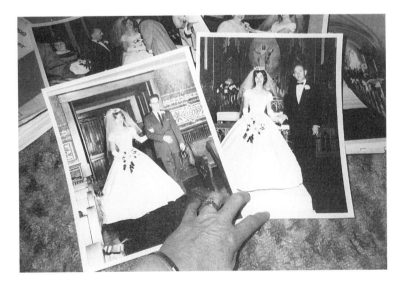

experience of being a nursing student and a nurse; stories of these nursing experiences are critical in helping to generate and understand nursing knowledge.

Sandelowski (1994) notes that nurses are increasingly revaluing narrative knowing—the knowledge transmitted in our nursing stories. Writing your stories can help you form new ways of understanding both your clients and yourself. Writing your stories for publication offers opportunities to communicate these concepts to other health professionals.

Process of Writing a Story

Although you may think of writing as a product, something to be read on a piece of paper, the *process* of writing is increasingly understood as an important learning strategy. Research in composition has provided evidence that writing is a complex process that is often oversimplified. The process of writing appears to enhance thinking, helping us process isolated bits of information and synthesize them into a coherent, verbal shape that can create for us new understandings (Sorrell, 1994a).

The writing of stories is sometimes referred to as "expressive writing." Expressive writing is a type of writing often written to oneself, such as in diaries, journals, or personal letters. It is believed by some to be the closest to the thinking process itself (Sorrell, 1994b). This type of writing can be a powerful strategy for helping you connect your past with your present experiences. Writing about memories of your nursing experiences and examining and reexamining the meaning of events that make up your nursing stories can help you come to new understandings.

Writing a client's story, or one of your own, is not simply a recounting of events. The process of writing a story of a critical incident in nursing practice, referred to by Benner (1984) as a paradigm case, involves thinking about the events in a new way and encourages connecting isolated bits of information from the incident into a cohesive story. This written story, in turn, serves as a case for reflection about the meanings embedded in the concrete experiences of your clients and yourself.

Many of our most profound experiences—witnessing a birth, suffering with a loved one, comforting someone who is dying—cannot be adequately expressed through technical, scientific writing. Skillful writing of stories, however, can allow the power of these experiences to emerge.

As you read the stories in this text, think about why you like certain ones. Is it the focus of the story that is appealing? How does the writing style help to make the story effective? Both the topic and the style of writing are important for conveying important information through stories. The most effective stories are often referred to as "never again" stories—stories that stand out in a person's mind because they illustrate an experience that is extremely important to that individual. These are the types of stories that you want to write about because they will help capture insights that are important for nurses to understand in planning therapeutic interventions. Table 4–1 provides some guidelines to help you write effective stories.

Writing effective stories takes practice—writing and rewriting and more rewriting—but it is worth the effort when you realize the power that your story can have! The following story, written by a junior baccalaureate student, helps us understand how surprisingly difficult it can be in community-based nursing to do something that at first seems very simple—to locate a client in her home for a visit.

A COMMUNITY CLINICAL EXPERIENCE

What I chose to write about happened to me over a course of the entire time we have been in our community clinical so far. That has been seven weeks. I have had great experiences. Not always, though. Sometimes things haven't gone so well. One challenge that I've found during the course of the semester is locating a patient. Part of the requirement for the community clinical is that we each must have two patients to visit in their homes. One patient is prenatal. The other can be anything. I was assigned a prenatal patient at the beginning of the seven-week clinical. I called the number that the health department gave me

Table 4-1

Guidelines for Writing Your Story of a Health-Care Experience

Think about your own experiences with one of these ideas:
Describe an incident related to health care that stands out in your mind because it went exceptionally well and made a real difference in your life.

Describe an incident that stands out in your mind because there was a frustrating breakdown in providing effective health care.

Describe an incident related to health care in which you made a mistake.

Describe an incident related to health care that was a special challenge.

Describe an incident that you think illustrates the essence of what nursing is about.

(Adapted from Benner, 1984)

Use these guidelines for writing your story:
Write in the first person, using simple phrases, just as you would tell it to a friend. Include important details that help the reader understand the context, or background, in which the experience occurred. Try not to include unnecessary details that distract the reader from the main story line. Describe why the incident is "critical." State what concerns, thoughts, and feelings occurred during the incident.

Stories are often only one to two pages. Think about how you want your story to begin and end. If you present too much background information, especially at the beginning, your readers may lose interest before they get to the main message of the story. Try to begin your story in an interesting way that makes the reader want to continue reading. Also, end your story in a way that leaves the reader thinking about the message of this "never again" story.

so I could set up an appointment to come visit her. I forgot to say that she lives in an area that I knew was of low income. When I called the number, the person to whom I was speaking was a child and the only individual who spoke English in the house. After about fifteen minutes of trying to ask if I could speak with Sandy, the child finally understood me but told me that she didn't live at that house anymore. I explained who I was and why I was calling. The child said she would show me where she lives if I came over there. I asked if I could call her at her new house, but the child told me she didn't have a phone there and any phone calls she gets are at this number. I preferred to speak to her herself, so I asked if she would be back the next day to visit and the child said yes. I was frustrated! I had been excited about my first home visit and I had thought it would be really easy to organize — I would call Sandy up, we would set up a time, and I would visit her. It seemed really easy before I made this phone call.

The next clinical day I located her chart and asked one of the nurses who was fairly familiar with her about the phone number. I told her that the number in the chart was not the number where I could reach her, and she did not even have a phone where she lives now. I thought it would be good to know when she was at the clinic last so I asked when she had been in for her last prenatal visit. Maybe I would be lucky and I could meet her in the clinic so we could set up a time that way. I was in luck. The nurse said that she had been in two days before but she had gotten a

Purified Protein Derivitive (PPD). After the PPD, she had been given a card telling her when to be back, and that date happened to be the day I was trying to locate her. Perfect! So all I had to do was show up at the PPD reading and wait for her.

I looked up the time that PPDs would be read. The scheduled reading time was for 3:00 and I was sitting right up at the front desk with the clerks when that time came. Lo and behold, 10 minutes later she came in with her mother! I talked to her and explained who I was, that I was a nursing student getting experience in community nursing. I said that I would like to visit her soon so we could talk about her pregnancy. We set up a time for the visit and I walked away relieved. I finally talked to her—and in person!

The day of our appointment, I knocked on her apartment door with my bag of "goodies" clutched in my hand. I was all set to talk about what she would expect during the delivery of her baby. A teenage boy answered the door. I asked if Sandy was available and he told me that she had left an hour ago with her mom and wasn't sure when she would be back! My heart sank. After all the work I did to try to track down my patient and set up this visit, she wasn't there. Keeping my professionalism, I introduced myself and gave him a note. I told him that I was a nurse and I would like to visit with Sandy. I said that I would be back a week later and gave him the time. My only hope was that she would get that note.

I didn't have any more patients to see that day so I went back to the library to study. At post conference that day I was crushed. I explained what happened and my instructor told me that if she did not show up next week, I would have to get a new patient. I did not want a new patient! I had worked so hard for so long, and I was not going to give up yet. I had worked too hard to give up now. Just then a nurse from the health department came in and asked which one of us was following Sandy. Quickly I spoke up; maybe this could be a clue! She told me that she had her baby the day before. So that is why Sandy wasn't at home that day! I could not help but laugh. What an experience this was. I told my instructor what happened and she was happy too that I had found out what happened. I also told the others in my post conference.

So the next week I knocked on her door arriving right on the scheduled time and an older woman (her mother) answered. I asked for Sandy and as I did, she peeked around the corner. Sandy was home! She invited me in and right away I saw her beautiful baby son asleep in a little car seat.

I learned a great deal about community nursing through this whole incident. Working with the community is not always going to be easy; home visits may not always go as planned and pa-

tients are not going to always be available according to our schedules. This is not like working in the hospital at all. In the hospital, the nurses call all of the shots. In the community, the nurses are working on the patients' territories. Every day is different; every day brings new challenges.

Process of Rewriting a Story

You can make a story more effective through careful attention to the style of the writing. The preceding story, "A Community Clinical Experience," leaves us with a message, but too much detailed information distracts the reader from the main point of the story. Often, some minor changes, such as taking out unnecessary details or clarifying some details, can make a story more effective.

The rewritten version of "A Community Clinical Experience" follows. Do you think it is more effective this way? What changes make it a more memorable story? What suggestions do you have for helpful changes?

A SURPRISING CHALLENGE

Who would think it would be such a challenge to locate a patient? At the beginning of the clinical I was assigned a prenatal patient, Sandy, who lived in an area that I knew was low income. I called the number the health department gave me to set up an appointment to visit her, but a child answered; she said she was the only one in the house who spoke English. I tried for 15 minutes to explain that I wanted to speak with Sandy. Finally, I understood that Sandy didn't live there anymore and didn't have a phone at her new house. I was frustrated! I had been excited about my first home visit and thought it would be simple to organize—I would call Sandy, set up a time, and visit her. It had seemed really easy!

The next clinical day I told one of the nurses that the number in Sandy's chart was not current and that she did not have a phone where she now lived. I asked when she had been in for her last prenatal visit. I was in luck. The nurse said that she had been in two days before but she had gotten a PPD and was scheduled to return to have it read that day. Perfect!

The scheduled PPD reading time was for 3:00 and I sat at the front desk to wait. Lo and behold, 10 minutes later Sandy came in with her mother! I explained who I was and said that I would like to visit her soon so we could talk about her pregnancy. We set up a time for the visit and I walked away relieved. I finally talked to her—and in person!

The day of our appointment, I knocked on her apartment door with my bag of "goodies" clutched in my hand. I was all set to talk about what she could expect during the delivery of her baby. A teenage boy answered the door and told me that Sandy had left an hour ago with her mom, and he wasn't sure when she would be back! My heart sank. After all my work to track down my patient, she wasn't there. Keeping my professionalism, I introduced myself and gave the boy a note saying that I was a nurse and I would return next week at a specific time to visit with Sandy. My only hope was that she would get that note.

At postconference the next day I was crushed. My instructor told me that if Sandy did not show up next week, I would have to get a new patient. I did not want a new patient! I had worked so hard for so long, and I was not going to give up yet. Just then a nurse from the health department came in and said that Sandy had her baby the day before. So that was why Sandy wasn't at home that day! I could not help but laugh.

The next week I knocked on the door, arriving right at the scheduled time, and Sandy's mother answered. I asked for Sandy and as I did, she peeked around the corner. She invited me in and right away I saw her beautiful baby son asleep in a little car seat.

I learned a great deal about community nursing through this whole incident. Working with the community is not always going to be easy; home visits may not always go as planned, and patients are not going to always be available according to our schedules. This is not like working in the hospital at all. In the hospital, the nurses call all of the shots. In the community, the nurses are working in the patients' territories. Every day is different; every day brings new challenges.

Writing Your Story for Publication

You may not want to invest the extra time and work needed to write a story for publication, but it can be a very satisfying experience. If nursing students and nurses do not share their insights from listening to clients' stories, from listening to stories from their peers, or from their own "never again" stories in a public forum, then the knowledge inherent in these stories will remain isolated with the few individuals who have been involved in the storytelling. A variety of nursing journals publish stories written by nursing students and nurses. Some journals targeted to the layperson may also publish this type of story. Frequently, journals publish *Author's Guidelines* in specific issues of the journal; these guidelines provide helpful suggestions for how to write your story. If the guidelines are not included in the journal itself, you can request that they be sent to you.

If your story is rejected by a publisher the first time, try not to become discouraged. It is unusual to have a story accepted the first time without any changes. The editor may provide helpful feedback and suggestions on how to improve the story. Too many writers become discouraged at this point and do not invest the extra effort to revise the story. Instead, find a peer or teacher who has had experience with writing for publication and ask him or her to review your story and the editor's comments to help with revisions. Editors say that writers who do not give up and who are willing to follow suggestions for revision are often successful when they resubmit the story. Who knows, your story could be published in a nursing text like this!

A student wrote the following story for a classroom assignment. She later sent it to a nursing journal to be considered for publication. Can you identify characteristics that the editor saw in the story that made it effective for publication? Although this story describes an experience in an acute-care setting, it has important implications for nurses in community-based practice. What are some of these implications?

REFLECTIONS: NEW YEAR'S EVE

The cheering crowd and bleating horns reverberated from the TV set on the wall, signaling the start of the new year. The rhythmic swish of the respirator contrasted with the cacophonous sound on the television. The tiny body lay motionless on the white sheets. A big white bandage on her head—the result of tonight's earlier craniotomy—overpowered the small, fragile face. Even the tracheal suctioning elicited no attempt at a cry from this tiny being. I knew this night in the pediatric ICU would be long.

As I checked her vital signs, questions filled my mind. How did this small toddler spend this evening? Who caused these bruises and the cigarette burns on her back? What other tortures has she endured? I fought to keep my objectivity and professionalism; I wanted not to care. We spent the quiet hours of the new year together, and I sang lullabies. I stroked her arms. I shared quiet thoughts. I felt warm tears run down my cheeks.

I tried to imagine this child in a better place and time. What would she look like in a party dress at a birthday celebration? Did she ever have a happy birthday? I wanted to help. It was 4 A.M. when her mother arrived. She was a distant woman, with stringy hair, dirty clothes, and no socks. She sat at the bottom of the crib, opened a coloring book, and began to color and sing. Hers was not a song of hope, but of unrelated words. She never went near her daughter; never asked what was happening. I wanted to know more. I tried simple questions. But she just colored, and colored.

It's 5 A.M. and now my little Jane Doe has a name: Amanda. She is just 2 years old. She has a brother named Darryl, her mother says. Social Services thinks he's missing. The mother tells me he's with his father in South Carolina. Darryl is 1 year old.

It is 6 A.M. and the new year has been cruel to Amanda. She is having seizures. The doctors attempt to stabilize her condition. I hold Amanda's hand. I say silent prayers. Why can't we help this child?

The sun is rising. Amanda's life has ended. The doctor tells her mother, who just leaves. The pediatric intensive care unit (PICU) is quiet and hushed now. The doctor writes in the chart. I do the postmortem care. I pick up this warm body, now wrapped in a shroud, and my body trembles as I carry her to the morgue.

The weeks following are filled with depositions to police officers, social workers, and lawyers. Amanda's mom denies ever abusing little Amanda. The judge believes her. Amanda's brother is still missing.

Amanda becomes just a sad memory—until the morning the unit resident brings in the newspaper. There on page 3 is a story about Darryl. Yes, it's true: Amanda's brother is also dead. The body of a battered and bruised little boy was found inside a suitcase at a vacant lot. Amanda's mother is being questioned. The resident and I just embrace and cry. How could our world have lost sight of these two precious little lives?

The years have passed and here I stand again in an ICU, looking down upon a tiny motionless body on white sheets. Once again, a big, white bandage on a child's head—the result of tonight's craniotomy—overpowers a fragile face. The respirator's rhythmic swish fills the silence. The tracheal suctioning elicits no response. I remember Amanda. But I know this little girl's name: Alissa. Alissa's mom is at her bedside, stroking her arms, singing her lullabies, and sharing quiet thoughts. Alissa has fallen out of a third-story win-

dow. This time, the mother shares with me her feelings of guilt, her love for her child, her promises for the future. And we cry.

She holds her daughter's tiny hand within her own to pass on courage and strength. Love floods the room. Alissa begins to respond, first to the suctioning and then to the human voices. She tries to smile when her mother speaks to her. I feel tears on my cheek. We have helped this child; Alissa will recover.

Through all my years of nursing, I have learned one lesson: caring hurts. I used to believe that this hurt would make me lose my objectivity, but that was naive. Hurting provides perspective. I have stopped believing that I alone can change the world or reverse the fate of small lives like Amanda's. Instead, the sorrow and hopelessness of losing patients has made me more introspective and aware of my feelings. I still think about Amanda and her brother. Now, I also allow myself to think of all the Alissas whose lives I have touched. Nursing can make you cry. (Hahn, J. (1998). American Journal of Nursing, 98(12), 49. [reprinted with permission]).

CONCLUSION

Storytelling can be a creative and powerful nursing intervention when caring for clients in community-based practice. Remember, stories have been used for centuries as a valuable means for communicating a special kind of knowledge. Although health-care professionals for many years dismissed "anecdotal" evidence and stories as a useful means of gaining knowledge about clients, preferring to rely on "hard" numerical data, stories are increasingly seen as a unique and valuable way to know our clients and ourselves.

Given the pressures and real time constraints that nurses face in their daily work, it may seem unrealistic to incorporate stories into your practice. It may seem that there is just not enough time for this type of intervention. You may be surprised, however, at how little time it takes to use storytelling with your clients. It can serve as an excellent source of information for your care plan and offer therapeutic benefits for your clients. It is important for nurses to gain skills in both listening to and telling stories, as well as in writing stories. Future research can help to evaluate present strategies and identify new ones for using storytelling as a therapeutic nursing intervention in community-based nursing practice.

Active Learning Strategies

1. Use the guidelines in Table 4–1 to write *your* story about some experience that is important to you. It could be an experience in nursing school with a client, peer, or faculty. If you prefer, write about an illness that you or a person you know has experienced. Describe how the experience affected you. Write your story in Box 4–9. Then read the story aloud to a classmate and ask what she or he learned from your story. Also ask for suggestions to make your storytelling more effective.

2. Interview a friend, family member, or neighbor who has had an experience with a health care professional. Use the guidelines in Table 4–1 to write a story that illustrates the experience. Tell the story from the client's point of view, as if you are telling her or his lived experience. Write the story in Box 4–9. Discuss how the story could help you to plan therapeutic community-based nursing interventions.

3. Go to the public library and look at the various children's books available. Identify different characteristics of stories for different age groups. What forms of stories do you think are best for very young readers? What types of stories do adolescents prefer? How does this information relate to the use of stories in understanding health for these age groups?

4. Select a community-based site where nursing care is provided, such as a managed care agency, a school, a church, or a community support group. Are nurses using stories to assess their clients' problems? How are the nurses obtaining the information they need to plan the nursing interventions?

References

Banks-Wallace, J. (1999). Story telling as a tool for providing holistic care to women. MCN: American Journal of Maternal Child Nursing, 24(1), 20–24.

Benner, P. (1984). From novice to expert: Excellence and power in clinical nursing practice. Menlo Park, CA: Addison-Wesley.

Canales, M. (1997). Narrative interaction: Creating a space for therapeutic communication. Issues in Mental Health Nursing, 18(5), 477–494.

Chelf, J. H., Deshler, A. M. B., Hillman, S., & Durazo-Arvizu, R. (2000). Storytelling: A strategy for coping with cancer. Cancer Nursing, 23(1), 1–5.

Clark, M. C., & Standard, P. L. (1997). The caregiving story: How the narrative approach informs caregiving burden. Issues in Mental Health Nursing, 18, 87–97.

Coles, R. (1989). The call of stories. Boston: Houghton Mifflin.

Crisp, J. (1995). Making sense of the stories that people with Alzheimer's tell: A journey with my mother. Nursing Inquiry, 2(3), 133–140.

Draucker, C. B. (1998). Narrative therapy for women who have lived with violence. Archives of Psychiatric Nursing, 12(3), 162–168.

Eide, B. L. (1996). The place of stories in the practice of medicine. The Journal of the American Medical Association, 276(13), 1098.

Evans, B.C. & Severtsen, G.M. (2001). Storytelling as cultural assessment. Nursing and Health Care Perspectives, 22(4), 180–183.

Emden, C. (1998). Theoretical perspectives of narrative inquiry. Collegian: Journal of Royal College of Nursing, Australia, 5(2), 30–35.

Fiumara, G. C. (1990). The other side of language: A philosophy of listening. New York: Routledge.

Gibb, H., Morris, C.T., & Gleisberg, J. (1997). A therapeutic programme for people with dementia. International Journal of Nursing Practice, 3(3), 191–199.

Good, B. J., Del Vecchio, & Good, M. J. (1994). In the subjunctive mode: Epilepsy narratives in Turkey. Social Science Medicine, 38(6), 835–842.

Gordon, S. (1997). Life support: Three nurses on the front lines. Boston: Little, Brown & Co.

Hahn, J. (1998). Reflections: New Year's Eve. American Journal of Nursing, 98(12), 49.

Kirkpatrick, M. K., Ford, S., & Castelloe, B. P. (1997). Storytelling. An approach to client-centered care. Nurse Educator, 22(2), 38–40.

Lawlis, G. F. (1995). Storytelling as therapy: Implications for medicine. Alternative Therapies, 1(2), 40–45.

Post, S. G. (1995). The moral challenge of Alzheimer disease. Baltimore: Johns Hopkins University.

Sandelowski, M. (1994). We are the stories we tell: Narrative knowing in nursing practice. Journal of Holistic Nursing, 12(1), 23–33.

Sorrell, J. M. (1994a). Writing as inquiry in qualitative nursing research: Elaborating the web of meaning. In P. L. Chinn (ed.), Advances in methods of inquiry for nursing (pp. 1–12). Gaithersburg, MD: Aspen.

Sorrell, J. M. (1994b). Remembrance of things past through writing: Esthetic patterns of knowing in nursing. Advances in Nursing Science, 17(1), 60–70.

Steffen, V. (1997). Life stories and shared experience. Social Science Medicine, 45(1), 99–111.

Vezeau, T. (1993). Storytelling: A practitioner's tool. MCN: American Journal of Maternal Child Nursing, 18(4), 193–196.

Box 4-8	Student Learning Activity

Your Story

Use this space to write *your* story. The guidelines in Table 4–1 will help you to get started. Write about an experience that stands out in your mind as important to you—one in nursing school or with one of your clients.

Box 4-9   Student Learning Activity

A Client's Story

Writing a story from a client's point of view helps you to see the lived experience of an illness from her or his eyes. Interview a friend, family member, or neighbor about an encounter with the health-care system in the community. In the space provided, write this client's story in a way you think she or he would write it. The guidelines in Table 4–1 should help you to write an effective story.

CHAPTER 5

Health Promotion, Risk Reduction, and Disease Prevention in the Community

Marie Peterson Kodadek

LEARNING OBJECTIVES

1) Define health promotion, risk reduction, and disease prevention.

2) Discuss research related to health promotion, risk reduction, and disease prevention.

3) Identify three factors that influence the success of a health-promotion program.

4) Design four health-promotion activities for individuals, families, or groups to use at three different types of community agencies.

Health promotion, risk reduction, and disease prevention are three concepts that may help guide your community-based nursing clinical experiences. Health-promotion activities can be as simple as taking blood pressures at a grocery store or as complex as planning a community health fair. Risk-reduction activities may range from suggesting simple exercises to a group of seniors at a senior center to teaching skin-care techniques to perform during diaper changing at an infant day-care center. Disease prevention may involve distributing brochures listing clinic hours for flu shots to area businesses or the actual administration of the flu shots to clients.

Definitions of health promotion, risk reduction, and disease prevention may vary among health professionals and clients. However, it is important to be aware of both your perspectives and your client's perspectives on these concepts. One useful definition of health promotion is that it is proactive decision making at all levels of care to assist clients in changing their lifestyle toward a state of optimal health (Edelman & Mandle, 1994). Disease prevention means not only preventing the development of a disease, but also in a broad sense, limiting the progression of disease at any stage. It is also important to help your clients identify risks for illness or injury so that they can make important decisions to maintain or improve their health status by taking risk-reduction actions (Edelman & Mandle, 1994).

Healthy People 2010 (Public Health Service, 2000) outlines national health goals for the country, stressing the health-promotion aspects of the recommendations. The premise is to provide guidance for practitioners who are interested in improving the health of both the local community and nation. Health promotion, risk reduction, and disease prevention are all intertwined. Programs and interventions that stress one area of the guidelines, such as health promotion, should also impact the other areas. For example, a health program on nutritional sources of calcium for seniors will help improve their present health status, and seniors who implement the program will also slow the rate of calcium loss resulting from the aging process (risk reduction). The American Nurses Association (1995) states that more care activities are taking place in the community. Your clinical experiences in the community will prepare you to participate in these activities.

One of the reasons that you are given the opportunity to explore various learning sites is because the current *Essentials of Baccalaureate Education* standards of the American Association of Colleges of Nursing (1998) state that "health promotion requires knowledge about health risks and methods to prevent or reduce these risks" (p. 21). As nursing students, you will need knowledge that encompasses not only the disease process but also strategies on keeping individuals, families, and small groups healthy as well. Junior nursing students can focus on small-group health needs, and senior nursing students can focus on the health needs of the community as an aggregate. Nursing students are in a unique position to provide health-promotion programs and interventions to a variety of individuals and groups in the community. You are learning new skills, and the health programs and interventions provide a structured environment, with faculty support, to practice those skills. You also have a unique opportunity to provide a service to the community. You can form partnerships with community agencies to provide health programs based on needs-assessment data. As your knowledge

base increases, the health-promotion projects should also become more complex. Therefore, junior and senior nursing students may work at the same clinical site, but be involved in different aspects of a health-promotion project. The individual and family enter and exit many groups and communities over a lifetime. You need to develop strategies that address the health-care needs of individuals across the life span. Your challenge is to provide guidance and resources for individuals and families regarding health-promotion, risk-reduction, and disease-prevention activities. The *Essentials of Baccalaureate Education* (1998) stresses that the nurse and nursing student must use a multitude of technologies to accomplish this task, from the Internet to community partnerships.

Helvie and Nichols (1998) state that primary health-care needs have a prominent place in a nursing curriculum. Maltby and Robinson (1998) state that in Australia, health promotion and disease prevention should be strands in the nursing curriculum. Health-education programs should be offered in a variety of locations, from beaches to office buildings. Often, you, as students, will learn about health promotion firsthand; the research for the various health programs provides you and the client with new information. Oesterle and O'Callaghan (1996) state that nursing educators must revise curricula if nurses are to be prepared to practice in the changing health-care environment. Primary health-care needs must be incorporated in all aspects of the curriculum. Acute-care settings should not be the only agencies used for student learning. Students need to be exposed to various settings in which primary health care is the prominent focus. Some students need to be convinced that their role in the community can be more challenging than their role in the fast-paced acute-care setting. You will find that many technologies are performed in homes and outpatient facilities. New mothers gavage feed their infants in the home, and IV treatment therapies are continued in the home setting.

LEVELS OF PREVENTION

You may want to organize the teaching projects you plan to implement for individuals, families, and groups in the community into three categories: primary, secondary, and tertiary levels of prevention. Craven and Hirnle

(2000) define primary, secondary, and tertiary levels of prevention as the following: "Primary prevention is preventing [the] disease or condition before it occurs[;] secondary prevention applies to early detection of a disease process or specific conditions[;] and tertiary prevention refers to rehabilitation situations after the disease or disability has occurred, where the goal is to minimize residual dysfunction" (p. 665). The goal of intervention is to look at the health needs of individuals and families with developmental milestones in mind. As these milestones are achieved, health-care interventions need to change for individuals and families to maintain their levels of health.

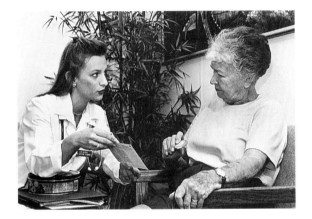

Many of the teaching projects you design will focus on primary prevention. The classes for new parents on safety in the home, the importance of nutrition, hand washing for school-age children, noise levels in cafeterias and workplaces, and the necessity of weekly exercise programs are a few examples. Some primary levels of prevention education involve "hands-on interventions," especially giving injections. You can participate in flu clinics and immunization clinics. More adults are interested in starting the hepatitis B vaccine series. Often, you can present a class on the dangers of hepatitis and then give the first injection in the series at the end of the class. Secondary prevention projects and activities might include classes on self-breast and testicular exams (the American Cancer Society has great handouts), nutrition classes for new diabetic clients, weight reduction and smoking cessation classes to groups with cardiovascular

disease, and weight-bearing exercises for women during the perimenopausal period to help prevent osteoporosis. Tertiary prevention measures are supportive and restorative. They often include services to individuals with a chronic illness. You may be able to teach classes or help with weight-bearing exercises after an amputation or total hip replacement. You can teach stress-reduction classes to individuals after a stroke or a myocardial infarction. You may teach coping skills to substance abusers in a rehabilitation program. You may be able to teach exercises to parents that use play for teaching developmentally delayed children. The primary, secondary, and tertiary levels of prevention will help you plan health-promotion activities for individuals, families, and groups with a variety of health needs and issues. Box 5–1 provides space for you to list projects appropriate for each level of prevention.

Box 5-1	Student Learning Activity

Projects for Levels of Prevention

Think about clients you have cared for during your clinical experiences. List at least one project you can undertake for these clients for each level of prevention.

Primary prevention:

Secondary prevention:

Tertiary prevention:

COMMUNITY COLLABORATION RESEARCH

Zotti, Brown, and Stotts (1996) define the community-based nursing experience as nursing-guided care provided to individuals, families, and groups in their own environment. This leads to various kinds of partnerships and an awareness of the resources in the community. The goal is to promote health by using the values within the community, remembering that a community is a composite of multiple subpopulations defined by common characteristics. A community can be a neighborhood, an entire town, a school, a prison, or a workplace, or it may be a group of persons that share similar characteristics such as culture or religion. Community-based practice or experiences should imply a broad-based involvement of services to all community members, including those to whom a particular offering may be targeted. Community involvement ensures that health-promotion priorities are unique to that community. There should be equal partnership between the private and public institutions in the community. The nurse should assess the health needs of the community and collaboratively set health priorities with these institutions. Of all the members of the interdisciplinary teams of providers, the nurse should be a central participant and is best suited to helping groups set priorities and evaluating health interventions. Community-based health-care strategies should be grounded in the framework of primary health care. When members of the community collaborate with the nurse, they are empowered to take an active leadership role in setting goals, developing programs, and evaluating outcomes concerning the health of the community.

Health-promotion Research

Health promotion usually involves providing information and informed choices so that healthy individuals can achieve optimum health (Redland & Stuifbergen, 1993). Health-promotion, risk-reduction, and disease-prevention activities are influenced by the individual's, family's, and community's definition of health. The environment or community also must develop or be supportive of healthy behavior concepts. The individual, family, and community all define health differently at different times. That is one of the challenges facing health-promotion programs. For example, if parents do not engage in preventive dental care themselves, they are unlikely to bring their 1-year-old child to the dentist to begin preventive care.

According to Redland and Stuifbergen (1993), nursing and related disciplines have studied health-promotion behaviors, but there is no standard analysis of the data with the survey methods that were used. Health promotion and preventive health are used synonymously. Many of the studies focus on changing a particular behavior, such as smoking or overeating, or address the problem of motivating individuals to maintain the healthy behavior. The studies stress that the relapse problem is twofold: declining participation in a program and failure to integrate the new behavior into one's lifestyle. Redland and Stuifbergen (1993) found in their review of studies that women, older adults, and those with higher education levels report a greater number of health-promoting behaviors and engage in a healthier lifestyle. The research also states that the reasons the individual has for engaging in health-promotion behaviors, regardless of demographic characteristics, might be the most important factor in determining whether the healthy behaviors continue. Motivation for the continuance of a healthy behavior needs to be assessed. Conrad (1988) found that participants in a weight-loss program did not necessarily transfer healthy behaviors to other aspects of their lifestyle (e.g., some of the participants still smoked). Conrad concluded that individuals need to find inner strength to maintain healthy behaviors.

Botelho and Skinner (1995) state that the traditional advice-giving approach might not be the most effective method for changing health behaviors. Behavioral scientists have introduced cognitive-behavior approaches to

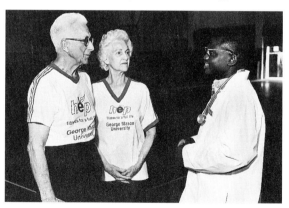

many health-promotion and disease-control programs. Motivating the individual and the family to change health behaviors using autonomy and support gives the individual and the family skills to change their health behaviors and to maintain these changes. Nurses can help individuals, families, and communities define health as wellness, not just absence of disease. Many motivational techniques have helped individuals and families maintain and improve their health. These include such techniques as contracting, self-control, and controlling cues, behaviors that can be fostered by the general environment and community. For example, such things as healthy food choices advertised in the newspaper and billboards that either discourage smoking or promote the use of seat belts are all ways that the environment supports health promotion, risk reduction, and disease prevention.

Shields and Lindsey (1998) stated that health should be a positive concept in our lives. Health promotion should focus on the personal and also on the social resources in a community. Health should be viewed as a resource of everyday life, and the community itself should be evaluated as a resource. The community may have health resources, but are these resources available to everyone in the community? Are there restrictions on the resources, such as geographical or eligibility criteria? Shields and Lindsey quote Mc Knight's definition of community: "Community is about relationships, not a place" (p. 25).

The experience of community changes over time, which becomes a challenge when planning health-promotion programs. A young, childbearing community might over time become a community of seniors, or rural health concerns may develop into urban health concerns. Shared emotions may also influence health-promotion programs. Urban communities may find it is more of a challenge to agree on health-promotion programs because of negative groups within the community, for example, gangs or groups that do not feel empowered (e.g., the homeless). Some communities have instituted informal group meetings to rebuild a needed sense of community and incorporate the sociopolitical aspects of the community into health-promotion programs. You, as students, must formulate your own definition of community, which will influence the skills and strategies you employ when de-

signing and offering health-promotion programs. Shields and Lindsey (1998) state that "if community health promotion practice is to embrace divergent reasoning, with many different and contradictory strategies, practitioners must be willing to tolerate a high degree of ambiguity and uncertainty in their daily practice" (p. 28). Instead of focusing on the universal problem and being unable to find a solution, the nurse or nursing student may focus on small health-promotion problems, the resolution of which may solve a piece of the universal problem. Health promotion involves changing belief patterns and values of both the individual and community; this takes time. Individuals and families may need help to compose their own picture of health, which will continue to evolve. Nurses need to involve the community in consciousness raising and advocacy for health-care programs that meet the needs of the community. According to Wickizer and associates (1998), community-based programs for preventing disease and promoting health rely on interventions like community-wide health education and screening, dissemination of information through mass media, and actions to change laws or regulations that affect health. Factors that lead to program success are the level of community involvement, support from sponsoring agencies, and the fit of the program with the sponsoring agency.

Risk-reduction Research

Risk reduction usually targets a specific area of concern to the individual or the community, such as adolescent pregnancy, cancer, weight gain, cardiovascular disease, promiscuous sexual behaviors, injuries, or substance abuse. Personal choices for behavior can create risk factors for certain diseases. Often, health information related to risk factors is presented in health education classes, health fairs, peer modeling, or alternative choices such as drug- and alcohol-free sponsored events. Botelho and Skinner (1995) stress the importance of motivating the individual or family to change health behaviors to decrease health risks and increase preventive health behaviors. Luepker and associates (1994) studied the morbidity and mortality resulting from coronary heart disease in three pairs of Minnesota communities for 13 years. The secular education in the communities and the trends toward healthy living choices were ongoing in the communities studied. The authors concluded that the study's intense educational program, both individually and through mass media programs, did not significantly reduce the morbidity and mortality rates. Bablouzian, Freedman, Wolski, and Fried (1997) evaluated the effectiveness of a community-based childhood injury prevention program in which high-risk pregnant women received information about hazards in their home. At the conclusion of the study the participants had significantly reduced four safety hazards in their homes; thus this program did provide risk reduction for the study participants.

Ulione (1997) studied the effects of a nurse-directed health-promotion program at a day-care center. The researcher evaluated the health of the children using the Child Health Assessment Inventory once a week for 4 weeks. The health-promotion program, consisting of signs and symptoms of childhood illnesses, infection control, injury prevention, and simple first aid, was taught to the day-care staff. At the conclusion of the educational program, the children's health was evaluated for 4 weeks. The statistical analysis showed that there was a significant decrease in the number of upper respiratory illnesses and accidental injuries. This is an excellent teaching program for both beginning nursing and senior nursing students. The staff at many day-care centers are amenable to student teaching. They often request that the teaching occur during the children's nap time, when the staff can devote their attention to the information presented.

Willis, Williams, and Rozell (1994) used a collaborative model with students and the community-health nurse. The students rated their own health risks, then the community-health nurse helped them identify groups at risk for the same health problems. The students designed and implemented teaching projects for these groups. The students' analysis of their own health risks helped them apply health-promotion and risk-reduction concepts to their teaching material.

Disease-prevention Research

Disease prevention usually focuses on providing identified groups at risk for a particular problem with alternatives to

maintain or improve their health. There is some overlap between health-promotion and disease-prevention activities. Shields and Lindsey (1998) state that nurses need to assess the health of the community. These data will enable the health planners to implement health programs that address the disease patterns and risk factors present in the community. It is helpful, when a clinical site is chosen for a learning environment, to review the disease patterns and risk factors prevalent in the community being served. Primary prevention is the focus of health-promotion activities, but unexpected results may occur. For instance, the senior center's exercise class for mobility may reduce the risk factors for individuals or families by changing the exercise activities of members with coronary heart disease. The same exercise class may lead to discussion groups on exercise led by community members and result in development of a walking path that benefits all groups within the community.

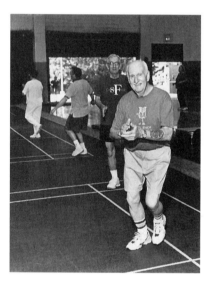

Flynn (1998) states that a primary goal for the future is to eliminate health disparities. The population is becoming more diverse and there are now more populations at risk, including the uninsured and underinsured. Individuals are able to live longer both with and without chronic health concerns. There are more health services available in the community, and the media provides health information to a wide range of individuals and families. Flynn (1998) reviewed research studies that support community-based nursing practice that addresses disease-prevention and health-promotion services in a community, focusing on the "at risk" populations—elderly, women, school-aged children, the homeless, the prenatal poor, and rural populations. Community-based nursing practice can improve the health of the community through home visits and the workplace. Flynn (1998) states that community-health nursing practices must be communicated to the community through the media as well as word of mouth. A combination of both approaches provides communication to both the individual and the community at large as a resource for health promotion. In Box 5–2, list key words and databases appropriate for research.

Box 5-2   Student Learning Activity

Research on Health Promotion, Risk Reduction, and Disease Prevention

How can you identify current research related to health promotion, risk reduction, and disease prevention? List key words that you can use to locate these studies:

What databases can you search to identify research on these topics?

STUDENT-DESIGNED HEALTH-PROMOTION PROJECTS

Jossens and Ferjancsik (1996) developed a pilot project involving nursing students, school nurses, and elementary students. Students taught health-education classes in elementary schools. They also participated in other school activities such as vision and hearing screening, involvement in the family life curriculum, planning and presenting information at a community health fair, and developing health-educational materials for Mexican children. The responses of the school nurses were positive. The school nurses stated that the nursing students were an asset to the health-promotion activities during the school year. Kyba, Hathaway, and Okimi (1997) established a collaborative community health education project between a science and history museum and a university school of nursing. Nursing students were involved with the museum's public education program that focused on health promotion, disease prevention, and risk reduction of diseases. The students were docents in the museum's traveling exhibits called "discovery carts." These "hands-on" carts were used to provide didactic learning and visualization of health-related topics (e.g., digestive system, drug abuse, good nutrition, dental care, or exercise). In the Body Hall the nursing students developed and updated various exhibits. They also participated in Kids Corner Television and the museum health fair. These unique clinical experiences provided the nursing students with an opportunity to distribute health-promotion material and collaborate with other professionals and visitors to the museum.

Getting Started

This section provides ideas on how to get health-promotion projects started in the community. Some of the suggestions have already been tested with other nursing clinical groups. The first step for a nursing student clinical group is to define the community of service. You and your clinical group have to explore the community, perhaps by performing a "windshield survey," simply driving around the neighborhood. If this is your first involvement in health-promotion activities in the community, you will need extensive guidance from a faculty member. Because you live in a community, you may find learning experiences that the faculty are unaware of. Often, students are not sure what are considered health-promotion activities. One easy way to explore some of the choices for health-information teaching is to visit a drugstore, especially one that specializes in home health-care products. You can look at the "health" items on the shelves and list all of the products that are unfamiliar. You may sort the items into body system categories, like sunblock and fungal agents for skin and antacids for the gastrointestinal system. Then decide what health behaviors may be implemented so that the product will not be needed or why a product is necessary (e.g., sunblock). This activity helps students focus on a manageable health-promotion project such as skin protection at the beach or skin cancer. This activity may also help you target a population, for instance, parents with preschoolers or seniors with hearing loss. You may also do comparative shopping for certain items. You may be amazed at the price range for particular items, and this activity also provides an additional community resource for clients when they ask where to purchase certain items. This is helpful when parents on a limited budget ask where to purchase formula and diapers or what store carries batteries for hearing aids.

Toy Store Ideas

You may also make trips to large chain toy stores. Focus on the aisles that contain products for infant safety and newborns. You may feel overwhelmed by the volume of products and decide to categorize the items into "need to have" and "nice to have." This activity helps students narrow the focus of their presentations on health promotion and infant safety classes to parents attending childbirth classes. You may also want to present a similar class to teen mothers groups sponsored by the health department. Students have discovered that they must amend the number of "need to have" items because of budget and space constraints. After this particular experience, students are able to analyze the differences between the groups and focus on the essential infant health and safety needs of a new family. As nursing students, you will realize that teen mothers historically have had limited resources for obtaining needed supplies. One group of nursing students developed a list of various community agencies and businesses that provide infant safety items free or at a minimal cost. You may do the same thing in your community. Box 5–3 provides space for you to write your ideas about shopping for infant and children supplies.

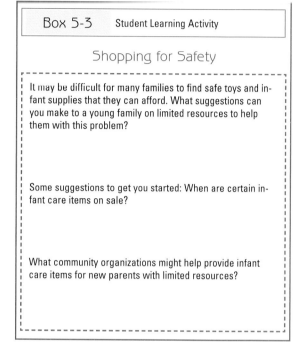

Box 5-3   Student Learning Activity

Shopping for Safety

It may be difficult for many families to find safe toys and infant supplies that they can afford. What suggestions can you make to a young family on limited resources to help them with this problem?

Some suggestions to get you started: When are certain infant care items on sale?

What community organizations might help provide infant care items for new parents with limited resources?

Fast-food Restaurants

You may spend time in fast-food restaurants looking at consumers' food choices and parenting behaviors. This experience helps students focus on particular nutrition topics relevant to families with small children. The analysis of parenting interactions with children in fast-food establishments helps students design health-promotion projects delineating age-appropriate developmental behaviors. Developmental age health-promotion projects have been successful. One group of students taught mothers four simple games they could play with their children while they were eating. This increased the children's food consumption (nutrition) and decreased the mothers' frustration level (stress). The students also taught a class on the attention spans of children at different ages. The students used grocery shopping as an example. They taught the mothers to involve the children in the purchase of one healthy food item per aisle; this activity amused the children and provided the parent with a more relaxed trip to the store.

The following story describes one student's experience with teaching mothers about safety in the home:

A student who liked details decided she wanted to teach household safety to a new mothers' play group at a community center. She obtained permission from the director of the center to speak to the group. The mothers stated they would appreciate any help in trying to childproof their homes. The student started her literature review, visited toy stores, and prepared her lecture. When she was practicing her lecture, she realized she had enough information for a 4-hour presentation. This was way beyond the hour meeting time allotted for the presentation. She was in her apartment, frustrated with the amount of material she was cutting out of her lecture, when she dropped her pencil. In her search for her pencil, she ended up on her hands and knees looking under the sofa and a chair. She found quite a collection of misplaced items in both places. Then she started to laugh. She had the answer to her information dilemma. The next day, after she had presented some information, she asked the mothers to close their eyes and visualize what dangers they would find in their homes if they searched each room on their hands and knees. The nursing student was amazed at the items the mothers mentioned when they described just one room of their homes. The mothers shared a wealth of information with this simple exercise, which touched on most of the information the student had found in the literature. By the time class was over, the mothers had a new list of things to do at home that included items other than dusting.

Elementary Schools

If an elementary school is your community-based site, you are fortunate. Elementary schools are a great site for health-promotion, disease-prevention, and risk-reduction teaching. You can coordinate your health-promotion teaching with the community-health nurse, school nurse, or classroom teachers. In some areas, the community-health nurse may provide you with a list of requests for specific health-promotion topics to be covered in a particular school. In other areas, the entrance to the school population is through the principal. If you are lucky and the school has a nurse, she or he can serve as a rich source of information concerning the school population and local health problems. The school nurse is usually more than willing to help plan and implement health-promotion projects and often has props from other teaching projects. If you choose the school population for your projects, you will be asked to teach on a variety of topics on personal hygiene, from hand washing to use of deodorants. The kindergartners, first-graders, and second-graders love to see the germs that are still on their hands after they wash with water alone and how the number of germs decreases after soap is used to wash. The fifth- and sixth-graders have many questions on personal hygiene, from what deodorant to use to how often they should take a shower. You can teach classes on nutrition, first aid, bike safety, stranger awareness, dangers of drugs, and dental health. Most dentists are willing to donate toothbrushes and toothpaste for the classes. You can call a dentist and request toothbrushes and toothpaste for a health education class, specifying the date of the class and the number of students. The American Dental Association also provides free information for classes. Any local dentist has the association's address and telephone number. Most Head Start programs have an established dental teaching unit that has many charts and ideas for classroom projects. Often, teachers do not have the time to develop and present the entire topic, so they are appreciative when you offer the program. The dental health classes can be fun for both you and your students. Depending on the time frame, you may be able to use dye tabs to show students areas they have missed while brushing their teeth. This exercise is always a big hit with the kindergarten students. You can provide an individualized brushing chart, with stickers, to encourage the students to brush at least twice a day.

Nursing students have had success teaching elementary students about the dangers of overexposure to the sun and the use of sunscreen when playing outside, including sports activities. Some skin-care manufacturers provide samples as well as written material for use in classes. In a letter to the manufacturer, list your objectives for the class and the number and ages of students. Sometimes they include printed material as well as samples. However, they usually need at least 1 month's notice between request of the items and the delivery date, so allow for this when planning presentations. You may be able to make home visits to families to reinforce health education information. Some nursing students have provided in-home education concerning the control and eradication of head lice and ringworm. You may also be able to continue teaching topics to the student and family at home that have been started in the school clinic with the student and the family at home.

The following story describes how one student dealt with a potentially sensitive problem:

A junior nursing student had spent two weeks in an elementary school clinic where she met Jamie, age 7. Jamie was crying and scratching her head as she walked in the door, and the nursing student asked her what was wrong. Jamie stated that the kids were laughing at her again because she had to go home. The school nurse examined Jamie's head and discovered lice. She later told the nursing student that this was the fifth time that Jamie had been sent home for head lice. The mother continued to state that she washed Jamie's head with the lice shampoo and combed her hair. The nursing student asked Jamie's mother if she could visit her at home to discuss the treatment of head lice. When the student arrived at the home she was greeted by the mother, Jamie, and Jamie's younger sister. Jamie's mother outlined all the things she had done to treat Jamie's head lice. After a lengthy discussion, the student discovered that the mother had completely cleaned Jamie's room, but failed to clean the rest of the house. She didn't understand that the nits could be transferred to other objects in the home (e.g., car, bike helmet, stuffed animals, and clothes). Jamie's mother treated the house, other family members, the car, toys, and even the family dog. She was as frustrated as Jamie. (Literature states that dogs do not contract or transmit head lice.) The student saw Jamie at the end of the semester, and was rewarded with a big hug because she had taught Jamie's mom how to get rid of the "little bugs."

Health Fairs

Health fairs provide a unique opportunity to reach a number of people. You can participate in health fairs for middle school, high school, and college students. Through planning and implementation of the health fairs, you may interface with the school administrators, PTA representatives, parent groups, and the health team for a particular county. You can provide table posters depicting health information. Often poster subjects depend on the planning committee and the age of the audience. You may want to provide samples of products to emphasize the health information presented on the posters. For example, one poster on sun protection listed the dangers of sun exposure. Nursing students obtained samples from different sunblock manufacturers to hand out to participants. The students wrote letters to four national skin-care vendors listing the other vendors they were contacting and asking them if they would like to have their products included in the examples depicted on the poster display. All four vendors sent samples of their products. A poster about healthy foods listed foods for athletes to eat before a sports event. The nursing students researched different sports drinks and nutrition bars and were able to provide samples for the participants. The students also obtained bagels and fruits to give to the participants as examples of healthy foods by visiting local grocery stores and bagel shops and asking for their day-old items, which would have been discarded anyway. The stores only requested that their name be displayed at the bottom of the poster, and the students picked up the bagels at the close of business the night before the Health Fair. The health fair participants read the information on nutrition while eating their bagel. One enterprising group of students used a computerized dietary analysis for individual participants based on a five-day diet recall. This particular activity is work-intensive because the results must be interpreted individually for each participant. Students have also provided education on drunk driving and drug abuse at the fairs, including walking the line with special glasses that simulate alcohol impairment. Many of the props for this display may be obtained from Mothers Against Drunk Driving. An easy but popular poster display concerns vision, hearing, and blood pressure screening. High school students routinely visit this area. You can secure space for a vision test using the Snelling chart. You need only a table, chairs, a simple form to record values, a stethoscope, and a sphygmomanometer for a mini-blood pressure clinic. All ages of students are intrigued by their blood pressure. You can also obtain gifts and certificates from local merchants to give away during the health fair to encourage attendance.

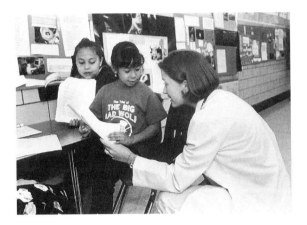

Prisons

Prisons are a unique place to offer health promotion. You can provide a variety of programs in this environment. The students and faculty need to be aware of the risks and safety precautions. The nurse at one prison was worried about the noncompliance of inmates with their tuberculosis (TB) medication. The nursing student provided a program on the treatment and spread of the disease. In another prison environment, the health staff was concerned about the increasing number of pregnant women in the population. The nursing student provided a program on normal pregnancy to the health team and was invited back for a program on high-risk pregnancies. This led to mini-classes for the pregnant inmates on healthy behaviors during pregnancy. Teaching in this environment requires careful consideration of the interventions suggested. Even reading material may be allowed only in the library, not in the individual cells. Some of the props normally used to teach the classes are not allowed in the prison; the students learn to improvise. One prison found a more secure room in which to hold the classes. One inmate discovered she was pregnant with her first child while she was in prison. Because she would still be serving her sentence on her delivery date, the inmate was very appreciative of an opportunity to learn about her baby and the delivery process.

Occupational Health

Occupational health nurses may request that you provide health information to employees. You may provide programs on healthy foods to decrease cholesterol, appropriate clothing for the workplace (e.g., no loose sleeves in an industrial environment), hand washing, exercise during the lunch hour, stress-relieving techniques, and normally expected tests (e.g., mammogram) during a physical exam. You will find this a valuable learning experience, because the audience always asks questions, and you can perfect your ability to answer them on the spot. You may also be able to do individual teaching when you call participants back with information they requested. Another possibility is to teach first aid classes for employees, often at the specific work site. Because of time constraints, these classes should be short and only focus on one item. Often, employees have questions about what to do if someone faints or falls in front of them before the health-care worker arrives. You must obtain supervisor support, so that employees have release time to attend the classes, which can be held as brown bag seminars in specific office areas. Usually, you can obtain meeting space for classes; however, space can sometimes be a challenge, and you may need to explore the use of the lunchroom.

Shelters

Nursing students have provided a range of health information and direct care to families living in shelters or safe homes. You must build in time to verbalize your feelings and concerns for the clients you meet in these situations. Many nursing students are motivated after these interactions to find any and all community resources that might help this population. They even have obtained funds from a local bank to buy toys for the women's shelter. You may offer classes on self-breast exam, immunizations, finger foods, toilet training, hand washing, household remedies for the common cold, infant safety, stranger danger, and how to choose a health-care provider. The needs of this group vary often from day to day, and you will learn about the "teachable moment," which may only be five minutes. This is a needy group; they may or may not be able to articulate their health-promotion needs, and you must explore needs with them after a trust-building period.

Senior Centers

Other places you may provide health-promotion and disease-reduction information are senior centers and senior adult day-care centers. You may be approached by the directors of the centers or by family members. You can always ask permission to survey the participants concerning their health concerns. Design survey questions to reflect both health-promotion and disease-reduction information needs. With this valuable information, you can design the classes and activities around the topics identified in the survey. When clinical groups tried this technique, the seniors also critiqued the students' teaching techniques, which was a valuable lesson on the special needs of this particular group. The students learned that they had to speak clearly during the presentation, the visual material should be in big print, and handouts were always welcomed. The seniors liked to compare the information they obtained in class with other resources. Some of the seniors took the information to their health-care providers for changes in medication and treatment regimen. After one of the student-taught classes on exercise, a senior brought the information handout on exercise to her health-care provider and requested physical therapy for an old fall that had resulted in stiffness in one leg. The health-care provider read the handout and prescribed a month of physical therapy. In a month's time, the senior's mobility had improved. Another senior had arthritis. The student cited research on a new medication that, although expensive, reduced inflammation and therefore increased mobility and decreased pain. The senior took the research article to her health-care provider, and within 4 months of beginning the medication, the senior, who had been confined to a wheelchair, was walking with a cane. Another lesson the students learned is that the seniors appreciate the little things in a program. The exercise class is a good example. The students asked the seniors what kind of music they wanted played and how loud. The students wore clothes similar to those of the seniors, so they could adapt the exercise to the clothes

(e.g., leg lifts and arm raises). For example, the students didn't realize the constraints of raising the arms above the head while seated in a chair, wearing a dress made of fabric that has no give. In Box 5–4, list exercises that you could design for frail older adults.

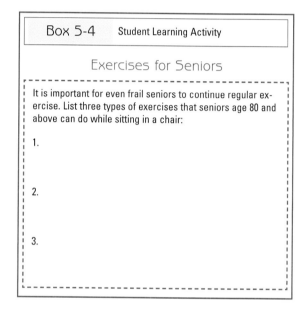

Box 5-4 Student Learning Activity

Exercises for Seniors

It is important for even frail seniors to continue regular exercise. List three types of exercises that seniors age 80 and above can do while sitting in a chair:

1.

2.

3.

You may want to initiate a dance hour or a dance class for the seniors who are mobile. When you partner the seniors, you can assess their mobility and enjoy the program at the same time. You may also be able to perform some technical interventions like flu shots and TB testing. The seniors will evaluate your injection technique. Often you will hear "That didn't hurt at all" or "I didn't know you were finished." This experience helps build confidence in your ability to perform the technique. Seniors are often patient and usually don't move during invasive procedures as children do. You will find that the seniors will approach you on a one-to-one basis so that you may answer their questions or explain some health-care concern. The students who have done health-promotion programs with senior groups stated that their self-confidence grew during the semester because the seniors saw them as experts. You need to listen to the seniors' storytelling and jokes. Often, just listening to and paying attention to one senior tends to attract a group, and then everyone is interacting. You need to also consult with the activities directors at the different senior sites. Our students were able to provide a health-promotion activity to a group gathered for a planned social or art activity. One week the students helped with medication regimen. During the planned art activity, the group made little boxes that the students suggested could be used to keep all medication in one place. Another time, when the activity was about gardening, the students talked about precautions against falling outside. The students noticed that the senior women enjoyed making wreaths with flowers and ribbons, so they linked this activity with hand exercises. They devised different hand and wrist movements the seniors could do while making the wreaths. The activities director still starts this program with five minutes of hand exercises.

The following story describes one student's change of attitude that came about through working with "old people" in her clinical practicum:

A nursing student at the beginning of the clinical experience stated that she didn't like old people. Her grandmother had always frightened her. The student was always willing to make the posters and research the topics for health education, but she never directly related to the seniors. On the day of wreath making, Mrs. P. was having a terrible time cutting the silk flowers. The activities director asked the closest student to her, which happened to be the student who didn't like old people, to help with the cutting. Mrs. P. remarked to the student that she reminded her of her granddaughter, who lived far away. Mrs. P engaged the student in conversation for most of the hour. During postconference, this student shared with the group that seniors were not her favorite, but maybe this clinical would not be so bad.

CURRENT RESEARCH

Health promotion focuses on both maintaining and improving health status. Current health-promotion literature addresses research that studies the behaviors a person or community can employ to help keep themselves and the community healthy. Scales (1999), of the Search Institute in Minneapolis, suggests that developmental as-

sets should be used to help young people validate their well-being. Therefore, if young individuals see their value in the community, they are more likely to participate in healthy behaviors. The World Health Organization emphasizes that health promotion is a process to facilitate people increasing their control over, and improving their health (Breslow, 1999). Callahan, Koenig, and Minkler, (1998–1999) describe some of the obstacles the public faces in its pursuit of a healthy society: limited health maintenance organization dollars, uninsured populations, and the political tension between the individual and common good. *Healthy People 2010* outlined both personal and community health-promotion and disease-prevention objectives. The School Health Policies and Programs Study listed multiple components of the school health program and found that the health-education portion of the program needed improvement (Small et al., 1999). The increasing emphasis and value the public has placed on health promotion has enabled the community-health nurse to expand that role and include more health-promotion programs and activities that benefit the community as a whole (Dixon, 1999).

The risk-reduction literature focuses on how to manage an illness or reduce the impact of the disease on the individual or family. One study (Gregory, 2000) focused on the learning needs of children with asthma. This study found that the school nurse can provide information relevant to the management of asthma in the school setting. The school nurse featured in this study reported that the students enrolled in the program increased their knowledge and management of the disease.

Disease prevention often means avoiding specific diseases that affect health. Disease-prevention literature has shifted from studies about reduced exposure to environmental contaminates to those behaviors that can prevent or delay illness (Breslow, 1999). The public often reads about the diseases that mass immunizations curtail and not the healthy behaviors that prevent diseases. The School Health Policies and Programs Study examined multiple components of the school health program and found that many of the programs focused on disease prevention. The authors concluded that the program was successful in regard to injury prevention, nutrition education, substance use prevention, HIV and sexually transmitted diseases prevention, and tobacco use prevention behaviors (Small et. al., 1999).

CONCLUSION

Health promotion, disease prevention, and risk reduction are important concepts to consider when planning clinical nursing experiences. Increasingly, nursing practice has shifted from acute-care to community-based focus. Your educational experiences will also reflect that shift. Your nursing interventions, which may be in the form of health-promotion projects, should address the changing health-care needs of individuals and families across the life span. The research states that for individuals and families to change their health practices, they must be motivated to change their behaviors. Health-promotion concerns need to be evaluated and prioritized by the community. You need to assess the resources the community has to offer for health-promotion, disease-prevention, and risk-reduction projects. There are many settings in which you can provide health promotion. Schools, community centers, prisons, senior centers, health fairs, and industry are just a few examples. The possibilities are endless. As groups change in the community, so do their health-care needs.

Active Learning Strategies

1. Work with a partner to identify three nutritious foods that preschool children can eat each day.

   What food groups are they in?

2. Think about a client whose baby who has just started to crawl. List four safety hazards in a living room for a child who can crawl. How can these hazards be corrected?

3. Discuss with your classmates three first aid topics that are beneficial to teach in the workplace. Do coworkers need any special training or education?

4. You are going to help with the planning of a Health Fair for senior high school students. List seven health topics that should be addressed at the health fair. Identify two health topics that should have an interactive display.

References

American Association of Colleges of Nursing. (1998). The essentials of baccalaureate education for professional nursing practice. Washington, D.C.: American Association of Colleges of Nursing.

American Nurses Association. (1995). Scope and standards of population-focused and community-based nursing practice. Washington, D.C.: American Nurses Association.

Bablouzian, L., Freedman, E. S., Wolski, K. E., & Fried, L. E. (1997). Evaluation of a community-based childhood injury prevention program. Injury Prevention 3(1), 14–16.

Botelho, R. J., & Skinner, H. (1995). Motivating change in health behavior: Implications for health promotion and disease prevention. Primary Care, 22(4), 565–589.

Breslow, L. (1999). From disease prevention to health promotion. The Journal of the American Medical Association, 281, 1030–1033.

Callahan, D., Koenig, B., & Minkler, M. (1998–1999). Theory, policy and social issues. Promoting health and preventing disease: Ethical demands and social changes. International Quarterly of Community Health Education, 18, 163–180.

Conrad, P. (1988). Health and fitness at work: A participant's perspective. Social Science Medicine, 26, 545.

Craven, R., & Hirnle, C. (2000). Fundamentals of nursing. Philadelphia: Lippincott.

Dixon, E. L. (1999). Community health nursing practice and the Roy Adaptation Model. Public Health Nursing,16, 290–300.

Edelman, C. L., & Mandle, C. L. (1994). Health promotion throughout the lifespan. St. Louis: Mosby.

Flynn, B. C. (1998). Communicating with the public: Community-based nursing research and practice. Public Health Nursing, 15(3), 165–170.

Gregory, E. K. (2000). Empowering students on medication for asthma to be participants in their care: An exploratory study. Journal of School Nursing, 16, 20–27.

Helvie, C. O., & Nichols, B. S. (1998). Reconceptualization of community health nursing clinical for undergraduate students. Public Health Nursing, 15(1), 60–64

Jossens, M., & Ferjancsik, P. (1996). Of Lillian Wald, community health nursing education, and health care reform. Public Health Nursing, 13(2), 97–103.

Kyba, F., Hathaway, W., & Okimi, P. H. (1997). Health promotion in a museum: A collaborative community partnership. Nurse Educator, 22(4), 32–35.

Luepker, R. V., Murray, D. M., Jacobs, D. R., Mittlemark, M. B., Bracht, N., Carlaw, R., Cron, R., Elmer, P., Finnegan, J., Folsom, A., Grimm, R., Hannan, P., Jeffrey, R., Lando, H., McGoven, P., Mullis, R., Perry, C., Pechacek, T., Pirie, P., Sprafka, M., Weisbrad, R., & Blackburn, H. (1994). Community education for cardiovascular disease prevention: Risk factor changes in the Minnesota health program. American Journal of Public Health, 84(9), 1383–1393.

Maltby, J. J., & Robinson, S. (1998). The role of baccalaureate nursing students in the matrix of health promotion. Journal of Community Health Nursing, 15(3), 135–142.

Oesterle, M., & O'Callaghan, D. (1996). The changing health care environment: Impact on curriculum and faculty. Nursing and Health Care: Perspectives on Community, 17(2), 78–81.

Public Health Service. (2000). Healthy people 2010: National health promotion and disease prevention objectives. Washington, DC: U.S. Government Printing Office.

Redland, A. R., & Stuifbergen, A. K. (1993). Strategies for maintenance of health-promoting behaviors. Nursing Clinics of North American, 28(2), 427–442.

Scales, P. C. (1999). Reducing risk and building developmental assets: Essential actions for promoting adolescent health. Journal of School Health, 69, 113–119.

Shields, L., & Lindsey, E. (1998). Community health promotion nursing practice. Advances in Nursing Science, 20(4), 23–35.

Small, M. L., Kann, L., Warren, C. W., Collins, J. L., & Kolbe, L. J. (1999). Progress in attaining the national health promotion and disease prevention objectives for schools. Journal of Health Education, 30, S58–S64.

Ulione, M. (1997). Health promotion and injury prevention in a child development center. Journal of Pediatric Nursing, 12(3), 148–154.

Wickizer, T., Wagner, E., Cheadle, A., Pearson, D., Beery, W., Maeser, J., Psaty, B., Von Korff, M., Koepsell, T., Diehr, P., & Perrin, E. (1998). Implementation of the Henry J. Kaiser Family Foundation's community health promotion grant program: A process evaluation. The Milbank Quarterly, 76(1), 121–128.

Willis, S., Williams, R. D., & Rozell, B. R. (1994). Teaching health promotion: Motivating students through collaboration. Journal of Nursing Education, 33(6), 281–282.

Zotti, M. C., Brown, P., & Stotts, R. C. (1996). Community-based nursing versus community health nursing: What does it all mean? Nursing Outlook, 44, 211–217.

CHAPTER 6

Cultural Competence as a Foundation for Community-based Nursing Practice

Charlene Yvonne Douglas

LEARNING OBJECTIVES

1) Describe the demographic changes occurring in industrialized countries.

2) Define culture and cultural competence.

3) Discuss the components of cultural competence at the individual nurse and health system level.

4) Provide guidelines for avoiding cultural pitfalls when working with clients from selected populations.

5) Interpret research findings that indicate a lack of cultural competence and the effects on patient outcomes.

6) Provide examples of individual and family cultural assessment tools.

Demographic changes in all industrialized countries have resulted in new levels of diversity within populations. Immigration across borders and population shifts within geographic areas have presented health-care providers with new challenges. These immigration patterns are resulting in populations that are diverse in terms of race, ethnicity, culture, language, and religion. Health-care providers and organizations must implement funda-mental changes to meet the health-care needs of this diverse population. This new diversity requires the skills of "cultural competence" to bridge the gaps between nurse and clients (National Center for Cultural Competence [NCCC], 1999).

This chapter discusses the changing population composition of the United States and Canada and the health-care challenges that are presented by these changes. The concepts of culture and cultural competence are examined, along with their impact on the nurse-client relationship and the care delivered by health-care systems. General guidelines for culturally competent interactions with selected populations are discussed, and a sample tool for cultural assessment is provided.

DEMOGRAPHIC CHANGES

The total U.S. population is projected to grow from 275 million in 2000 to 300 million by 2010 and 350 million by 2030. Although these figures seem to indicate a rapid rate of growth, the percent change in population that they represent is slower than at any other time in the 20th century. The projections assume that the rate of immigration into the United States will remain constant, but the rate of **natural increase** (births minus deaths) will slow as a result of the aging U.S. population. The increased number of aged individuals will result in a higher number of deaths (NCCC, 1999; Bureau of the Census, 1996).

International Projections

Italy—Demographic Changes

The population pyramids in Figures 6–1, 6–2, and 6–3 are projections for the male and female populations of Italy, the United States, and Canada. The pyramid for Italy is constricting. Currently, two people die for every child that is born in Italy, with families averaging less than two children each. As in the United States, Italy has a large segment of the population that is aging, but unlike the United States, Italy has a low level of immigration. This has resulted in a low rate of natural increase. This low rate of birth and an aging population is resulting in a high **dependency ratio.** The dependency ratio indicates how many children (0 to 17 years) and elderly (65 years and older) there are for every 100 people of working age, 18 to 64 years. A rising dependency ratio strains a country's ability to provide pensions for the aged and health care for all of its dependents, including children.

United States—Demographic Changes

The most significant shift in the age composition of the United States will be the aging of the baby boomers, per-

sons born after World War II, from 1946 to 1964. Currently, about 13 percent of the population is over 65 years of age. By the year 2030, 20 percent of the population will be 65 years of age or over. The most rapidly growing age group will be the 85+ population, which will double its current size by 2025 and increase fivefold by 2050.

This aging trend, coupled with a relatively stable number of children under 18 (kept stable largely through immigration) will contribute to an increased dependency ratio.

The population profile of the United States from 2000 to 2050 is presented in Table 6–1. The U.S. Census projects that from 1997 to 2050, less than half of the population growth will occur in the combined black and white non-Hispanic populations. The groups with the greatest rates of growth will be the Hispanic and Asian/Pacific Islander (AAPI) populations.

Immigration will be the major factor in future population growth. The U.S. Census Bureau projects a net immigration (number of persons entering the United States minus the number leaving) of 820,000 persons a year, composed of 350,000 Hispanics, 226,000 Asian/Pacific Islanders, 186,000 non-Hispanic whites (largely from Europe), and 57,000 non-Hispanic blacks.

The Hispanic-origin population will contribute the largest number of persons to the total population. However, through 2020, the Asian/Pacific Islanders will be the fastest growing race/ethnic group. By the year 2000, Asian/Pacific Islanders will number 11 million, which will double by 2020 and triple by 2040. The Native American, Inuit, and Aleut populations will grow primarily by birth. These populations will grow steadily, but slowly.

Canada—Demographic Changes

Less densely populated countries, such as Canada, are also experiencing population changes fueled by immigration. Table 6–2 presents Canada's demographic profile for 1998 and a projected profile for the year 2010.

The rate of natural increase (births minus deaths) is slowing over time, and natural increase accounts for only one-half of the annual rate of population growth. Immigration is thus powering Canadian population growth. The number of international migrants has grown precipitously in the last two decades.

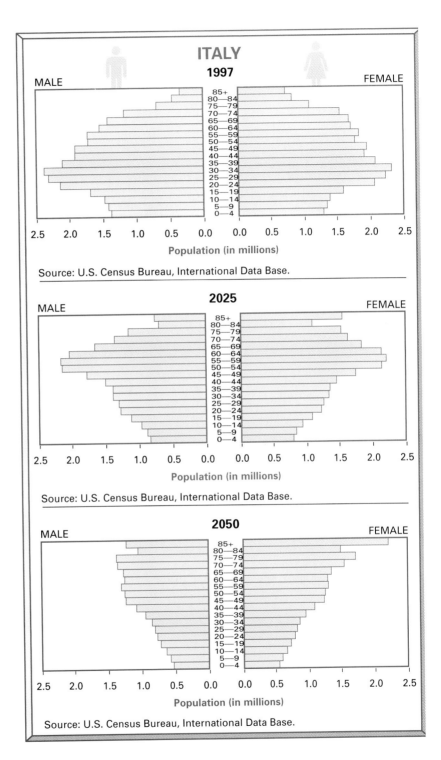

Figure 6–1 Population Pyramid for Italy: 1997, 2025, and 2050

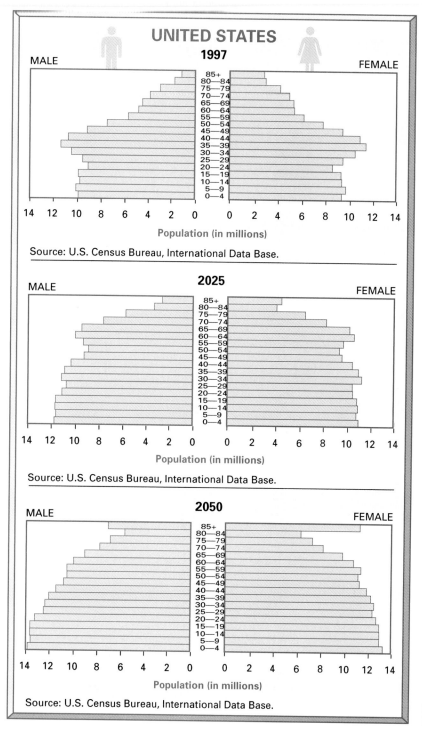

Source: U.S. Census Bureau, International Data Base.

*Figure 6–2   Population Pyramid for
United States: 1997, 2025, and 2050*

Table 6–1

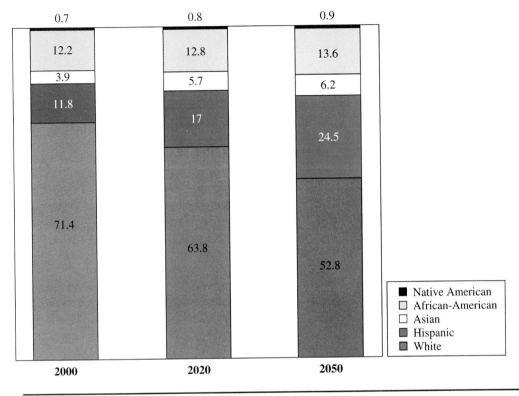

Source: *Population Projections of the U.S. by Age, Sex, Race, and Hispanic Origin: 1995–2050.*

The countries of origin for these immigrants are clearly documented in Canadian records, with specific countries and religious groups catalogued. Table 6–4, listing selected populations, shows the pattern of increase among all ethnic groups migrating to Canada. As in the United States, nurses in Canada will be caring for clients whose diversity is expanding to form new mosaics.

NURSING POPULATION DATA

The nursing population in the United States does not begin to approximate the diversity in the general population (see Figure 6–4). In addition to displaying competence in technical skills and developing a scientific knowledge base, nurses must become competent in caring for clients from ethnic and racial backgrounds that are very different from their own.

Nurses bring their own cultural heritage as well as the heritage of biomedicine into the professional setting. The U.S. health-care system has long valued *fighting* disease. *War* was declared on cancer, cells were *killed* for the greater good of the body, and death was the ultimate *defeat*. Alternative medicine has become popular in the United States, with a corresponding demand for alternative treatments and practitioners. Demand for alternative practices has made inroads into standard medical care and changed some of the focus of traditional medicine toward working with the body. Hospice care treats the dying process as the final transition in the life span, with a focus on comfort and the absence of pain. These changes demonstrate how a culture, in this case medicine, changes and adapts in response to larger societal changes.

The nurse-client relationship includes the interaction of three cultural systems: the culture of the nurse, the

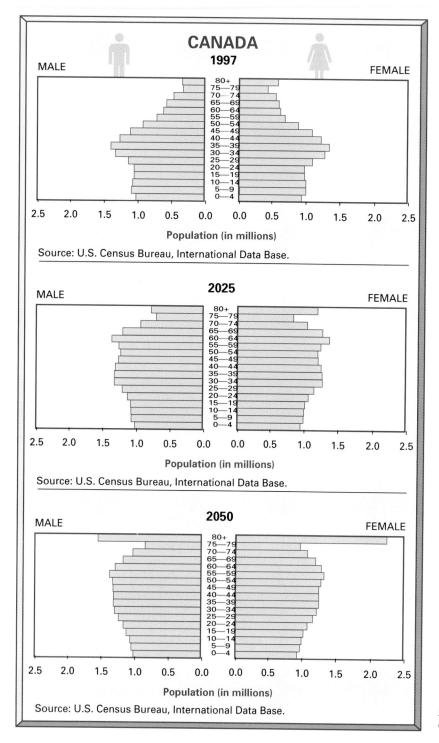

Figure 6–3   Population Pyramid for Canada: 1997, 2025, and 2050

Table 6-2

Demographic Profile of Canada

	1998	**2010**
Births per 1000 population	12.0	11.0
Deaths per 1000 population	7.0	8.0
Rate of natural increase (percent)	0.5	0.3
Annual rate of growth (percent)	1.1	0.8
Life expectancy at birth	79.2	80.7
Infant deaths per 1000 live births	6.0	5.0
Total fertility rate (per woman)	1.7	1.6

Source: U.S. Census Bureau, International Data Base

Table 6-4

Immigration Patterns for Selected Groups in Canada

POPULATION GROUP	**1971**	**1981**	**1986**	**1991**
Polish	316,425	254,000	222,260	272,810
Ukrainian	580,660	530,000	420,210	406,645
Dutch	425,945	408,000	351,765	358,180
Chinese	118,815	289,000	360,320	586,645
Jewish	295,945	264,000	245,860	245,840
Black			11,580	214,265

Source: U.S. Census Bureau, International Data Base

Table 6-3

YEAR	**TOTAL POPULATION**	**NUMBER OF INTERNATIONAL MIGRANTS**
1983-84	24,593,000	38,144
1991	28,118,000	4,947,645

Source: U.S. Census Bureau, International Data Base

culture of the client, and the culture of the setting (American Nurses Association [ANA], 1998).

CULTURE

To the layperson, the word *culture* may denote an appreciation of classical music and fine art, but culture is much more inclusive. **Culture** is "the integrated pattern of human behavior that includes thoughts, communication, actions, customs, beliefs, values and institution of a racial, ethnic, religious or social group" (National Technical Assistance Center for Children's Mental Health [NTAC], 1989, p. 13). Culture shapes how people view their world and how they structure their families and communities. Culture is learned from earliest childhood within the family (a process referred to as **enculturation**), is shared by the majority of the members of the culture, and may change in response to societal change. Culture is not the result of biological inheritance (Health Resources and Services Administration, 1996; Purnell & Paulanka, 1998; ANA, 1998).

Every interaction and life experience has a cultural component. The behaviors and beliefs learned at an early age that persist into adulthood achieve the status of "truth." Eating may involve a knife, fork, and spoon—or chopsticks. Rules governing behavior are referred to as **norms.** There may be norms governing the interaction of children and adults: Children may be required to use titles of respect when addressing adults; some children were taught to look at adults when speaking, whereas others may have been taught to look down. Cultural

Distribution by Racial/Ethnic Group
March 1996

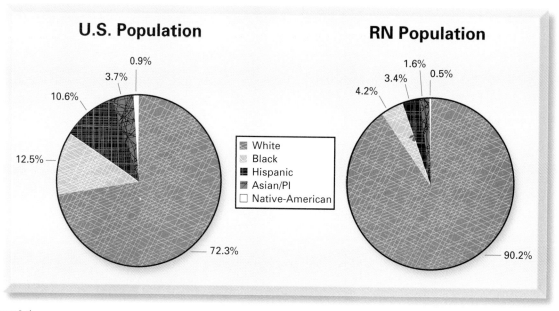

Figure 6–4

Source: Bureau of Health Professions (2000)

understanding is typically established by the age of 5 (Lynch & Hanson, 1998).

Culture is not limited to client groups. Despite our racial and ethnic diversity, nurses share a common and very powerful culture—biomedicine. This culture dictates our worldview. What makes a "good" nurse? Is it scientific knowledge, organization, or technical competence? The "answer" is based on the values held by the profession. **Values** are principles and standards that have meaning and worth to individuals, groups, or communities. Cooperation is valued over competition in some cultures, whereas the opposite is true in others. Appearance is another value closely held within cultures. The cultural aesthetic may dictate a preference for a broad nose or narrow, straight hair or curly, specific standards of dress, or thin bodies (Lynch & Hanson, 1998). Box 6–1 gives you an opportunity to discuss the nursing culture.

Box 6-1	Student Learning Activity

Nursing Culture

Nursing has its own culture. List here some of the norms and values that you believe are inherent in the nursing profession.

Norms:

Values:

Culture refers to socially transmitted beliefs, institutions, and behavior patterns, whereas **ethnicity** refers to a common history, a shared culture or religion, or a separate sense of identity. Ethnicity is often confused with **race,** which refers to biologically related people. The term *Hispanic* is an ethnic designation that refers to people with a common Spanish heritage. Hispanics can be of any race. The U.S. Census differentiates racial categories as follows: Hispanic, non-Hispanic white, or non-Hispanic black. Individuals identifying themselves as Hispanic can have features that range on the physical continuum from black to white.

The term *ethnic* may provoke negative feelings because it indicates separateness from the majority, but it is important in defining cultural context. Most Americans cannot visually distinguish a Protestant from a Catholic, but that ethnic difference is clear and powerful in Northern Ireland. The holiday traditions of three white American families may be very different, even if they all identify themselves as "white American." Consider the differences in food and holiday traditions if the grandmothers serving the families immigrated from Italy, Germany, and France; the differences are *ethnic* differences. The U.S. Census racial groupings (black, white, Hispanic, Native American, and Asian/Pacific Islander) are a mixture of race, ethnicity, and geographic location (ANA, 1998). There are at least 106 ethnic groups and more than 170 Native American groups in the United States (Julia, 1996; Spector, 1996).

Ethnocentrism is the almost universal tendency of human beings to believe that their way of thinking, behaving, and believing is the only correct way. Ethnocentrism can be a major barrier to providing culturally competent care. An ethnocentric mind-set interprets behavior different from its own as strange and unenlightened, and therefore wrong. Another cultural pitfall is **stereotyping,** an oversimplified opinion or belief about a group of people (Purnell & Paulanka, 1998). Stereotyping can result from a single piece of misinformation about a group of people. However, stereotyping can also result when someone with a great deal of cultural knowledge fails to appreciate the diversity between members of the same group or the diversity between generations.

Diversity between generations is often the result of acculturation and assimilation. **Acculturation** is the intermeshing of the cultural threads of the ethnic and mainstream groups, which reduces the friction between groups. This adaptation can include learning the language or speech pattern of the mainstream, changing the spelling of a name (usually to make it less ethnic), or actually changing a name to be more mainstream. The degree of acculturation of an individual depends on a number of factors, including age (the young acculturate more quickly), generation (since immigration), social support, socioeconomic opportunities, length of time in the new country, personality characteristics, and life experiences (Julia, 1996).

Because it is adaptive, acculturation is generally seen as positive. In matters of health, this is not always true. Successive generations of Japanese immigrants who moved to Hawaii, then to California, have experienced increased rates of heart disease. This change has been attributed to a change in diet as the generations moved toward the mainland and acculturated their eating patterns from the fish and rice staples of Japan. Diets of Japanese persons with heart disease are more typically "American," high in beef content and saturated fats.

As Mexican-Americans have become more Americanized, their infant mortality rates have begun to rise. As behaviors learned in the Hispanic culture have changed (e.g., community support of pregnant women and a low incidence of smoking and drinking during pregnancy), pregnancy outcomes have worsened (Julia, 1996).

Acculturation is adaptation, whereas **assimilation** is an actual change that occurs when an old set of traits is relinquished through interaction with the new society. Assimilation involves cultural adaptation, psychological adjustments, and social integration. The assimilation of European immigrants in the United States is more complete than for groups who are racially different from the mainstream. The degree of residential segregation or concentrations also influences the degree of acculturation and assimilation. If groups can maintain entire communities that support their activities of daily living (businesses, stores, worship facilities, newspaper and TV programs in their language, and large numbers of people

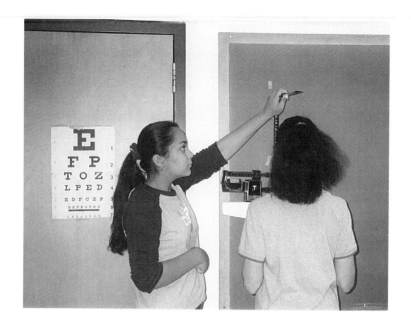

with which to interact), the pressure to become part of the mainstream is lessened (Julia, 1996).

Cultural Competence

Cultural competence goes beyond cultural sensitivity. It can be defined as the ability to care for culturally diverse populations by incorporating knowledge of their culture into clinical practice, into health education, and at key points of patient contact. Knowledge related to ethnicity, culture, and acculturation is important so that stereotypical assumptions are not made, which always compromise the nurse-client relationship. Nurses need accurate information about the norms of the ethnic and cultural groups that are part of their clinical practice. These norms will impact on the nurse-client interaction and the determination of health priorities and practices (ANA, 1998; Association of Asian Pacific Community Health Organizations, 1996).

Cultural competence in clinical practice is not a discrete endpoint, but a career-long commitment that nurses enter into with themselves, their patients, and their communities. This process requires self-reflection and self-critique for nurses committed to being lifelong learners and reflective practitioners. There is a danger of settling into a false

sense of security in one's own training and knowledge, as shown in the following real-life experience:

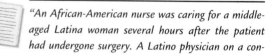
"An African-American nurse was caring for a middle-aged Latina woman several hours after the patient had undergone surgery. A Latino physician on a consult service approached the bedside and, noting the moaning patient, commented to the nurse that the patient appeared to be in a great deal of postoperative pain. The nurse summarily dismissed his perception, informing him that she took a course in nursing school in cross-cultural medicine and 'knew' that Hispanic patients over-express the pain they are feeling. The Latino physician had a difficult time influencing the perspective of this nurse, who focused on her self-proclaimed cultural expertise. The nurse's notion of her own expertise actually stereotyped the patient's experience, ignored clues (the moaning) to the patient's present reality, and disregarded the potential resources of a colleague who might (albeit not necessarily) be able to contribute some relevant cultural insight" (Tervalon & Murray-Garcia, 1998, p. 118–119).

As a model of practice, cultural competence involves individual health-care providers, agencies, and health-care systems with the capacity to respond to the unique needs of different populations. The rationale for cultural competence in health care includes, but is not limited to, the following:

- The perception of illness and disease and their causes varies by culture.
- Diverse belief systems exist related to health, healing, and wellness.
- Culture influences help-seeking behaviors and attitudes toward health-care providers.
- Individual preferences affect traditional and nontraditional approaches to health care.
- Patients must overcome personal experiences of biases within health-care systems.
- Health-care providers from culturally and linguistically diverse groups are underrepresented in the current service delivery system (NTAC, 1992; NCCC, 1999).

A nurse who is culturally competent is able to think, feel, and act in ways that acknowledge, respect, and build on ethnic, cultural, and linguistic diversity. There is an underlying assumption that *all* individuals and groups are diverse, with their own cultural heritage. To be culturally competent, a nurse must demonstrate knowledge and understanding of the client's culture, accept and respect cultural differences, and adjust the nursing care provided to be congruent with the client's culture. At the same time, the nurse must be consciously aware of his or her own culture without letting his or her culture exert undue influence on clients from other backgrounds (Purnell & Paulanka, 1998). Box 6–2 provides you with an opportunity to discuss your own culture.

Box 6-2   Student Learning Activity

Culture Sharing

Think about your own culture that you bring to nursing. Write three characteristics of your culture that you would want others to consider if you were a patient with a chronic illness.

The first step of the journey toward cultural competence is cultural self-awareness. When nurses can identify their own ethnic roots, they can determine how their values, beliefs, customs, and behaviors have been shaped by culture. It is common for Americans to identify with many different countries of origin in Europe, thus escaping any identification with a specific ethnic heritage. The designation of being from Europe is a source of amusement for many Europeans, who clearly understand that Europe is a continent, not a country, and each country is unique in many different ways (Lynch & Hanson, 1998).

The harsh toll taken on the lives of early immigrants from Europe fostered a desire for a quick, and hopefully total, assimilation into America. Many family names were "Americanized" at Ellis Island, the U.S. point of immigration in the last century. Other families changed their own names to be more "American," worked to lose their accents, and changed their diets and dress to be more mainstream. This level of assimilation has led many Anglo-European groups to feel that they have no definable culture outside of the United States. America, as a separate culture, has indeed emerged. There are several cultural forces that have come to define Americans, and they include:

1. Insistence on choice
2. Pursuit of seemingly impossible dreams
3. Obsession with "big" and "more"
4. Insistence on immediate gratification
5. Acceptance of mistakes
6. Urge to improvise
7. Fixation on what is new (Lynch & Hanson, 1998, pp. 53–54)

As we explore our own personal cultural background, it is important, as nurses, that we not lose sight of our place in the culture of biomedicine. Part of the discomfort and frustration of caring for diverse clients is that they may not share the values that are inherent to our belief in the traditional biomedical approach to health and illness—the biologic basis of disease, physiology, and pathophysiology.

INDIVIDUAL PRACTICE LEVEL

It is important to have an overview of ways in which values, beliefs, and behaviors differ across cultures. Difference

Table 6-5

Cultural Continuum

Extended family and kinship networks	Small unit families with little reliance on the extended family
Interdependence	Individuality
Nurturance of young children	Independence of young children
Time is given	Time is measured
Respect for age, ritual, and tradition	Emphasis on youth, future, and technology
Ownership defined in broad terms	Ownership—individual and specific
Differentiated rights and responsibilities	Equal rights and responsibilities
Harmony	Control

does not imply that one set of behaviors is normative and, therefore, correct, whereas another set is deviant and, therefore, wrong. It may be more helpful to view culture as a continuum. Table 6–5 presents sample end points of the cultural continuum.

CULTURAL ASSESSMENT MODELS

Gathering data on clients and families is one of the first steps to working in a culturally competent manner. Lynch and Hanson (1998) have a family assessment tool focused on family structure, child-rearing practices, perceptions and attitudes, and language and communication style. Giger and Davidhizar (1995) are nurse researchers who have developed a comprehensive cultural assessment model (Figure 6–5) focused on the "Culturally Unique Individual." Questions related to both models are at the end of this chapter (Lao Family Community of Minnesota, 1997).

TRANSLATORS

A March 1997 survey by the Census Bureau found that 1 in 10 persons in the United States is foreign born (Bureau of the Census, 2000), and the 1990 Census found

that 28.3 million people speak a language other than English at home (Bureau of the Census, 1996). When clients do not speak the mainstream language, they are separated from both the culture around them and the culture of biomedicine (Roat, 1999).

Housekeepers, groundskeepers, and dietary workers are often not appropriate interpreters for health-care situations. Issues of confidentiality make this an obvious statement, but the use of these ancillary personnel as translators is a daily occurrence in the health-care setting. Children and family may not be familiar with the appropriate names for body systems, medications and treatments, and physical symptoms, and again, confidentiality is breached. Professional interpreters reserve the word *translation* for written work and *interpretation* for the verbal exchange of one language for another. Medical interpreters must be multilingual and multicultural. Their work as interpreters must encompasses the culture of the "source" (patient) and the culture of the "target" (nurse, physician, or social worker) to enhance communication (Purnell & Paulanka, 1998; Roat, 1999).

Medical interpreters must also have a basic understanding of the Western biomedical model to find ways to express words, ideas, and physical processes that may have no equivalent in the target language. Misunderstandings can be dangerous, even fatal. Interpreters may need to advocate for clients unfamiliar with the U.S. health-care system to ensure that they receive all of the services that they require. Given these demands, it remains important that the interpreter *facilitate* not *take control of* the communication between patient and provider. Interpreting for clients requires sensitivity and a willingness and ability to respect the autonomy of the client-provider interaction, intervening when necessary but basically remaining in the background to help patients and providers communicate clearly (Roat, 1999).

Among all population groups, there are linguistic differences. Length of time in the United States, degree of education, and acculturation account for some of the variation. When speaking with clients who are not fluent in English, speak clearly but not more loudly than normal and look for nonverbal cues that signal a lack of understanding, such as glazed eyes, looking off to one side, or shifting uncomfortably. Simplify all explanations, using simple words, but not broken English.

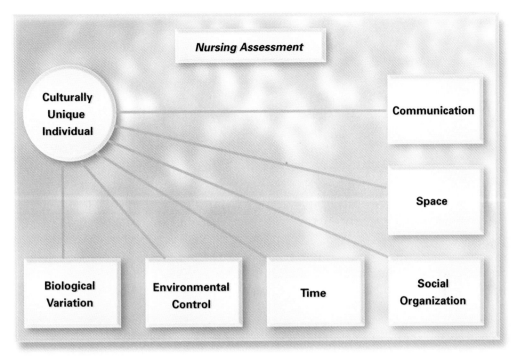

Figure 6–5   Giger and Davidhizar's Transcultural Assessment Model

Source: Giger and Davidhizar, 1995, used with permission

Barriers to Communication

A community interpreter has a very different role and responsibility from a commercial or conference interpreter. She [or he] is responsible for enabling professional and client, with very different backgrounds and perceptions and in an unequal relationship of power and knowledge, to communicate to their mutual satisfaction. (Roat, 1999, p. 16)

There are many potential barriers to mutually satisfactory communication. They include linguistic barriers, barriers of complex language, experience with healthcare concepts and procedures, cultural barriers, and systemic barriers (Roat, 1999).

Linguistic barriers are simply differences in language and dialect. Some providers use complex language understood by those with a formal education, but not by someone with a limited education. This level of language is referred to as **register.** Providers may also refer to body systems, physical problems, and procedures pertinent to

Western medicine, but there may not be comparable words or meanings in other systems of care. Cultural barriers may result in different expectations of behavior that affect communication and the quality of care. Finally, systemic barriers such as the complexity of the healthcare system and systemic problems such as racism may create barriers to effective care (Roat, 1999).

Roles of the Interpreter

The pyramid in Figure 6–6 depicts four common roles for interpreters. As you proceed up the pyramid, the interpreter becomes more involved in the communication itself, and the role of the interpreter becomes more complex and invasive. The most appropriate role for the interpreter is the least invasive. Interpreters, however, must be able to move from role to role.

Being a **conduit** is the most common and basic role for the interpreter. One language is simply translated into

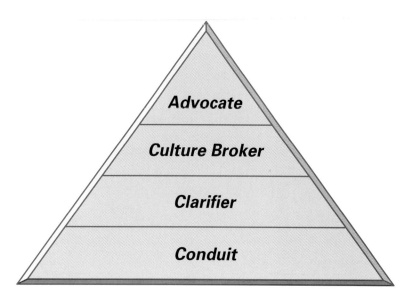

Figure 6–6   Roles of the Interpreter

*Adapted from Roat, C.E. (1999). Bridging
the gap: A basic training for medical
interpreters (3ʳᵈ Ed). The Cross-Cultural
Health Care Program: Seattle, WA. (used
with permission).*

another without adjustments. In the role of **clarifier,** the interpreter facilitates understanding by adjusting register and making word pictures for terms that have no linguistic equivalent. When cultural differences lead to a misunderstanding between the client and provider, the interpreter becomes a **cultural broker** by providing a framework for understanding the message. As an advocate, the interpreter takes action on behalf of the client outside of the interpreted interview. Examples of advocacy include giving information to the client or connecting the client with other clinic staff whose responsibility it is to resolve the client's issue.

Clinical Considerations

It is important to use interpreters whenever possible, allow time for interpretation, use same-age and same-gender interpreters whenever possible, and maintain eye contact with both the client and the interpreter to get feedback and read nonverbal cues. Speak slowly without exaggerating mouthing, use as many words as possible in the client's language, and use empathic nonverbal communication especially when you do not know the client's language. Social class differences between the client and the interpreter may interfere with the communication; information considered superstitious or unimportant may

not be conveyed (Purnell & Paulanka, 1998). Political considerations can also serve as a filter for interpretation. If both client and interpreter come from a country suffering upheaval and they would consider themselves political enemies at home, the interpretation may be affected.

SPECIAL POPULATIONS

The following sections discuss specific racial and religious populations. Their demographic profiles are presented and general guidelines for nurse-client interactions are offered. Guidelines are not definitive statements, and diversity within populations is always an important consideration. Different populations present with different risk factors and different disease processes. The accompanying table (Table 6–6) is a brief summary of the leading causes of death, organized according to race and ethnic group.

A common thread in many special populations is the use of non-Western treatments, herbs, and actual medications. Many alternative therapies have successfully been used in conjunction with Western medicine to the client's benefit. However, there are documented reports of serious drug interactions and overdose effects between Western and non-Western medications. Examples are numerous and include the use of the plant foxglove (the

Table 6-6

Leading Causes of Death by Race and Ethnic Group, 1996

RANK	WHITE, NON-HISPANIC	AFRICAN-AMERICAN	LATINO	NATIVE AMERICAN	ASIAN-AMERICAN
1	Heart Disease	Heart Disease	Heart Disease	Heart Disease	Heart Disease
2	Cancer	Cancer	Cancer	Cancer	Cancer
3	CVD	CVD	AUI	AUI	CVD
4	Chronic Lung Disease	HIV/AIDS	CVD	Diabetes	AUI
5	AUI	AUI	HIV/AIDS	CVD	Pneumonia and Influenza

AUI = Accidents and Unintentional Injuries
CVD = Cerebrovascular Disease

Source: National Center for Health Statistics, 1998
Office of Minority Health, 1998

original source of digoxin) in addition to medically pre-scribed Digoxin, and St. Johns Wort used in addition to a prescribed antidepressant. Box 6–3 gives you the oppor-tunity to research other serious drug interactions.

Box 6-3	Student Learning Activity

Alternative Health Care Effects

Identify here at least two non-Western treatments, herbs, or medications that have been reported in the news recently to have caused serious drug interactions or overdose effects.

1.

2.

Hispanics

Persons of Hispanic origin are an ethnic group and may be of any race. The ethnic origin for Hispanics is the country of Spain, and can mean either peoples descended from Spain or peoples colonized by Spaniards. This group is cur-rently the second-largest minority group in the United States, with a population of 29 million, or 11 percent of the population. The projected census for the year 2000 pre-dicted a Hispanic population of 31 million persons. The countries of origin for Hispanics in the United States in-clude Mexico (62 percent), Puerto Rico (13 percent), Cen-tral and South America (12 percent), and Cuba (5 percent). Other Hispanic peoples constitute 8 percent (Office of Mi-nority Health Resource Center [OMHRC], 1998).

The word *Hispanic* was created by U.S. demographers. The growing Spanish-speaking segment of the popula-tion needed an identity more specific than "Other." Indi-viduals commonly referred to as "Hispanic" most commonly refer to themselves as **Latino** or **Hispano.**

The ethnic diversity within the Latino population is an important consideration in delivering culturally compe-tent care. About 70 percent of Latinos are U.S. born, and

Countries of Origin for Hispanics in the U.S.

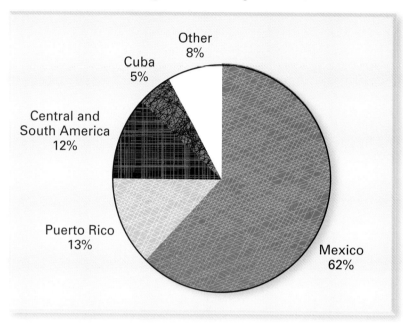

Figure 6–7   Countries of Origin for Hispanics in the U.S.

Source: Office of Minority Health Resource Center, 1998.

approximately 30 percent are foreign born. A Latino client may be an 11th-generation Mexican-American, a first generation Salvadoran with no resources who is fleeing military persecution, or a first-generation Chilean with a college education. Knowledge of the client's social and economic circumstances greatly enhances the nurse's cultural competence, making interventions more effective (Zambrana, 1994; Zambrana & Dorrington, 1998).

Because of the diversity of the Latino subgroups, the spoken and written Spanish of the U.S. Hispanic population varies according to country of origin. The U.S. government and major volunteer agencies, such as The American Cancer Society, are working to develop a standard written Spanish to be used in official documents and health education materials. However, clients who do not speak or read English may or may not be literate in Spanish. Furthermore, the language of the materials provided may not be the Spanish language of their country of origin.

Cultural Considerations

The *process* of an interaction is usually more important to Latino clients than the outcome. An informal and relaxed time of exchange is necessary before nursing tasks or education begins. When working with Latino clients, it is important to reevaluate your general style of interaction with clients and modify actions that might be perceived as "hurried." Latino clients may use a form of communication called "indirectas," which discourages frank exchanges with care providers and minimizes the report of side effects of medications or treatments. If both husband and wife are present, speak to the husband first. The following actions may offend your Latino clients:

- Appearing hurried or impatient.
- Using a harsh or authoritarian tone of voice.
- Declining a beverage or food offering.
- Laughing at or dismissing a cultural artifact or ritual. (Lynch & Hanson, 1998; Tirado, 1995).

Knowing the class and economic background of the family, as well as their immigration status, is helpful to tailor effective actions. Currently, only 30 percent of the U.S. Latino population are recent immigrants, and many are documented. **Undocumented immigrants** is a more professionally accepted term than *illegal aliens*. If your clients are undocumented, be very clear that your role as a nurse does not require you to report to the Immigration and Naturalization Service (referred to as *La Migra*). Familiarity with community resources is vital to the referral process in community-based work. Identify the Latino community resources that support client well-being, health, and empowerment. Box 6–4 helps you think about culturally considerate health care.

Box 6-4   Student Learning Activity

Hispanic Cultural Values

List four actions you could do as a nurse to provide health care that is considerate of Hispanic clients' cultural values.

1.

2.

3.

4.

African-Americans

A challenge for professionals who work with African-American clients is working outside of the stereotypes of this population. *Time Magazine* notes that although 26 percent of poor Americans are black, the percentage of stories on poor people in *Time, Newsweek,* and *U.S. News & World Report* that were illustrated with black people was 69 percent (Time, 1997). The rates of poverty are greater for African-Americans (26 percent) than for non-Hispanic whites (8.2 percent), and African-Americans constitute only 12 percent of the population. The total number of whites living in poverty is 15.8 million,

whereas blacks in poverty number 9 million. When working with *any* population living in poverty, it is important not to equate poverty with dysfunction. Many impoverished families, from all racial and ethnic backgrounds, manage to provide strong, nurturing care for their children and foster strong family bonds (Bureau of the Census, 1996, Lynch & Hanson, 1998).

Cultural Considerations

It is helpful to use titles (Mr., Mrs., Ms.) and last names unless given permission to do otherwise. Young nurses may make the mistake of addressing clients by their first names, believing that they are forming a special bond. Clients are not immediate friends; it may seem intrusive and presumptuous to use first names, regardless of clients' race or ethnicity. There is an inherently different base of power when a professional interacts with a layperson. Clients may not approve of the nurse's familiarity, but may feel inhibited from or afraid to confront a professional charged with their health care (Lynch & Hanson, 1998).

Extended kinship bonds may be in effect with multiple generations in one home. This can be a powerful resource, but it may also result in unclear boundaries. For example, a grandmother could begin to take over the care of her adolescent daughter's infant. Social support networks such as church, neighbors, and friends may be available as resources, if permitted by the family, to supplement formal referrals (Lynch & Hanson, 1998).

"Certain words have negative and inflammatory associations when used by the wrong people. Lavalle, who is African-American, was the primary nurse for four 16-year-old Black gang members. She had developed a good relationship with them and treated them like her own children. When one got out of line, she would simply say, 'Boy, keep your mouth shut and go somewhere and sit down.' They usually complied.

One day, Susan, an Anglo nurse, tried the same tactic with one of them. It was time for Earl to go to physical therapy, but he was giving Susan a hard time. She assumed from his smile that he was joking. Finally, she tried Lavalle's approach, 'Come on boy,' she said. 'I'm not kidding with you. You have to go to therapy.'

Earl flew into a rage and started swearing at Susan. Lavalle had to help calm him down. Susan was confused. He had never responded that way to Lavalle. She had not considered that the term boy is inoffensive when used by one Black person speaking to another but is highly insulting when used by Caucasians because of its origins among slave owners.

. . . Many people know that boy is highly insulting to a Black man, but few are aware that the term gal has similar connotations for many Black women. Black slave women were called gals which explains why several Anglo nurses reported receiving cold and hostile glares from African-American nurses whom they innocently referred to as gals." (Galanti, 1997, pp. 18–19)

Asians/Pacific Islanders

According to the 1990 census, Asians composed 2 percent of the U.S. population. This group comes from more than

20 different countries. The most common countries of origin are China, Japan, Korea, Cambodia, Vietnam, and Laos. Pacific Islanders make up less than 1 percent of the U.S. population, but they have great ethnic and cultural diversity. Hawaiian, Samoan, Guamanian, and Tongan are the four most common Pacific Islander groups. Although there are Pacific Islanders in every state, the majority live on the West Coast or in Hawaii, New York, and Washington, D.C.; 60.7 percent of Asian-Americans and Pacific Islanders are foreign born. By the year 2010, the AAPI population in the United States will increase by more than 100 percent. The wide variety of spoken languages and dialects are barriers to accessing primary-care services, and this factor has hindered the development of printed health education and health promotion materials. Even within a single country, the languages can vary widely. For example, there is no language called "Chi-

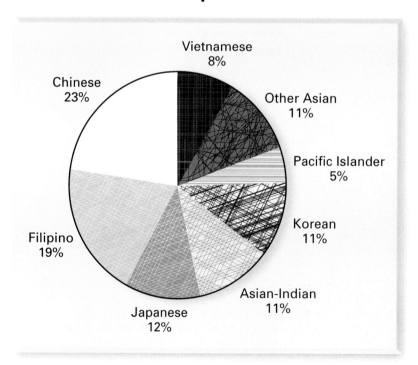

U.S. Asian and Pacific Islander Population 1990

Figure 6–8   U.S. Asian and Pacific Islander Population 1990

Source: Association of Asian Pacific Community Health Organizations, 1996

nese"; Mandarin and Cantonese are China's primary languages, but the country's 1 billion people speak numerous distinct dialects. Regardless of the skill of the interpreter, there are medical terms in Chinese that do not have precise relationships in Western medicine (OMHRC, 1998; Healthy People 2000, 1991; Tirado, 1995).

Cancer is the leading cause of death for Chinese and Vietnamese. Korean stomach cancer rates are five times the rate of the total population, and liver cancer rates are highest for Vietnamese. Deaths from cerebrovascular diseases are increasing for both male and female AAPI populations.

Cultural Considerations—Chinese

Chinese clients tend not to challenge questions or recommendations from health-care providers because of personal modesty and as a sign of respect. This deference can make obtaining an accurate health history difficult. Clients may be hesitant to correct a provider's misunderstanding. Grandmothers are often the decision makers for children and must be included in any health-care discussion or education. There is often a tendency for family members to hide an older patient's condition (particularly parents) from the patient. Newly emigrated Chinese patients may be likely to use traditional medicines and treatment along with Western treatment. Ad-

verse consequences have resulted from mixing agents drawn from the two medical traditions. Finally, Chinese patients often expect that treatment (e.g., injection, prescription) will accompany a physician visit. For nurses delivering community-based care, this translates into the need for a skill intervention (e.g., blood pressure, weight screening) when providing health education.

Cultural Considerations—Hmong

The Hmong are a tribal people originally from Southern China who eventually emigrated to northern Burma, Thailand, Laos, and Vietnam. Following the war in Southeast Asia, the Hmong fled to Thailand. Beginning in the 1970s, the Hmong began to resettle in countries willing to accept them as refugees. Australia, France, and the United States were primary destinations. Minnesota was a main resettlement center. With the closing of the Thai refugee camps in 1997, the primary wave of immigration from Thailand has stopped, but a secondary wave of Hmong migration to Minnesota from other U.S. cities has occurred as families reunite and other Hmong relocate to benefit from resettlement resources and favorable economic conditions (Lao Family Community of Minnesota, 1997). The word *yes* does not always mean "yes" to the content of a question; it often means, "Yes, I respect that you asked a question." *No* is

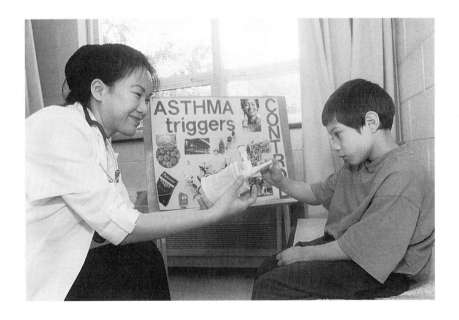

considered disrespectful; avoid questions that are answered with a simple yes or no. Women may not be used to shaking hands, and the behavior of looking someone in the eye is considered rude or bold. Even as the Hmong adapt to Western culture, looking someone in the eye remains difficult.

The Hmong believe the soul resides in the head, and only certain elders have the right to touch a person's head. Do not touch an adult Hmong's head without permission, and do not pat a child on the head. A visit from the spiritual leader (shaman) should be encouraged and supported for hospital inpatients. When ill, the Hmong prefer plain (not spiced) foods and soups, and women who have given birth prefer warm or hot fluids. Many clients may use herbal medications. If possible, get a list of herbal remedies to be used and give the list to a pharmacist to ensure that the herbs will not interact with prescribed medication.

Cultural Considerations—Koreans

The Korean-American population has more than doubled over the last decade, making it one of the fastest-growing Asian-American groups. Koreans have immigrated to the United States in three waves. The first wave arrived between 1898 and 1905 when 8000 plantation workers and 1000 "picture brides" immigrated to Hawaii. The Oriental Exclusion Act of 1924 banned all Asian immigration until after World War II. The second wave arrived between 1945 and 1980 and included over 14,000 wives of American soldiers, Korean children orphaned by the war who were adopted by Americans, and students who came to continue their education. The third and largest wave occurred after the 1965 Immigration and Naturalization Act. All quotas limiting immigration were abolished, and a preference system was instituted for Korean relatives of U.S. citizens and for professionals with skills needed in the United States (Association of Asian Pacific Community Health Organizations, 1996).

According to the 1990 census, 52 percent of Koreans do not speak English fluently. Interpretation support for many Asian groups is a significant part of their ability to access health care. Family is all-important in the Korean culture; during pregnancy, for example, everything the mother does and eats is for the good of the baby. "Tae Kyo" is a set of rules for safe and easy childbirth that protects from disease and influences infant development.

Certain foods are avoided. Reading an intellectual book during pregnancy results in a wise child, whereas swearing and gossiping adversely affects the child's personality. There are special terms of honor to address elders in Korea, and there is a traditional ceremony at age 60 to celebrate the completion of a person's first cycle of life on earth. Many older Koreans who immigrate to the United States suffer significant psychological distress as they adjust to a society where elders are not honored.

Yang and Um are two great contrasting forces that control life in the Korean tradition. These are based on the Chinese concepts of Yin and Yang. These forces are the basis of remedies such as eating certain "cold" foods to lower a fever, instead of taking aspirin. Levels of depression are higher among Koreans than other ethnic groups. Many Korean families start small businesses, and the success or failure of those businesses may affect the survival and future of multiple generations. In many Asian cultures, psychological problems carry a social stigma and may be expressed somatically by having constant headaches, difficulty sleeping, or gastric distress. It should be noted that stomach cancer is the leading cause of cancer death in Korea, and in the United States, the incidence of stomach cancer is significantly higher in the Korean population (Figure 6–9).

Native Americans, Eskimos, and Aleuts

The official Indian Health Service designations of these special populations are American Indians, Alaskan Eskimos, and Aleuts. These groups have their origins in any of the indigenous, or original, peoples of North America who maintain cultural identification through tribal affiliation or community recognition. According to the U.S. census data for the year 2000, Native Americans and Alaskan natives number 2.4 million persons, or .88 percent of the U.S. population (Bureau of the Census, 2000). Diabetes, heart disease and stroke, and infant mortality disproportionately affect American Indians (Bureau of the Census, 1995).

More than 500 different American Indian tribes are recognized throughout Alaska, Canada, and across the continental United States. The amount of Indian blood necessary to be considered a tribal member varies across tribes. Within the continental United States, American Indians most often refer to themselves as Native Americans. The largest American tribe is the Navajo, with

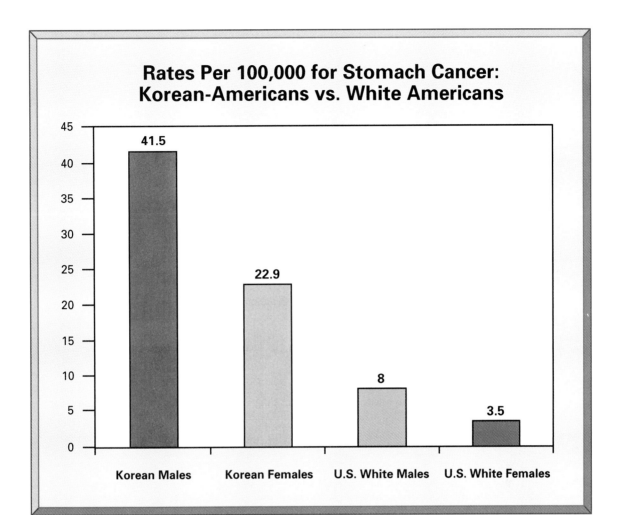

Figure 6–9   Rates per 100,000 for Stomach Cancer: Korean-Americans vs. White Americans

Source: Association of Asian Pacific Community Health Organizations, 1996.

200,000 persons. The Indian people of Canada and Alaska are composed of several tribes unfamiliar to most Americans: the Tsimshian, the Haida, the Tlingit, and seven small tribes in the Athapascan language family.

The Navajo (Din[11])

Instead of a handshake, Navajo (or Din[11]) extend their hand and lightly touch the hand of the person they are greeting; this is considered a "weak" handshake by Western

standards. Because the Navajo do not share their thoughts and feelings with those outside of the clan, it takes a long time for nontribal providers to build trust. Talking loudly is considered rude. The Navajo are comfortable with long periods of silence and may take what seems like a long time to give a response to a question. It is considered immature to answer a question too quickly and it is rude to interrupt. Acceptable personal space is much greater for Native Americans than for most Westerners (Giger & Davidhizar, 1991; Purnell & Paulanka, 1998).

The clan system (family identification) is an integral part of Navajo life. In introductions, the mother's clan is mentioned first, then the father's clan. A child is *of* the mother's clan and born *for* the father's clan. The maternal and paternal grandfather's clan can also have an impact on a child's identity. The community provides assistance to clan relatives. The elderly clan members who have remained on reservations are faced with the challenges of growing older in remote areas with very limited support. Many Native American young people have left the reservations in search of education and job opportunities.

There are many traditional practices related to pregnancy and childbirth. Clothes are not purchased for the baby before birth, the placenta may be buried to show the child's connection to the earth, and mothers massage their babies as a form of bonding. Contrary to the Western practice of maintaining eye contact as a sign of connection, among the Navajo eye contact is considered rude and possibly confrontational. Even among friends and across socioeconomic levels, eye contact is not maintained. Traditional healing ceremonies restore mental, physical, and spiritual balance. Do not assume that any Native American family *is* or *is not* practicing their tribal religion or using traditional healing ceremonies. Unless the family volunteers information, do not ask questions about these ceremonies. On a home visit, ask the family if this is a good time to visit. If the family says "no," do not enter the house because they could be conducting a ceremony; reschedule the visit. On reservations, it may be necessary to travel great distances to obtain health care. Even if cars are available for appointments, money for gasoline may not be. Whenever an opportunity for patient contact occurs (e.g., emergency room, a child accompanying an adult on a visit) the need for primary care should be determined and services such as immunizations should be offered (Lynch & Hanson, 1998; Purnell & Paulanka, 1998).

The Eskimo

The Eskimo people live along the Bering Sea, the Arctic Ocean coasts, and the lower Yukon and Kuskokwim river regions. Archaeologists believe that the ancestors of the Eskimos migrated across the Bering Strait from Asia

10,000 to 15,000 years ago. The Eskimo population refer to themselves as Inuit, or "Real People." Culturally distinct groups within the Inuit include the Yup'ik, the Inupiat, or the Inuvialunit, depending on the region.

In the spoken language of the Inuit, they refer to themselves and others in the third person. When referring to himself or herself, an Inuit says, "Someone is hungry" or "Someone is going hunting." Translators are helpful, but because there is no vocabulary for future events or abstract concepts, health-care discussions must be kept simple and concrete. Avoid the use of idioms such as "out in left field," because they have no meaning to Inuits.

Inuits tolerate periods of silence more easily than Western people typically do; in fact, it is considered rude to fill periods of silence with chatter. An Inuit may seek out health care and just sit for a period of time before discussing the reason for the visit. Many younger Inuits have adapted to Western society by being more verbal, but more traditional Inuits are sometimes perceived as passive, which is an untrue interpretation. Inuits also use nonverbal communication extensively, such as raised eyebrows for yes and a wrinkled nose for no. When Inuit clients perceive insincerity or discrepancy between verbal and nonverbal language, distrust develops between nurse and client, and further communication is blocked (Giger & Davidhizar, 1991).

The Aleuts live in the Aleutian Islands and the Alaskan peninsula. The Aleuts and Inuits are closely related because the ancestors of the Aleuts also emigrated from Asia thousands of years ago. However, the Aleuts have their own unique customs, traditions, and language. After contact with Russian fur traders in 1750, the Aleut population declined because of sickness and harsh treatment—traders exploited their hunting skills. Before contact with foreigners, the Aleut population numbered between 12,000 and 25,000; today about 8,000 Aleuts remain (Giger & Davidhizar, 1991).

Arab-Americans

Arabs are the inhabitants of the Arab World, 22 countries in the Middle East and North Africa, with a population of 180 million persons who speak Arabic. The majority of Arabs are Muslims, but there are a large number of Arab Christians in Greater Syria (Lebanon, Syria, and

Palestine), Iraq, and Egypt. Ramadan is a month-long holy celebration at the beginning of the calendar year, when everyone observes fasting during the day. During this celebration, clients may even resist taking medications. Adjustments may be made for medical conditions (i.e., diabetes) or nursing mothers. Some Muslim women wear long dresses and scarves to cover their bodies and sometimes cover their faces except for their eyes. Community organizations provide points of contact, support, and activity for the Arab community. Mosques, unlike churches and synagogues, are not used for socialization and community activities. Arabs attend mosques to pray, and then they leave; even weddings are not held in mosques. There are no spiritual leaders within each mosque similar to a priest, pastor, or rabbi (Cross Cultural Health Care Program [CCHP], 1996; Purnell & Paulanka, 1998).

Cultural Considerations

The most respected health-care provider is a middle-aged to elderly male physician, with a prominent position at a hospital. For maternal care, however, Arab women prefer midwives. Nurses are seen as helpers rather than professionals, and their suggestions and advice may not be taken seriously. Nurses who encourage self-care may be perceived as incompetent, lazy, or uncaring. Newly immigrated families may need to be educated about the role of the nurse in their care; in the Arab World, physicians respect each other and not necessarily other health-care providers (CCHP, 1996; Purnell & Paulanka, 1998).

When clients visit a physician, they expect medication and relief from symptoms. If no medication is given, an explanation should be offered. Although clients may discuss at length any ordered lab tests or procedures, they will comply with medications and procedures. Once patients feel better, they often do not return for follow-up. Family members may be used frequently as interpreters, and Arab clients look to other interpreters freely for support. Muslims do not eat pork, and some only eat Halal meat (slaughtered according to Islamic tradition). Hospital inpatients may not be aware that they can order religiously appropriate meals. It is in the Arab tradition to circumcise newborn boys (CCHP, 1996).

Mental illness remains a stigma within the Arab community. Patients with mental health conditions do not typically seek professional help and may have no support system to help deal with their mental illness. Individuals with disabilities are cared for within the family unit and may be shielded from the public to "protect" the family member. The family may require support in accessing professional rehabilitation services (CCHP, 1996; Purnell & Paulanka, 1998).

 "Mustafa Mourad, a Muslim Arab, was admitted to the oncology floor. A few weeks earlier, he had been diagnosed with extensive colon cancer. His family kept him at home until he went into a coma. Upon admittance, it was determined that he was a "no code," but little else had been discussed. There had been no time to develop rapport. Six to ten family members were at his bedside throughout the night.

At 2 A.M., the daughter ran to get the nurse—he had stopped breathing. When the nurse confirmed that he had no pulse, several family members began to cry and wail loudly. The nurses tried to comfort them, but Mr. Mourad's son pulled them away. Soon the entire family joined in the wailing. The son asked the staff not to interfere, stating that the loud display was part of the grieving process. He added that it was necessary in order for his father's soul to be released.

The problem was that it was 2 A.M., and the wailing and crying were disturbing all the other, non-comatose patients, who were pushing their call buttons. They were angry, concerned, and frightened, and wanted to know what was going on. When the nurse asked the patient's son to have them please soften the noise, he became angry and accused her of being disrespectful. . . .

The doctor from the emergency room arrived nearly an hour later [to officially declare the death]. When he requested they stop their wailing, they complied. He arranged to have the body moved to the chapel where they could continue their mourning without disturbing the other patients. The physician also instructed the nursing staff not to call the mortuary until told to do so by the family, which they did at 10 A.M. the next morning.

There are a number of cultural elements displayed in the Moustafa case. No plans had been made with the mortuary regarding the impending death because to do so would interfere with the will of Allah. The most disturbing element of the case for the staff was the loud crying. Wailing is an important cultural ritual. The nursing staff, unaware of this, was totally unprepared.

Another cultural aspect was the fact that the family ignored the requests of the nurses but complied with those of the physician. Arabs have a great deal of respect for authority—of physicians, not nurses. This is accentuated by the greater respect the culture has for men.

In this situation, the physician demonstrated an important understanding of cultural diversity and suggested a solution (moving to the chapel), which allowed the family to continue their ritual without compromising other patients. It is important to work within the culture rather than impose solutions from without" (Galanti, 1997, pp. 110–111).

CULTURALLY COMPETENT HEALTH-CARE SYSTEMS

A culturally competent health-care system is based on a set of underlying values. Understanding these values guides the practice of individual health-care members as they interact with clients and their families:

- Culture represents an important force in shaping behaviors, values, and institutions.
- Cultural has an impact on service delivery.
- Natural systems (e.g., family, church, healers, etc.) serve as primary mechanisms of support for minority populations.
- "Family," as defined by each culture, is the primary and preferred point of intervention.
- Concepts of "family," "community," and so on differ for various cultures and subgroups.
- Taking the best of both worlds enhances the capacity of all.
- Values of minority groups may conflict with dominant society values,
- Process may be as important as product.
- Diversity within cultures is as important as diversity between cultures. (NTAC, 1989)

Diversity includes age, gender, race, and ethnic background. A culturally competent health-care provider must use the skills of cultural competence to navigate through personal and societal biases related to diversity, to provide the best possible health care.

Cultural Assessment Tools

Because the family is considered the point of intervention for culturally competent care, the "Guidelines for the Home Visitor," shown in Table 6–7, have been adapted from Lynch and Hanson (1998) for use as a family assessment tool.

Research Considerations in Culturally Competent Care

The absence of cultural competence can allow bias to negatively affect patient care. A groundbreaking study in the *New England Journal of Medicine* found that blacks and women with identical complaints of chest pain are less likely than whites and men, respectively, to be referred by doctors for cardiac catheterization (Schulman, et al., 1999). Because the study was tightly controlled for confounding factors, the authors concluded that racial and sex bias accounted for the different referral rates. According to Dr. David Satcher, U.S. Surgeon General, "This study deals with a very serious problem. It shows that the same problems that affect relationships in other segments of society affect the doctor–patient relationship. Blacks are 40 percent more likely to die from heart disease than Whites . . . this could be one factor" (Kamat, p. 6).

Davidhizar and Bechtel (1999) carried out a study of public-health nurses using the Giger and Davidhizar Transcultural Assessment Model, shown in Table 6–8, to explore the needs of residents in the Colonias settlements. These settlements along the U.S./Mexican border are reflective of developing communities because many of the residents lack basic educational and work opportunities found in most other parts of the United States. Because the residents of the Colonias are primarily Hispanic, it was important to develop, implement, and evaluate health-care interventions in a culturally sensitive manner. The Giger-Davidhizar Model was found to provide a useful framework for assessing individuals in this community. The researchers believe that this model can facilitate the identification of essential components of the Colonias' culture and the collaboration of care through community outreach partnerships.

Table 6-7

Guidelines for the Home Visitor

PART I—FAMILY STRUCTURE AND CHILD-REARING PRACTICES

Family composition
- Who are the members of the family system?
- Who are the key decision makers?
- Is decision making individual or done in a group situation?
- Is decision making individual or group oriented?
- Do family members all live in the same household?
- What is the relationship of friends to the family system?
- What is the hierarchy within the family? Is status related to gender or age?

Primary caregiver(s)
- Who is the primary caregiver?
- Who else participates in caregiving?
- What is the amount of care given by mother versus others?
- How much time does the infant spend away from the primary caregiver?
- Is there conflict between caregivers regarding appropriate practices?
- What ecological/environmental issues impinge on general caregiving (e.g., housing, jobs, etc)?

Child-rearing practices

Family feeding practices
- What are the family feeding practices?
- What are the mealtime rules?
- What types of foods are eaten?
- What are the beliefs regarding breast-feeding and weaning?
- What are the beliefs regarding bottle feeding?
- What are the family practices regarding transitioning to solid food?
- Which family members prepare food?
- Is food purchased or homemade?
- Are there any taboos related to food preparation or handling?
- Which family members feed the child?
- What is the configuration of the family mealtime?
- What are the family's views on independent feeding?
- Is there a discrepancy among family members regarding the beliefs and practices related to feeding an infant or toddler?

Family sleeping patterns
- Does the infant sleep in the same room/bed as the parents?

- At what age is the infant moved away from close proximity to the mother?
- Is there an established bedtime?
- What is the family response to an infant when he or she wakes at night?
- What practices surround daytime napping?

Family's response to disobedience and aggression
- What are the parameters of acceptable child behavior?
- What form does the discipline take?
- Who metes out the disciplinary action?

Family's response to a crying infant
- Temporal qualities—how long before the caregiver picks up a crying infant?
- How does the caregiver calm an upset infant?

PART II—FAMILY PERCEPTIONS AND ATTITUDES

Family's perception of health and healing
- What is the family's approach to medical needs?
- Do they rely solely on Western medical services?
- Do they rely solely on holistic approaches?
- Do they use a combination of these approaches?
- Who is the primary medical provider or conveyer of medical information?
- Do all members of the family agree on approaches to medical needs?

Family's perception of help-seeking and intervention
- From whom does the family seek help—family members or outside agencies or individual?
- Does the family seek help directly or indirectly?
- What are the general feelings of the family when seeking assistance—ashamed, angry, demanding, view as unnecessary?
- With which community systems does the family interact (educational/medical/social)?
- How are these interactions completed (face-to-face, telephone, letter)?
- Which family member interacts with other systems?
- Does that family member feel comfortable when interacting with other systems?

(Continued)

Table 6-7

Guidelines for the Home Visitor cont'd

PART III—LANGUAGE AND COMMUNICATION STYLES

Language

To what degree:
- Is the home visitor proficient in the family's native language?
- Is the family proficient in English?

If an interpreter is used:
- With which culture is the interpreter primarily affiliated?
- Is the interpreter familiar with the colloquialisms of the family members' country or region of origin?
- Is the family member comfortable with the interpreter? Would the family member feel more comfortable with an interpreter of the same sex?

- If written materials are used, are they in the family's native language?

Communication styles
- Does the family communicate with each other in a direct or indirect style?
- Does the family tend to interact in a quiet manner or a loud manner?
- Do family members share feelings when discussing emotional issues?
- Does the family ask you direct questions?
- Does the family value a lengthy social time at each home visit unrelated to the early childhood services program goals?
- Is it important for the family to know about the home visitor's extended family? Is the home visitor comfortable sharing that information?

Table 6-8

Giger and Davidhizar's Transcultural Assessment Tool

Culturally unique individual
- Client's cultural and racial identification
- Place of birth
- Time in country

Biologic variations
- Body structure
- Skin color
- Hair color
- Other physical dimensions
- Enzymatic and genetic existence of diseases specific to populations
- Susceptibility to illness and disease
- Nutritional preferences and deficiencies
- Psychologic characteristics of coping

Environmental control
- Cultural health practices
- Efficacious
- Neutral
- Dysfunctional
- Uncertain
- Values
- Definition of health and illness

Time

Use of:
- Measures

- Definition
- Social time
- Work time
- Time orientation (future, present, past)

Social orientation
- Culture
- Race
- Ethnicity
- Family (role, function)
- Work
- Leisure
- Church
- Friends

Space
- Degree of comfort observed (conversation)
- Proximity to others
- Body movement
- Perception of space

Communication
- Language spoken
- Voice quality
- Pronunciation
- Use of silence
- Use of nonverbal

Scaz (1999) carried out a descriptive study to examine the features of transcultural education programs for registered nurses in Pennsylvania home-health agencies. The study included a random sample of 195 home-health agency administrators, who were asked to complete a questionnaire describing needs of the agency related to transcultural education programs and current perceived cultural barriers to the delivery of care. Seventy-five percent of the agencies indicated an intent to take action to reduce barriers to the delivery of care.

CONCLUSION

In the future, as immigration patterns continue to change, health-care providers and organizations need to be increasingly aware of changes needed to meet the health-care needs of diverse populations. As a nurse providing care in the community, you need to be aware of the characteristics of culturally competent care. Using information in this chapter related to cultural values of specific ethnic groups and cultural assessment tools, you will be able to offer to your clients nursing care that is sensitive to their unique cultural needs.

Active Learning Strategies

1. Talk to your classmates about your differing perceptions of the term culture. Make a list of the most common shared meanings. Note the differences between your classmates' views of the meaning of culture. Discuss how these differences impact care for your clients.

2. Think about the clients you have cared for this semester. What characteristics did you need to consider to provide culturally competent care?

3. Pair up with a classmate who is from another ethnic group. Discuss how you each have encountered various barriers to communication.

4. Interview someone in your community from an ethnic group different than yours. Ask this person to describe his or her perceptions of how culture influences the care he or she receives within the health-care system.

References

American Nurses Association. (1998). Culturally competent assessment for family violence. Washington, D.C.: Author.

Association of Asian Pacific Community Health Organizations. (1996). Pocket guide to medical interpretation. Oakland, CA: AAPCHO. (www.aapcho.org)

Bureau of Health Profession. (2000). Workforce personnel factbook. Washington, DC: Author.

Bureau of the Census. (1996). Population projections of the United States by age, sex, race and Hispanic origin: 1995–2050. Washington, DC: U.S. Department of Commerce. (www.census.gov/population/www/projections/natsum-T3.html)

Bureau of the Census. (2000). Population by race and Hispanic/Latino status. Washington, DC: U.S. Department of Commerce. (www.census.gov/statab/www/part1a.html)

Cross Cultural Health Care Program. (1996). Voices of the Arab communities. (www.xculture.org/resources/download/arab.pdf)

Davidhizar, R., & Bechtel, G. (1999). Health and quality of life within Colonias settlements along the United States and Mexico border. Public Health Nursing, 16(4), 301–306.

Galanti, G. (1997). Caring for patients from different cultures: Studies from American hospitals (2nd ed.). Philadelphia: University of Pennsylvania.

Giger, J. N., & Davidhizar, R. E. (Eds.). (1991). Transcultural nursing. St. Louis: Mosby.

Giger, J. N., & Davidhizar, R. E. (Eds.). (1995). Transcultural nursing (2nd ed.). St. Louis: Mosby.

Health Resources and Services Administration. (1996). Guidelines to help assess cultural competence in program design, application, and management. (www.bphc.hrsa.dhhs.gov/omwh/omwh_3.htm)

Healthy People 2000. (1991). National health promotion and disease prevention objectives. Washington, DC: Department of Health and Human Services.

Julia, M. (1996). Multicultural awareness in the health care professions. Boston: Allyn and Bacon.

Kamat, M. R. (1999). Blacks, women less likely to be referred for high-tech cardiac tests, according to study. Closing the Gap: Office of Minority Health, p. 6.

Lao Family Community of Minnesota. (1997). Cultural Competency. (www.laofamily.org)

Lynch, E. W., & Hanson, M. J. (1998). Developing cross-cultural competence. (2nd ed.). Baltimore: P.H. Brookes.

National Center for Cultural Competence. (1999). Policy Brief 1: Rationale for cultural competence in primary health care. Washington, DC: Georgetown University Child Development Center.

National Technical Assistance Center for Children's Mental Health. (1989). Towards a culturally competent system of care. Vol. 1. Washington, DC: Georgetown University Child Development Center.

Office of Minority Health Resource Center (OMHRC). (1998). Sources of health materials. Washington, DC: OMHRC.

Purnell, L., & Paulanka, B. (1998). Transcultural health care: A culturally competent approach. Philadelphia: F. A. Davis.

Roat, C.E. (1999). Bridging the gap: A basic training for medical interpreters (3rd ed.). Seattle: The Cross Cultural Health Care Program.

Scaz, L.C. L. (1999). A descriptive study of current transcultural education programs for registered nurses in selected Pennsylvania home health agencies. Journal for Nurses in Staff Development, 15(3), 120–125.

Schulman, K. A., Berlin, J. A., Harless, W., Kerner, J. F., Sistrunk, S., Gersh, B. J., Dube, R., Taleghani, C. K., Burke, J. E., Williams, S., Eisenberg, J. M., & Escarce, J. J. (1999). The effect of race and sex on physician's recommendation for cardiac catheterization. New England Journal of Medicine, 340(8) 618-619.

Spector, R. E. (1996). Cultural diversity in health and illness (4th ed.). Stamford, CT: Appleton & Lange.

Tervalon, M., & Murray Garcia, J. (1998). Cultural humility versus cultural competence: A critical distinction in defining physician training outcomes in multicultural education. Journal of Health Care for the Poor and Underserved, 9 (10), 117–125.

Time. (1997). Numbers. 150(9) 25.

Tirado, M. D. (1995). Tools for monitoring cultural competence in health care. Report to the Office of Planning and Evaluation Health Resources and Services Administration. San Francisco: Latino Coalition for a Healthy California.

U.S. Census Bureau, International Data Base. (www.census.gov)

Zambrana, R. E. (1994). Latino/Hispanic families and children: Vulnerability as a function of sociocultural and socioeconomic status barriers. Paper presented at the Institute for Educational Transformation on April 28, 1994.

Zambrana, R. E., & Dorrington, C. (1998, January/February). Economic and social vulnerability of Latino children and families by subgroup: Implications for child welfare. Child Welfare, Vol. LXXVII, #1.

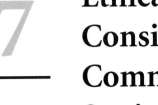

CHAPTER 7

Ethical and Legal Considerations in Community-based Settings

Mary Cipriano Silva

LEARNING OBJECTIVES

1) To identify key ethical and legal terminology.

2) To analyze seven ethical theories.

3) To analyze four ethical and legal principles.

4) To apply key ethical and legal terminology, ethical theories, and ethical and legal principles to community-based nursing situations.

DEFINITIONS RELATED TO ETHICS

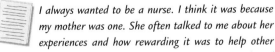

I always wanted to be a nurse. I think it was because my mother was one. She often talked to me about her experiences and how rewarding it was to help other people. Well, when I was assigned to my first community-based nursing clinical, I was to teach a wife who was caring for her dying husband about how to change his dressing. That did not bother me because I was well prepared to do a dressing change,

but, you know, I had never been around a dying patient. He was so thin and he was coughing a lot. He had radiation treatments for cancer of the stomach and was in terrible pain. I felt so sorry for him. His wife told me that, because of the pain, she was giving him double the pain-relieving medication from what the doctor had ordered. I was so scared, because I didn't know what to say or what to do. I went to the home to change a dressing, which I did, but I didn't know what to do about the other unexpected problem. I was afraid the wife would get into trouble with the doctor or the law if someone found out about the medication, and I didn't know whether what she was doing was ethical.

I wanted to get out of there, but I didn't. My mother made it all sound so easy, but sometimes it's not!

Nursing Student

Most nursing students can identify with the student in this story. She went into a home to simply change a dressing, which she was well prepared to do and with which she had no difficulty. At issue, however, was the unexpected nursing problem that she encountered, a situation that often occurs in community-based nursing. These unexpected nursing problems may center on the ethical and legal aspects of nursing care, which are often more difficult to manage than the technical aspects. Would you agree? The purpose of this chapter is to focus reflection on the ethical and legal aspects of client and family care and how they are often interrelated in community-based nursing. (This story will be revisited in the last part of this chapter, so keep thinking about it as we proceed.)

Your Definitions

Before definitions to important terms related to ethics are given, write in Box 7–1 how you would define the terms listed.

Box 7-1   Student Learning Activity

Your Definitions

What is ethics?

What is an ethical dilemma?

What is morality?

What is moral distress?

Definitions from Other Sources

Many definitions for the terms in Box 7-1 exist in the nursing, health-care, philosophy, and other literature. The following definitions are food for thought, a beginning point from which you can continue to build your own definitions—definitions that you are committed to and can defend.

Ethics

Ethics is that branch of philosophy that focuses on what one ought to do in matters of good and evil or right and wrong. It also entails a systematic problem-solving process that leads to a decision that can be morally justified through virtuous behavior and application of ethical theories, principles, values, professional codes of ethics, accurate facts, and so forth. Therefore, ethics involves both knowledge and critical thinking skills. Another term for critical thinking skills is *mindful thinking* or, in the case of ethics, *ethical mindfulness* (Weston, 1997). Weston discusses three obstacles to ethical mindfulness:

1. Dogmatism—Dogmatism presents an obstacle to ethical mindfulness because it circumvents one of the essential characteristics of ethics—open-ended thinking. Open-ended thinking means that you are willing to listen (and I mean listen!) to more than one side of an issue. In the ethics courses I teach, students often tell me how much they learn from viewpoints different than their own. Remember, to mindlessly assert and reassert a position on ethical issues is neither good ethics nor good thinking.

2. Rationalizing—Another obstacle to ethical mindfulness is rationalizing. Rationalizing is grasping for straws in an effort to save face instead of using sound reasons. Weston (1997) calls rationalizing "unintelligent opinions" (p. 6) or "self-deception" (p. 10). Have you ever cheated on an exam and justified your behavior by saying that you cheated because everyone else does? That is rationalizing.

3. Relativism—The third obstacle to ethical mindfulness is relativism. Relativism is the belief that any ethical position is as good as any other, or that ethical positions are no one's business but your own.

Boxes 7–2 through 7–4 will give you the opportunity to apply your understanding to the obstacles to ethical mindfulness discussed previously.

Box 7-2	Student Learning Activity

Dogmatism

How dogmatic about ethical matters do you believe you are? Write down two issues related to ethics about which you believe you are dogmatic.

Box 7-3	Student Learning Activity

Rationalizing

How often do you rationalize ethical matters? Write down two incidents related to ethics in community-based nursing in which you have used rationalization. (We all use it sometimes!)

Box 7-4	Student Learning Activity

Relativism

Can you think of counterarguments to the two examples of relativism stated in point 3? Try to use examples from your community-based nursing experiences.

Ethical Dilemmas

Ethical dilemmas are those situations in which a person feels that he or she both ought to and ought not to make a decision about a moral matter. The feeling is one of inner conflict and struggle because, regardless of the decision made, the decision is only partly morally acceptable. Sometimes, the nurse may even have to choose between two undesirable options. Here is what one student said about such a situation:

 I was assigned to observe a nurse midwife deliver a baby in the mother's home. At first, everything went well and then, suddenly, both the mother's and the baby's conditions changed for the worse. I suddenly had a terrifying thought: "What if they weren't able to save both of them; it might be either the mother or the baby." I thought, "What a terrible ethical decision to make!" Fortunately, through quick thinking on the part of the nurse midwife, both the mother and the baby were saved.

Complete Box 7–5 to explore this dilemma further.

Box 7-5	Student Learning Activity

Ethical Dilemma

What would be your feelings in the situation? If the situation had indeed continued to worsen, what ethical course of action would you have taken and why?

Morality

Morality usually refers to well-established and accepted rules of right and wrong that are culturally passed from one person or group to another. An example of a moral statement is "You ought not to break promises." With morality, the values and principles of a society are articulated and followed; thus morality has a social-cultural orientation.

Completion of Box 7–6 helps you to expand your understanding of morality.

| Box 7-6 | Student Learning Activity |

Morality

What are some strengths of the preceding definition of morality?

What are some problems with the definition?

Moral Distress

Moral distress is painful psychological feelings related to an ethical situation in which ethical standards are compromised and the nurse (or other members of the health team) feels powerless to do what she or he believes is the right thing.

What do research studies tell us about the phenomenon of moral distress? Powell (1997) conducted research on "The Lived Experiences of Moral Distress Among Staff Nurses." She interviewed 10 nurses who had experienced moderate to high moral distress when caring for patients for whom recovery was not possible or death was impending. Some of the themes that emerged from her data were that the nurses felt as if they were on a moral crusade (patient advocacy role), had unresolved feelings about the situation (some for many years after the incident), and had a different moral orientation and decision-making

process than the physicians (which at times caused the doctor/nurse relationship to become adversarial).

To illustrate, regarding the theme of unresolved feelings, here is what two nurses had to say:

The hopeless feeling, oh God, to see that man cry every time you turned him, every time you had to change his dressing off his backside and then he would choke on the vent. Every time you would suction him, he would turn purple. . . . He wanted you to stop. And I would think, why am I doing this? Why am I doing this to this man, knowing he was not going to get out of there? (Powell, 1997, p. 114)

I felt guilty sometimes for doing the care because it was hurting the patient. Like when we turned him, or anytime you held him, he got a bruise or his skin tore. I can hear myself telling him I am so sorry, over and over again. But how many times can you say you're sorry? Because you still have to do what you have to do. . . . I was glad that he did not live. . . . (Powell, 1997, p. 115)

Box 7–7 gives you an opportunity to discuss these stories.

| Box 7-7 | Student Learning Activity |

Moral Distress

How did the preceding two stories make you feel? Write down your thoughts.

What would you have done if you were the nurse?

Although the nurses who related the two preceding situations experienced moral distress, this outcome does not always occur. Whether working in a hospital or in a community-based setting, nurses often experience feelings of satisfaction when they have advocated successfully for a person or a family about ethical issues.

ETHICAL ASPECTS OF COMMUNITY-BASED NURSING: ETHICAL THEORIES

As already noted, ethics involves knowledge—knowledge about ethical theories, principles, values, professional codes of ethics, and accurate factual information. We begin with six ethical theories: virtue-based theory, consequence-based theory, duty-based theory, rights-based theory, communal-based theory, and caring/feminist-based theory.

Virtue-based Theory

Since the times of Plato and Aristotle, virtue-based ethics (also called character ethics) has focused on the question of "Who ought I morally to be?" Who a person morally ought to be is based on a person's moral virtues. Moral virtues are internal character traits that, taken individually or as a whole, predispose a person not only to moral goodness but also to act in a virtuous way.

According to Beauchamp and Childress (1994), another factor is important to virtue-based ethics—motive. In other words, the proper motive must accompany the good or right action for the action to be virtuous. Examples of virtues are courage, honesty, truthfulness, and fairness. Can you think of other virtues? Examples of proper motives are acting in a certain way because a person wants to help another or to ease another's suffering.

According to Beauchamp and Childress (1994), "It is possible to be disposed to do what is right, to intend to do it, and to do it, while also yearning to avoid doing it" (p. 64). Under this condition, the act may be a good one, but the person performing the act is not exhibiting a moral virtue. For example, you are assigned to a homeless shelter to assess the health needs of that specific community, and you want to do an excellent assessment. In fact, you do so, but at the same time, you harbor feelings of disgust toward the homeless. According to virtue-based theory, your ac-

tions may be good and commendable but, in this situation, you are not virtuous. Completion of Box 7–8 will expand your understanding of virtue-based theory.

Box 7-8	Student Learning Activity

Virtue-based Theory

Can you think of a community-based situation in which you were virtuous? What made you virtuous in that situation?

Can you think of a community-based situation in which you were *not* virtuous? What made you lack virtue in that situation? How could you change that behavior? Jot down your thoughts and also talk to another student about your thinking.

Consequence-based Theory

How often have you heard the expression "the greatest good for the greatest number"? This expression is important for two reasons. It refers to an ethical theory known as utilitarianism (based largely on the writings of the 19th-century philosopher John Stuart Mill), and it also refers to a basic tenet of community-*health* nursing in which, unlike community-*based* nursing, "individual rights may be sacrificed for good of [the] community" (Zotti, Brown, & Stotts, 1996, p. 212). As you know, individual choices and rights are core values of community-*based* nursing. We address the preceding premise later in the chapter.

Utilitarianism is called a consequence-based theory because actions are assessed as right or wrong according to the weight of their consequences. Simply put, the right act is the one that produces more good than bad consequences for all persons affected by the act or for the persons most affected by the act. Usually the persons most affected by the act are the client and his or her family. For example, if you are assigned to a community-based family planning clinic whose funding has been severely cut, the consequences of this action will affect the morale of the staff, including yourself, at the very least. Most likely, however, the consequences of the cut-back will affect the clients the most because they will not be able to receive the same quality of care as they did before the funding cut.

If you profess to be a utilitarian, this means that you have committed yourself to thinking about and balancing consequences and only consequences to determine right or wrong actions. This is why utilitarianism is often referred to as an ethical theory that is based on a single principle (known as the *principle of utility*). Virtues, duties, or rights, for example, are not a part of utilitarian thinking because they are not grounded in consequences. Completion of Box 7–9 will expand your understanding of consequence-based theory.

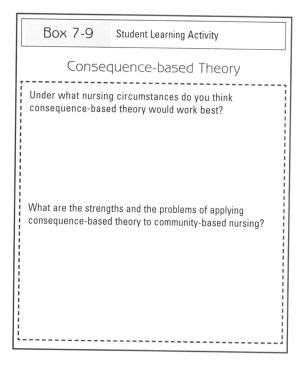

Box 7-9   Student Learning Activity

Consequence-based Theory

Under what nursing circumstances do you think consequence-based theory would work best?

What are the strengths and the problems of applying consequence-based theory to community-based nursing?

Duty-based Theory

How often have you heard the expression, "It's your duty"? This expression forms part of the basis for an ethical theory known as *deontology*. Deontology is an ethical theory in which characteristics of a person's actions other than, or in addition to, their consequences, make an act right or wrong. Examples of characteristics other than consequences are virtues or obligations.

A person who ascribes to deontology is called a deontologist. Some deontologists would not include consequences as a part of deontology, whereas other deontologists would. Deontology, then, is a much broader theory than utilitarianism because it accommodates many more principles and concepts than utilitarianism.

Many of the conceptualizations of duty-based theory are associated with the writings of Immanuel Kant, an 18th-century philosopher. Three aspects of his writings are worth pondering (Kant, 1785/1981).

1. The categorical imperative—One version of this imperative is that you should never treat other persons as only a means to an end. For example, if during a community-based clinical experience in a senior center, you choose to socialize with a senior only because that person reminds you of a loved grandparent, you would be using that senior as only a means to the end of meeting your own psychological needs.

2. A good will—An action of good will is motivated to take the right action regardless of consequences. For example, when making a community-based home visit motivated by good will, you tell the client who asks you that she is dying of cancer. You tell the truth because you believe strongly in respecting the client as a person regardless of the consequences. (Note that utilitarians may also tell her the truth or they may not; their response depends on the consequences.)

3. Duty—A duty, according to Kant, is an obligation that all persons morally ought to keep, for example, truth telling. Unlike virtue theory, discussed previously, Kant finds actions that are performed out of moral duty, although one may prefer *not* to do them, to be morally praiseworthy. For example, when assigned to an outpatient clinic that serves persons with human immunodeficiency virus (HIV) and acquired immunodeficiency syndrome (AIDS), you follow through with your assignment even though you may prefer not to do so because of your unresolved feelings about HIV/AIDS.

Completion of Box 7–10 will expand your understanding of duty-based theory.

```
┌─────────────────────────────────────────────────────┐
│  Box 7-10     Student Learning Activity               │
│  ┌─────────────────────────────────────────────────┐ │
│  │                                                   │ │
│        Duty-based Theory                              │
│  ├ ─ ─ ─ ─ ─ ─ ─ ─ ─ ─ ─ ─ ─ ─ ─ ─ ─ ─ ─ ─ ─ ─ ─ ─ ┤ │
│  Under what nursing circumstances do you think       │
│  duty-based theory would work best?                   │
│                                                       │
│                                                       │
│                                                       │
│                                                       │
│                                                       │
│  What are the strengths and the problems with         │
│  applying duty-based theory to community-based        │
│  nursing?                                             │
│                                                       │
│                                                       │
│                                                       │
│                                                       │
│                                                       │
└─────────────────────────────────────────────────────┘
```

Rights-based Theory

Rights are justified claims that groups or individuals can make on society or on each other (Beauchamp & Childress, 1994). For example, a group right might be for the group to claim a right to health care, and an individual right might be for the health-care client to claim a right to safe nursing care. As a nursing student, you also have rights. For example, you have a right to refuse to give nursing care to a client, whether in a hospital or a community-based setting, if you know the care would harm the client (e.g., to give a wrong medication or a wrong dosage of a medication). But keep in mind that rights are justified (not capricious) claims or demands. *Justified* means that the claim is based on relevant and appropriate knowledge and reasoning.

Thus a *moral* right is a claim that is based on *ethical* theories, principles, concepts, rules, precedents, and a defensible line of moral reasoning. In the case of your right to refuse to give nursing care that would cause you to administer a wrong medication or dosage, your justification

is based on the moral principle, "Do not harm any client," and not on a capricious principle such as "Do not harm only white clients."

Many issues surround rights-based theory, such as "Are rights absolute or not?" and "For every right, is there a corresponding obligation?" Questions such as these are beyond the scope of our discussion, but an explanation of how rights-based theory became important in nursing is within our scope. I address two factors that increased its importance: The American Nurses Association's (ANA) 1985 *Code for Nurses with Interpretive Statements* and the American Hospital Association's (AHA) 1970 *Statement on a Patient's Bill of Rights*.

In the 1985 *Code for Nurses* (and earlier *Codes*), rights language is used. The second provision of the *Code* states, "The nurse safeguards the client's right to privacy by judiciously protecting information of a confidential nature" (ANA, 1985, p. 1). In the interpretive statements of the *Code*, a right to privacy belongs to the person, and the *Code* considers it to be "an inalienable human right" (p. 4). Notice, however, that when confidentiality is concerned, the nurse acts judiciously. That is because, by law, not all information that a patient tells you can be kept confidential (e.g., venereal diseases must be reported to the state health department). Nevertheless, apart from the law, the *Code* stipulates that only those health-care providers who are directly involved with the care of the client should have access and only on a need-to-know basis regarding the client's care.

In 1970, the AHA formulated the first Patient's Bill of Rights, which has continued to serve as a basis for similar patients' bills of rights since that time (Davis, Aroskar, Liaschenko, & Drought, 1997). The Patient's Bill of Rights, although originally written for hospitalized patients, also has relevance for community-based nursing. Some of these rights focus on the right to considerate care, the right to know about the nature of one's illness, the right to privacy and confidentiality, and the right to continuity of care. Regardless of the community-based settings in which you are assigned, these patients' rights should be upheld unless compelling ethical or legal considerations dictate otherwise.

Completion of Box 7–11 will expand your understanding of rights-based theory.

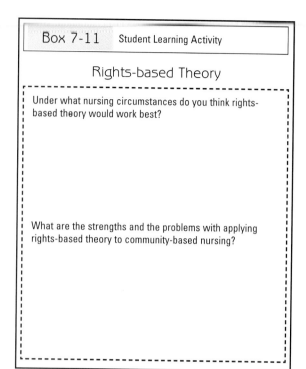

Box 7-11   Student Learning Activity

Rights-based Theory

Under what nursing circumstances do you think rights-based theory would work best?

What are the strengths and the problems with applying rights-based theory to community-based nursing?

in community-based nursing is strong and supports autonomous decision making by the individual and family; the principle of autonomy in community-health nursing is less strong, and the tenet, "The greatest good for the greatest number" dominates.

During your community-based nursing experiences, you may experience tensions among consequence-based ethical theories, rights-based ethical theories, and communal-based ethical theories. You will feel the tug between the needs of the individual and his or her family (whom you serve as an advocate) and the needs of the community, especially when resources are scarce (Aroskar, 1998). Completion of Box 7–12 will expand your understanding of communal-based theory.

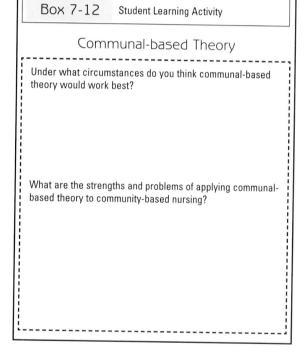

Box 7-12   Student Learning Activity

Communal-based Theory

Under what circumstances do you think communal-based theory would work best?

What are the strengths and problems of applying communal-based theory to community-based nursing?

Communal-based Theory

Simply put, communal-based ethical theory focuses on the community and its collective communal values. There is an emphasis on what is good for the community as a whole instead of what is good for individuals who make up the community. According to Beauchamp and Childress (1994), "The importance of traditional practices and the need for communal intervention to correct socially disruptive outcomes are standard themes in communitarian thought" (p. 81).

Consider some of the differences between community-based nursing and community-health nursing (Zotti, Brown, & Stotts, 1996). By so doing, you can anticipate ethical and other conflicts between the two. The goal of community-based nursing is to manage health conditions and to promote self-care among individuals and families; the goal of community-health nursing is to help a community maintain its health. The client in community-based nursing is the individual, family, and small group; the client in community-health nursing is the population or aggregate. The principle of autonomy

Caring and Feminist-based Theories

Although the caring and feminist-based theories are at times presented separately, there are links between them (Silva & Kroeger-Mappes, 1998). Both theories reject morality based on rules and instead stress response to others through relationships or connections with them. Both theories typically focus on a need to respond to others, to view caring (in all its dimensions) as a moral imperative, to resolve conflicts through communication, to focus on everyday real ethical problems, rather than on abstract theories and principles, and to care for and value self and others so that neither is harmed.

However, there are some important distinctions. According to Silva and Kroeger-Mappes (1998), "Many moral theorists argue that the ethic of care is a *feminine* ethic rather than a *feminist* one" (p. 8). Whereas a feminine ethic may include the preceding components of an ethic of care, feminist ethics also usually go beyond them. Feminist-based ethical theories are usually concerned with the worthiness of women's moral experiences (at least as worthy as men's) and the social-cultural-political environments that wrongly oppress women. Feminist ethicists are concerned that the voices of women be heard both in theory (in conceptualizations about ethics) and in practice (in actions that will make a positive difference in the valuing of women by themselves and by others). For both of these goals to occur, genuine caring among all people must occur. Now, reflect on some research that focuses on caring and uncaring.

Juethong (1998) investigated caring and uncaring behaviors that 24 Thai nursing students reported experiencing with their instructors. She collected her data through audiotaped interviews with the students. I am going to share one caring and one uncaring story with you, both of which deal with a medication error. As a student nurse, you may be able to identify with both of these students.

CARING STORY

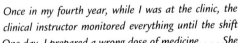

Once in my fourth year, while I was at the clinic, the clinical instructor monitored everything until the shift was over. One day, I prepared a wrong dose of medicine. . . . She gently asked me at the medicine counter "What are you doing?" So I replied, "I was preparing [a] medical injection for a patient." Then the instructor rechecked the medicine and found that it was a wrong dose. . . . The instructor did not criticize me, instead she asked me to re-prepare the medicine. She did not discuss my mistake. . . . I still remember this experience. She impressed me very much. (Juethong, 1998, p. 97)

UNCARING STORY

During my second year, we practiced antibody [vaccine] injection at an OPD [out-patient department]. . . . I incorrectly interpreted the information on the record and injected 0.5 cc of antibody instead of 0.25 cc to the patient. . . . I did not know what to do. I was afraid to tell this incident to the clinical instructor in charge because she was a very strict person. I decided to relate the incident to a clinical nurse instead. . . . The clinical nurse reported this to a physician and the clinical instructor. . . . The clinical instructor kept asking me, "Why didn't you inform me by yourself?" "Why did you inform the clinical nurse first instead of me?" I told her that I was personally afraid of her. I was afraid of being severely punished by her. The instructor accused me of being a coward for not accepting my own mistakes. (Juethong, 1988, p. 126)

Completion of Box 7–13 will expand your understanding of caring and feminist theory.

Box 7-13	Student Learning Activity

Caring- and Feminist-based Theory

Under what circumstances do you think caring theories would work best?

Under what circumstances do you think feminist-based ethical theories would work best?

What are the strengths and problems of applying caring and feminist-based theories to community-based nursing?

Table 7-1

Ethical Theories: Focus and Applications to Community-based Nursing

ETHICAL THEORIES	FOCUS	APPLICATION TO COMMUNITY-BASED NURSING
1. Virtue-based	Character traits	Student nurse uses compassion when caring for a client with AIDS who is dying at home.
2. Consequence-based	Consequence of actions	Student nurse weighs all the positive and negative consequences of lying to a client about having cancer when the family doesn't want the client to know.
3. Duty-based	Obligations	Student nurse views it as a duty to treat the women in a homeless shelter with respect.
4. Rights-based	Individual's claims	Student nurse advocates for a prisoner's right to have a kidney transplant.
5. Communal-based	Community as a whole	Overall, is not applicable to community-based nursing; is applicable to community-health nursing.
6. Caring-based	Connectedness of relationships	Student nurse spends considerable time carefully listening to family problems of a Vietnamese parishioner.
7. Feminist-based	Connectedness of relationships and social-cultural-political environments that oppress women and their lower their moral worth	Student nurse attends community meetings that seek to empower women who are widowed and who have never worked outside of the home.

Table 7–1 summarizes the seven ethical theories just discussed. Let us next turn our attention to knowledge about four important ethical principles of respect for autonomy, beneficence, nonmaleficence, and justice and how the law interfaces with them.

ETHICAL AND LEGAL PRINCIPLES

Ethical and Legal Aspects of the Principle of Respect for Autonomy

The ethical principle of respect for autonomy contains two major ethical and legal concepts: the concept of respect for persons and the concept of autonomy.

The Concept of Respect for Persons

What do you think of when you are asked to respect persons (clients)? Can you think of an example when you

respected a client during your community-based experiences? Can you think of an example when you (or someone else) did not respect a client during your community-based experiences? What was the outcome of each experience?

Although respect for persons can be defined in many ways, one definition that may be helpful to you follows: Respect for persons (clients) means the ability to identify, appreciate, and give due consideration to other persons' (clients') values, perspectives, and judgments. It encompasses such character traits as empathy, compassion, a nonjudgmental attitude, a lack of arrogance about knowing what is in the client's best interest, and a commitment to not use clients as merely a means to your own ends. When you respect your clients, among other actions, you address them properly, you individualize their care, and you respect their wishes as long as they do not harm themselves or others or break the law. You deny them respect when you, among other actions, feign listening or concern, ignore reasonable requests, address them in a dismissive way, or talk about them inappropriately.

Ludwick and Sedlak (1998), based on research findings, reported a story about two beginning student nurses who cared for a 79-year-old, hard-of-hearing and confused Czechoslovakian woman who had fallen at home. One student expressed how she felt about the other student's care:

Throughout the entire feeding and the rest of the morning, Kathy talked to MB with some sort of accent and broken English. She told me later she did this because working in a nursing home she had a foreign patient who seems calmed when she speaks to him in that way. I could not help but be annoyed when she did this though, because it seemed degrading in a way. Like she was treating MB as a child. It is like talking extremely loud to a person who does not speak English. Thinking that somehow the loudness will help them understand better, forgetting that they simply can't understand. . . . (Ludwick & Sedlak, 1998, p. 17)

Box 7–14 gives you an opportunity to discuss the story above.

Box 7-14	Student Learning Activity

Respect for Persons

Write down all the ways Kathy showed lack of respect for the client.

How would you have handled the situation with Kathy? Discuss the situation with your classmates.

In contrast to the preceding story, the ANA *Code for Nurses* (1985), in its first provision, states that "the nurse provides services with respect for human dignity and the uniqueness of the client, unrestricted by considerations of social or economic status, personal attributes, or the nature of health problems" (p. 1). The interpretive statements associated with the provision emphasize several important points (ANA, 1985, pp. 2–4):

1. Nurses have a moral obligation to respect the individuality of human existence.

2. Clients have the moral right to decide what will be done to their persons when nurses plan and implement their care.

3. Nurses have an obligation to know and support clients' moral and legal rights.

4. Nurses should actively work to ensure clients' individual rights.

5. Nurses have a moral obligation to provide care to clients without prejudice related to such factors as race, gender, lifestyle, and sexual orientation.

6. Nurses' high-quality nursing care should not be limited by such factors as whether the care is acute or chronic, whether the care is in the hospital or community, or whether the patient's health problem is common or stigmatized.

Think about the preceding six points and I think you will agree that respect for persons is a cornerstone of ethical and legal nursing practice.

The Concept of Autonomy

The word *autonomy* is derived from the Greek language and means self-governance. One way you can think about autonomy is by considering autonomous persons. Autonomous persons have the capacity for self-governance (i.e., they can reason, comprehend, and possess the ability to make independent decisions). A second way you can think about autonomy is by considering autonomous choice. Persons who possess autonomous choice go beyond the capacity for self-governance and exhibit the ability to make choices (e.g., they can formulate options about, such as whether they want to stay in their own home, move to a condominium, or move to an assisted-living facility). A third way you can think about autonomy is by considering autonomous actions. Persons who perform autonomous actions go beyond capacity and choice (for they possess both) and carry out (act on) their choice(s) based on

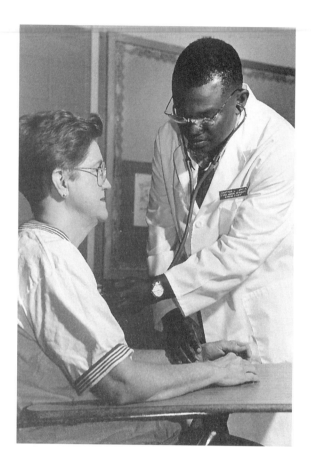

capacity. However, keep in mind that autonomous persons do not always act on their capacities or choices because they choose not to or because their freedom has been constrained in some way that prevents them from acting as they choose (e.g., a poor, uninsured person may have the capacity to make good choices about health-care practices, but cannot act on these choices because of lack of money).

The Ethical and Legal Principle of Respect for Autonomy

The preceding sections have put forth a discussion about "respect for persons" and about "autonomy." In your everyday practice in community-based nursing, how can you conceptualize the principle of respect for autonomy? Here is one way to think about it. As an autonomous student nurse (or as an autonomous client), your capacities,

choices, and actions belong only to you. However, the respect shown to you comes from outside you, from another person. Put another way, the principle of respect for autonomy focuses on how autonomous persons should be treated. They should be treated in such a way that they are free to choose and act without having controlling constraints placed on them by others (except under those conditions previously noted—harm to self or to others). The key here is *morally justified noninterference.*

Here is Sally's story about her experience dealing with these concepts when, as student nurse on a home visit, she discovered that a 40-year-old female, MC, was having heavy menstrual bleeding, was passing large blood clots, and was pale.

I was assigned to a faith community. We worked with the parish minister, who would provide us with the names of parishioners who had requested home visits. MC was a 40-year-old woman who had been married for 10 years. She and her husband had undergone fertility tests and procedures, but MC had not been able to get pregnant. She called C, the parish minister, saying she was very depressed and thought that talking with a nursing student might help her to deal with her sadness. Before I went on the home visit, I knew that MC had been diagnosed with fibroids and had a recent history of heavy menstrual bleeding. But what I saw on this visit disturbed me. MC showed me her bed where she had been resting; there was a large area of bright red blood. I immediately took her pulse and blood pressure. Her pulse was over 100, although her blood pressure was normal for her. I consulted with my instructor on my cell phone, and we, along with MC, agreed that she should be transported to the emergency room of City Hospital. My instructor gave me permission to accompany MC. Once there, MC was diagnosed with bleeding due to the fibroids, and the surgeon-on-call said a hysterectomy was indicated within the next several hours. But to my surprise, MC said, "No, I won't go to surgery without first talking to Dr. B! She is my family doctor and also a good friend of mine." But Dr. B. was tied up for two hours. I began to ask the patient questions to determine her decision-making capacity; it seemed intact. The surgeon-on-call said that she would wait two hours but no longer. Fortunately, Dr. B. showed up just in time, and MC was taken to surgery for a hysterectomy. But I kept wondering what would have happened if Dr. B. hadn't shown up!

Box 7–15 gives you an opportunity to discuss the story on the preceding page.

Box 7-15   Student Learning Activity

Respect for Autonomy

In what ways did the care providers show respect to MC (respect for persons principle)?

Was the surgeon-on-call morally or legally justified in postponing the surgery for two hours (noninterference principle)?

What do you think might have happened if Dr. B. had not shown up? What ethical and legal factors would you think about?

An Ethical and Legal Application of the Principle of Respect for Autonomy

The following ethical and legal application to consent and informed consent relates to respect for autonomy and is primarily based on and adapted from Hall's (1996) book. (Hall is both a registered nurse [RN] and a lawyer.) Both in ethics and in law, the concepts of consent and informed consent are primarily grounded in respect for client autonomy. A good example of this is a law passed in 1914; it said that all adults of sound mind have a right to decide what can happen to their own bodies. (In the United States, persons age 18 and over are considered adults.) This law came about because a hysterectomy was performed on a woman when she had consented only to a pelvic exam. Consent law protects persons from a battery (unwanted touch) suit. Battery suits usually occur when consent is not obtained for medical procedures or surgeries.

Consents can be written, spoken, or implied; however, if a lawsuit should arise, written consent affords the best ethical and legal protection to health-care providers, including

nursing students. The consent that you are probably the most familiar with is informed consent. Let's discuss now some of the ethical and legal aspects of informed consent.

The legal standard used most frequently today regarding informed consent is: "What would a reasonable person in similar circumstances need to know to make an informed decision?" (Hall, 1996, p. 229). Implied in that question is that persons have the competence (capacity if using ethical terminology) to make an informed decision. What persons can you think of who would not (or who would not at certain times) meet the competence/capacity criterion?

If you thought of minors as one category, you are correct. Know your state law regarding specific consent statutes related to minors, because each state has its own statutes. Sometimes minors can give consent if they are considered mature minors or are emancipated (e.g., are married or are in the military). If minors are not emancipated, their parents (or the parent with custody) or their guardians can usually give or refuse consent for the child.

As a nursing student, you must use good judgment regarding informed consent with minors. Sometimes the ethical and legal principle of respect for autonomy can be overridden by another important ethical and legal principle: You must act in the best interest of the child. For example, if a young child were to die because the parents believed only in "natural" remedies rather than modern science, you cannot idly stand by and watch the child die. According to Hall (1996),

> The child is the nurse's patient, to whom the nurse's advocacy is owed. If parents refuse treatment, especially when the refusal could result in harm to the child, the nurse's duty to the patient requires that she [or he] take steps to protect the patient; at a minimum to involve the agency's management and the patient's doctor. (p. 231)

As a nursing student in a community-based practice setting, you also should notify and inform your instructor. Although not detailed in Hall's book, the ANA (1985) *Code for Nurses with Interpretive Statements* takes a strong stand on situations such as the preceding:

> Nurses are accountable for judgments made and actions taken in the course of nursing practice. Neither physicians' orders nor the employing agency's policies relieve the nurse of accountability for actions taken and judgments made (p. 9).

Always remember that laws meet minimum standards of morality, whereas ethics meet higher or the highest

Table 7-2

Application of the Ethical and Legal Principle of Respect for Autonomy: Questions Frequently Asked by Nurses about Informed Consent

QUESTIONS	ANSWERS
1. What is informed consent?	1. Informed consent is both an ethical and legal concept based on respect for autonomy that allows competent adults to make decisions about their bodies and about their health care. It can be written, spoken, or implied and applies not only to research and surgical procedures but also to all care that nurses and other health-care providers render, regardless of setting. It is also a dynamic concept that can change over time.
2. What are the most important components of informed consent?	2. The most important components of informed consent include a voluntary client's capacity to understand the risks, and so forth about the procedures/care/studies to be done, as well as the client's ability to make a decision about the disclosed information and understand its consequences.
3. What happens if a client does not have the capacity to understand or make a decision?	3. Under these circumstances, a proxy consent is obtained from other persons. These persons may be guardians, family members, or nurses or other health-care providers if there are no guardians or family available. If a nurse obtains consent for a medical procedure, the law will hold that nurse to a medical standard.
4. What are the nurse's responsibilities in the consent process?	4. The nurse serves as an advocate and intermediary for the client who does not comprehend the consent process or cannot make a decision about it. She or he reports this situation to the appropriate health-care providers and, if needed, to management. If the consent is for a nursing study or procedure, the nurse must ensure that all important components of the consent have been met (see point 2, preceding).
5. What is the meaning of a witness signature on a consent form?	5. The witnessing of a client's consent form means that the nurse saw the client signing the consent, thus verifying that the client is who she or he says. It has nothing to do with the adequacy or inadequacy of the consent process.

standards of morality. Therefore, as a nursing student, you should think about ethics *before* you think about law. Hall (1996) gives a good rule to follow: "The ethics incorporated into good nursing practice are more important than knowledge of the law; practicing ethically saves the effort of trying to know all the laws" (p. 2).

Table 7–2 presents important questions to consider in applying the principle of respect for autonomy in community-based nursing.

Ethical and Legal Aspects of the Principle of Beneficence

Bene is a Latin word for "good," and *ficence* is a Latin word for "to do or make" (Hall, 1996, p. 106). Thus beneficence translated means "to do good." The doing of good is an

important ethical and legal principle in nursing; it requires an other-regarding focus. That other-regarding focus is primarily the clients who nurses and student nurses serve. Beneficence is required of nurses; it shows clients that we care for and about them. According to Hall (1996), nurses are professionals at caring and, thus receive pay to care; furthermore, nurses have an ethical and a legal duty to care. If nurses fail the ethical duty to care, they may experience moral distress. If nurses fail the legal duty to care (i.e., promote the client's life), they may experience malpractice suits.

Principle of Beneficence

Before returning to malpractice issues, I want to explore the principle of beneficence more deeply. Think about your most recent community-based clinical experience and jot down all the ways you cared for or about your client(s). Because beneficence in nursing is so ingrained into our value system, we often take for granted the good that we as nurses and student nurses do. Here is an opportunity for you to congratulate yourself for a job well done!

In addition to Hall's (1996) notion of beneficence as a legal duty, other perspectives exist. The promotion of good, the prevention of harm, and the removal of harm are terms typically found in ethics books to define the principle of beneficence. Examples of beneficence are also found in codes for nurses. Excerpts from the International Council of Nurses' (1973) *Code for Nurses: Ethical Concepts Applied to Nursing* that address beneficence are:

- The fundamental responsibility of the nurse is fourfold: to promote health, to prevent illness, to restore health and to alleviate suffering. (p. 1)
- The nurse shares with other citizens the responsibility for initiating and supporting action to meet the health and social needs of the public. (p. 2)

Beneficence, Advocacy, and the Code for Nurses

Beneficence is also addressed in the ANA's (1985) *Code for Nurses with Interpretive Statements*. Provision 3 states that "the nurse acts to safeguard the client and the public when health care and safety are affected by incompetent, unethical, or illegal practice by any person" (p. 6). In the interpretive statements for provision 3, one of the most important sentences in the *Code* occurs. Provision 3 states, "The nurse's primary commitment is to the health, welfare, and safety of the client" (p. 6). Certainly the principle of beneficence is operating here! Let's ponder a situation that you may face in your community-based nursing assignment.

Based on research, Ludwick and Sedlak (1998) reported this account of a beginning nursing student who, by her actions, promoted the good of a client.

My patient was in a bad mood and came across in a mean way. . . . He said, "Well, come on and hurry this [taking of vital signs and grooming] up!" . . . I felt so rushed and so nervous. . .he constantly questioned what I was doing and told me in a mean tone whether he thought I was doing it right or not. . . . One important decision I had to make was how to act. I wanted to provide the care needed and be responsive to him even if he came across in a mean way. . . . (p. 15)

The student goes on to say that she remembered something that one of her instructors had said: A nurse provides good care no matter how mean a patient is. The student kept this in mind, explained everything she was doing, and was nice to the patient. By the end of her time with him, the patient was relaxed and complimentary of her. When the student walked out of the room she "felt wonderful" because she had promoted the welfare of this client (Ludwick & Sedlak, 1998). Box 7–16 allows you to discuss the story above.

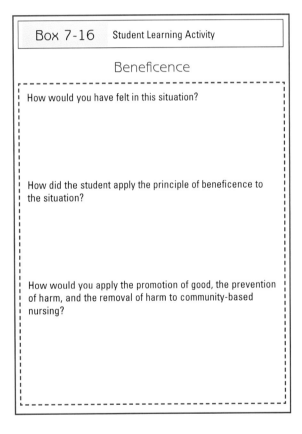

Box 7-16	Student Learning Activity

Beneficence

How would you have felt in this situation?

How did the student apply the principle of beneficence to the situation?

How would you apply the promotion of good, the prevention of harm, and the removal of harm to community-based nursing?

The ANA (1985) *Code for Nurses with Interpretive Statements* states that the nurse serves as an advocate for the patient. The preceding story also shows how a beginning nursing student was able to assume this role through caring. In a recent study on advocacy, Chafey, Rhea, Shannon, and Spencer (1998) interviewed 17 practicing nurses from three different community-based systems to ascertain how they defined the advocacy role and what they believed enhanced or impeded this role. Results were as follows:

1. Advocacy was defined by four major characteristics: coordination, intervention, empowerment, and interpersonal relatedness. All of these four characteristics took place within each of the three community systems and were focused on enhancing the welfare of the client (beneficence). Let's emphasize interpersonal relatedness here because this was the advocacy role that our beginning nursing student used, and it was the role that the study authors said "remained the cornerstone of nursing advocacy" (Chafey et al., 1998, p. 49). One nurse in the study said, "being there, being a listener, a confidante. . . many times they'll talk to us and tell us things that they wouldn't tell anybody else" (Chafey et al., 1998, p. 48). Another client-centered nurse said, "I guess there has to be genuine interest and concern, not so much in the issue as in the person. Part of advocacy would be accessing information or resources, because it's hard to advocate for somebody on an issue if you don't know what's going on" (Chafey et al., 1998, p. 48).

2. Some of the factors that enhanced advocacy were personal values and beliefs such as religious convictions, professional values and ethical/legal considerations such as clients' rights, and personality traits such as strength of conviction and persistence.

3. Some of the factors that impeded advocacy were unprofessional physician behavior such as intimidation, yelling, or throwing objects; lack of institutional support that threatened job security; personality conflicts with clients; and lack of commitment or self-confidence. From the preceding study, you should be able to identify examples of how the principle of beneficence was either honored or dishonored.

An Ethical and Legal Application of the Principle of Beneficence

The following discussion of malpractice as it relates to beneficence is primarily based on and adapted from Hall. Hall (1996) identifies four essentials for malpractice: "The nurse must have had a *duty* to another person and must have *breached* the standard of care which *caused* an *injury* to the person" (p. 110). Now examine each of these necessary components for malpractice as stipulated by Hall (1996), while keeping in mind that malpractice law enforces the principle of beneficence.

1. Duty—Does the nurse, while on the job and receiving payment for the work, have a legal duty of beneficence to clients? The answer is yes. This duty is imposed because it is inherent in the practice of nursing to do good; thus nurses must both ethically and legally assume this duty. (If you were not acting in your professional capacity as a nurse, the principle of beneficence as interpreted by the law usually would not apply). Payment for work done on one's job appears to be an important variable that affects liability for malpractice regarding the doing of good. However, an exception to the duty of beneficence exists when the nurse, while on the job, is unable to foresee unexpected circumstances (e.g., a patient's visiting relative has a heart attack).

2. Breach of the standard of care—Having established that the nurse has both an ethical and legal duty of beneficence, the second essential of malpractice liability is breach of that duty. According to Hall (1996), "The definition of breach for nurses is failure to act as a reasonable, prudent nurse in that circumstance" (p. 113). In other words, a nurse violates the duty of beneficence by failure to meet the standard of accepted nursing practice in a particular situation (e.g., the nurse does not use side rails for a client who needs them). The law does not care about the nurse's work situation (e.g., short staffed or any other negative circumstance) because the patient didn't cause it.

   Examples of standards or evidence that may be used to determine malpractice include:
   - Nurses or physicians who give testimony as expert witnesses
   - Protocols or standing orders
   - Books that specify how to use equipment
   - Nursing journals that focus on good practice
   - Joint Commission on the Accreditation of Healthcare Organizations (JCAHO) standards
   - ANA *Code for Nurses with Interpretive Statements*
   - American Nurses Association's (ANA) and other nursing organizations' standards
   - Nurse practice regulations and statutes (statutes are weighty and establish both the duty and the standard of care).

3. Injury—The third essential of malpractice liability is injury, usually substantial injury. In injury cases, it is the plaintiff (the individual who initiates the lawsuit) who has the burden of proving the case. If the plaintiff cannot prove that injury has occurred, liability does not exist. Damages for physical injury are easier to prove than for psychological injury. For example, it is harder to prove that a nurse verbally abused a client than to prove that a nurse injured a client's nerve while giving an intramuscular injection.

4. Causation—According to Hall (1996), "causation is [usually] established when it is proven that (1) the patient's injuries would not have occurred *but for* the nurse's failure to act as a reasonable prudent nurse; and (2) the nurse could *foresee* that failure to act in such a way would result in injury..." (p. 118).

Regarding point 1, if in your community-based nursing experience you fail to report obvious physical abuse of a minor child, you will have violated both the ethics and law of beneficence. Regarding point 2, if in your community-based nursing experience with a family over several visits you can foresee a pattern of abuse of a minor child but do nothing with your assessment, you will have violated both the ethics and law of beneficence.

Ethical and Legal Aspects of the Principle of Nonmaleficence

Definition and Code for Nurses

The principle of nonmaleficence historically has been associated with the phrase *primum non nocere*, which means, "Above all do no harm." In contemporary health-care ethics, the principle of nonmaleficence is often referred to simply as the "do no harm" principle. This principle is explicitly stated or implicitly implied in all the ethical theories described earlier (see Table 7–1).

Nonmaleficence, however, is different from beneficence. The former focuses on obligations not to harm others whereas the latter focuses on obligations to help others (Beauchamp & Childress, 1994). An example of the violation of the principle of nonmaleficence in community-based nursing is when a nurse (or her or his representative) does not turn a client and therefore causes bedsores, whereas an example of beneficence in community-based nursing is when a nurse promotes the client's welfare by teaching the client about diabetes. Usually your strongest obligation is to do no harm to the client, but when harms are minimal, beneficence may take priority. For example, when you give an antibiotic by intramuscular injection, you cause minor trauma (harm) to the skin, but the minor trauma is for the greater good of the client's well-being (prevention of infection).

The principle of nonmaleficence is noted in various parts of the ANA (1985) *Code for Nurses with Interpretive Statements.* The *Code* addresses the nurse's role in safeguarding the client's safety and health. If illegal, incompetent, or unethical practice is performed by a health-care institution or health-care provider, the nurse has an obligation to initiate appropriate professional action. The *Code* also addresses the institution's role in safeguarding the client's safety and health. The institution should have established processes in place to handle illegal, incompetent, or unethical practice, and the nurse has a responsibility to know about and act on the processes if needed.

Ethical and Legal Applications of the Principle of Nonmaleficence

The following discussion of the law's point of view on harming others, as well as legal and ethical safeguards to protect clients, is primarily based on and adapted from Hall (1996). To help you better understand the language of law as it relates to nonmaleficence, see Table 7–3.

The following are some viewpoints on the ethical and legal principle of doing no harm. Let's begin with an analysis of intentional torts. Intentional tort means a state of mind about the outcomes of a voluntary action or failure of action that involves both the desire for the outcomes (injury) to occur and the knowledge that the outcomes (injury) most likely will occur (Brent, 1997). As a nurse or student nurse, if you *did not intend* to injure your client (e.g., a medication you gave the client caused unexpected injury), you are neither liable under civil law nor ethically culpable. However, if you *did intend* to injure your client and *acted on this intent,* you are both legally and ethically culpable.

Here is an example. Suppose, as part of your community-based experience, you are assigned to care for a client who is suffering from biochemical depression of such magnitude that the client wants to commit suicide. You are an empathic nurse and you feel the client's pain and desperation. He tells you that over time he has accumulated a sufficient number of barbiturates to kill himself. He asks you to bring him the barbiturates *(which I know in reality you would not do, but you do here for the sake of the example),* and in your presence, he takes the pills and dies. Under these circumstances, your behavior is both unethical and illegal.

Table 7-3

Definitions of Important Legal Terms Related to the Principle of Nonmaleficence

TERMINOLOGY	DEFINITIONS
1. Breach of Contract	1. "When one party to a contract fails to perform, without a legal justification, any major promise or obligation under the contract" (Brent, 1997, p. 556).
2. Tort	2. "A civil wrong other than a breach of contract, where the law will provide a remedy by allowing the injured person to seek damages" (Brent, 1997, p. 565).
3. Defamation	3. "A tort which occurs when an individual's good name or reputation is damaged because of something that is written (libel) or said (slander) about the person that is untrue" (Brent, 1997, p. 558).
4. Assault	4. "This tort protects an individual's interest in the freedom from the apprehension of harmful or offensive contact. There is no requirement of an actual touching of the plaintiff; the intent to spur apprehension and the resultant fear that contact might occur in the victim satisfies this requirement" (Brent, 1997, p. 556).
5. Battery	5. "This tort protects an individual's interest in freedom from an affirmative, intentional, and unpermitted contact with his or her body, any extension of it (e.g., clothing), or anything that is attached to it and identified with it. Unlike assault, actual contact is essential" (Brent, 1997, p. 556).
6. False imprisonment	6. "Freedom from a restriction of one's choice of movement" (Brent, 1997, p. 559).
7. Negligence	7. "Conduct that falls below the standard established by law for the protection of others against unreasonable risk of harm" (Brent, 1997, p. 562).
8. Fraud	8. "Conduct involving an individual falsely representing a fact (by conduct, words, false or misleading allegations) or concealment of that which should have been disclosed to another person" (Brent, 1997, pp. 559–560).

Source: Brent, N. J. (1997). Nurses and the law: A guide to principles and applications. Philadelphia: Saunders.

Having discussed intentional torts in general, I now concentrate on three specific torts and their ethical and legal implications.

1. Assault—A simple legal definition of assault is "fear of immediate harm from a battery" (Hall, 1996, p. 167). (See Table 7–3 and point 2.) Assault deals with threats to do harm that are believable and believed by the client. Typically, assault and battery occur together. Your tone of voice and the language used are important here; they could make a difference between what is perceived as an immediate assault and what is not. Kind, gentle words do not constitute an assault; shouting and swearing place you in jeopardy. The nurse or student nurse who commits an assault is ethically wrong and legally culpable.

2. Battery—Battery is considered the most common intentional tort in health-care. A simple legal definition of battery is unwanted or harmful touching without the client's consent. Keep in mind that the contact made by touching does not have to be direct; battery can occur if, for example, unwanted equipment touches a patient who has not given consent for a procedure. As a nurse, you cannot force care on any client—whether in the hospital or in your community-based practice. Your best protection against battery is consent. Be sure that you always tell your clients what you are going to do to them that involves or affects their person. Be sure that they understand and give at least their verbal consent. One exception: There is usually implied consent for routine care for voluntary treatment; nevertheless, good nursing

practice entails informing clients of your intended care and assessing their consent to that care. The nurse or student nurse who commits battery is ethically wrong and legally culpable.

3. False imprisonment—As defined in Table 7–3, a simple legal definition of false imprisonment is "restriction of one's choice of movement..." (Brent, 1997, p. 559). What you need to remember is this: *You should not restrict the client's choice of movement without good reason!* Good reason means sound nursing, moral, and legal justification(s) for any restrictions. Also remember that clients who believe that they cannot leave a facility, for example, can sue for what they perceive to be false imprisonment. Competent patients legally are allowed to leave a hospital or community-based setting against a nurse's or doctor's advice. Competent discharged patients legally are allowed to leave a hospital or community-based setting without first paying their bills. To hold a patient in these situations constitutes false imprisonment. The nurse or student nurse who imposes false imprisonment is ethically wrong and legally culpable.

The best legal defense that nurses' clients have against assault, battery, false imprisonment, and other torts is *licensor.* Licensor enforces both the legal principles of nonmaleficence and "punishes failure to uphold the value of doing good, by seeking to assure that only capable people perform tasks that might harm" (Hall, 1996, p. 192). The power to license belongs to the states; a state can prohibit (by not licensing) any person who does not meet educational or other standards to practice in a certain profession or trade.

The best ethical defense that nurses' clients have against assault, battery, false imprisonment, and other torts or harms is the ANA (1985) *Code for Nurses with Interpretive Statements.* Provision 4 of the Code states that "The nurse assumes responsibility and accountability for individual nursing judgments and actions" (p. 7). The interpretive statements stress the ethical value that clients are entitled to nursing care of the highest quality and that the individual nursing licensor is the legal mechanism used to minimally enforce the ethical value. Beyond the minimum standards, nursing must regulate its own practice and, in addition, individual nurses must be accountable for their own practice. *Standards of Nursing Practice* also assist the nurse with this accountability. Therefore ultimately good patient care that supports the ethical and legal principle of nonmaleficence is in your hands.

Ethical and Legal Aspects of the Principle of Justice

Some examples of words for justice are *fairness, equitableness, entitlement,* or *rightfulness.* Simply stated, justice means giving individual persons or groups what is due them or what they can legitimately claim. What is due to individual persons or groups can be rewards, punishments, or burdens. If, for example, you performed your community-based nursing assignments well, you believe (or you should believe) that you deserve a "reward" such as positive feedback from your instructor and a good grade. However, if you did not show up for many of your community-based clinical assignments because of capricious reasons, you believe (or you should believe) that you deserve a "punishment" such as negative feedback from your instructor and a poor grade.

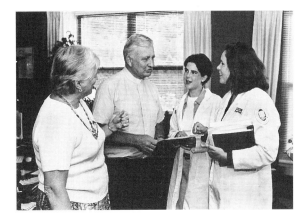

Types of Justice

In health care, one principle of justice that typically focuses on distribution is known as *distributive justice.* According to Davis and associates (1997),

> How we are to distribute burdens and benefits when not all will benefit from the required decisions [is an ethical matter]. Such decisions range from determining the number and kind of nursing home beds in a given geographic area to deciding who should get what levels of nursing care in a hospital that is downsizing or in a home care agency that provides care for people with a variety of health problems. (p. 53)

A second type of justice is known as *fairness.* According to Rawls (1971), "Injustice. . .is simply inequalities that are not to the benefit of all. . .while the distribution of wealth and income need not be equal, it must be to everyone's advantage" (p. 62). What is Rawls saying? He is saying that inequalities in a society are acceptable if everyone in that society benefits, including the least-advantaged members, such as the homeless or those with severely diminished physical or mental capacities. For example, if advantaged persons or groups in a community (including nurses and doctors) were given incentives to help disadvantaged persons or groups, both groups would benefit.

Keep in mind that the implications of both distributive justice and Rawls' concept of justice focus more on population-based assessments and policy development in public-health-based nursing practice rather than in community-based nursing practice. Nevertheless, it is important for you to begin to think about your community-based nursing practice within a broader societal context. Why? Because in your community-based nursing practice, you most likely will encounter individuals and families who are poor and who are severely physically or mentally handicapped. You also need to begin to ask yourself who will pay for their health care?

A third type of justice that can be applied to either public-health-based nursing practice or community-based nursing practice is known as the *material principles of justice.* The material principles of justice are concerned with only relevant moral characteristics that serve as a basis for deciding what is due a person or family. What are examples of relevant moral characteristics of justice that you might encounter in your community-based clinical experience? They could include client or family need, effort, or ability to pay, to name a few.

For example, if parents need insulin for a young child but cannot afford it, that meets the criterion of moral relevancy regarding what is due the child. However, if the same parents need (think they need) an exotic toy for the child, that need cannot be morally justified because it does not meet the criterion of moral relevancy regarding what is due the child.

Ethical and Legal Applications of the Principle of Justice

The following discussions of the law's point of view on justice, as well as legal and ethical applications to clients'

care, is primarily based on and adapted from Hall (1996). An important point that Hall stresses about justice is the tension that occurs between persons who highly value social justice (focus on groups) and persons who highly value autonomy (focus on individuals). What may be fair for the group (e.g., a community) may be unfair to the individual (e.g., one citizen) and visa versa. For example, if you are an elderly person who happens to live in a community largely composed of young couples with children, and your community decides to financially support a child-care center, you probably will not be happy about this decision because it provides no benefit to you.

Hall (1996) warns against "assuming that *all* laws are *fair*. . .merely because they are laws" (p. 301). Although that which is ethical usually also is legal (e.g., most would say informed consent), that which is legal may not always be ethical (e.g., some would say abortion). According to Silva and Kroeger-Mappes (1998):

> The conflict between ethical and illegal and unethical and legal will probably always be with us. Ethics cannot be bounded by the law when ethical considerations override legal ones. Law cannot be held hostage to ethics in the sense that a law cannot be enacted to control every immoral act. (p. 16)

What, then, are some specific applications related to ethics and law? Here are two such applications for you to consider.

1. The right to a decent minimum standard of health care. In the United States, the vast majority of poor people are either underinsured or uninsured and are unable to obtain access to health care. Others have sufficient wealth to pay for health insurance, but cannot obtain it because they are considered to be in poor health, to have too many preexisting conditions, or to engage in high health-risk lifestyles. Still others experience gaps in health insurance as they await new jobs. Beauchamp and Childress (1994) refer to these groups as the uninsured, the underinsured, the uninsurable, and the occasionally insured. And, of course, there are the fully insured. Think about yourself, your classmates, your friends, your clients, and other people you know. What categories do they fall into?

   Hall (1996), rather than focusing on a decent minimum of health care, discusses the economics of illness care law. She raises the following question, which I would like you to think about: Does a natural conflict exist between good economics (cost savings) and good client care? Certainly ethical, legal, and economics issues are all intertwined. However, regarding health care, the economic, ethical, and legal issues primarily focus on the availability of illness care. The effects of law and economics on illness care are primarily determined by demand (what health-care clients want), by supply (what resources are available, including the quality of nursing care), and by cost (what work and money are available to be spent for care). Keep in mind, however, that to mandate illness care as a legal entitlement profoundly affects economics and can result in the government providing health care. The operating ethical principle here is the material principle of justice of "to each person an equal share of health care." Would this be a just system?

2. The allocation of scarce health-care resources. Logically following from point 1, the right to a decent minimum of health care, is the allocation of scarce health-care resources. Whereas public-health-based nursing practice focuses on such topics as allocation decisions within all aspects of a societal budget and allocation decisions within a health and a health-care budget, community-based nursing practice focuses on the allocation of scarce health-care resources for the individual and family. For example, if you are responsible for the care of a client in his or her home who is receiving dialysis while waiting for a kidney transplant, you may question why this client is on a waiting list as opposed to another client.

This brings us to another question: What ethically relevant criteria might be used in determining the distribution of scarce organs? Some criteria that have been identified include a client's age, ability to pay, lifestyle, health, donor to recipient match, past contribution to society, future contribution to society, likelihood of successful outcome of the procedure, willingness to comply with the medical regimen required after receiving a scarce organ, social-family structure, and lottery. Which of these criteria can be morally justified? Why?

Consider Sally's story.

I was assigned to assess two male clients in the community, who were both receiving dialysis and awaiting a kidney transplant. After my assessment, I thought both were in equal need of the transplant. They were both in their 50s, their health status was similar, they both were married and had good family support systems. Neither of them smoked or drank. Well, when I went to visit Mr. HB, he was so excited because his doctor had told him he was next on the list to receive a kidney. I was happy for Mr. HB, but it got me to thinking about why Mr. HB selected over Mr. WC. Then I started to get upset and then angry because the only difference I could see between the two clients was that Mr. HB was "upper middle class" and had good health insurance and Mr. WC was poor and had no health insurance.

Box 7–17 gives you the opportunity to apply the distribution of scarce resources to the above situation.

Box 7-17   Student Learning Activity

Distribution of Scarce Resources

Do you think Sally was justified in being upset in this situation? If so, why? If not, why not?

What if one of your loved ones needed a kidney transplant? What criteria would you consider to be morally relevant and why?

Ethical/Legal Decision-making Frameworks

Many examples of ethical frameworks exist in the nursing literature. Familiarize yourself with several of them so that eventually you will be able to internalize a framework that will work best for you. This process should not be difficult because most ethical frameworks follow the steps of the nursing process. Although fewer frameworks exist that combine both ethics and law on an equal footing, usually something about law is incorporated into ethical frameworks and something about ethics is incorporated into legal frameworks.

Criteria and Frameworks

Regardless of the framework used, there are criteria that will help you to assess that the framework is valid (Silva, 1990).

1. Adequacy: The framework addresses content relevant to ethics, law, professional codes, and legal statutes.
2. Consistency: Use of the framework on different occasions yields similar outcomes in similar situations.
3. Coherence: The framework is logical and internally consistent.
4. Comprehensiveness: The framework can offer guidance in a variety of ethical and legal issues.
5. Practicality: The framework works well to resolve everyday ethical and legal issues in practice. (p. 110)

Here are two articles in the nursing literature that help to think through ethical and legal decision making. The first article, by Aroskar (1998), discusses a community-based nursing situation in regard to the rights of a mentally impaired elderly client versus the rights of the community when the two are in conflict. The second article (Chally & Loriz, 1998) focuses on a six-step process for ethical decision making applied to three cases in a hospital setting. One case demonstrates a conflict between autonomy and beneficence; a second case focuses on justice; and the third case focuses on truth telling. What were the outcomes of these interesting cases? I leave that question to your curiosity; try to locate and read these two articles.

Now we work through an ethical and legal framework. I have added some comments and questions under each step for your consideration. The framework has the following five steps.

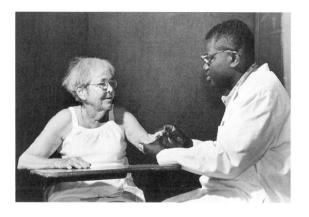

1. Collect and assess data. This is a critical part of the decision-making process because incomplete or erroneous data can lead to the wrong ethical or legal decision. You most likely will need data about the client's presenting problems that led to the ethical or legal dilemma, about family members' thoughts and feelings related to the dilemma, about roles and responsibilities of appropriate team members, about the mission and philosophy of the organizations or communities involved, and about any other relevant facts.

2. Identify ethical and legal issues. You need to be "on your toes" here because step 2 can be tricky. First, you need to sort through your data to make sure that you are indeed dealing with an ethical or legal dilemma and not another aspect of nursing care such as a communication breakdown not related to either ethics or law. Once you have settled this matter, you need to become clear on the exact ethical or legal dilemma. Is it a conflict between two or more ethical theories? Is it a conflict between ethical principles? Is it a conflict within a given ethical theory or principle? What about the situation makes it an ethical dilemma? What about the situation makes it a legal dilemma or a combination of both?

3. Consider actions based on ethics, laws, codes, statutes, and so forth. This is the step that may be new to you. You have learned much about certain aspects of nursing so far, but you may not have explored ethical theories, principles, laws, codes, statutes, and other relevant ethical or legal content. This type of content (all prior chapter content) is essential to your decision making because it constitutes the necessary knowledge base to make the right (morally defensible) ethical and legal decision(s). You need both a decision-making process *and* ethical and legal knowledge to make the right decision. Based on this knowledge, you can then determine various morally defensible options that you (or the health-care team) can take.

4. Take action. Although this step sounds straightforward, it may be difficult.

   Remember, you are trying to take the best action when an ethical dilemma exists, so you may feel torn about taking the action, although it is morally justified. At times you may have to take action when all options are ethically troubling. Under such circumstances, you have to take the action that is the most ethical, even if it is not easy. You are not obligated to take an action if it genuinely violates your conscience, but you cannot, under any circumstance, abandon your client. If you do so, there are both ethical and legal consequences to face.

5. Evaluate and document action(s) and outcomes. Once the action has been taken, it must be evaluated. Did the

action turn out as expected or did it backfire in some way? How has each person involved in the action responded? Planning an action and doing it, even if morally justified, are very different. Does the client, client's family, or any member of the health-care team, including yourself, need psychological support because of the action taken? Has the action(s) taken and the outcome been documented appropriately?

Research in Ethical and Legal Considerations for Community-based Nursing Practice

This chapter has provided several examples of research related to ethical and legal considerations that you may want to consider in your practice. You will also want to become familiar with the nine provisions of a new Code of Ethics for Nursing that were approved by the ANA House of Delegates in June 2001 (New Code of Ethics, 2001). In addition, a few additional articles are provided here to stimulate your thinking about research in this area.

Earlier in this chapter you were introduced to the concept of moral distress. Wurzbach (1996) studied the relationship between comfort as a concept and 15 RN's decisions about moral choices. For those RNs who felt uncomfortable (usually associated with decision-making uncertainty), Wurzbach used the term *moral discomfort* rather than *moral distress*. Nevertheless, nurses both in this study and a previous study conducted by Wurzbach described two areas of moral discomfort. One area related to the nurses' attempts to influence a client or family decision. The second area related to the phenomenon of the nurses "looking back" years later and still feeling uncertain about whether they had made the right moral choices. These feelings were accompanied by anger, sleeping difficulties, and lack of inner peace.

One study (Joudrey & Gough, 1999) explored how student nurses construct ethical values pertaining to their professional field. The setting for the research was a community college in central Alberta, Canada. A questionnaire containing 10 questions was used to provide qualitative data for the nonrandom sample of 110 students in the second year of their program. Data were collected over a 2-year period. Seventy-three students responded; all but four of these were female. Content analysis was used to analyze the data, and responses were compared and coded to identify common themes. The themes that emerged were centered on the caring ethic versus the curing ethic. The researchers used the following quote from one of the respondents to indicate the major finding of their study: "Nurses care and doctors cure." Many of the respondents saw the curing ethic of physicians associated with a narrow focus on the technical, medical aspects of patients, whereas the caring ethic of nurses was related to a more holistic approach to their patients. The second perceived contrast between caring and curing characterized nursing as focused on advocacy for patients, whereas physicians were characterized as motivated by other goals. One respondent summarized this view: "Nurses help to support persons with whatever decisions they make, where doctors at all cost want to preserve life." Although this was a small study, indicating the need for further research in this area, it is interesting that the researchers believed that they were able to identify clear distinctions between nurses and physicians.

Box 7–18 allows you to explore this research in more detail.

Box 7-18   Student Learning Exercise

Learning Ethical Values

The study described (Joudrey & Gough, 1999) is available online through several databases that feature full text. Locate the article to read it in more detail. Think about why the students may have seen such a contrast between ethical values of nurses and physicians. Was this value communicated to them through their education process? Was it a way of making the nursing students feel more professional? Write some of your ideas here about the meaning of this study.

Revisiting an Ethical Dilemma

I have now come full circle and want you to take another look at the situation with which this chapter began. I will discuss it within the five-step framework, previously discussed, as well as share some personal experiences. Here, again, is the beginning nursing student's story.

 I always wanted to be a nurse. I think it was because my mother was one. She often talked to me about her experiences and how rewarding it was to help other people. Well, when I was assigned to my first community-based nursing clinical, I was to teach a wife who was caring for her dying husband about how to change his dressing. That didn't bother me because I was well prepared to do a dressing change, but, you know, I had never been around a dying patient. He was so thin and he was coughing a lot. He had radiation treatments for cancer of the stomach and was in terrible pain. I felt so sorry for him. His wife told me that, because of the pain, she was giving him double the pain-relieving medication from what the doctor had ordered. I was so scared, because I didn't know what to say or what to do. I went to the home to change a dressing, which I did, but I didn't know what to do about the other unexpected problem. I was afraid the wife would get into trouble with the doctor or the law if someone found out about the medication, and I didn't know whether what she was doing was ethical. I wanted to get out of there, but I didn't. My mother made it all sound so easy, but sometimes it's not!

Nursing Student

Box 7–19 allows you to explore the ethical dilemma above.

1. Collect and assess data. This story is adapted from my own first clinical experience in a hospital. The task I was assigned sounded easy: feed a patient. But the patient was dying (and I had never seen a dying patient), was in an oxygen tent, and was only partially conscious. The patient even had trouble taking liquids. I was frightened the patient would choke or, even worse, that I might somehow kill the patient. I was so traumatized by this first clinical assignment that I almost left nursing.

   The student in the preceding situation, like myself, was taught a skill with which she felt comfortable, but she was unprepared to deal with the other situational factors for a first clinical experience. The point is that the student's instructor should have collected

| Box 7-19 | Student Learning Activity |

Ethical Dilemma

If you were the student nurse in the preceding situation, what would you have done and why?

What are your thoughts on mercy killing? Discuss with your classmates.

Why is the differentiation of the nurse as a professional versus a private citizen so important?

and analyzed the data about the patient's situation to determine its appropriateness before placing a beginning nursing student into the situation.

Because the student was afraid and seemingly overwhelmed, her ability to collect and assess data was impaired. Also, her lack of knowledge about ethical and legal nursing dilemmas impeded her ability to know what questions to ask to collect and assess data about the potential ethical and legal dilemma. Examples of data collection and assessment questions might have been: (a) What was the cause of the client's cough? Was the cough increasing the client's pain? If so, was there medication ordered to control the cough? (b) Why was the pain management so ineffective? Did the wife talk to the doctor about this problem? What pain-relieving medication was the client receiving? What was the anticipated outcome of doubling the dosage of that medication? (c) What was the client's state of mind? What was his wife's state of mind? Did her husband know that she was giving him double the prescribed dose? When did the wife last talk to the doctor about the medication? And so forth. The point to be made here is the critical importance of seeking factual information before identifying whether or not an ethical or legal issue exists.

2. Identify ethical and legal issues. Part of the reason the student was so scared was that she knew that she was unable to identify ethical and legal issues. Most likely the reason for this lapse was that she had not yet received content related to these types of issues in her nursing courses. To compound the issue, the student had run into a type of ethical and legal issue that was more complex, because different morally and legally justified opinions exist. An ethical issue concerned whether the wife was violating the ethical principle of nonmaleficence (do no harm) by giving her husband twice the prescribed dosage of medication. A legal issue was whether the wife was breaking the law by giving her husband twice the prescribed dose of medication.

3. Consider actions based on ethics, law, codes, statutes, and so forth. Possible morally and legally justified actions the student nurse could have considered include one or more of the following:

   • Consult with her instructor.
   • Collect more data from the client, the client's wife, the client's record, and so forth.
   • Determine if the doctor and the client knew what the wife was doing.
   • Talk to the wife about what she was doing and why.
   • Determine if the wife was informed about various alternative methods to decrease pain and, if not, inform her of such.
   • If she had not done so, encourage the wife to discuss the medication issue with the doctor.
   • Spend time listening to the client.
   • Make sure the client was as physically comfortable as possible.
   • Seek out community resources (with wife's permission) that could help the wife cope better with her husband's illness and dying.

4. Take action. Regarding ethics, was the principle of nonmaleficence violated? If the wife's motive was only to relieve her dying husband's suffering, her action most likely could be morally justified if consequence-based thinking was used, but not if duty-based thinking was used. If her motive was to kill him because she could not stand to see him suffer anymore and he was unaware of her plan, her action most likely could not be morally justified (especially if all other reasonable options had not been tried). From a legal point of view, verdicts vary depending on the situation. Some juries would not find the wife guilty of murder by reason of tempo-

rary insanity even if killing him were her motive. The basis for these juries' decisions was that the wife's motive was mercy.

If the person who was giving the double dose of medication was a nurse or a student nurse, the motive was to kill the client, and the client died, she or he would be legally culpable for violating the doctor's order and for murder. The nurse would be morally culpable also for violating the ANA's (1985) *Code for Nurses with Interpretive Statements,* which states that "the nurse does not act deliberately to terminate the life of any person" (p. 3). Keep in mind, however, that the ANA (1985) *Code* also states that "the nurse may provide interventions to relieve symptoms in the dying client even when the interventions entail substantial risks of hastening death" (p. 4). Whether the wife or a nurse, motive is an important consideration. However, the nurse must remember that while rendering client care she or he is acting in a professional role and not as a private citizen coping with the same problem with a family member.

5. Evaluate outcomes and document actions taken. Outcomes could be:

   • Medication killed client
   • Medication relieved client's pain but did not kill him

   Whatever the outcome, the nurse must document it.

SUMMARY

Community-based nursing practice may raise unique ethical dilemmas for nurses. Often, the nurse interacts with clients in their homes or in a community setting where the usual support systems to aid in decision making may be absent. It is important to think about the ethical and legal situations you may encounter as you care for clients in the community. Think about how you would define the various terms in this chapter. Discuss with others how you might apply different ethical theories, ethical and legal principles, and ethical and legal decision-making frameworks provided in this chapter. It is also important to stay current with research addressing ethical and legal problems in community-based practice. With thoughtful attention to these ethical and legal concerns, you can be an effective advocate for your clients in the community.

Active Learning Strategies

1. In the community-based setting where you are practic-ing, do you know what your ethical and legal obligations are if a client should die? Do you know if your client has a living will? A durable power of attorney for health-care decisions? Where are they located? Write the answers to these questions and share them with your clinical group. If you do not know any of the answers to these questions, find them.

2. Make a list of the three types of justice that you have en-countered in a community-based setting. Compare your list with a classmate.

3. Reflect on justice as a moral concept. What thoughts come to mind?

4. What types of health-care coverage, if any, do your community-based clients have? How do the economic laws of demand, supply, and cost affect your clients' health-care coverage? What ethical principles of justice apply to your clients' health-care coverage?

References

American Hospital Association. (1970). Statement on a pa-tient's bill of rights. Chicago, IL: Author.

American Nurses' Association. (1985). Code for nurses with in-terpretive statements. Kansas City, MO: Author.

Aroskar, M. A. (1998). Administrative ethics: Perspectives on pa-tients and community-based care. Online Journal of Issues in Nursing. Available at http://www.nursingworld.org/ojin/topic8/topic8_4.htm

Beauchamp, T. L., & Childress, J. F. (1994). Principles of bio-medical ethics (4th ed.). New York: Oxford.

Brent, N. J. (1997). Nurses and the law: A guide to principles and applications. Philadelphia: Saunders.

Chafey, K., Rhea, M., Shannon, A. M., & Spencer, S. (1998). Characterizations of advocacy by practicing nurses. Journal of Professional Nursing, 14, 43–52.

Chally, P. S., & Loriz, L. (1998). Ethics in the trenches: Decision making in practice. American Journal of Nursing, 98(6), 17–20.

Davis, A. J., Aroskar, M. A., Liaschenko, J., & Drought, T. S. (1997). Ethical dilemmas and nursing practice. Stamford, CT: Appleton & Lange.

Hall, J. K. (1996). Nursing ethics and law. Philadelphia: Saunders.

International Council of Nurses. (1973). Code for nurses: Ethi-cal concepts applied to nursing. Geneva: Author.

Joudrey, R., & Gough, J. (1999). Caring and curing revisited: Student nurses' perceptions of nurses' and physicians' ethical stances. Journal of Advanced Nursing, 29(5), 1154–1162.

Juethong, W. (1998, Summer). Thai baccalaureate nursing stu-dents' caring and uncaring lived experiences with Thai nursing instructors. Unpublished doctoral dissertation, George Mason University, Fairfax, VA.

Kant, I. (1981). Grounding for the metaphysics of morals (J. W. Ellington, Trans.). Indianapolis: Hackett. (Original work pub-lished in German in 1785.)

Ludwick, R., & Sedlak, C. A. (1998). Ethical issues and critical thinking: Students stories. Nursing Connections, 11(3), 12–18.

New Code of Ethics. (2001). Nine provisions of a new Code of Ethics for Nursing. (www.ana.org/ethics/chcode.htm)

Powell, R. M. C. (1997, Fall). Lived experiences of moral distress among staff nurses. Unpublished doctoral dissertation, George Mason University, Fairfax, VA.

Rawls, J. (1971). A theory of justice. Cambridge, MA: Belknap Press of Harvard University Press.

Silva, M. C. (1990). Ethical decision making in nursing adminis-tration. Norwalk, CT: Appleton & Lange.

Silva, M. C., & Kroeger-Mappes, J. (1998). Ethical frameworks into the 21st century. In J. Dienemann (Ed.), Nursing adminis-tration: Managing patient care (2nd ed., pp. 3–22). Stamford, CT: Appleton & Lange.

Weston, A. (1997). A practical companion to ethics. New York: Oxford University Press.

Wurzbach, M. E. (1996). Comfort and nurses' moral choices. Journal of Advanced Nursing, 24, 260–264.

Zotti, M. E., Brown, P., & Stotts, R. C. (1996). Community-based nursing versus community health nursing: What does it all mean? Nursing Outlook, 44, 211–217.

8

Differentiating Nurses' Scope of Practice in the Community

Joyce Hahn

LEARNING OBJECTIVES

1) Differentiate the roles of health professionals involved in community-based practice.

2) Discuss how the nurse's role within the collaborative process benefits the patient and family.

3) Identify the components of the nurse's role in the community nurse organization.

4) Examine the significance of research and the nurse's role in community-based practice.

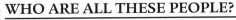
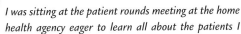

WHO ARE ALL THESE PEOPLE?

I was sitting at the patient rounds meeting at the home health agency eager to learn all about the patients I would be visiting. I heard the "team leader" talk about the first patient. This going to be exciting to learn about the patient before the home visit. But then she asked the "case manager" to lead the report. This first patient was an elderly woman with a hospital discharge diagnosis of "CVA." I tried to recall all I had ever heard and learned about stroke patients. As I listened, I heard reference to the "PT," "OT," "ST," and the "dietitian" involved in the case. It was suggested that the "MSW" speak with the County Social Worker.

The second patient was experiencing confusion and now the plan of care would include a "patient sitter" and a "nurses' aide." The remainder of the patient rounds continued with a repeat of similar initials. They almost sounded like alphabet soup as I struggled to keep up with all the abbreviations in my notes.

Who are all these people? Are they health-care professionals? Who requests their services? Do you ask the patient first? Is there a fee for the patient to pay to see these people? Do these professionals go to the patient's home or does the patient go to them? I was very confused.

Excerpt from a nursing student's journal

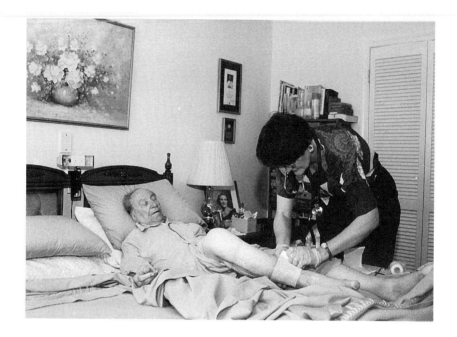

In the community-based practice setting, the student nurse comes into contact with many different providers of health care. Together, these health-care professionals from several different disciplines work toward one common goal: the goal of holistic health care, to treat the patient as a whole in a combined effort to restore optimal health and to promote wellness. This holistic practice considers the physical, emotional, social, economic, and spiritual needs of the patient. Together all these health professionals are referred to as the health-care team. A health-care team can consist of one or more of the following professionals: nurses, advanced practice nurses, case managers, nurse aides, physicians, physician assistants, dentists, social workers, dietitians, respiratory therapists, physical therapists, occupational health therapists, speech therapists, chaplains, and at times, alternative care providers. The types and numbers of available members of a health-care team depends on the size, location, and purpose of the specific community-based organization.

This chapter identifies and explores the roles of the health-care team and the nurses' collaborative interaction within this team. As secondary and tertiary care and prevention moves into the community, it is the nurse who is becoming the coordinator and patient advocate for accessing available services for clients. Understanding the roles of all the health-care providers available within community-based practice will clarify how the collaboration and coordination of care occur. Box 8–1 allows you to expand your knowledge of the healthcare team.

Box 8-1	Student Learning Activity

Health Care Team

List three members of the health-care team you might encounter in a community-based practice organization.

What is the common goal of the health team?

HOW CAN NURSING HISTORY RELATE TO TODAY?

What does Florence Nightingale and her work, "Notes on Nursing: What It Is and What It Is Not," have to do with community-based nursing in the 21st century? And what about Clara Barton and Lillian Wald, can their work in the 1800s really have anything to do with working in the community today? What is all this nursing theory and philosophy about? How can I be expected to understand and use it?

Questions from a student nurse

THE PAST IS THE PRESENT

The questions asked by this student nurse are relevant to developing an understanding and working knowledge of community-based nursing practice. Historically in the United States, nursing began as community-based nursing. Florence Nightingale is well known for " Notes on Nursing: What It Is and What It Is Not," published in the 1850s. This sentinel work addressed the difference between "health nursing" and "sick nursing" (Buchholtz & Klainberg, 1998). Nightingale's definition of health nursing spoke to nursing care outside of the hospital walls aimed at keeping healthy persons free of disease. Doesn't this sound a lot like the preventive medicine model of today? Her sick nursing definition was directed at persons with disease and nursing efforts to restore health. Doesn't this sound familiar as well?

The work of Clara Barton is well documented for her Civil War efforts working in the battlefields with soldiers. Clara worked to protect her soldiers from the rampant communicable diseases that existed in the battlefields and the camps. Her work can certainly be visualized as outside hospital walls and "in the community." Clara's work led to the founding of the American Red Cross, a non-profit agency that to this day aids victims of disaster. And yes, nurses work at this agency and have outreach into the community.

Lillian Wald was an outspoken activist in the late 1800s who is credited with being the first "home-care nurse." Her privileged societal position allowed her to be heard as the champion of patient health rights in her time. Her New York City district nursing model bears a striking similarity to nursing work still practiced in the community. Lillian Wald's model is the cornerstone of the community nurse organization model of the 1990s. She developed what we now call case management.

These bright and motivated change agents, our nursing role models of the past, laid the foundation for community-based nursing practice. What we now examine is how far from these original models we have progressed as nurses in the community. You will see a striking resemblance to these women as you work in the community. You will find that the energy, dedication, and outspoken activism for patient rights are alive today in the modern community nurse. Look for it and become a part of this energy. It's worth it.

Box 8–2 will help you identify the contributions of past nursing leaders.

Box 8-2   Student Learning Activity

Nursing Leaders

List three nursing leaders of the past.

List their contributions to community health.

MODERN COMMUNITY-BASED NURSING PRACTICE

The role of the nurse in community-based practice evolves and changes based on the needs of the community and the health-care environment. Today's nurse may indeed visit patients in their homes, wellness clinics, community centers, schools, occupational health settings, ambulatory care settings, long-term care facilities, day-care centers, hospice centers, crisis centers, or just about anywhere the need arises. The community may be urban, suburban, or rural. The role of the nurse varies with the needs of the client. The nurse's practice will be collaborative, and this collaboration will depend on the resources available to be part of the health team.

Health-care Team Members and Roles

The health-care team or health professionals come from different disciplines and use their collaborative skills to treat the patient as a whole and work toward the common goal of wellness. Which health-care professional is part of this team depends on patient needs, availability of resources, and the patient's participation in a plan of care.

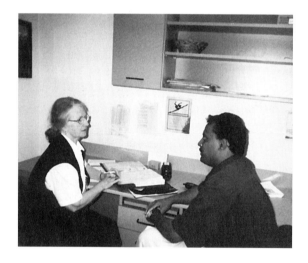

Registered Nurse

The registered nurse (RN) is the primary health provider for the patient. This role is dynamic and changes with the patient's needs. Within this role are multiple responsibilities, which include care provider, educator and counselor, role model, patient advocate, case manager, collaborator, discharge planner, case finder, change agent, and leader (Helvie, 1997).

As a **care provider,** this role includes assessing, planning, implementing, and evaluating care for the patient

and family. In the role of **educator and counselor,** the nurse provides the patient with the information and knowledge to make wise choices. This education may extend to the family and community. The nurse in the community serves as a **role model** for other health professionals in the community. Positive, caring, calm, and purposeful nursing actions gain the respect and trust that is the basis for care. The **patient advocate** role is an exciting community role. Traditionally the nurse (think back to Florence, Clara, and Lillian) has been at the forefront of health change. The nurse may be an advocate on a family level, on a community level, or even on a national political level. In the role of advocate, the nurse may help the clients obtain the skills necessary to advocate for themselves. The **case manager** role incorporates a health care delivery process that aims to provide quality health care and decrease fragmentation with a cost-effective approach. The nurse uses the nursing process to assess the patient's needs and coordinate the activities of the health-care team to achieve these needs in a financially responsible manner. As a **collaborator,** the nurse interacts with the patient and the health-care team to best meet the patient's need. This may be within the patient's own family or within the community. The **discharge planner** role is twofold. First, there is planning for the hospital discharge. This involves identifying the immediate needs of the patient, including durable medical equipment necessary in the home (e.g., wheelchair, commode, crutches, etc.). This role includes identification of community resources available to this patient such as meals-on-wheels, home-health services, part-time homemaker services, volunteers, and religious support. At some point in the outpatient community setting the patient may be discharged from the services of the agency or support group with whom the case manger is affiliated. In this case, arrangements need to be made to transfer care or prepare the patient and family for self-care and continued wellness. The **case finder** role involves identifying and finding the patients who meet the agency protocols for health-care intervention. The nurse as a **change agent** and **leader** is another dynamic role. To bring about the change necessary, the nurse must influence behavior in a positive way. This might mean dietary teaching to diabetics or wellness classes in health clinics. Box 8–3 focuses on nursing roles.

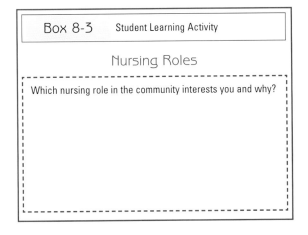

Box 8-3   Student Learning Activity

Nursing Roles

Which nursing role in the community interests you and why?

So Many Different Titles

"I want to understand what nurses do in the community but there are so many titles. How do I know who does what and when?"

Registered nurses in the community can be as specialized and educated as the nurses working in the acute-care hospital setting. Many specialized nurses are certified in their specialty area and hold advanced degrees. The availability of nurses with special skills depends on the community setting and the patient population served by the particular agency. The titles often define the specialty practice. For example, the **gerontological nurse** works with the elderly, and the **oncology nurse** works with patients diagnosed with cancer. **Maternal** and **child health nurses** follow patients at home or in a clinic during and after pregnancy. The **child health consultant** works as a facilitator in child-care centers and links professional health-care programs and services with the agency or program where the child is enrolled. The **wound care** and **ostomy nurse** works with the patient population with ostomies and wounds needing care outside the hospital setting. The **infusion therapy nurse** follows the patient population with intravenous (IV) therapies needed outside the acute-care setting. The **hospice nurse** is involved with patients in a hospice center or a patient's home working with the patient and the family to deal with terminal illness. **Psychiatric** and **mental health nurses** are found in

clinics, home health and mental health agencies, and long-term care facilities. A **parish** or **religious nurse** works with patients within a specific religious community. The **case manager** (sometimes called a **team leader**) may be a nurse who is working for an insurance company, hospital, outpatient facility, or agency to coordinate the care of multiple disciplines and services for the patient. The **home-health nurse** visits patients in their homes. **Occupational health nurses** follow patients within their workplace. Counties and cities often have **public health nurses** working in a department of health for wellness counseling and immunization follow-up as well as tracking communicable illness. **School nurses** care for children in educational settings who may have acute, chronic, or emergency health needs. All these nurses may be known as generalists (having an undergraduate degree) or Clinical Nurse Specialists (CNSs) or Nurse Practitioners (NPs) (both have earned graduate degrees and specialty certification). Together, this broad spectrum of nursing practice can be called Community Health Nursing. Box 8–4 contains an exercise on using resources.

Box 8-4   Student Learning Activity

Using Resources

You are a director of a child-care center and not a health professional. Several infants in your center have diarrhea. One infant's mother has just received a call from the pediatrician. Her infant has been diagnosed with giardiasis, a communicable disease. Which community nursing resource would you call and why?

Licensed Practical Nurse

The licensed practical nurse (LPN) or licensed vocational nurse (LVN) has limited educational training and works directly under the supervision of a registered nurse. Tasks performed by an LPN or LVN are subject to state and local agency regulations.

Nurses' Aide or Clinical Technician

This unlicensed member of the health-care team provides care related to daily hygiene. This includes giving a bed bath or assisting with a shower, changing linen, providing mouth care, shaving, and basic ambulation such as from the bed to the bathroom or to a chair. A nurses' aide works under the supervision of a registered nurse in community clinics or in home-health settings. Nurses' aides have vocational training provided from their employer or technical institutes. Individual states offer certification exams on completion of basic education modules.

Patient Sitter

This is another unlicensed member of the health-care team. The role of this person is to stay with the patient to provide for safety. A patient sitter might be necessary for a confused patient or a patient suspected of inflicting harm to himself or herself. This health-care team member works under the supervision of a registered nurse.

Social Worker

Also known as a licensed medical social worker (LMSW), the social worker provides counseling for major life crises to include terminal illness and family problems. A social worker is a master's prepared practitioner who assists in locating appropriate community resources, which might include obtaining equipment such as a wheelchair, helping to find volunteers, or arranging for transportation to clinics or physician offices. Social workers are a valuable resource in finding financial resources to cover medical costs (Christensen & Kockrow, 1994).

Respiratory Therapist

A respiratory therapist is trained in the therapeutic measures necessary for the care of patients with respiratory problems. There are two levels of respiratory care practitioners: the Certified Respiratory Therapist (CRT) and the Registered Respiratory Therapist (RRT). A respiratory technician completes a 12-month college study program and is then eligible to take a credentialing exam to become a CRT. Respiratory therapists are required to complete either a two-year associate degree or a four-year bachelor's program and are eligible to take a national certification exam. The credentials of RRT are awarded after successful completion of the credentialing exam. A respiratory therapist is knowledgeable about all oxygen therapy devices, including artificial mechanical ventilators and accessory devices used in inhalation therapy. Respiratory therapists administer many tests of pulmonary function necessary to follow a patient's respiratory progress (Kozier, Erb, Berman, & Burke, 2000).

Physical Therapist

The physical therapist (PT) assesses and treats patients with musculoskeletal problems. The physical therapist evaluates safety in the home and works with the patient and family to establish safe ambulation patterns when using assistive devices (walkers, canes, or wheelchairs). The goal is to restore optimal muscle function or to prevent further disability.

Occupational Therapist

The occupational therapist (OT) works with the physically challenged patient to obtain optimum functioning in the activities of daily living (ADLs). Specially fitting devices and strategies are used to perform these skills.

Speech Therapist

The speech therapist (ST) is trained to help hearing-impaired patients speak more clearly, to assist clients who have had strokes to relearn how to speak, and to work with children and adults to modify speech patterns and disturbances. Speech therapists also help diagnose and treat swallowing problems in patients who have had a head injury or a stroke (Taylor, Lillis, & LeMone, 1997).

Dietician

The registered dietitian (RD) works with patients to adapt specialized diets for the patient's individualized needs. The dietitian is knowledgeable about nutrient and food requirements necessary for therapeutic healing.

Pharmacist

The registered pharmacist (RPh) is responsible for dispensing patients' medication and keeping track of all the medications prescribed by various physicians. This role also includes the responsibility of informing the physician and other members of the health-care team when drug or food interactions are likely to occur.

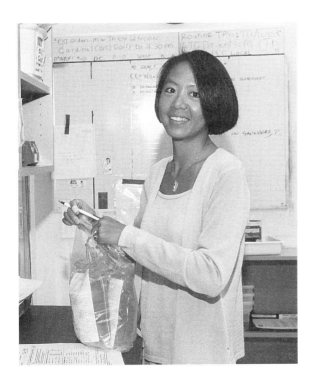

All these members of the health-care team work under the direction of the patient's physician. Together they work collaboratively to provide a total care package of holistic health for the patient in the community. Box 8–5 will help you review health-care team members.

Box 8-5	Student Learning Activity

Health Team Definitions

Return to the first story "Who are all these people?" Review the initials and define the members of the health-care team mentioned.

EXPANDING OPPORTUNITIES AND ROLES

Thinking back to my student nurse days, I never dreamed I would find myself in a community setting. Our education was based on the medical model of the hospital and the "nursing tasks" each patient needed. Of course, we knew about clinics in the city hospitals for the indigent patients but not for the "real patients" because they came to the hospital. Patients were admitted with diagnoses of "fatigue," "urinary tract infections," and to give families "a break" from caring for their elderly family members. A usual stay for any patient was certainly a week or more. Times have changed and so have the nursing opportunities to reach out and touch our patients. Community-based nursing practice allows nurses to make a difference in their patients' lives, not only during an acute episode, but also on a daily basis. This is what nursing and caring is really about.

Innovation and putting the patient first has always been the way of nursing. If you want to talk about innovation just look at Community Nursing Organizations (CNO). The American Nurses' Association (ANA) has supported a demonstration project of community and home health-care services for Medicare beneficiaries since 1992. This innovative idea for nurses to case manage with strong emphasis on prevention and education was really ahead of its time. These Community Nursing Organizations still exist today and are effectively providing good-quality patient care and meeting the government's capitation needs. Nursing is about changes resulting in better patient care and outcomes. I can only imagine what today's student nurses will achieve in their careers. My advice is look to the community. The community is where you will find the growth and satisfaction in our nursing future.

Thoughts from a Community Health Nurse

COMMUNITY NURSING ORGANIZATIONS

The CNO demonstration model was designed to provide community nursing and home health-care services for Medicare beneficiaries and was initiated through the 1987 Omnibus Budget Reconciliation Act. The CNO model features a nursing care delivery model with the core components of managed care. The two basic elements of the CNO are nurse case management and partial capitation payments. This CNO model was intended to promote timely and appropriate health-care services with a strong emphasis on prevention and health education. The CNOs combine the benefits to the patient of individual preventive and chronic care with the positive aspect of managed care financing for the Medicare system. Four CNO sites implemented the demonstration projects in Arizona, Illinois, Minnesota, and New York in 1992 (ANA, 1999).

The CNOs were originally planned more than a decade ago with the goal of taking the patient back into the community and to provide for the needs of the patients at a lower cost. The patients are positive in their response to the CNO experience. Some of the enrollees have described it as an extra insurance policy. The patients continually identify that the nurses' listening skills, clinical knowledge, ability to support patients in decisions, and providing information and clinical monitoring are highly valued (Burtt, 1998). There are three other CNOs—the Healthy Seniors Program of Carondelet Health Network in Arizona, the Healthy Seniors Project at the Living at Home Block Nurse Program in Minnesota, and the Carle Clinic Association CNO in Illinois. All of these programs provide a package of Medicare benefits to include skilled nursing care, home-health aides, social work, physical therapy, speech therapy, occupational therapy, durable medical equipment, ambulance services, and outpatient therapies. The models are all reimbursed on a capitated pay-

ment plan. This plan sets a fee per patient based on the variables of the patient's age, sex, previous home-care use, and functional status (Burtt, 1998).

All the CNOs focus on health promotion and disease prevention and do individualize services to meet the needs of the patients. Recent additions to the New York CNO site include alternative and complementary therapies such as therapeutic touch, biofeedback, and visualization therapy to promote comfort. Advance practice nurses deliver all these modalities. The Arizona-based CNO offers a variety of holistic services as well, ranging from herbal remedies to t'ai chi (Burtt, 1998). The RNs in the CNOs have the opportunity to reach out and treat the patients as a whole in an effort to restore optimal health and promote wellness.

Case management (a revival of the Lillian Wald approach to care) is the centerpiece of the CNO model. The case management responsibility lies within the nurse consultant's role at the CNO. This case management role is intended to integrate, coordinate, and advocate for patients, families, and groups needing extensive services. The coordination of care is the basic component of case management. Within the CNO, the nurse consultant actively coordinates the health-care needs of the members and has the authority to authorize the CNO services available, including preventive care and education. The nurse consultant brings the personal touch to an otherwise impersonal system (Storfjell, Lloyd, Mitchell, & Daly-McCormack, 1994).

The Health Care Financing Administration's (HCFA) Program of All-Inclusive Care for the Elderly (PACE) and the Social Health Maintenance Organization (SHMO) demonstrations have also shown results in prevention of high-cost hospitalization and other institutionalizations. The PACE program offers services at community adult day health centers and are coordinated by an interdisciplinary team of health professionals led by nurse case managers. The SHMO demonstration project also is a community-based program offering long-term care services for the frail elderly population. Under this nurse case-managed plan, the patients are provided with Medicare A and B benefits, prescription drug coverage, benefits for eyeglasses and hearing aids, and up to $1,000 per month in home community-based service benefits. The SHMOs have been effective in reducing nursing home use and reducing caregiver burden. Nurse case

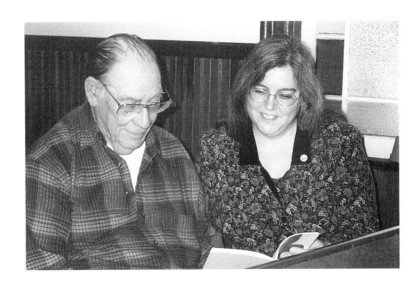

management is the cornerstone of these two demonstration projects (ANA, 1999).

The CNO, PACE, and SHMO models provide us with examples of how nurses in the community can work to provide compassionate and competent care outside the hospital medical model. These three demonstration projects continue to be funded by HCFA because nurse case management has the side benefit of being cost effective in the delivery of community-based care. Box 8–6 helps you discuss community case management models further.

Box 8-6	Student Learning Activity

Case Management Community Models

Identify three nurse case management community models with federal government funding.

List the two basic elements of the CNO model.

RESEARCH, NOT ME!

Say research to me and my mind goes fuzzy. I'm going to be a nurse not a statistician. Why should I care about research in the community? I want to take care of people not numbers. How impersonal can you get? What's the purpose anyway?

A nursing student's view of research

THE VALUE OF NURSING RESEARCH IN THE COMMUNITY SETTING

Research is a very valuable tool in nursing practice. It is through nursing research that dollars can be allocated toward a project that actually improves patient care. This could be through increased nursing services or longer clinic hours or a new clinic or facility. The primary purpose of the Visiting Nurse Service of New York CNO is to assess the impact of both a capitated reimbursement approach to payment of community-based services and a nurse-managed model of care (Storfjell-Lloyd, Mitchell, & Daly-McCormack, 1997). The evaluation of the program has been an essential concern from the beginning. Keep in mind that federal funding supports this project and is necessary for the CNO to exist for the patients to receive community-nursing service. This CNO developed a computer information system that can track both the clinical and the financial data. This allowed the CNO to look back at the first three years of operation and identify the community trends, the cost of services, and staffing patterns and to develop management and marketing (enrollment) strategies. Based on the analysis of their research, the CNOs were given federal funding to continue.

Research can identify how well a new process is working. In an effort to consolidate costs and maintain quality services, eight counties in New York implemented some form of cluster care (shared aide) for Medicaid clients receiving home care between 1982 and 1989. Cluster care was designed to be cost effective, efficient, and caring. The Gray's Home Care Satisfaction Scale was used to gather the information necessary for this study (Gray & Sedhom, 1997). The findings of this research study showed that the patients receiving the traditional care had a higher level of satisfaction than the patients receiving the cluster care. The implications from this research demonstrate to policy makers the need to further evaluate this new "cluster" concept based on the patients' dissatisfaction. It is important to remember that this study only reflects the "cluster" care concept in the beginning stages. This study pointed out areas that needed to be improved and modified with this new delivery of care model. It also demonstrated that patients need education and more understanding of the new process to adapt to the change. Now this study can be used as a baseline to evaluate future studies.

Another interesting community-based study involves student nurses. This study looked at outcomes in an academic nursing center and the patient satisfaction with the nursing student's services. The nursing students were providing home visiting services to improve access to care for vulnerable populations in the community (Lindsey, Henly, & Tyree, 1997). The faculty and staff of the University of North Dakota Nursing Center surveyed the patients at the end of each semester. The results reported an overwhelming satisfaction with all aspects of the care provided by the nursing student.

Research is not just data collection using computers or surveys. It goes beyond the numbers to the analysis of what is really happening. The results of research can increase funding, continue programs, validate programs, provide insight into new change, or assist at developing future change. Research is vital in community-based nursing practice to demonstrate the impact of nursing on patient care.

The nurse researcher is responsible for designing and implementing the research project. This researcher role is an advanced practice role. All nursing staff within the agency or facility may be involved in the collection of data and patient contacts. The results of the research study are shared with all the nursing participants. Research is a positive way to change and improve patient care in the community.

Box 8-7	Student Learning Activity

Client Example

To help you put all of the information in this chapter together, use your knowledge of the community-based practice roles of the nurse and apply it to the following case study. As a case manager (team leader), what services and supplies would you recommend for this patient and why?

Case study

Mrs. B. is an 88-year-old woman who has had a stroke. She was hospitalized for one week and is coming home with her daughter. This is a new living arrangement for Mrs. B., who has always had her own home and has been independent in her daily life. She is aphasic. The nursing staff at the hospital reports difficulty swallowing. Mrs. B. can use a walker with assistance, but her daughter's home has many levels and staircases.

SUMMARY

Community-based nursing practice involves collaboration with multiple health professionals in a variety of settings. All of these settings are outside hospital walls and are defining new directions for both patient care delivery systems and the role of the nurse. Exciting new demonstration projects such as CNOs are validating the usefulness of the nurse as a case manager to facilitate cost-effective but quality care for the patients. Research has shown that patient satisfaction is high when nurses (and nursing students) are involved with community-health services. Box 8–7 contains a client example to help you apply the information you learned in this chapter.

Active Learning Strategies

1. Think about a patient you have worked with in the community. What community-health professional roles did you see involved with that patient's care? Can you suggest other interventions with additional community-health professionals?

2. You are visiting an elderly patient with the home-health nurse. This patient sits in a chair and stares at the floor, not making eye contact. Is it appropriate to ask the gerontological nurse working at the home-health agency to make a visit to assess this patient? Make a list of background assessment information to use in your collaboration with the gerontological nurse.

3. Go online and search "case manager." See how many differing roles under this title you can find in the community setting.

4. If you could design a community-based agency or facility, what would it look like? Who would you hire and why? How would you fund this professional service? Contact a local community-based program and ask about their start-up planning.

References

American Nurses Association (ANA). (1999). ANA recommendations on Medicare reform. (On-line), Available at: http://www.ana.org/pressrel/medrpt/medrpt2.htm

Buckholtz, S., & Klainberg, M. (1998). An historical perspective of community health nursing. In M. Klainberg, S. Holzemer, M. Leonard, & J. Arnold (Eds.), Community health nursing: An alliance for health (pp. 23–36). New York: McGraw-Hill Nursing Core Series.

Burtt, K. (1998). Issues Update. Nurses step to forefront of elder care. American Journal of Nursing, 98(7), 52–54.

Gray, Y. L., & Sedhom, L. (1997). Client satisfaction: Traditional care versus cluster care. Journal of Professional Nursing, 13(1), 56–61.

Helvie, C. (1997). Advanced practice nursing in the community. Thousand Oaks, CA: Sage.

Kozier, B., Erb, G., Berman, A. J., & Burke, K. (2000). Health care delivery systems. In B. Kozier, G. Erb, A. J. Berman, & K. Burke (Eds.), Fundamentals of nursing: Concepts, process, and practice (6th ed., pp. 93–97). Upper Saddle River, NJ: Prentice Hall Health.

Lindsey, D. L., Henly, S. J., & Tyree, E. A. (1997). Outcomes in an academic nursing center: Client satisfaction with student services. Journal of Nursing Care Quality, 11(5), 30–38.

Storfjell, J. L. (1994). Community focus and case management (CNO orientation, pp. 47–53). New York: VNA of NY.

Storfjell-Lloyd, J., Mitchell, R., & Daly-McCormack, G. (1997). Nurse-managed healthcare: New York's community nursing organization. Journal of Nursing Administration, 27 (10), 21–27.

Taylor, C., Lillis, C., & LeMone, P. (1997). Community based healthcare. In C. Taylor, C. Lillis, & P. LeMone (Eds.), Fundamentals of nursing: The art and science of nursing care (3rd ed., pp. 181–187). Philadelphia: Lippincott-Raven.

CHAPTER 9

Community Resources

Pamela A. Avent
Christena Langley

LEARNING OBJECTIVES

1) Understand the value of client referrals to community resources.

2) Identify factors influencing the use of resources in health care.

3) Recognize the variety of resources available within each of the three levels of prevention.

4) Describe the referral process.

5) Reflect on five questions to ask when assessing the match between client and referral.

6) Discuss the characteristics of an effective referral.

7) Consider the potential barriers to clients' use of resources.

8) Describe the attributes the community-based nurse needs in order to be an effective resource manager throughout the referral process.

Nursing students are often surprised to find that clients have different priorities regarding the services they need to improve their health. It is also difficult for nursing students to comprehend how time consuming and challenging it is to locate appropriate resources for their clients. It takes much time and effort to become familiar with resources available for various populations and to assist families in building a structure of community support (Zerwekh, 1997). Little has been written about the process of becoming familiar with community resources, evaluating their potential value to clients, and following through with the referral process, although these activities are a central piece of community-based and public-health nursing care.

This chapter will help develop the critical-thinking skills involved in locating and evaluating community resources and their value to clients across the continuum of acute care, long-term care, and community-based settings. As you read the rest of the book, you may want to come back to this chapter, because you will find examples

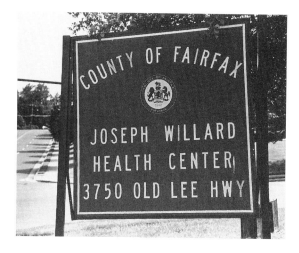

throughout the book that prove the necessity of knowing the community and how to access its resources.

Traditionally, nurses working in acute-care settings assist clients in locating resources in the community through discharge planning, and public-health nurses rely on multiple agencies to assist in meeting clients' needs. Now that nurses are working in so many different community-based settings, they are responsible for knowing a whole network of agencies and services available in the community. The nurse and other health-care workers link clients to appropriate services through effective referrals. Successful linkages provide the needed support to the client and family to improve their overall health. A community with many resources offers support throughout the life span, thus helping the population to

achieve optimal health; the community with few resources that are scattered and disconnected is inefficient in helping its population achieve its full health potential. Nurses must be knowledgeable about services offered by their agencies as well as the other resources available within the community and how to access them to serve clients' needs. This facilitates a seamless health-care system so that clients can move between home, acute care and long-term care, and outpatient services with as little disruption of their lives as possible.

The use of resources through the referral process impacts a client's health by improving the continuity of health care through various agencies, that is, from the hospital to rehabilitation or home to support group. Our health-care system is designed to treat acute problems and is concerned with cost effectiveness. Community-based care has expanded our health-care system to reach clients in their homes, schools, churches, and places of recreation and work. The appropriate use of resources decreases fragmentation, improves the quality of care, and promotes cost-effective outcomes (Dickerson, Peters, Walkowiak, & Brewer, 1999).

It is not as easy as it sounds for a nurse to use community resources. It is a highly complex task that requires the various skills of coordination, referral, delegation, and client advocacy. It is a service performed by people of various disciplines, including social workers, physicians, dietitians, and physical therapists, as well as nurses. Nurses are often in the best position to oversee a continuous plan of care because they provide primary care, have an ongoing relationship with the client, supervise the paraprofessionals, and collaborate with other members of the health-care team regarding the clients' health needs. The nurse needs to assess what clients know and what their past experiences using community resources have been. The nurse can best ascertain the client's and family's knowledge of their needs, as well as their previous experiences with the referral process. Although the nurse is in the best position to understand clients' needs, it is not the sole responsibility of the nurse to obtain the resources needed. It is a shared responsibility with an open-systems approach for the nurse and the client's family. When someone is appointed the primary case manager, it is not only her or his job to find resources for the client but also to be sensitive to the constant change occurring within the open system.

FACTORS INFLUENCING THE USE OF RESOURCES IN HEALTH CARE

The face of health care is changing as we embark into the 21st century. First, the explosion of medical technologies has changed the life expectancy of several vulnerable groups including low-birth-weight infants, children with special needs, adults with chronic illnesses, and the elderly. Individuals who once might have died now live long lives, even with illnesses once considered life threatening. The treatment of illnesses has changed from intermittent, episodic care to care distributed over time through health-promotion and disease-prevention activities, management of chronic illness, and home and long-term care. Rather than treating single illnesses in isolation, the health-care delivery system is managing chronic conditions over time for people of all ages. Health services must offer health promotion as well as sick care to individuals, groups, and communities. The increased longevity within the population has placed an increasing demand on community resources to meet the needs of the population within communities. Resources are used to treat illness, manage diseases, and promote health. As we live longer, it stands to reason that communities will consume more resources. As health-care providers, nurses must have not only a basic knowledge of resources, but must also consider cost-effective means when using them. Because this is a dynamic process and the resources change frequently, one of a community-based nurse's most important tasks is the maintenance of a current "Rolodex" of resources. As one student described:

> *Since the utilization of resources is so much a part of their daily job, sometimes when I ask for help from the staff, they quickly list all the resources needed and how to get them. I feel overwhelmed to try to sort out the information that will help my client. The nurses can tell me the relative pros and cons of several different agencies. I have to sort them out with my client and come to a decision as to what's best for her to pursue.*

In addition to the changes in the longevity of the population, clients spend less time in hospital settings and return to their homes more quickly with additional needs for services from their home. This increase in clients with medical home-care needs has tightened the relationship between acute-care nursing and community-based nursing so that each relies on the other to assist in smooth transitions for clients.

A third major change affecting the need for community resources is the continuing influx of immigrants to the United States. This has shifted the focus of health-care delivery from individual health needs to population-focused health care. As a nation, we are more aware of the impact of the overall health status of groups entering the country from various parts of the world. The community is only as strong as the general public's health. Consequently, the general welfare of the community is sometimes more important than an individual's needs. Health promotion and disease prevention is a major focus when working with these specific immigrant populations. New immigrants often require health screening, as well as treatment, because they often come from countries where health standards are different from those in the United States. Many immigrants are trying to cope with the challenges of the Western health-care system as well as language barriers that may prevent access to needed services (Hunt & Zurek, 1997). The Western biomedical belief system clashes with other worldviews about the cause and treatment of illness as well as the meaning of health (Hunt & Zurek, 1997). We must use our resources wisely for the good of the whole population. It is a delicate balance that swings between sickness and health. Referrals to appropriate resources provide a positive push toward optimal wellness. Box 9–1 gives you an opportunity to categorize community resources.

Box 9-1   Student Learning Activity

Categorizing Resources

How would you categorize resources in your community in relation to health promotion, disease prevention, and care of people with acute and chronic health conditions?

DEFINING RESOURCES

Prevention is a key concept of community-based nursing (Hunt & Zurek, 1997). Resources that include community and support services can be identified at each of the three levels of prevention. Examples of community resources by level of prevention appear in Table 9–1. What other examples can you think of in your community?

At first, one might think that health promotion would not be included in the prevention of disease, but anticipating or averting health problems is a major part of community-based practice. Health-promotion activities are included within the level of primary prevention. Health-promotion activities are positive approaches to increasing the level of wellness within a community. Promoting health is an active process that includes assisting clients to a level of well-being that maximizes individual potential. Nursing has a social responsibility within its realm of practice to engage in health promotion, which focuses on improving the health behaviors of individuals and families. Many health-promotion practices are directed toward raising the level of health of the general

community (Hunt & Zurek, 1997). To achieve this improvement, the nurse relies on community resources. Often at this level of prevention, the community-based nurse needs organizations that provide speakers and educational materials such as pamphlets, videotapes, and other teaching tools to assist with programs offered during health-education sessions.

The community resources that are related to the primary level of disease prevention are those that focus on the promotion of health and the prevention of illness. These may include health departments providing immunizations; private physicians and nurse practitioners providing physical examinations; community service agencies, such as those providing smoking cessation classes, car seats at reduced cost, or furniture and baby equipment for a new family member. All health-care settings that provide environmental protection, alcohol and drug prevention programs, fitness classes, and well-child care are included in this primary prevention level.

At the secondary prevention level, resources include those programs and facilities that provide early identification and treatment of an existing health problem or disease. This includes mammography centers, private

Table 9-1

Community Resources According to Level of Prevention

LEVEL OF PREVENTION	MATERNAL AND YOUNG CHILDREN	ADULTS	OLDER ADULTS
Primary prevention	Head Start immunization clinics	American Heart Association American Cancer Society Adult immunization clinics	Nutrition counseling Fitness programs Recreation programs
Secondary prevention	Child Find school screening programs	Planned Parenthood Mammogram vans	Hospital wellness clinics Nursing home screenings
Tertiary prevention	Child development programs Early intervention programs Lions Club Furniture/clothing closets (Goodwill Industries, Salvation Army) Shelters	Group homes Support groups Alcoholics Anonymous Food pantries Psychiatric social centers Sheltered workshops	Meals-on-Wheels Senior day care and respite programs Rehabilitation centers

doctors offices or clinics that provide scoliosis screening, vision and hearing screening, tuberculosis (TB) screening at health centers, and human immunodeficiency virus (HIV) testing with counseling at health departments. Screening centers for early detection of diabetes or testicular cancer, blood pressure screening, and chiropractors, as well as those providing prenatal care, are also in this secondary prevention group of resources. When the nurse refers clients to services at this level, she or he must keep in mind the possible need for additional resources if the testing or screening outcome is positive. For example, when you refer a high school student to the health department for free pregnancy testing, you must also anticipate her need for follow-up services that include maternity care, pregnancy termination, adoption options, family planning, or possibly testing and treatment for a sexually transmitted disease.

Tertiary prevention actually minimizes disability and maximizes recovery after an illness. Resources to meet these needs include acute-care facilities, private and public clinics, churches, financial and legal aid, and housing services. Rehabilitation activities such as those found in self-help groups, speech therapy, and mental health groups are all a part of the tertiary prevention aspect of health care. Some community resources may fall into more than one category. For instance, the American Cancer Society provides smoking cessation groups that are part of secondary prevention resource, yet it also provides a service called Reach to Recovery that helps breast cancer survivors at the tertiary or recovery level of prevention. These levels of prevention are merely a model to organize the particular resources within a general framework.

All of the previously mentioned resources are services that help people to maintain their lifestyle or to solve problems that interfere with their self-care or well-being. They offer the much-needed assistance to clients and families at times when total self-sufficiency is not possible. This may often occur during difficult economic times or in a health crisis. One could say that these services "prop up" the individual or family until they can become self-sufficient. Resource services are not always health related, and are not always obvious to clients or families. These support services may be more difficult to identify within a community than the services directly related to

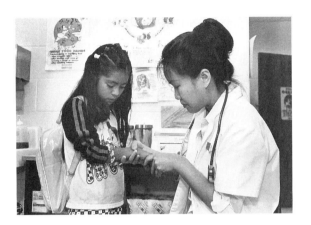

a client's health-care needs (Hunt & Zurek, 1997). Therefore the community-based nurse must spend a good part of his or her time seeking out and evaluating available community resources. These community resources provide an important piece of continuity within the health-care system.

Support-care service providers may include churches; financial aid; legal services; housing; protective services for children and older adults; day care; group homes; food services; self-help groups; physical, occupational, music, art, and alternative health therapists; and mental health services. These support services may be more difficult to identify within a community than the traditional health-care services but are equally important to improving clients' health (Hunt & Zurek, 1997). These types of services may be funded by both private and public monies. Also within this group of health-care providers are the home-health agencies, numerous agencies offering alternative health therapies, health departments, outpatient departments, and screening facilities. Churches, schools, and neighborhood centers are also part of the support care providers network. As one student stated:

 It really surprised me that there were so many organizations out there ready to help. One just needs to contact them and get the ball rolling to help the client.

Box 9–2 gives you the opportunity to link clients with community resources.

Box 9-2   Student Learning Activity

Community Support

Think about the clients with whom you are working in the community. Discuss the kind of support needed from service providers to ensure quality care.

Table 9-2

Steps in the Referral Process

- Establish the need
- Set objectives for the referral
- Explore the resources that are available
- Have the client make a decision concerning the referral
- Make the referral to the selected service
- Supply the agency with needed information
- Support the client and family in pursuing the referral

Source: Hunt, R., & Zurek, E. (1997). Introduction to community based nursing. Philadelphia: Lippincott Williams & Wilkins, p. 302.

In the rest of this chapter, we give more details on how to refer clients to community resources with successful outcomes.

THE REFERRAL PROCESS

The referral process consists of working with clients to locate and access resources to meet their needs. The referral process can be defined as assisting individuals, families, groups, and organizations to use necessary resources available to prevent or resolve problems. Table 9–2 delineates the steps in the referral process. Referral may be used to enhance a client's self-care capabilities to assess resources (Stanhope & Lancaster, 1996). The purpose of the referral is to share/communicate information with the service-provider agency so that clients' specific needs are met and coordinated. The information that is shared is the sum of the assessment, nursing diagnosis, and plan of care. During the referral process, information about the medical, social, environmental, and financial aspects of the client's situation is exchanged between the caregiver (it is not always a nurse) and the service-providing agency. Community-based nurses maintain a file system of the resources with which they have had success. This can be a database on computer, on a Rolodex file, or any other systematic method for retaining the pertinent information for use in the referral process.

After defining and locating the community resources within a certain area, the nurse is now ready to refer the

client or family unit to the specific community service. When making a referral for a client to a community agency or to a community service, the student should ask very specific questions to assess if the client and the desired service are a match. Does this liaison between client and agency have a good chance for a positive outcome? These questions may include:

What are the eligibility requirements for services?

How does the client contact the agency for services?

Does a client need an appointment to obtain services?

Are there specific days that services are offered?

What is the cost of service?

Does the service accept payment from a third-party payer?

Can specific financial arrangements be made that will not hurt the client's credit rating?

Is there a translator available on site?

Is there information about the service in languages other than English?

Do these services offer culturally competent care?

Where is the service located?

Is there public transportation available? Is parking available?

Is there accessibility for the disabled?

What are the consequences if the client does not keep the appointment? (Can there be a second or even a third chance for services?)

The referral process is for the benefit of the client and to effectively help meet the client's needs. It also helps coordinate care among service organizations providing that care. The ultimate goal of the referral process is the strengthening of the client's or family's capacity for self-help through a network of community support (Zerwehk, 1997). The following are characteristics of an effective referral:

The referral is individualized. Each referral must work for the specific client, taking into account each individual's needs, culture, and resources. What works for one client may not be right for another. This is why the nurse's ongoing family assessment is crucial to the referral process. The nurse should always observe what's happening and how the situation is changing over time.

The referral is practical and can be accomplished in a timely manner. Consider the client's finances, time, and personal responsibilities. Does the client view this resource as a real priority? Is the client ready to address the health-care need at this time? Does the client's work and other responsibilities allow the time needed to satisfy the referral process?

The referral is made together with the client and/or family and the organization providing the care. Is there a duplication of services? Be sure the family is not already being seen by a similar service or agency. Has the family been involved in the process of initiating the referral? Is the purpose of the referral clear to the resource agency and family? Is the expected outcome of the referral shared by all involved?

The referral has reliability. The community resource has been carefully evaluated and proved suitable for clients. The nurse needs to ensure that the client is

handled in a timely, courteous, and professional manner before making subsequent referrals. A follow-up evaluation after each referral is essential to the process of referring clients (Hunt & Zurek, 1997).

Remember, the client always has the right to refuse a referral. It is his or her right to say no to any part of the health-care plan. After all, it is the client's life and the client's health. This can sometimes be frustrating for the nurse who initiated the process. One nursing student summed it up in this manner:

I couldn't believe that even when I told the client exactly what to do, and how to contact the resource, he didn't follow through. He didn't seem to understand how much work had gone into getting this appointment.

A FRAMEWORK FOR THE REFERRAL PROCESS

When considering the use of resources, the community-based nurse can use the traditional, epidemiological questions as an outline to guide efforts in the community: Who? What? Where? When? How?

Who? Who is in need of a referral to a community resource? Is the referral for one individual or is it for an entire family? Often, the community-based nurse is looking for a more complicated service, such as a primary-care provider for several children, one of whom may have a chronic illness like asthma.

In a more general sense, who really needs the use of resources within the health care arena? All clients do! To meet the needs of clients and their families, a nurse cannot assume that there is a single profile of a person who uses resources. All clients need different resources at different times throughout the life span. The nurse needs to be open minded when planning care. For example, a middle-class professional woman with an alcoholic husband may have education and financial support, but she may be in need of many other services. These may include resources such as Alcoholics Anonymous (AA), a battered woman's support group, temporary shelter, legal aid assistance, or nutritional counseling. It is not easy to be open minded because we bring our own histories with us to each situation. This is where objectivity comes into play. We must work with the client to outline the plan, not just decide what we feel are the needs of this situation.

The nurse also needs to consider the total assessment of the client or family. Is this someone that can make calls independently to seek out services, or go to the library and use the Internet to find information? Or is this a client who needs much more guidance in the specifics of how to access services? As one student explained:

 My client was really afraid to make the phone calls! She said she didn't know what to ask and was concerned that the person at the other end would get impatient if she didn't ask the "right questions." Together we wrote down a set of questions to ask. That seemed to give her the confidence to make the calls. . . .

Again, in answer to the question, who needs resources? Everyone does!

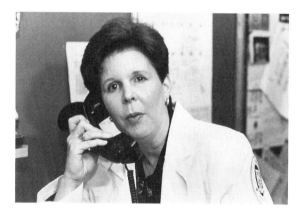

Many times, people in crisis feel very alone and isolated from other parts of the community. It needs to be clearly understood that we are not alone, but part of a much larger society, a community that can help find the resources to begin to solve the problems at hand. Nursing students are often surprised by the number of useful resources they find while assisting their clients.

Box 9–3 allows you to brainstorm a wish list of community resources.

What? What does the person or family need? Remember, this means what the client or family feels they need.

Box 9-3	Student Learning Activity

Community Resource Wish List

Create a "wish list" of community resources within your own community (do not include resources already in existence).

The nurse also has ideas about services and resources that may be helpful, but the client must be in agreement for the process to be successful. What is the goal that has been agreed on by all involved?

Other "whats" to consider:

- What skills does the client have that enable him or her to participate in the referral process? (Can he or she communicate to get the housing, electricity, or phone?

- What are the specific cost, location, accessibility, and hours of operation? It is crucial that what the client needs is congruent with what the agency offers. Suppose you are working with a young mother with two toddlers. The mother tells you that she often loses her temper with the children and feels she needs help understanding toddler behavior. You know that there is an excellent parenting class offered weekly at the local community center. The class includes the children, so there is no need for outside child care, but this mother has limited English. Her native language is Farsi. The teachers speak only English. You'll need to help this mother find someone who is bilingual to go with her, or you'll need to help her find a different source of parenting information.

- What resources are useful to the nurse or nursing student but are not useful to the client? You might want to go to the American Cancer Society to find pamphlets to teach adults the warning signs of cancer, but you would not send a client with colon cancer alone to find educational materials.

Where? Where do you find these specific tools to help clients meet their needs? In most areas of the United States, there are many different types of resources. Many

organizations such as the Cancer Society and Lung Association have local, state, and national resources that offer
educational materials and program information as well
as direct services. There are private, voluntary, and religious organizations that provide many services. Sometimes it is overwhelming for a student to decide where to
begin:

*When I began this endeavor, it really helped that my
teacher pointed me in the right direction. A little bit of
guidance seems to go a long way, and I felt more comfortable seeking added information on my own, once that I felt
familiar with the task.*

Health services in the United States are often provided
by independent agencies. Hospitals, nursing homes, and
rehabilitation programs offer their own specialty health
care, but leave the clients to find other resources by themselves. The local health-care delivery system must plan,
implement, and pay for services needed within a community. Many times the force that drives the health system is budgetary and determined by a combination of
local, state, and federal funds as well as private monies.
When private providers do not meet the needs of a community, government and charity groups are left to bridge
the gap. Many urban localities or small rural areas may
not have adequate funding to provide some aspects of
health care. In many localities, the community-based
nurse needs to become familiar with private providers
who donate hours and services to the provision of care
for the indigent.

Nurses must be creative and use resources from multiple locations. It is very important that nurses be familiar
with the resources available to them within their agency
or locality. It is also important that nurses learn about
their communities and how they relate to the changing
local, state, and national priorities. One way to stay current with health-care programs and resources is via the
Internet.

To take advantage of the superhighway of health-care
information on the Internet, you need a search engine or
directory, plus sites to access. In other words, you need
the web addresses of the medical and nursing sites.
Therefore you need to have some idea of what you are

seeking to be successful in this medium (Hodson-Carlton
& Dorner, 1999). For example, you might be looking for
resources for a family with a child with cerebral palsy.
There may be multiple headings that may or may not lead
you to the specific resource needed by that family, but
with some time and effort you can locate many possibilities. Then you must narrow the focus. Once you find
these sites, you should place a marker at each location so
that you can retrieve the information more easily the next
time you need it. Table 9–3 provides web sites and search
engines as well as web addresses. These are examples of
sites that will take you to health information, services,
and resources by specific topic. Allow enough time (at
least 1 hour) to browse and search for the specific information needed.

Another tried-and-true method for finding resources
is to use the Yellow Pages. This telephone directory is
filled with information that is cataloged by name in alphabetical order or by subject or topic. Most local and
state government information is listed in special sections
of the telephone book. All school addresses and phone

Table 9-3

Directories and Search Engines

SITE	ADDRESS
Alta Vista	*http://www.altavista.digital.com*
CliniWeb	*http://www.ohsu.edu/cliniweb/ search.html*
Lycos	*http://www.lycos.com*
Matrix	*http://www.slackinc.com*
MedWeb	*http://www.medweb.emory.edu/ MedWeb/*
Yahoo	*http://www.yahoo.com*
MedHelp International	*http://medhlp.netusa.net/index.htm*
1-800 Numbers for Client Support Organizations	*http://infonet.welch.jhu.edu/ advocacy.html*

numbers are also found there, as well as private hospitals and voluntary agencies. This may seem like a simple approach to finding resources, yet it is a perfect beginning method to obtain information. Problems arise when there is a language barrier. Most of the phone books are in English; therefore a command of the language is imperative when soliciting information from this source. Telephone books are generally organized by specific towns or counties. The location of the resource must be known to access it. Frequently, it is necessary to look through several phone books to find all of the desired information.

When? Timing is everything. The client has to be ready to accept and use the resources available. The nurse may be ready with all the information needed about the resource, but the client may have other priorities. The client must be willing and able to address the health-care need. The ideal situation is to have the client and the family participate in the referral process. They are then involved in the decision making and can choose the services they prefer. This should help to ensure a positive outcome in the referral process. Sometimes the nurse must negotiate with the client and family about what has to be accomplished before the client is ready for the referral to be made.

How? How are these resources accessed? The nursing process is very helpful when planning for referrals to resources. Develop specific nursing diagnoses from your assessment, then your plan will follow. Following a structured method allows you to decrease your subjectivity with the particular situation and to practice objectivity. For example, some member of your own family may have battled alcohol, and you were not satisfied with group AA. Perhaps you have a negative history and bad feelings toward that particular resource. Nevertheless, you cannot share your previous experience with your client. You must practice objectivity and make the referral to that agency if appropriate. This situation is not about you, but about your client and his or her needs. Objectivity must be practiced when choosing resources.

This is where common sense and practicality are extremely important. It is imperative to know if the agency has the ability to translate in the native language of the client referred. The resource selected must be appropriate for the transportation available to the client. That is to say, that if Mrs. G. has to take three buses to get to the clinic for her appointments, her compliance is highly unlikely. If clients have to make complex transportation arrangements for multivisit clinic referrals, it is highly unlikely that they will be able to follow through and attend the clinics, even if their own well-being is in jeopardy. Use of resources is a complex process.

So far, the *hows* of accessing information that we have discussed have been within the paper arena. However, there is another method that involves person-to-person contact, or networking. This personal resource to seek and network is a social skill. It is based on the ability to communicate and interact with others. Networking is developed through family, peer, and community relationships. It occurs when information is shared with members of the network. In the referral process, networking is actually the sharing of information about a particular problem and how it is solved. For example, it can mean information about a community service that provides rides for clients to a health-care facility, free of charge. In this case, the ride must be accessed through a church group, and there is no age requirement or time constraint. This information was obtained through a discussion a nurse had with her neighbor, who works at the church. She was networking by talking about her need to find an inexpensive way to transport her clients to a specialist.

Another way to network is to go to a meeting with other community service providers and have a "lunch bunch," where information is exchanged about what services are offered. Many church groups have day care, clothes closets, food pantries, and transportation services. They also provide language and computer classes, holiday gifts for indigent families, and senior day care. There are also various service clubs, such as the Lions Club, that specialize in eye care programs.

BARRIERS TO SERVICE

Why don't these people comply? Why don't they do what we tell them to do? Sometimes I feel that this is a waste of time and money. Why can't they help themselves? Even though we tell them about great services that will accept them as clients, they don't follow through. . . .

Sometimes, despite the best efforts of the community-based nurse and the willingness of the resource service to help, clients are unable to avail themselves of what is offered. This is frustrating to the health-care providers who have worked so hard to put the referral together. Some of the most common barriers to following through with the referral process include:

- Eligibility issues
- Transportation issues
- Time
- Language
- Uncertainty
- Powerlessness, lack of problem-solving skills

Most of the clients who we encounter in community-based settings have multiple needs and lack the resources to meet these needs. Nurses must be flexible to work effectively with a wide variety of clients and staff. There are sometimes roadblocks to the clients' use of resources, even though they are available and acceptable to the client. If the resources are not accessible, they will not be used. Look at some of the most common barriers that make resources inaccessible for the client's use:

1. Eligibility issues: Each system or agency has specific requirements for the use of services. There may be income limits, geographic requirements, or age eligibility. Any of these criteria may limit the client's use of a certain service. In the public domain, clients who want health department clinic services must meet both income and service area criteria. Often clients who have immigrated to the United States are fearful of becoming known to official agencies, even if their immigration status is legal. They have come from environments where there was danger in being known to the government, and they are reluctant to believe that it is different in this country.

2. Transportation issues: Often, health-care facilities are not accessible by bus, which makes it very difficult for clients to meet their appointments. Communities offer rides, but there may be financial or time constraints. Personal cars are often being used by other family members for work and are not available for health-care appointments. The family priority is working so that they can meet their most basic needs of food and shelter. Community-based nurses need to explore all of the possible transportation resources and maintain them as part of their ongoing resource file to help overcome this very basic and extremely prevalent barrier to services.

3. Time: Our health-care system, as well as many voluntary and charitable organizations, is based on an appointment system. Our culture also dictates specific times for services. It is not a "free time, come whenever you can" system. Many clients come from different cultures that are not time driven. This causes a problem when accessing services. The clients come late and do not understand that they missed their appointed time, which is the only space in which they can be seen. They do not see why 30 minutes or 1 hour makes a difference. They came on the correct date and do not understand when they are turned away. There are also very few evening or night services available. This is in direct conflict with families who do shift work. Employers are not always understanding of the need to leave work for a family member's appointments.

4. Language: Language may be a very difficult hurdle for clients because the system may expect the client to either understand and speak English proficiently or provide an interpreter who does. At times, the nurse may think that the client understands the information, because he or she continually nods, as if in agreement. However, that is not necessarily what this behavior means. Health-care providers must continually clarify communications with the client. The nurse can use pictures to aid in overcoming the language barrier. There are language banks that provide interpreters. Many organizations use their own employees to help clients with information in English.

5. Uncertainty: Being uncertain is not knowing what to expect from a situation. It occurs when one is unable to predict certain events. This is a barrier to some clients using resources because it contributes to fear of possible outcomes. Clients may think that parts of the health-care system are linked to the immigration department. Because many clients are undocumented, this misunderstanding hinders their compliance. If they are fearful, they will not follow through on the plan, even if they agreed to do so.

6. Powerlessness/lack of problem-solving skills: Many clients feel helpless when interacting with the health-care system. The organization is foreign, the language is foreign, and they may feel a lack of control. These feelings may manifest themselves in passivity and an inability to make decisions and take action. The nurse needs to support clients to see that they do have power to affect their own lives. Clients do have authority over their health. They are not hopeless.

The nurse must work with the client to identify potential barriers and help the client to learn strategies to overcome them. Remember that it is also the client's responsibility to learn resources and independently use them. Suggest that the client call on family members, friends, and church and inquire what help they may offer. The nurse solves problems with the client and helps form a list of possible resources that may provide needed services. Many clients are unable to outline a plan of action and decide what to do without help. They feel overwhelmed by their situation, and this impacts their ability to look at the problem realistically. The nurse is influential in the development of independence and self-care for clients and their families through teaching and reinforcing positive problem-solving skills.

BEING AN EFFECTIVE COMMUNITY RESOURCE MANAGER

Several attributes are important to develop as a community-based nurse responsible for working through the referral process with clients. Consider the following:

• Your Organizational Style:

Do you consider yourself as very organized or as chaotically organized? Think about the organizational pattern that best represents you. It is very helpful to maintain some type of file system when using resources. It is not helpful to attempt to store information mentally, without any written documentation. Your mental list of resources would very quickly overcome your memory!

Identify your organizational methods and style, and use them consistently. One nurse may choose to use an index card system for a resource file. Another may use a three-ring binder, and a third might opt to maintain a resource record on the computer.

• Consistency:

Are you consistent in your approach to new situations? One should always follow the nursing process when assisting clients with the use of resources. Always follow through on your plan with the client. Follow a pattern and use consistent thinking. Make the assessments, plan the strategies, implement the actions, and always evaluate the outcomes. Recognize your inconsistencies. An experienced community-based nurse states:

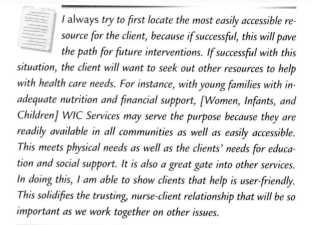

I always try to first locate the most easily accessible resource for the client, because if successful, this will pave the path for future interventions. If successful with this situation, the client will want to seek out other resources to help with health care needs. For instance, with young families with inadequate nutrition and financial support, [Women, Infants, and Children] WIC Services may serve the purpose because they are readily available in all communities as well as easily accessible. This meets physical needs as well as the clients' needs for education and social support. It is also a great gate into other services. In doing this, I am able to show clients that help is user-friendly. This solidifies the trusting, nurse-client relationship that will be so important as we work together on other issues.

• Ability to Acknowledge Feelings:

How do you feel about the resource? How do you think the client will respond to this particular resource? Have you or the client had a negative experience with this organization in the past?

Do you already have an answer before you begin the process? (You are thinking: "This will never work" or "They won't ever follow through!") These feelings are your emotions, and they should not be ignored. Nurses as well as clients have feelings that must be recognized and handled. These feelings and prejudices can be barriers to the successful use of resources. Always keep an open mind when helping clients through the health-care system. Remember that each of us is different. What you might personally desire in a resource may not be right for someone else. Talk through the process with your clients to ensure success.

• Recognition of Past Experiences:

Everyone has used resources in the past either for themselves, family members, or neighbors. Nurses bring some knowledge to the client, even if it is personal. This is an arena that can build on your previous knowledge and experience. Using resources is a chance to develop skills that can be shared with others. This is an opportunity to increase the quality of life for your clients, as well as changing you from a beginner to an expert. It is important to build on what we know, expanding our knowledge base.

In addition to those attributes discussed previously, certain interpersonal skills are helpful to community-based nurses as they work with their clients to find and use appropriate resources in the community. Using resources calls on nursing students to understand their own temperament as well as that of their clients. Here are a few questions that may help you to understand yourself and your client as you proceed with using resources or when making referrals:

1. How do you react to new situations? If you are fearful or anxious in new situations, you must overcome this. By getting to know a variety of resources and the people who staff them, you will become more comfortable and better able to serve your clients.

2. Do you leap into new situations enthusiastically or are you cautious, weighing each aspect? Timing is essential, and the nurse must consider that procrastination ruins more good intentions than any other factor. If you can begin the process today, then do it. On the other hand, it is important to think through the nursing process as you work with clients to get some idea of the likely outcomes of one type of referral versus another. Always consider: What is the immediacy of the situation? How does the client view the immediacy?

3. Is the idea of change typically upsetting? It is important to look at this from your viewpoint and from the viewpoint of your client. Change is difficult, and when you ask clients to embark on a new path, such as acting independently, it is not always smooth.

4. Have you set too many goals in a short time? Is this resource about you or your client? Is it about getting the job done and being finished with this case? One or two goals for one visit is enough. Do not give too many directions or make them too complex; otherwise, you run the risk that none of your instructions will be followed. How likely is the client to follow through, especially if the family is overwhelmed by too many suggestions at one time? The multicultural aspect of community-based nursing demands that the nurse be familiar with the client's culture, particularly its frame of reference to time and goal setting. Nurses must remember that time-driven dates and appointments are characteristic of industrialized, Western society and may not be valued in the same way by people of other cultures.

5. Do you tend to be trustworthy when people ask you to do something or to follow through? It is extremely important that nurses follow through with what has been promised to clients in the time frame in which it was presented. This is part of building the trust relationship that is so important in community-based care, in which nurses work with clients over long periods of time. It is also important for nurses to allow clients time to do their part in securing resources so that they become more independent in self-care.

Remember: Ask yourself these questions when working with clients. Your answers will affect the relationship you will establish with your clients. The nurse-client interactions determine the success of the outcomes.

In addition, certain factors related to the client also must be considered. Client reactions serve as important indicators of whether the referral process will reap positive benefits. Clients may be fearful of new responsibilities. Following through on referrals to community resources requires a good deal of self-reliance and independence that can be very daunting. They are sometimes doubtful about their abilities to follow through with self-care plans. Talk with them about this. Ask about their past reactions when they have had to do something new. If they have followed through in the past, you are probably on safe ground. However, if they have been nonadherent, you must pay close attention, because they may have doubts and will not follow through with the plan or referral process. After all, this plan should be designed and implemented by the nurse and client in collaboration.

Clients need to accept the current plan for the use of resources as outlined, despite their doubts, fears, or previous experiences. Nurses need to accept clients as they are and work from there. The decisions made about using resources impacts the life of the client and their family in ways that are sometimes known only to them.

It is also crucial for the community-based nurse to follow the results of the client contact with the resource, thereby closing the loop of the referral. Was it a successful encounter? What kind of reception did the client or family member receive? Were they satisfied with their experience, and do they understand what needs to be done next?

The essence of the relationship between the client and the nurse is trust. Checking the outcome of the referral helps to foster that trust. In addition, the nurse may need to follow up with a worker at the resource agency to determine the worker's impression of the outcome of the referral. It is also important to thank the helping agency for the assistance provided to the client. This provides valuable information to the community-based nurse about whether client referrals to a particular resource agency are appropriate so that the nurse knows whether this agency can be used again for other clients with similar needs.

TIPS FOR SUCCESS

Now that you have a good idea of why community-based nurses need to be familiar with the referral process and the resources available, as well as how to locate and access these resources, let's review a few basics that enhance the likelihood of successful outcomes with our clients:

1. Network by asking peers and others working in your setting which agencies or services they have used successfully to help with a particular problem; in other words, say, "I have a client with sickle cell anemia. What resources do you know of for a family dealing with this problem?"

2. Be an effective resource manager by building your own resource list. Use the telephone book, community resource guides, and Internet sites to locate potential referrals. Use index cards or a computer file to keep the information organized and in alphabetical order so you can easily access it for future use or in networking.

3. Be sure to call or visit each of your listed resources to be sure that the services are still available. Information in the telephone book and on the Internet is not always current. Find out what criteria are needed to qualify for the resource. Do clients need to bring financial information to qualify? Does the agency require appointments or does it offer drop-in services? Does the agency offer transportation? Child care?

4. If you are considering referring clients to a hotline, it may be significant to know where the hotline is located. Some hotlines are able to refer clients to specific local services and others provide more generalized counseling and information. It can be frustrating for clients to place telephone calls and not reach the type of services they need.

> *Most of the people that we visit are "multiproblem families." They have so many needs . . . sometimes it's really hard to know what to do first . . . to decide which resource is most important to get them to first.*

Read the case study in Box 9–4 and answer the questions.

Box 9-4	Student Learning Activity

Client Situation

As a community-based nurse, you receive a referral from the prenatal clinic to visit Yolanda Garcia because she has missed several maternity clinic appointments and has no telephone. She speaks little English and lives with her boyfriend in a two-bedroom apartment that they share with two other families. She is in her seventh month of pregnancy and has no other children.

You begin your visit with a brief review of her health, and you find that her blood pressure is 180/86, and her ankles are swollen. The fetal heart rate is 140 beats per minute, strong, and regular. Yolanda complains of a headache that has lasted about 4 or 5 days; she denies double vision. She complains of constant thirst and frequent urination. She is unsure of her weight gain and complains of fatigue.

The four-room apartment is clean yet crowded. Each bedroom is inhabited by one family with four members—a mother, a father, and two preschool-age children. Yolanda sleeps on the couch in the living room. There is no place set aside for the forthcoming newborn. A little girl is playing on the living room floor and appears to be unable to walk, although Yolanda says she is 3 years old. Yolanda also tells you that the girl was born in Mexico and has lived in the United States for 6 months with her parents, who are both unemployed and undocumented.

- What do you see as the major health problems? How would you prioritize these problems?

- What kinds of resources need to be arranged or organized so that Yolanda can be evaluated medically?

- What factors do you need to consider in planning referrals for Yolanda?

- How will you address the missed clinic appointments?

The number one priority in this situation is medical evaluation for the symptoms that suggest Yolanda may be experiencing eclampsia. Although Yolanda may not understand the potential seriousness of these symptoms, it is crucial that the nurse help her to see the urgency of her need for medical attention. What are the factors that lead you to this nursing diagnosis? They include the elevated blood pressure, her headache, swollen feet, polyuria, and fatigue.

Yolanda also explains that she was given an appointment at the clinic for 10 A.M., but the buses she needed to get to the clinic only run in rush hour. Therefore she could not ride the bus and her boyfriend took the car for his job. A taxi ride to the clinic costs $15.00, and this was money she did not have. She did not understand that she could call the clinic for help with transportation. Who speaks Spanish at the clinic? Who can Yolanda call to confirm the appointment and get transportation in Spanish? Who should Yolanda see in the clinic? These are the questions that Yolanda needed help to answer.

There are other obvious problems in this situation that are not related to the immediate priority of our identified client. The nurse should leave the door open for further investigation as well as further interventions. The following are some possible problems that may need to be considered:

- Inadequate housing
- Unreliable transportation
- 3-year-old with possible developmental delays
- Nutritional status of the family
- Language barriers

It should be noted that the nurse must be attuned to the whole picture from the client's viewpoint. Many clients must have the proposed plan broken down into a step-by-step progression to attain the goal. This is called individualizing the care plan. Clients often appreciate a concrete approach in a complex situation. The K.I.S.S. rule applies here: keep it short and simple. People have lived in this situation for a time, and the situations do not need to be changed overnight. Small steps are critical for the achievement of positive outcomes.

For example, you first need to discuss the problem list with the family members to understand their priorities. They may tell you that they feel extremely inhibited by their inability to speak English. The most important resources would then center around English as a second language classes, which are often available for free in churches, adult education centers, and community centers. In addition, you want to share names of community resources that have interpreters available. At the same time, you want to provide specific information for a maternity evaluation through the local health department, assuring the mother that the provider will be able to converse with her in her native language. You could also help connect Yolanda and her family with Women, Infants, and Children (WIC) services to begin the process of improving the family's nutritional status.

Community-based nurses may feel frustrated when clients are not as receptive to referrals and resources as the nurse feels they should be:

Don't they realize how much work it takes to get them these services? This help does not fall from the sky! They should be grateful for the help we find for them. I just don't understand.

Box 9–5 provides an example of a client situation to help you to test your knowledge of community resources.

The nurse neglected to ask the client whether she wanted a bed. She did not seek collaboration with the client for the plan. She thought that the family would want and use all of the furniture. If she had asked about sleeping arrangements, she would have discovered that in Ms. Ling's culture, there is a belief that evil spirits live under beds. Ms. Ling will probably never sleep on a traditional frame bed that sits off the floor. This is an example of not getting all the facts, assuming values, and not questioning or discussing cultural differences.

The nurse assumed that the client's backache was caused by sleeping on the floor, when, in fact, she had been lifting heavy boxes. She did a family assessment, but did not communicate with her client. She did not accurately assess the need for resources. Remember to ask the question "Who?" and to think about the client and the whole family. Include in your assessment the social, physical, and emotional, as well as cultural, aspects of the client. When the nurse became annoyed with the client's behavior, it was negative for the nurse–client relationship.

Box 9-5   Student Learning Activity

Client Situation

There has recently been an influx of immigrants from Southeast Asia, and the community-based nurse has been working to get physical evaluations and other health services for the members of the Ling family. The nurse has home-visited Ms. Ling several times to complete the family assessment. During these visits, she noticed that Ms. Ling sleeps on the floor on a bamboo mat. The apartment is sparsely furnished. The nurse located some secondhand furniture from a nearby community church and worked very hard to get the furniture moved to the apartment. After 3 weeks, another community agency donated a bed. The nurse was very excited about the bed, because she felt it would help with Ms. Ling's lower back pain. During the next scheduled home visit, she noticed the unassembled bed, with the straw mat lying on the floor next to it. The nurse asked, "Don't you like the bed? Did you have trouble putting it together? Do you think it will be uncomfortable?"

The nurse was distressed. Didn't Ms. Ling know that others could use the bed if she didn't want it? The nurse thought to herself, "How ungrateful of her. After all that work!"

• How would you address this problem?

• Who has the problem, the client or the nurse?

• Which resources would most benefit the client?

• What questions would you ask the client?

• What will you tell Ms. Ling when you visit her again?

What happens when the resource is not used? It must be remembered that it is the client's choice to use or not to use a resource. The nurse must live with the decision and not impart a negative attitude toward the client or family.

By carefully answering the commonsense questions of who, what, when, where, and how, and by taking into account circumstances such as feelings, history, and barriers, the nurse should be able to share resources with clients with positive outcomes. These questions highlight the core of the referral process. They help evaluate the process and the outcomes of care. They enable the nurse to center on a concern for the total well-being of the client and family. The referral process involves the client, the family, and all caregivers interacting toward a common goal in the communication process. It is an open system that is ongoing. There is a continuing collaboration among various team members as well as different health-care providers. All members involved must have an open communication system that results in appropriate options for the client and, hopefully, decreases the duplication of services among the different systems involved.

As the resource manager, the community-based nurse is a partner in the client's corner to help obtain the desired outcome. You are not alone in locating resources. You are merely the facilitator for the client or the family in need. Choices about the use of resources belong to the client. You cannot make an individual or family do something they do not wish to do. Noncompliance may reflect a person's or family's effort to control the situation to meet personal needs. Today's nurses need patience and persistence to ensure success in the referral process and use of community resources.

NURSING RESEARCH IN COMMUNITY RESOURCES

Research opportunities abound for inquisitive nurses interested in exploring the impact of the referral process and the use of community resources on client outcomes. Although the current literature suggests that the referral process and the location and evaluation of community resources with clients are crucial components of community-based and population-focused nursing (Armentrout, 1998; Clark, 1999; Hunt & Zurek, 1997), little has been written to document the impact of these resources on client outcomes. This is partially because of the nature of community services as they are distributed over time and influenced by multiple variables, making it difficult for the researcher to isolate the impact of a particular resource. Another challenge in this type of research is the difficulty separating the outcome from the process used and the characteristics of the nurses and other providers acting on behalf of their clients (Chan, Mackenzie, Ng, & Leung, 2000).

A review of the literature reveals three populations that have been studied in relation to their changing health needs and the effectiveness of referrals to community services in meeting those health needs: elderly clients wishing to remain independent, chronically mentally ill patients, and high-risk teenage mothers and their infants. Through interviews with elderly clients maintaining their own homes, Krothe identified formal and informal care resources that the interviewees considered essential to their independence (1997). In another report, the author outlined the work done in Oregon to redirect funding to create a "long-term care service network" to support senior and disabled citizens in maintaining independent living (Dietsche, 1996). Both authors report the satisfaction of the clients and improvement in their health when services were accessible to them.

As discussed at the beginning of this chapter, changes in the structure and reimbursement mechanisms of the health-care system have resulted in more chronically ill patients leaving institutions and living in the community. Clients with chronic mental illness are no exception. Salem reported on the need for a diversity of service and resource options that are selected with input from the clients for this group to be successful in community environments (1990). Similarly, the case management model was found to be more effective with community-based schizophrenic clients when the case manager worked closely with other providers to ensure continuity and a diversity of services (Chan et al., 2000).

Finally, much research has been done in the area of interventions that are most successful with very young parents and their infants. Although the findings are somewhat conflicting, there is evidence that home visitation by nurses to these clients can reduce the number of subsequent pregnancies, the use of welfare, and child abuse and neglect (Olds et al., 1997). As part of the pre-natal and early home-visitation program, multiple resources and services are offered to these young women and their children through collaborative planning with the nurse. Similarly, women enrolled in an intensive early intervention program that included home visits and referrals to other services had reduced rates of premature birth and low-birth-weight infants (Koniak-Griffin, Anderson, Verzemnieks, & Brecht, 2000). In both studies, the researchers were careful not to directly relate the outcomes to any one part of the process. The overall impact of increased contact with the nurse and other health services through referral and health education was positive and worthy of replication studies. Clearly, there is a great need for continued research.

Active Learning Strategies

1. As an exercise to aid in understanding resources, choose a community agency of interest to you, for example, the American Heart Association. Find the funding source. Then ask how much money is spent on patient education or research. How much money is devoted to services? How do community members access the services? Finally, what are the services provided by this agency to you, the nurse?

2. You are home visiting an elderly widower who is no longer able to cook his meals each day. He has asked you to find him someone to cook for him or deliver meals to him. Your community has an active volunteer service called "Meals-on-Wheels." You arrange with your client for him to receive meals daily. Construct a survey form to assess his satisfaction with this service. List at least five questions that you would need to ask your client to evaluate the quality and reliability of the service.

3. Use the telephone directory to find hotline numbers for a client experiencing a manic episode, a woman being abused by her husband, a college student who has been raped, and a teenager with an alcohol dependency problem. How accessible are the hotlines? How do they respond to the calls that they receive?

4. Think about a resource that you have personally used as a student or as a health-care consumer that was particularly helpful to you or a family member. What was it about the resource that made it such a positive experience? How did you first find out about it? To who else would you recommend it? (Think about both private and public sector agencies.)

References

Armentrout, G. (1998). Community based nursing: Foundations for practice. Stamford, CT: Appleton & Lange.

Chan, S., Mackenzie, A., Ng, D., & Leung, J. (2000). An evaluation of the implementation of case management in the community psychiatric nursing service. Journal of Advanced Nursing, 31(1), 144–156.

Clark, M. J. (1999). Nursing in the community: Dimensions of community health nursing (3rd ed.). Stamford, CT: Appleton & Lange.

Dickerson, S. S., Peters, D., Walkowiak, J., & Brewer, C. (1999). Active learning strategies to teach case management. Nurse Educator, 24(5), 52–57.

Dietsche, S. (1996). Oregon's long-term care system—from nursing facility to community-based care: An evolution. Nutrition Reviews, 54(1), S48–S50.

Hodson-Carlton, K., & Dorner, J. L. (1999). An electric approach to evaluating healthcare web resources. Nurse Educator, 24(5), 4–5.

Hunt, R., & Zurek, E. (1997). Introduction to community based nursing. Philadelphia: Lippincott Williams & Wilkins.

Koniak-Griffin, D., Anderson, N., Verzemnieks, I., & Brecht, M (2000). A public health nursing early intervention program for adolescent mothers: Outcomes from pregnancy through 6 weeks postpartum. Nursing Research, 49(3), 130–138.

Krothe, J. S. (1997). Giving voice to elderly people: Community-based long-term care. Public Health Nursing, 14, 217–226.

Olds, D. L., Eckenrode, J., Henderson, C. R., Kitzman, H., Powers, J., Cole, R., Sidora, K., Morris, P., Pettitt, L. M., & Luckey, D. (1997). Long-term effects of home visitation on maternal life course and child abuse and neglect. Journal of the American Medical Association, 278(8), 637–643.

Salem, D. A. (1990). Community-based services and resources: The significance of choice and diversity. American Journal of Community Psychology, 18, 909–915.

Spradley, B., & Allender, J. (1996). Community health nursing concepts and practice. Philadelphia: Lippincott Williams & Wilkins.

Stanhope, M., & Lancaster, J. (1996). Community health nursing: Promoting health of aggregates, families and individuals. St. Louis: Mosby.

Zerwehk, J. V. (1997). Opening doors to public health nursing: A guidebook. Fairfield, CT: T. S. Media.

CHAPTER **10**

Alternative/ Complementary Health Practices— A New, Yet Old Area for Community-based Nursing Practice

Mary Anne Noble

LEARNING OBJECTIVES

1) Develop a beginning understanding of the history and current status of alternative health treatments and modalities.

2) Explore the underlying theories and principles of selected alternative therapies and modalities.

3) Understand the nursing profession's contributions and participation in the field of alternative health.

4) Develop beginning assessment and evaluation guidelines for advising patients as they seek alternative health treatments.

A BEGINNING STORY

Nancy, a new graduate nurse, was working in a community mental health center. As a nursing student, she did clinical work in a similar setting, so she was prepared for the types of patients and their mental health problems. What she wasn't prepared for were the many questions and concerns of both patients and families that she now had to address as a graduate nurse. For instance, one patient who tended to take his antidepressant medications inconsistently because of both cost and side effects asked her about using St. John's Wort. He felt that because it was a natural substance, he would feel better taking it. He was also concerned about having a "record" with his insurance company and possibly with his employer. He was currently not taking all his prescribed medication and was substituting some St. John's Wort. Nancy knew little about herbal medications, and she was not sure how to find out more.

Two family members of different patients asked Nancy about using acupuncture in one case and ayurvedic medicine in another.

Their concerns were similar. In the case of acupuncture the wife knew that acupuncture was based on an energy and meridian theory, and she thought that it might be helpful in treating her husband's addiction problems because a friend of hers found some success with acupuncture. This woman was discouraged that her husband's progress with conventional psychiatric treatment was so slow and unreliable. In the other case, a husband was wondering if he should try ayurvedic medicine for his wife because he had heard it was an ancient comprehensive system of medicine for mental and physical illnesses. He, too, was discouraged by the slow, unpredictable progress his wife was making with conventional psychiatric treatment. In both cases, Nancy knew nothing about these alternative therapies. They were not covered in her basic nursing program. Her only knowledge of these therapies was through the popular press, which she considered unreliable at best.

Finally, a mother and father approached Nancy about their schizophrenic teenage son. They were very disheartened as they witnessed what seemed to be becoming a chronic condition. They had done some reading and talking to friends, and they had come to the conclusion that their son might have a "spiritual" problem as a result of soul loss. They wondered if they should consult a shaman who was skilled in soul retrieval, or if they should look into more conventional spiritual therapies that focused on prayer and the laying on of hands. Nancy was at a total loss to advise these parents. On one hand, she knew that there were fraudulent New Age therapies to which vulnerable patients and families were victims. On the other hand, she knew that spirituality and healing was a fast-growing and respected area.

It is for reasons such as these that nurses in all community areas need some knowledge in the rapidly growing field of alternative health. This knowledge has not yet been adequately integrated into most nursing curricula. This chapter provides introductory information for this rapidly evolving area of interest.

BACKGROUND

The field of alternative and complementary health and medicine is a natural field for nursing, and furthermore, it is almost entirely community based. The theoretical underpinnings of alternative health (the most popular term) propose that health and illness are complex inter-

actions of the mind, body, and spirit. Furthermore, it proposes that many aspects of clients' health experiences are not subject to traditional scientific methods.

From the days of Florence Nightingale, nursing has voiced the importance of the body/mind/spirit in illness and health. Nursing has always had a holistic, multidimensional approach to health and illness. Furthermore, the terms holistic nursing and holistic care are not new and date back at least 20 years, if not longer. In addition, nursing has objected to the mechanistic and materialistic view of the human being, as was so long the model in Western medicine. To nurses, the human being was always more than the sum of his or her parts. This view partly stems from the fact that nursing has been a profession that frequently deals with dying patients and their families, and from the understanding that illness is not always curable—hence the concept of care and healing.

Nursing has long recognized a nonmaterial reality. The mind and spirit, by definition, are nonmaterial. Nursing has been defined as both an art and a science. Although the art role has not been as well developed or recognized, it nonetheless represents the intangible and intuitive role that lends itself, with difficulty, to scientific investigation and that is so important in the field of alternative medicine.

With these thoughts in mind, then, nursing has a pivotal role to play in the emerging field of alternative health and medicine. Nurses in all specialties or fields and in all settings can participate in this field of health care. Some traditional nursing roles and functions are a vital part of alternative modalities. Take touch, for instance. Nurses have always touched patients, often for comfort, as in the time-honored back rub. The field of therapeutic or healing touch, pioneered by nurses, is an example of an alternative modality that is an extension of this traditional nursing role.

Alternative medicine has been defined as those treatments or therapies that are not traditionally taught in medical schools and not covered by health insurance. Sometimes the field is referred to as those treatments or modalities that are unproven or experimental. This picture is rapidly changing; the curricula of many medical schools now include alternative medicine (otherwise known as complementary or integrative medicine, as some authorities prefer). Both acupuncture and chiropractic treatments are now covered by some insurance carriers. Nonetheless, alternative medicine continues to be a field that does not lend itself readily to scientific study or investigation and is therefore not easily embraced by many hard-core scientists. However, this field is embraced by more and more persons in the Western world. Alternative medicine's increasing popularity is evidenced by the fact that the entire November 11, 1998, issue of the Journal of the American Medical Association was devoted to the field. The Office of Alternative Medicine at the National Institutes of Health perhaps first legitimized the field in this country in the last decade. Just at the end of 1998, the Office was elevated to a Center. Its new name is the National Center for Complementary and Alternative Medicine.

Much of what we consider to be alternative medicine comes from the Eastern world, from which there is a substantial literature; unfortunately, this literature is not written in English. Alternative medicine also traces its roots to folk medicine, Native American medicine, Shamanism, and psychic healing. The history of alternative medicine is very much tied to religious and spiritual practices, and in many cultures the healer was a religious practitioner.

There are several important points to stress in this rapidly emerging field. The first is that there is no unifying basic theory for the vast array of treatments or modalities except, as noted previously, that health and illness are considered to be complex interactions among the body, mind, and spirit. There is a definite distinction between the mind and the spirit—the spirit is the eternal aspect of the human being, and the spirit can indeed be ill even when the body and mind appear to be healthy. Health and illness are considered mysterious processes, and the healer (or alternative practitioner) does not claim to have all the answers. Many modalities use an energy theory, and the source of that energy is often seen as coming from God, although the use of the word *God* is frowned on by some authorities. Other words or terms are used such as *Force* or *Universal Energy.*

Another important point to stress is that as a result of the increasing popularity of the field, there is increasing fraud and quackery. Guidelines for assessing practitioners and treatments are presented later in this chapter. It is very important for nurses at all levels and in all specialties to take a critical viewpoint of the field so that they can counsel and refer patients as they seek treatment.

Finally, it is important to stress that many alternative health-care practitioners have little or no formal or academic education in their specific practice, yet they are effective and legitimate. They may have learned their therapeutic practice informally or through an apprenticeship. However, if a practitioner is well educated, especially with a graduate degree, he or she is likely to be that much more credible and will be able to communicate and teach both patients and the public. As the field grows, education, certification, licensing, and credentialing are increasingly important. Box 10–1 allows you to practice assisting a client to resolve a dilemma.

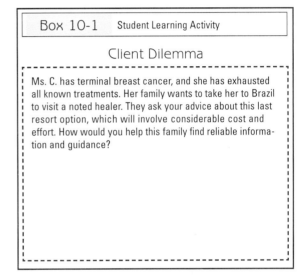

Box 10-1   Student Learning Activity

Client Dilemma

Ms. C. has terminal breast cancer, and she has exhausted all known treatments. Her family wants to take her to Brazil to visit a noted healer. They ask your advice about this last resort option, which will involve considerable cost and effort. How would you help this family find reliable information and guidance?

With these introductory thoughts, then, it is obvious that alternative medicine is here to stay. A recent poll indicated that 42 percent of Americans use some form of complementary and alternative medicine (CAM). This was an increase from 33 percent reported in 1993 (Eisenberg et al., 1998). It is important for the nurse to have at least introductory information about the major alternative therapies.

Definitions

The terms alternative health or alternative medicine are most frequently used. Most journals in the field also use these terms. Recently, the term complementary medicine has emerged. Many physicians prefer this term because this approach views alternative medicine as complementary to conventional medicine. However, for much of the world, this is irrelevant because what we define as alternative medicine is primary medicine for them. In other words, they never use conventional medicine. *Unorthodox* medicine, *Eastern* medicine, *Holistic* medicine, and *Integrative* medicine are other terms in use.

Conventional medicine is often called allopathic medicine or Western medicine to denote that it is primarily practiced in the Western world. Sometimes it is also referred to as the dominant medicine. Broadly, and perhaps too simply, the tools or methods used by conventional medicine are synthetic drugs, surgery, radiation, and the psychotherapies. The psychotherapies have never been fully accepted by all of conventional medicine, particularly in recent years, because mental illness and mental health problems are perceived to be primarily a brain dysfunction or a brain disease.

The tools or methods used by alternative medicine are almost too numerous to mention. They include material as well as nonmaterial methods. They include natural medicines such as herbs, needles, pressure, food, aroma, imagery, manipulation, touch, sound, color, light, thought, meditation, and prayer. Lately, there has been an emphasis on energy that is not measurable by ordinary means and that does not respond to the laws of time and space. If you tend to become skeptical at the outset, it is important to emphasize that there is considerable evidence for this approach in field theory and in quantum physics.

Table 10–1 presents a list of alternative modalities from *Alternative Therapies in Health and Medicine,* which is the most prestigious journal in the field and which is scientifically and research based.

As stated in *Alternative Therapies,* alternative therapies or modalities are not limited to those in Table 10–1. The focus of the journal is the scientific investigation of alternative therapies, and there are many other therapies about which there is very little literature.

Description of Selected Alternative Therapies with Nursing Implications

At this point it may be helpful to describe a few of the more commonly used alternative therapies, particularly because nurses may be involved either by participating or by referring patients.

Acupuncture

Acupuncture is an ancient therapy that originated in China perhaps as long as 5000 years ago. It was part of a system known as traditional Chinese medicine and is based on the belief that health requires a balanced flow of vital life energy known as *chi*. The life force circulates along energy pathways called meridians, and each meridian is associated with specific organs or functions. Illness and imbalance result when chi stagnates or is blocked or weakened. Acupuncturists restore the flow of chi by inserting very thin needles along critical acupuncture points. Ultimately, the theory behind this treatment is that acupuncture stimulates the body's natural healing abilities. The treatment is generally painless or very nearly so. Acupuncture is thought to treat a wide variety of conditions, and there is much disagreement among practitioners as to its use. However, most practitioners recognize that pain responds well to acupuncture (Holistic and Metaphysical Resource Book, 1997).

Acupuncture is gradually becoming accepted in this country, and some major insurance companies cover treatment. Education, licensing, and credentialing vary widely from state to state (Leake & Broderick, 1999). Many physicians become licensed by completing 200 hours beyond their basic medical education. Other acupuncturists complete a master's degree in acupuncture after completing a bachelor's degree in one of a variety of fields. A doctor of oriental medicine (DOM) has a completely different educational pathway that is often combined with Chinese herbal medicine. A nurse can usually become an acupuncturist by completing a master's degree in acupuncture after first obtaining a bachelor's degree in nursing. Such is the case in one of the interviews featured later in this chapter. Acupuncture can become a natural extension of the nurse's basic role.

Ayurvedic Medicine

Ayurvedic medicine is a very ancient and comprehensive system of healing that originated in India. It is thought by some scholars to be the oldest system in existence. It regards physical and mental health as the foundations for a creative and spiritual life.

Table 10-1

Alternative Treatments or Modalities as Reported in Alternative Therapies in Health and Medicine

Anthroposophy	Manipulation
Ayurveda	Massage
Behavioral medicine	Meditation
Bioelectromagnetic therapy	Mental healing
Biofeedback	Mind-body therapies (including behavioral and educational aspects)
Biofield	
Biologic/pharmacologic treatments	Naturopathy
Chinese medicine (including acupuncture, acupressure, *qi gong*, and traditional)	Nonlocal therapies
	Nutrition
Chiropractic medicine	Osteopathic medicine
Craniosacraltherapies	Placebo
Creative therapies (including art, dance, drama, and music)	Psychoneuroimmunology
Diet	Psychotherapy
Environmental medicine	Reflexology
Health promotion	Relaxation
Herbal remedies	Religion
Homeopathy	Spiritual/transpersonal healing
Hypnotherapy	Touch
Imagery	Tibetan medicine
Indigenous medical practices (including Native American healing practices and shamanism)	Vitamin treatments

Critical to this system of medicine are the three mind-body types of *Vata*, *Pitta*, and *Kapha*. Dietary habits, sleeping habits, and lifestyle are major components in health and illness. The ayurvedic doctor or practitioner does a comprehensive assessment and works with the patient in these areas. Sometimes it is possible to find a physician who incorporates elements of ayurvedic medicine in his or her practice. Ayurvedic medicine can be indicated for a variety of health problems and can be combined with conventional medicine in a complementary manner. As with other forms of alternative modalities, ayurvedic medicine is increasing in popularity in this country (Holistic and Metaphysical Resource Book, 1997.).

Chiropractic Medicine

Chiropractic medicine originated in this country about a century ago. It is the largest alternative health profession in North America. It involves manual adjustments to the spinal column and musculoskeletal system to enable electrical impulses from the brain to travel through the nervous system. The theory of chiropractic medicine is that the nervous system coordinates the function of all other body systems. Subluxations or spinal misalignments can cause nerve interference, pain, and illness. Chiropractors take a health history, X-rays, and an evaluation of the spine. Patients usually lie on a table fully clothed for treatment while the chiropractor makes manual adjustments. Again, treatment is usually painless. It is very popular for back, neck, and shoulder pain as well as treatment for traumas and injuries. There is disagreement among practitioners, however, about its usefulness for other conditions (Holistic and Metaphysical Resource Book, 1997).

For years, chiropractic medicine was frowned on by conventional medicine. However, people have been going

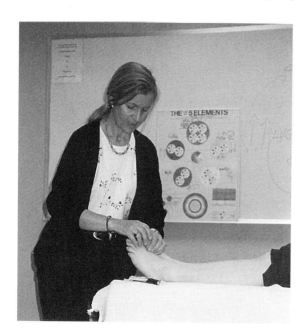

to chiropractors for years without telling their medical doctors. Many people are absolutely convinced of their worth and use them as practitioners for other conditions. Now many health insurance companies cover treatment, and chiropractors are gaining increased respect. According to a recent survey, the education and training of medical and chiropractic doctors share common areas in the clinical sciences (Coulter, Adams, Coggan, Wilkes, & Gonyea, 1998). A doctor of chiropractic is designated as DC. Again, nurses can and do become chiropractors, but then they provide chiropractic services not nursing. Box 10–2 provides an opportunity for you to list helpful advice about chiropractic services.

Box 10-2	Student Learning Activity

Client Example

Mr. B. has severe back pain and asks you about chiropractic medicine. What would you tell him? How might you help him find a reputable practitioner?

Herbal Medicine

One student told the following story:

I spent a major part of my childhood living in Marin County, California, in a suburb of the Bay area. One of my mother's favorite haunts was Chinatown in San Francisco, where she had a favorite shop that absolutely fascinated me. There were dead chickens and ducks hanging by their necks in the front window and glass jars filled with various kinds of teas and dried herbs. The smell of sandalwood incense permeated the shop, and I often felt like I was visiting another world when we went inside. Here I learned about Liang tea, a common Chinese remedy used to treat fever, and how to use crystallized ginger to make a tea to combat sinus congestion, sore throats, and coughs caused by colds. I can't remember one winter as a child when I did not have Tiger balm smeared over my throat and chest. My mother usually wrapped a washrag around my neck bandit style and fastened it with a safety pin to keep the warmth in. I can still smell that sweet camphor odor that engulfed our house during the winter months.

Perhaps no other alternative modality is as popular today as herbal medicine. There are numerous herbal and health food stores, and the claims for the effectiveness of herbs and food supplements are numerous. Some of these claims are fraudulent. It is difficult for the consumer and the health-care provider to assess and evaluate products. The nurse in all specialties needs to be as knowledgeable as possible about the use of herbs. A few simple points are worth mentioning. First, herbs and herbal medicines are not necessarily harmless just because they are natural. Second, herbs by the same name are not always equal; preparations and manufacturers can vary considerably. Third, herbal preparations can interact adversely with synthetic medicines and with food. And fourth, information regarding dosage, indications for use, side effects, and contraindications is not readily available. However, it is noteworthy that the first *Physician's Desk Reference (PDR) on Herbal Medicine* was published in December of 1998.

Box 10–3 provides an opportunity to list questions and advice related to one client's use of St. John's Wort.

Box 10-3 Student Learning Activity
Client Example
Mr. X. confides in you that he is taking St. John's Wort for his depression. What questions would you ask him, and what advice would you give him?

Homeopathy

A nursing student described her experiences with homeopathy:

I moved to Kaiserslautern, Germany, where I encountered a very new way of life. The folk medicine practices I discovered while living in Germany were often interlinked with the practice of homeopathy. Most of my German friends would often visit their local apothecary to obtain herbal substances that they would use in their homeopathic remedies, many of which had been passed down to them from their mothers. One of my elderly neighbors in the small village of Morlautern where I lived would go to the woods every spring and collect small buds from a particular pine tree. She would boil the buds in water, which she would drain off and use with sugar and other herbs to make a cough syrup for her family.

Homeopathy has been a respected alternative therapy or treatment for several centuries. For years it was a threat to conventional medicine, and it is currently more popular in England and other European countries than it is in the United States. Homeopathy defies the laws of chemistry, physics, and pharmacology. Homeopathic medicines contain substances that cause the very symptoms one wants to eliminate. The medicines are made by repeatedly diluting the active ingredient, and the more dilute a preparation is the more potent it is purported to be. The theory underlying homeopathy is called the Law of Similars, which maintains that "like cures like." In other words, getting rid of symptoms immediately may help the patient to feel better temporarily, but it won't help the healing process. Symptoms are not seen as the enemy or as the disease itself, but are signs of the body's effort to deal with the disease. Furthermore, symptoms are a part of the healing process and should be stimulated and supported rather than suppressed (Bruning, 1995; Chapman, 1999).

Homeopaths tend to spend a lot of time initially with their patients taking a detailed history and evaluating the patient holistically. They emphasize prevention and stress management. Homeopathy has been growing in this country in recent years, and common homeopathic remedies can be found in many drugstores and other health stores. A homeopathic medical doctor is designated by HMD or

DHt, and physicians often practice homeopathy under their conventional licenses. Many insurance plans also cover homeopathy (Chapman, 1999). Box 10–4 allows you to integrate and apply what has been discussed.

Box 10-4	Student Learning Activity

Client Example

Your client tells you that his neighbor took a homeopathic remedy for flu and that it was very effective. He asks you for the name of the remedy and whether you think it would be better for him than getting a flu shot. What would you tell him?

Spiritual Therapies

A nursing student shares an important memory:

One of my most memorable experiences in regard to folk medicine and healing occurred during my trip to the Santuario de Chimayo in northern New Mexico on Easter weekend. The town of Chimayo lies between the cities of Santa Fe and Albuquerque in the foothills of the Sangre de Christo Mountains. Every year during holy week people from all over the country come there to make their annual personal and collective pilgrimages. They come with faith that they or their loved ones will be healed. They light candles, touch the wooden saints, pray at the altar and most of all they come to obtain the sacred dirt that is housed within the church. The holy dirt is believed to have healing powers, and the walls surrounding the inside of the church are covered with crutches, statues of the Virgin Mary, paintings and photographs that have been left by those who have been healed. It is truly a wondrous place, and I felt very close to God as I walked through the church and around the grounds. I was surrounded by many other people who obviously felt the same way, as I learned that many of them continue to come to Santuario de Chimayo year after year to renew their faith and pray for healing.

Spiritual healing is a fast-growing area, perhaps the newest in the alternative health field. However, it is also probably the oldest therapy, and has been used in every culture throughout history in some form. Many alternative modalities such as the touch therapies, ayurvedic medicine, and meditation claim to have a spiritual focus or component. In fact, as stated earlier, the field of alternative health in general can be called spiritual because of the underlying recognition that the human being is body, mind, and spirit, and that reality is nonmaterial as well as material. Nurses are necessarily involved with aspects of the spiritual therapies because of their holistic heritage and because of their work with patients in critical care, hospice, and so forth. Two leaders in the field of spirituality and health are Dr. Larry Dossey and his wife Barbara Dossey, originally a critical care nurse. Their writings are crucial to nurses interested in this area. Another authority is Dr. Herbert Benson from Harvard University.

A number of spiritual assessment scales exist. Spiritual therapies also lean heavily on the cultural background of many groups of people. It is noteworthy that in many Asian cultures there is no dichotomy between health practitioners and religious or spiritual practitioners. Folk medicine and shamanism are two topics relevant to the nurse interested in this area.

Touch Therapies

The touch therapies include therapeutic touch, healing touch, reiki, pranic healing, and others. Therapeutic touch and healing touch originated in this country. Delores Kreiger, a nursing professor at New York University, is credited with developing therapeutic touch in the early seventies. The theories behind the touch therapies are very similar. These therapies work with the patient's energy fields and the aura that surrounds the body. The practitioner becomes centered or grounded and receives energy from the Universal Source or God (as is most frequently stated) and then channels this energy to the patient. The reiki practitioner actually touches and holds his or her hands on the patient, whereas the other therapies frequently do not. Intentionality is a critical factor for the practitioner; in other words, to be effective, the practitioner must have the positive intention to help the patient. Education and certification vary widely. Although therapeutic

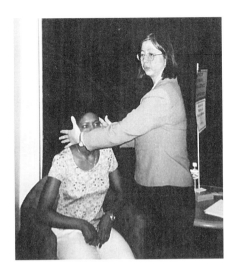

touch was scorned and ridiculed when it first became known, now many health professionals incorporate touch therapy in their practice. Nurses are probably at the forefront of this modality. The touch therapies are used to relieve pain and stress, to speed wound healing, to reduce inflammation, and for many other conditions.

Guidelines for Assessment

Following are guidelines or rules for assessing an alternative health practitioner or alternative health services, workshops, and literature. These guidelines are an outgrowth of professional and personal experience as well as the experience of students through the last 10 years. The list is not meant to be authoritative or dogmatic, because these dimensions do not exist in the field of alternative health or for that matter in conventional medicine either. Rather, they are simply suggestions based on some knowledge of the field.

1. Look for licenses, certifications, credentialing, and professional organizations to which the practitioner belongs. These often give credibility to the practitioner, and organizations provide a watchdog-like service.
2. Flyers sent through the mail, including coupons, and advertising in general are often a bad sign. These activities suggest that the practitioner may be desperate for customers and runs his or her practice primarily as a business.
3. Practitioners who have been in practice for a long time are likely to be credible. Quacks and fraudulent practitioners don't last long.
4. Referrals from satisfied patients are the best kind. This testifies to the effectiveness of the practitioner. Ask for these kinds of references.
5. Beware of practitioners who discourage questions from the patient. Look for practitioners who treat patients in a leisurely and relaxed manner. This reflects the underlying theory of alternative health in two ways. First, the interpersonal relationship is critical to the healing process. Second, practitioners are considered to be facilitators and enter into a partnership with the patient. They don't do procedures "to" the patient, but "with" the patient.
6. Beware of practitioners who feel threatened by other practitioners, including both traditional and alternative practitioners. They are afraid their cover is going to be blown.
7. Beware of practitioners who tell patients to follow their treatments to the exclusion of all others. Any reputable practitioner (both traditional and alternative) knows that health and healing are mysterious processes, and no one has all the answers. No one system has a monopoly on health and healing.
8. Beware of practitioners who tell patients not to follow or listen to their own thoughts, feelings, or rationality. A good rule to remember is that human beings were given intelligence for a reason.
9. Ask the practitioner for references or literature on the treatment in question. If he or she can't provide this, be suspicious. Scientific literature in respectable journals provides the best sources.
10. Beware of practitioners, including training courses, herbal supply houses, and so on, where the contact is only a phone number. A specific address is desirable, because one knows that the agency or practitioner is not totally secretive.
11. Beware of practitioners who treat all patients in the same manner, because any reputable health care practitioner knows that human beings are unique and different in their responses to health and illness.
12. Beware of unusual diagnostic procedures, particularly anything that seems inappropriate. This is likely to be fraudulent or quackery.
13. In checking literature on products or treatments, beware of language that makes claims like "miracle cures," "what your doctor won't tell you," "amazing new secrets," "secrets of the Amazon," and so on. The word *secret* is suspect because any practitioner who regards health as a secret is not

trustworthy. Even the word *cure* is suspect because absolute cure is not that simple.

14. Beware of practitioners who are unduly interested in making money. Although everyone has to earn a living, overemphasis on money suggests a lack of commitment, professionalism, and involvement.
15. Look for practitioners who are constantly upgrading their knowledge and skills and are attending workshops and continuing education programs.
16. In assessing literature, products, or training programs look for endorsement from reputable authorities and bibliographic citations.
17. When a practitioner becomes overly concerned with power or fame, or obsessed with his or her ability, then he or she becomes less effective.
18. Look for practitioners who truly "care." Much theory underscores this point. As Agnes Sanford said, "Only love can generate the healing fire" (Sanford, 1949).

Interviews with Alternative Health Practitioners

Following are interviews with four master's-prepared nurses practicing one or more alternative health treatments or modalities. Their stories are interesting and reflect how they got started along this path, the theory underlying their practice, the patients they treat, and how their practice complements conventional medicine and nursing.

Maureen McCracken, MSN, RN, CS

Maureen is a certified Healing Touch practitioner and instructor. Her practice is called McCracken and Associates, PC. Maureen received her BSN and MSN from George Mason University. While working for her master's degree, she focused on long-term care (the most relevant track in the program) and did a supplemental year at the Catholic University of America in family psychotherapy. She then became certified as a clinical specialist by the American Nurses' Association in Adult and Child and Adolescent Psychiatric and Mental Health Nursing.

Maureen became interested in healing touch or therapeutic touch in the mid-1970s while studying at George Mason University when she came across an article by Delores Kreiger. She then met a nurse at George Mason who demonstrated therapeutic touch. Maureen felt the effects of therapeutic touch on herself.

She began to practice therapeutic touch on patients when she worked at the National Institutes of Health for 5 years. She carefully documented her nursing interventions in her computer charting. Shortly afterward she became interested in other forms of alternative health, including homeopathy, as she sought treatment for her own fertility problems. Subsequently, she took all the courses on healing touch through Healing Touch International, Inc., which is endorsed by the American Holistic Nursing Association, and she has been teaching healing touch since 1994. Maureen also does psychotherapy as well as eye movement desensitization and reprocessing (EMDR), which is a procedure used in psychotherapy.

Maureen believes her nursing education prepared her for her career in healing touch in several ways. First, she believes that nursing has always stressed the holistic approach to the human being or the approach of mind, body, and spirit in both illness and health as well as emphasis on family and environment. She also took courses in cultural nursing, which, in addition to growing up overseas, gave her a different perspective on health and illness globally. She lived in Scotland, Germany, Israel, and Switzerland. In Switzerland she lived in a boarding school and witnessed a community approach to health, and in particular the use of herbs for the treatment of illness. Non-Western treatments and interventions were used and respected.

Healing touch, according to Maureen, can be used for a variety of conditions and patient problems. Prime uses are for pain, anxiety, and depression. Healing touch is helpful for many forms of mental illness including the manic phase of bipolar affective disorder, dissociative disorders, obsessive-compulsive disorders, and posttraumatic stress disorders. Healing touch can also be an adjunctive treatment to many chronic diseases including cystic breast disease, arthritis, fibromyalgia, diabetes, and hypertension. Healing touch accelerates wound healing such as lacerations and cuts. Of special interest is the fact that practitioners can use healing touch on themselves with good results.

The underlying theory of healing touch is that it influences the energy system of the person. Maureen believes that it affects the autonomic nervous system, particularly the parasympathetic branch, by putting the body in a resting state. Healing touch induces the relaxation state by decreasing heart rate, lowering blood pressure, and removing blocks from the energy field. When more people are involved in healing touch, the healing is greater. Maureen believes that certification, credentialing, and continuing education are very important for the healing touch practitioner. It is certainly possible for the practitioner to be effective without it, but in her case it means that her practice is reviewed by a panel, that she has had a mentor for a year, and that she must demonstrate to others what she is doing. This is congruent with the guidelines discussed earlier. These approaches enhance the credibility of the practitioner and help prevent the possibility (as often happens in the field of alternative health) that an occasional practitioner becomes so out of touch with mainstream practice as to become fraudulent or a quack.

Finally, Maureen believes that healing touch and alternative medicine in general should be integrated into conventional medicine. In fact, she believes that the two are already becoming integrated as evidenced by the number of medical schools addressing alternative medicine in their curricula. She believes that many doctors integrate various aspects of alternative health into their practice, illustrated in particular by the large numbers of both doctors and patients who believe that prayer is important to healing. She believes that allopathic medicine is far from having answers to many problems. In addition, clients often find that with conventional medicine the cure or treatment is often worse than the disease.

Peggy Brennan, MS, RN, CS

Peggy is a psychiatric clinical nurse specialist. As part of her practice she does hypnosis, guided imagery, visualization, healing touch, and neurolinguistic programming as well as traditional counseling and psychotherapy. She is a certified Practitioner of Hypnosis. Her patients are frequently referred to her by their primary-care physician; some are covered by traditional insurance plans and some are not.

The groundwork for these alternative treatments or modalities was laid in the beginning of Peggy's nursing education, or in "Basic Nursing 101," as she emphatically states. It was there that she was introduced to the concept

that humans are an inseparable whole—body, mind, and spirit. Her basic nursing program taught her that the patient is at the center of treatment and that the family is a part of this treatment. She learned that the patient is more than his or her pathologic condition and that practitioners must look beyond the pathology. After graduation she worked 1 year in critical care nursing, which only intensified her view on the holistic nature of the human being. Working in such close physical proximity to patients helped her to get to know them well. She believes that a practitioner cannot work with critically ill patients without being in touch with their spirit. After graduate school in psychiatric nursing, which strengthened her views and tendencies, she worked in liaison psychiatry as a consultant. Her work was with medically ill patients with a focus on psychiatric aspects of care, or as she likes to call it, "bridging the link between the body, mind, and spirit." These were patients with "life-changing events."

Although Peggy's nursing education launched her into a career in alternative health, the seeds for her career were sown much earlier. When she was in the fourth grade, she knew she wanted to be in the health field and most probably medicine. When she was in high school she realized that not many women went into medicine, and she felt that she did not have the confidence for this career. Medicine was considered a career for men; women were expected to be teachers, secretaries, or nurses. Consequently, she became a nurse.

Peggy believes that alternative modalities she practices are helpful or therapeutic for almost any condition. Hypnosis is useful for pain, anxiety, and depression or any habit the patient wants to change or modify. Healing touch is also helpful for depression, anxiety, and pain, including intractable pain. It can be used to manage the symptoms of chronic conditions such as cancer and heart disease. For example, healing touch can help patients with sleep problems and migraine headaches. The other alternative treatments have similar uses. Basically, physical conditions always have a psychological component because the human being is body, mind, and spirit.

Peggy believes the alternative modalities she uses are simply tools to assist the patients in management of their illness or problems. For instance, in hypnosis, the patient is put into a relaxed state and is able to be more in touch with his or her unconscious where creativity and ideas are generated. In the relaxed state the internal world opens up, and patients are able to experience their own internal resources. The solutions that are then generated come from within. This technique is not telling or doing to the patient but simply facilitating or empowering him or her. Peggy tells the story of an older woman preparing for hip replacement surgery. She helped this woman write a script to be given to the anesthesiologist so that he could read it to her. In a sense, this was a formula for relaxation and a speedy recovery. This technique is based on the theory that patients are able to hear (although not necessarily remember) while anesthetized, and that what they hear greatly affects them. The technique worked beautifully for this patient, and her recovery was facilitated by images and thoughts read to her during surgery. This created a language of the mind, which is so important to the notion of mind, body, and spirit involvement in health and illness. An interesting aside to the story is that Peggy got permission from the orthopedic surgeon for this intervention before she approached the anesthesiologist. This surgeon had experienced a negative reaction from one of his patients because of what that patient had heard during surgery. Thus the surgeon readily consented to this type of intervention.

Peggy shared another story related to the use of guided imagery and visualization. This patient, a woman, stated that she felt as though she always had a knot in her stomach, and she was anxious and depressed. When Peggy asked her to describe the knot she described it as a ball of yarn that was knotted and twisted with loose and dangling threads. Peggy helped her to change this image of a knot into a ball of yarn that was neatly wound and pleasant to view. In this situation, a new and pleasing image was created that helped to change the woman's feeling state and ultimately helped to change her behavior. These two examples illustrate the basic theoretical underpinnings of the field of alternative health.

Peggy believes that continuing education is essential to her practice. No one practitioner has all the answers and no one can work in isolation. Peer involvement and critique of skills is essential. Peggy also believes that theories and interventions associated with the Eastern culture are especially important in today's health world. In addition, she feels that nurses have a heavy responsibility to teach, as well as to continually learn, and continuing education

provides a forum for this task. In many ways, she views this as a spiritual experience.

Peggy believes that alternative health treatments or modalities should be integrated into conventional medicine. As she stated, both are inseparable parts of a whole, and one augments the other. She reflected on what life would be like without antibiotics and other treatments for acute illness. Alternative treatments are an adjunct to traditional treatments and the ones she uses augment psychotherapy. She believes that patients should have a choice in the treatment plan and should be made aware of what treatments are possible for their illness or problem. She likes the term, *complementary* medicine, instead of *alternative* because it poses fewer problems for working with conventional practitioners (i.e., complementary does not imply choosing one over the other).

Julie Rose Ruby, BSN, Mac, Lac, Dipl Ac, NCCAOM

Julie is a diploma school nurse who completed her BSN at George Mason University. She has since obtained a master's degree in acupuncture from the Acupuncture Institute in Columbia, Maryland. She attended school full-time for three academic years. Acupuncture is the primary modality she practices, and she also practices healing touch, zero balancing, and *qi gong.*

Julie relates that ever since she became a registered nurse, she always leaned toward holistic nursing. When she went back to school to obtain her BSN, this only reinforced her tendencies. She practiced in community health and more specifically in school health. She talks about working with the students who were clinic repeaters and was impressed that their problems seemed to originate from life experiences and were not just physical in nature. She finally decided to go into acupuncture after attending a weekend seminar at the institute. She found that the acupuncture school "spoke her language." She began to view health and illness conceptually as a matter of energy balance and imbalance. She started working on her master's degree in acupuncture in 1993 and graduated in 1995.

As a child, Julie read about Chinese culture and Chinese medicine. She read literature on the "Barefoot Doctor."

She said that unconsciously she was preparing herself for her work in acupuncture. She even used some of these thoughts and theories in her work in community health. For instance, she knew how to help children with certain conditions like asthma; she knew that illness and health was beyond the individual person, that it was holistic and included life's experiences.

When asked what kinds of conditions or patient problems acupuncture helps, Julie responded that acupuncture is for everyone; it is not just for symptoms. Acupuncture treatment can be health promoting as well as healing. Energy needs to be adjusted throughout life, and acupuncture treats body, mind, and spirit.

However, more specifically, Julie states that acupuncture is very effective for pain of all sorts. Specific conditions for which it is especially helpful are allergies, sinus problems, tinnitus, fibromyalgia, and back problems. It is also helpful for persons who have had surgery because surgery cuts through the meridians, and acupuncture helps the healing process. Julie took a continuing course on treating children with acupuncture and found it to be exciting and helpful in her career. Children should be treated when they are young to promote optimum health.

Acupuncture works, according to Julie, by balancing the chi, or energy. It is based on the theory of the electromagnetic fields and the meridians in the body. The use of the word healing is more appropriate than the use of the word treatment. The body heals the most recent injury or problem first. Acupuncture heals the imbalance, whether it is physical, mental, or spiritual. Chinese children may be healthier because of the routine use of acupuncture. In fact, Julie believes that she herself would not have needed surgery some years ago if she had been receiving acupuncture. To elaborate on the underlying theory further, energy and the meridians are associated with personal connections and relationships in life. Many times the patient has an insight after treatment into nonphysical aspects of his or her life, and true healing then begins.

Julie emphatically states that continuing education is imperative. She believes that with acupuncture, learning never ends. Furthermore, it is imperative for her licensure. She has taken many continuing education courses, both at the Columbia school and at the school in Bethesda, Maryland. The Bethesda school is based on traditional Chinese medicine whereas the Columbia school is based on the five elements of wood, fire, earth, metal, and water.

Julie believes that acupuncture should be integrated with traditional medicine and that both are complementary in nature. She believes that patients should have options in treatment, and that no practitioner should tell a patient what to do or where to go. All practitioners should present patients with choices, and patients should choose treatments or modalities based on personal choice and comfort issues.

In Virginia, state law requires that patients must be seen by a physician within 6 months of beginning treatment with an acupuncturist. This is not the case in Maryland. Also, insurance coverage is not based on the wellness model, but is based on the model of treatment for pain and other standard conditions. For the present, these regulations place restrictions on Julie's practice, but this may change with greater acceptance and use of acupuncture as well as with the other modalities in alternative health care.

Kathleen Tusaie-Mumford, MSN, RNCS

Kathie practices the modalities of hypnotherapy, relaxation, and imagery. She is a clinical specialist in psychiatric mental nursing, and she has an advanced certificate with Associate Trainers in Clinical Hypnosis. In the mid-1970s, before she went back to school for her master's degree, Kathie was working as the only nurse in a community mental health center. She was working with social workers, counselors, and psychologists. Her primary role at the time was medication management. However, she observed how hypnosis enhanced psychotherapy and that people were seeking training in it. She, herself, then took beginning, intermediate, and advanced courses over a period of 5 years. She found that this modality actually helped her in her work as well as in her own personal development. Later, she became interested in relaxation and imagery as other enhancement modalities. As she views all three treatments at this point in time, they are really extensions of the nurse's basic role. She credits that beginning work setting as a motivating factor in her work in alternative health.

Kathie's basic nursing education prepared her for her interpersonal work, but she also had tendencies or inclinations toward these treatments or modalities before this period Her nursing education helped her in that the ba sic preparation focused on the patient relationship. It was person-centered and reinforced her desire and ability to connect with people. However, she always had the ability to use her imagination to take her to different places. This ability was a natural skill in helping her to become interested in hypnosis, imagery, and relaxation. In other words, these treatments were "right" for her. She stated, "Although I have seen the benefits of therapeutic touch, therapeutic touch just did not feel right for my practice."

The modalities that Kathie practices can be useful to any patient. She believes that the overriding point to remember is that the use of these modalities is only limited by the nurse's skill and creativity. Very common and successful uses of this therapy are with pain associated with chronic medical conditions, such as with cancer patients. Kathie teaches students who are enrolled in anesthesia and nurse practitioner programs, and the students use these mind-body interaction strategies as adjuncts to their practice. Relaxation and imagery are especially appropriate for preoperative and postoperative situations. One of her students worked in a neurologist's office, and this student used relaxation and imagery successfully with a multiple sclerosis patient to decrease muscle tension and maximize ability to function. Also, these modalities are particularly good for people in crisis, including children. Kathie described several examples of successful use of alternative modalities. One was with a young man in the emergency room after an accident. In this case, she used hypnosis to help him through the crisis of necessary sutures and his phobic fear of needles. She believes hypnosis can be especially helpful for a number of emergency situations. Kathie also spoke of using hypnosis with a woman in crisis who was immobilized by grief after the death of her husband. There is still dispute as to whether hypnosis should be used for patients with depression— Kathie feels that it can, but that the techniques should be different to avoid increased withdrawal.

When asked about her opinion on the underlying theory or theories for the use of these treatments and modalities, Kathie stressed that there is much uncertainty as to why or how they work. She stated that there is obviously a mind-body connection. Related theories in which she puts some faith are the gate theory (in treating pain), energy transduction, an altered state of consciousness, and others related to the autonomic and endocrine systems. She stressed that in her experience with all treatments she works with patients to stimulate their own natural healing abilities.

In keeping her practice skills current, Kathie feels that it is extremely important for her to work with her peer group. She believes that peer supervision is particularly important. She feels that one needs to experience the treatment on oneself first to see what it feels like and to experience any fears related to it. She also believes that one should begin by first using the treatment on a patient with whom one feels comfortable and then discussing the case in supervision. Ongoing supervision and learning (workshops, reading, and so on) are necessary to maintain quality-effective practice. She was recently introduced to a new treatment called eye movement desensitization, and she is impressed by its effectiveness with trauma victims.

Kathie believes that alternative health treatments or modalities can be appropriate for any nursing practice. Ideally, it is not solely a conventional or alternative medicine but a combination, pulling the best from both. She stressed, as do many authorities, that traditional medicine obviously works best for acute conditions and that alternative medicine is often indicated for chronic conditions. She believes nurses should build up a strong referral system for their patients. She views all these treatments along a continuum, and this viewpoint is important for insurance reimbursement. Although insurance may not pay for hypnosis, it will often pay for cognitive therapy (of which hypnosis can be a form). It is this perspective that allows nurses flexibility to incorporate alternative treatment or modalities as a natural part of their work.

It is noteworthy that the four nurses described all found the alternative treatments and modalities that they practiced to be compatible and natural to the general field of nursing. Alternative health can be considered a natural extension of the basic nursing role in whatever specialty or area the nurse pursues. Perhaps many nurses have always been a part of this field but were reluctant to acknowledge their strengths and skills in this area at a time when medicine scoffed at all that was not "scientific and mechanistic."

In summary, alternative health and alternative medicine as a movement have important implications for nurses practicing in all areas, and especially in community-based practice. At the very least, nurses should understand the underlying broad theory of the field, which states that illness and health are complex interactions among the body, mind, and spirit. Furthermore, nurses should be knowledgeable about practitioners and referrals. They should encourage their patients to use reputable treatments and practitioners but at the same time to let their conventional doctors and nurses know what they are doing. Patients may not tell their health care provider about the use of alternative medicine because they are afraid of disapproval. Practitioners in both conventional medicine and alternative medicine must work together.

Perhaps nurses can help to bridge the gap between alternative and conventional health care modalities and ultimately can work to improve patient care. Perhaps nurses have been doing this from the very beginning, but have not given themselves credit or recognition. In many respects, the philosophy and theory underlying alternative health and medicine is part of the heritage of the nursing profession.

RESEARCH IN ALTERNATIVE/ COMPLEMENTARY HEALTH PRACTICES

Increasingly more research is being done in the field of alternative health. The National Center for Complementary and Alternative Medicine at the National Institutes of Health (NCCAM) facilitates research of unconventional medical practices. It also disseminates information to the public. Currently, acupuncture is being investigated for its use with many chronic conditions and in particular for its role in the alleviation of pain. Other treatments being investigated are herbal medicines and chiropractic medicine. A major illness being investigated is cancer: NCCAM has a Cancer Advisory Panel for Complementary and Alternative Medicine.

Alternative Therapies in Health and Medicine, a peer-reviewed bimonthly journal, publishes current research with a variety of alternative modalities. Review of the issues from March, May, and July of 2000 reveals that research on hypertension, hypnosis, homeopathy, herbal medicines, movement therapy, and prayer are reported.

The relationship of spirituality and health is a fast-emerging research area. The Institute for Health and Healing at the California Pacific Medical Center explores this subject, including the role of consciousness in health. It is evident that future research will continue to explore these and other alternative modalities.

Very little research has been done to survey the use of alternative therapies by nurses, either on themselves or on their clients. An interesting study was carried out by King, Pettigrew, and Reed (2000), in which the authors assessed nurses' self-rated knowledge level, perceptions of efficacy, use for self and clients, and referral patterns for common alternative and complementary therapies. A random sample of 2740 registered nurses living in Ohio were surveyed; this, however, represented only 2 percent of all registered nurses in the state. A response rate of only 17 percent suggests caution in interpreting findings of the study for changes in practice. It appears significant, however, that overall, the respondents held favorable opinions of complementary therapies and supported these therapies as an adjunct to traditional medical practices. Respondents reported that the most frequently used therapy with their clients was diet (38 percent), followed by prayer (30 percent). Conclusions of the study indicated that although nurses have positive opinions about alternative therapies, their knowledge level remains lower than their interest in the use of these modalities. This indicates a need for more education in the appropriate use of alternative and complementary therapies.

THE MIRACLE OF HAILEY

Kari, an American of Asian descent, tells this success story. She had endometriosis and a hormone imbalance, and she was not able to get pregnant. Her gynecologist put her on hormones, which made her feel terrible. She did not menstruate for a year. After two and a half years of trying with conventional fertility treatments, Kari was desperate.

Finally, with advice from her mother-in-law, Kari went to see Dr. C., a Doctor of Oriental Medicine. Dr. C. said that Kari's uterus was too cold. She prescribed warm liquids—juices and water. These liquids were hot or at room temperature. She could have absolutely no cold drinks, no caffeine, no sodas, no salads, no sprouts, no cold food, no melons, no lamb, no frogs. Near ovulation time, Dr. C. instructed Kari's mother-in-law to make scrambled eggs with green onion and shrimp for her. She also made her black chicken soup broth about once a week. Dr. C. prescribed herbs and teas, some of which smelled terrible. The ingredients of the teas varied, depending on the day of Kari's cycle. They included grains such as barley, seaweed, dried plums, and barks; there were about 20 different ingredients in total. Kari drank these teas every morning and evening.

In addition, Dr. C. prescribed acupuncture treatments. Kari had these treatments every other day. She remembers that the acupuncture needles were placed on her feet, ankles, stomach, hands, and liver area. Then she would have a heating pad placed on her stomach for about 15 minutes. These acupuncture treatments were for the purpose of assisting Kari's uterus to become warm and ready. She also took her temperature every morning as part of the treatment. Initially her temperature was not indicative of a balanced hormone level. But finally her temperature indicated an optimum low-high curve.

Kari was in treatment with Dr. C. for about 3 months. During this time, Kari had complete trust and confidence in Dr. C. She became pregnant, and Hailey, a beautiful, normal little girl, was born. As of this writing, Hailey is a happy, healthy two-and-a-half-year-old. Some added factors to this story are worthy of note. Kari relied on a book suggested by her sister-in-law, entitled How to Take Charge of Your Fertility. This book opened Kari's eyes to the signs indicative of when her body was fertile. She began to be much more conscious of her eating habits and the importance of organic gardening. She also became aware of how common household cleaning agents affect the hormones in the body. She stopped using many of them and began to use biodegradable cleaning products and baking soda or vinegar solutions.

This true story reflects a number of the underlying principles of alternative medicine. It reflects the theory of heat and cold and energy that is so well developed in Asian medicine. It reflects the effect of the power of the relationship between the patient and the doctor. And finally, it underscores the complex interaction of the body, mind, and spirit in both health and illness.

The following summary questions will give you an opportunity to reflect on the overriding principles of this chapter.

Active Learning Strategies

1. Can you describe several historical facts about the alternative health movement? How can or should nursing be involved in this field?

2. A patient asks you about homeopathic medicine. How would you help him or her find accurate information?

3. A patient asks you about the alternative health field in general. Can you describe some of the basic theories and principles?

4. A patient is confused about choosing an alternative health-care practitioner. She found a local magazine advertising unconventional treatments for a number of chronic conditions. How would you help her?

References

Bruning, N. (1995, January/February). The mysterious power of homeopathy. Natural Health, 85–89, 106, 108–110, 112.

Chapman, E. (1999). Homeopathy. In W. Jonas & J. Levin. (Eds.). Essentials of complementary and alternative medicine. Philadelphia: Lippincott Williams and Wilkins.

Coulter, I., Adams, A., Coggan, P., Wilkes, M., & Gonyea, M. (1998). A comparative study of chiropractic and medical education. Journal of Alternative Therapies in Health and Medicine, 4(5), 64–74.

Eisenberg, D. M., Davis, R. B., Ettner, S. L., Appel, S., Wilkey, S., Van Rompay, M., & Kessler, R. C. (1998). Trends in alternative medicine use in the United States, 1990–1997: Results of a follow-up national survey. Journal of the American Medical Association. 280(18), 1569–1575.

Holistic and metaphysical resource book. For Maryland, Virginia, and Washington, DC 1997–1998. (1997). Great Falls: Cliff.

King, M. O., Pettigrew, A. C., & Reed, F. C. (2000). Complementary, alternative, integrative: Have nurses kept pace with their clients? Dermatology Nursing, 2(1), 41–44.

Leake, R., & Broderick, J. (1999). Current licensure for acupuncture in the United States. Journal of Alternative Therapies in Health and Medicine, 5(4), 94–96.

Sanford, A. (1949). The healing light (8th ed.). St. Paul: Macalester Park.

CHAPTER # 11 Caring for Chronically Ill Clients in the Community

Francine Roberts

LEARNING OBJECTIVES

1) Provide an operational definition of chronic illness.

2) Identify assessment considerations for the chronically ill client in the community.

3) Describe effective approaches to managing care of the chronically ill client in the community.

4) Identify resources available to the chronically ill client in the community.

5) Describe effective approaches to meet needs of the caregiver of the chronically ill client.

CHRONIC ILLNESS

Students working with chronically ill clients find that there is no one definition for chronic illness. In preparing to write this chapter, I came across many definitions, but found one that seemed to best fit my perspective on chronic illness. Prince (1996) describes illness as a human experience involving loss or dysfunction. Chronic illness involves a permanent alteration in the client's way of life and a need for reappraisal of that life and what may be hoped for in terms of function and health. Persons who may normally ignore little aches and pains now become more aware of changes in their body functions. I consider it a chronic illness if the illness causes an individual to change his or her lifestyle to accommodate that illness and its treatment. This definition includes diseases that may not be thought of initially as chronic illness, such as

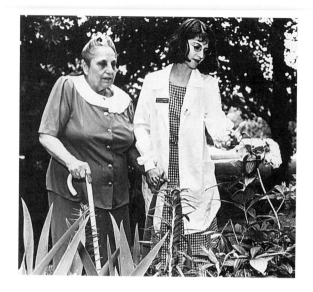

thyroid disease. Any disease that requires daily medication or treatment to keep the disease under control requires some type of nursing intervention. The individual with a chronic illness that requires minimal change in lifestyle may need less nursing intervention. The individual with considerable lifestyle changes may need a great amount of nursing intervention. The more the disease results in major changes in activities of daily living, the harder it may be for clients to continue their normal life, and the more nursing intervention may be needed.

Leidy (1990) states that chronically ill individuals increasingly experience stressors as distressors. Life, rather than seeming like a challenge, leaves the individual with a sense of pervasive helplessness. The more stressors that individuals experience in their lives, the more they may develop this feeling of hopelessness and depression. The inability to handle life's daily stress relating to illness and medical regimen can result in exacerbation of the disease or noncompliance with the medical treatment. The outcome may be poor management of health care. Appropriate nursing intervention can help individuals learn to handle their daily stressors and control their health care.

The nurse's challenge in working with chronically ill clients in the community is to determine what they view as appropriate functioning, maximize their abilities, and enable them to live with their illness, functioning at maximum capacity. To do this, it is important to determine the clients' perspective on their illnesses and what maximum functioning means to them. Being a skilled listener and interpreter of what the clients and their families are saying helps the nurse determine appropriate interventions with them. Part of the nurse's role is to empower the individual and family in controlling the medical regimen and health care. The nurse in the community has the unique opportunity to see clients and families in their own environment—the home—and not the environment that is most familiar to the nurse—the hospital. The nurse becomes the guest of the individual, rather than the other way around. It is a situation that can make the nurse feel less comfortable and not in control. This discomfort can be overcome, however, if you remember that you are knowledgeable about the disease and medical treatment, but the clients are the experts about themselves and their needs and wants. The nurse and client together make a complete picture.

This chapter does not focus on the specifics of the pathophysiology of disease because that information can be gained from other textbooks. This chapter focuses on seeing the needs of chronically ill individuals and caregivers in the community, helping them meet their needs, and guiding them through the health-care system.

How do you meet that challenge? There are several areas that you need to evaluate as you approach the individual with chronic illness. The first is education. This includes education about diagnosis, medical regimen, and suggested strategies to cope with both. Second, you must create an environment that develops trust and allows the individual and family to discuss feelings and concerns regarding the illness and the medical regimen. Third, the client and family need information about available services and resources in the community and how to access those resources. Fourth, you must guide and assist clients in fulfilling their roles, responsibilities, and self-care demands. Fifth, parents, spouses, and adult children, as well as the client, need guidance in advocating for themselves or their chronically ill family member. A final area of importance is encouraging and guiding the client to maintain social involvement to prevent isolation. Prince (1996) discusses the responsibility that the nurse has to try to understand the meaning of chronic illness from the client's perspective. Nurses are generally trusted caregivers and have the ability to influence behavior in a constructive way.

ASSESSMENT OF THE INDIVIDUAL IN THE COMMUNITY

Knowledge

The first area to assess is the clients' knowledge base regarding their illness. Never assume that because individuals have lived with a specific disease for years that they have accurate and complete information about their disease. They may have been taught at the time of diagnosis, which could have been 20 years earlier. With changes in health care, they could be operating on 21-year-old knowledge and may not be up to date with the newest information. It is also possible that at the time they were taught they were overwhelmed with the diagnosis and the amount of information they were given. In addition, they may not have retained all the information given or may have misinterpreted that information. The nurse must assess what the client knows currently about the disease and its effect on the body. Getting this information helps the nurse assess the knowledge of clients, how well they understand any previous information given them regarding their disease and the medical treatment prescribed for them. The nurse can gain useful information about the client's understanding of the medical regimen that has been prescribed and determine his or her knowledge of the prescribed drugs, their side effects, and the contraindications. Having the client explain what he or she knows about the disease, drugs, and other treatments helps the nurse assess for problem areas, areas of misunderstanding, outdated information, or misinformation. It may also give the nurse information concerning alternative therapies that the individual may be using to treat the illness. Getting this information can help the nurse begin to see the illness and treatment from the individual's perspective, providing the opportunity to explore the chronic illness experience together.

If clients share alternative treatments that they are using to treat their illness, the nurse can explore in more depth what they are using and how it might impact their prescribed medical plan. The nurse cannot overlook the amount of information that is available in the media and the influence this has on the client's health practices. If clients do not mention alternative treatments, it is important to ask if there are other things they are doing to help

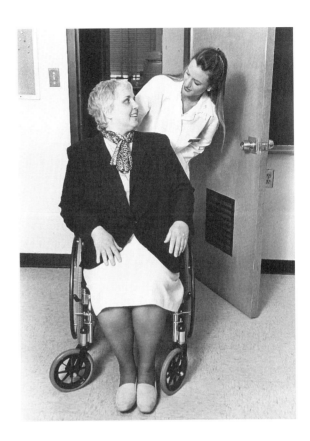

them manage their disease. In addition, cultural differences and ethnic practices can influence what the individual may be doing to treat the disease. When discussing alternative practices with clients, nurses should control their own responses to the information and not judge these alternative health practices based on personal feelings. The nurse must gain more knowledge about the practice to determine whether it might interfere with prescribed medical treatments. Nurses may have to learn more about alternative medicine, so that they can help clients and families blend the two treatment plans. Most individuals will not give up alternative practices, and if the nurse condemns them, clients may hide their use of alternative practices. The more open and nonjudgmental the nurse is, the more likely that a trusting relationship will develop. It is also important to find out if clients may be seeing an alternative healer as part of their cultural beliefs. The healer may be prescribing herbs or therapies that might interfere with what the physician is prescribing.

Turton (1998) found in his research of postmyocardial infarction clients that the type of information that clients wanted was in regard to symptom management and lifestyle factors. Other types of information identified in preferred order were: anatomy and physiology, activities, psychological factors, dietary information, and drug information. The postmyocardial infarction clients wanted to know how to live with their disease and how to adjust their lifestyle to the disease. In assessing knowledge, the nurse should remember that what is most important to the client and family is what should be discussed first. Keep in mind that this information may differ from what the nurse feels is most important. The nurse must implement teaching to answer those areas that are of most concern to the client and family and then give information that appears most essential.

Too often, as nurses we teach what *we* feel is most important. In working with cardiac clients I have developed a plan to teach them about their medication, the physiology of their disease, what the disease has done to their body, symptoms they should look for indicating problems, and needed dietary changes. When clients' information needs become the basis for the teaching plan, they want to know when they can go back to work and how soon they can resume normal functioning. If the things you have taught them do not answer their questions, they may choose to ignore or forget what you have given them. These clients may then be labeled as noncompliant because they are not doing what you told them to do, but have made a decision concerning their health behavior based on their needs and concerns. An example of this occurred when I was in graduate school:

In graduate school, while interviewing a man who recently had a myocardial infarction, we were discussing what he felt was important information that he needed. He started telling me about how he had been taught all about dietary changes. He talked about how he had been told to cut back on salt and fat in his diet. He then looked at me and said, "I was a prisoner of war in a concentration camp during World War II. I faced death every day I was in that camp and it doesn't frighten me. If I die because I continue to eat the types of foods I enjoy, I'm not afraid. If I have to quit eating these foods, I may as well be dead."

How could you argue with his reasoning? He knew and understood the consequences from a medical standpoint, but the possibility of dying was no threat to him. No one had taken the time to talk to the man about what he viewed as important information, approaching the teaching from that perspective. Box 11–1 gives you the opportunity to discuss the previous story.

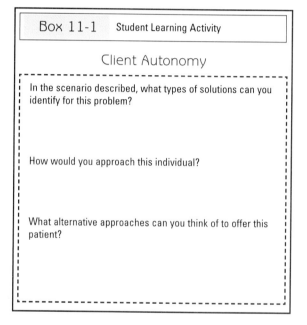

Box 11-1	Student Learning Activity

Client Autonomy

In the scenario described, what types of solutions can you identify for this problem?

How would you approach this individual?

What alternative approaches can you think of to offer this patient?

Individual Feelings and Needs Regarding Chronic Illness

Another area that must be assessed is the client's ability to adapt to illness and cope with necessary changes in lifestyle. This is an area in which the nurse can focus on getting the client to express feelings and concerns regarding the disease and treatment. The nurse must understand that lived experience, from the clients' perspective, is the best information and gives the greatest insight into how they are handling the medical treatment prescribed for them.

One study (McWilliams, Stewart, Brown, Desai, & Coderre, 1996) of individuals living with chronic illness identified ways those individuals promoted health while living with their disease. Included in their responses were four components: fighting and struggling, resigning oneself, creatively balancing resources, and accepting. Each of these areas focuses on how well the individual is able to maintain a lifestyle and continue living a normal life. Chronic illness can affect all aspects of the individual's normal lifestyle, and this can lead to depression, discouragement, and a feeling of helplessness. These feelings can result in clients failing to follow their prescribed treatment and medical regimen. They could become depressed and discouraged and want to give up on life.

One patient in the McWilliams et al. (1996) study reported his struggle with chronic illness in this way: "When you're cooped up, it's hard to keep positive. . . . I haven't been able to do hardly anything for a year. . . . I've got to keep struggling, I guess. . . . I try not to get discouraged, but you're sitting here and you get thinking, and the first thing you know you've got yourself all . . . worked up. . . . Life's a drag sometimes." (p. 5)

You can hear the discouragement in this statement. When talking to a client such as this, the nurse must listen and be sensitive to those subtle statements that tell how the person is feeling about the disease and its impact on his or her life. Continue to discuss this situation by completing Box 11–2.

Box 11-2   Student Learning Activity

Client Example

In the situation just discussed, how could the nurse respond and help guide the client to find some meaning in his life?

What information could help the nurse determine what is meaningful to the client?

The nurse must try to understand how clients are coping with their chronic illness. The nurse can do more to develop a care plan and determine what is an appropriate intervention when there is an understanding of what clients are experiencing as they live in their illness. This process takes time and is something that requires trust between the client and nurse. It does not occur in one visit, and the nurse must be patient, realizing it takes time to establish a relationship that will open communication to become aware of health-releated aspects of that client's life.

Stuifbergen and Rogers (1997) did research with individuals who had multiple sclerosis, exploring the meaning of health and well-being for them. Areas that the participants identified as part of health and well-being included family functioning to maintain independence, spirituality, work, socioeconomic security, and self-actualization. All of these areas are important and can play a part in the clients' ability to cope with their illnesses. A nurse should keep these areas in mind when talking to clients about their feelings concerning their diseases.

The first area identified in the Stuifbergen and Rogers study dealt with the need for clients to maintain independence. Clients who deal with chronic disease are forced daily to face the reality of the outcomes of those diseases. Many chronic diseases end with loss of mental or physical functioning or death. The more the nurse can do to provide clients with ways to continue to function within the home and community and maintain their independence, the more clients will keep a positive focus on their life. This may involve using health-care resources such as occupational therapy, physical therapy, or other health-care providers. The nurse must be creative in finding alternative approaches to helping clients maintain their lifestyle and to continue performing normal activities of daily living. Clients need to be aware of resources available in the community that clients can use to maintain their independence and normal lifestyle. In the McWilliams et al. (1996) study, an elderly woman was told that she needed to go to a nursing home. The doctor said, "What if they go into your home and find you dead in your chair?" The woman's response was, "It would be a happy dead. It would be my chair" (p. 1). This reflects her desire to remain in her home and to remain independent; this desire was stronger than her fear of death. The nurse must help clients focus on those areas they can control regarding their life while helping them to accept areas that cannot be changed.

The second area that must be assessed is spirituality. This area of nursing has been overlooked when working with clients. Recently the medical literature has published articles discussing the need for spiritual intervention, the power of prayer, and the effect of religious beliefs on the health and well-being of individuals who are ill. The nurse is in a unique position to assess the individual's spiritual beliefs. Working in the community provides an opportunity for the nurse to gain more information from clients and guide them to resources to help support them in times of stress. Often, clients have no immediate family to assist with their health care, and their religious group may act as their source of support. To overlook this area when working with the individual living with chronic illness is to cut the individual into pieces and ignore a part of the whole. Many clients whom the nurse contacts within the home may be living with a terminal disease. The nurse may be faced with questions from clients about personal views on life and death and what is going to happen to them. The nurse may be asked similar questions by family members who are trying to cope with the future loss of their loved one. In all of these situations, the nurse must be aware of personal feelings regarding life and death and be comfortable guiding the family and client to meet their spiritual needs, making sure that those areas that are important to them are being addressed. Nurses may even be asked to pray with clients and must be comfortable with this request. O'Neill and Kenny (1998) state that "in the past the nurse has depended on the clergy to work with patients in meeting their spiritual needs but with the emerging focus on holistic care it has reinforced the need for the nurse becoming principle provider of spiritual care" (p. 4) This means that the nurse works with the clergy to meet the spiritual needs and answer the client's questions.

The third area identified in the Stuifbergen and Rogers study (1997) was the desire of the individual living with chronic illness to continue productive employment. This is also a way for individuals to maintain independence. The nurse may be called on to identify resources available to help clients maintain their ability to work, possibly looking at alternative ways of completing their work responsibilities. For some clients, work may not be a job outside the home, but rather maintaining normal role responsibilities at home. A retired individual does not have a job, but may need to cook meals or take care of the lawn. This can be as important as going to a job for pay. The same applies to a mother with children at home and her need to maintain the roles of caregiver and nurturer for her family.

Coinciding with the ability to continue to work are the socioeconomic issues that go along with employment or nonemployment. The cost of health care for the person living with a chronic illness can become very expensive; if employment is lost, health insurance may also be lost. The cost of medications, treatment, and other health equipment can become overwhelming to a family and increase the feelings of helplessness.

The last area Stuifbergen and Rogers (1997) identified was that of self-actualization, which is part of all previously mentioned needs. Even if clients cannot work, they can find some sense of fulfillment, well-being, and control over their life. These areas can impact on one another and are a part of how clients respond to their illness and affect their motivation to maintain well-being. The ability to maintain one or more of these areas can give clients a sense of control over their lives and a sense of purpose.

Compliance is another area the nurse working with the chronically ill individual must address, because it can affect the client's feelings of independence and control. Nurses must be very careful when applying the label "noncompliant" to a client. Often, as nurses we tell clients our perspective of what they should do to control their disease process, but we do not take into consideration the individual's wants and needs. When these clients do not follow the care plan we have given them and continue to have difficulty controlling their disease or symptoms, we are tempted to label them as noncompliant. An example of this situation is found in a case study by Burkhardt and

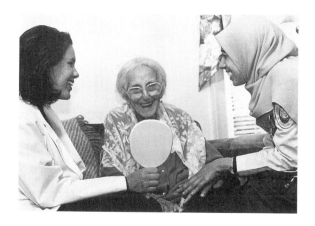

Nathaniel (1998). I often use this case study with students when discussing the principle of autonomy and clients making choices about their health care.

 Cora is a forty-five-year-old woman who looks years older than her stated age. She has a very limited monthly income and no health insurance. Cora smokes two and one-half packs of cigarettes per day. She has severe [chronic obstructive pulmonary disease] COPD with constant dyspnea and frequent exacerbations. The nurse who sees her at a local free clinic is interested in at least preventing further problems and speaks to Cora often about the importance of quitting smoking. The situation becomes very frustrating for all involved when Cora returns repeatedly for increasingly severe problems—having failed to quit smoking. Cora, of course, becomes labeled as noncompliant. During a particularly severe exacerbation, the nurse says to Cora, "You know you are committing suicide by continuing to smoke." Cora's reply is, "You don't understand. I live alone. I have no money, no friends, no family and will never be able to work. I know the damage I'm doing, but smoking is the only pleasure I have in life. (p. 43)

Continue to discuss this situation by completing Box 11–3.

Box 11-3   Student Learning Activity

Client Example

What do you think about Cora's position?

Do you feel that Cora's behavior was a lack of knowledge, or did she make a knowledgeable choice about continuing to smoke?

How would you handle the situation differently? Explain and discuss alternatives that might help Cora cope with her illness.

As a nurse, you have medical knowledge that the individual lacks, but that is only a part of the whole picture. The individual has a life to live separate from the medical field, and if the treatment plan does not fit into that lifestyle it will probably be ignored. In the preceding situation, the nurses had not been to Cora's home and did not understand her living situation. Many of the things discussed in this chapter play a part in this case, such as family support, independence, spiritual support, and self-actualization. The role the nurse plays in developing a care plan for a chronically ill client is that of negotiator. The nurse knows the disease, why the treatment plan was ordered, and the reasons behind the medication and treatments. Clients, on the other hand, know themselves and what is important to them and their lives. The nurse becomes the one that then works with the client and the medical doctors to develop a plan that meets both the client's personal and medical needs. It is not an issue of right and wrong, but one of finding the solution that leaves both parties feeling like they are winning and that the client is maintaining some control over his or her life. This process takes time and patience on the part of the nurse to learn about the client and how best to fit the medical treatment into the individual's lifestyle. This same process applies, whether you are working directly with the individual or with parents or the adult children of the client.

Community Resources

The nurse also must be knowledgeable about the sources available for the chronically ill individual in the community. One source available to more and more individuals is the Internet. Many people have access to computers, and if they do not have them in their homes, many public libraries have them for public use. On the Internet the client or family has access to many web sites that are related to health in general and sites that are specific to a disease. When I did a search on the Internet, putting in the words "health information," I received a list of 240 sites. These sites included discount places to buy vitamins, books, and other health products; sites that evaluate insurance programs; places to buy books about diseases; and sites that give information about illnesses and other medical advice including access to the National Library of Medicine. In many of these sites there are chat rooms where individuals can go to talk to others living with the same type of disease. One young woman described her experience with accessing the Internet for information when she was feeling frustrated about the control of her disease:

> *A couple of weeks ago, late at night, I was having pain from an ovarian cyst, and it worried me. Since I couldn't call my doctor, I got on the web to see if I could find out anything about concerns I had. Since I knew I have polycystic ovary syndrome (PCOS), I started by searching for that syndrome on Yahoo! Well, I had no idea how much information was out there! Yahoo alone had extended files and links for any syndrome I could name. The search led me to a couple of articles about new drugs used for treating PCOS, and each of these articles mentioned that the new drug treated the insulin resistance that leads to PCOS. Insulin resistance? I was shocked. When I was diagnosed 10 years ago, or even when I had blood work done 5 years ago, no such connection with insulin was mentioned. The articles also mentioned that the insulin resistance could, of course, lead to diabetes. The links on these sites also made me realize that many other "cysters," as they call themselves, were out there and could share information with each other—and with me! I looked at some bulletin boards and a newsgroup devoted to women with PCOS and was stunned to find they all had so many of the symptoms of my everyday life that I had never associated with PCOS (unstable blood sugar, inability to lose weight, very strong sugar cravings at certain points of their cycle, low energy, anxiety . . .). But the great thing was a lot of them had found a solution to all of these problems in a change of diet. To counteract the insulin resistance, they had tried low-carbohydrate diets, and were all very happy—losing weight, gaining energy, avoiding blood sugar problems. I've been keeping up with these support sources on a daily basis now, and already my life has changed. I feel more in control of my body and my health than I have in 10 years. I understand better the signals my body sends me, and I know that it's even more important than I ever thought it was to keep my weight down and my general well-being up.*

This young woman found information that she was able to put into use in her life and improved her health by controlling some of her symptoms. The nurse must be aware that the client may have information with which the nurse is unfamiliar. This places the nurse in the position of needing to increase his or her knowledge about the disease as well as knowledge about the Internet. As nurses become more comfortable with the resources available, they will be more comfortable in meeting the challenge of working with informed consumers. Nurses must be comfortable admitting to the client that they are unfamiliar with the new content and stating that they would like to review it and learn more about it. Then they need to be able to go to the Internet and the literature to search for more facts to increase their knowledge and to prepare them to counsel the client. This type of situation requires the nurse to be in a constant learning mode so that he or she can help the individual evaluate the information they have obtained from the Internet or other sources. Nurses must update themselves on new research in the medical arena as well as on the Internet so that they are prepared to guide the individual in evaluating that information and its usefulness to their health care. The nurse must be aware that some information out there can be good and useful and other information may be harmful if used by clients. Table 11–1 provides examples of useful Internet sites.

Other resources available in the community are organizations specific to the particular diseases, such as the American Diabetic Association, the American Cancer

Table 11-1

Examples of Internet Sites

Discovery Health Online: www.discoveryhealth.com

Search eLibrary: www.elibrary.com

Ask Doctors Questions about Health: www.askphysicians.com

Health A to Z: www.healthatoz.com

American Heart Association: www.amhrt.org

HealthGate Medical Information: www.healthgate.com

NCI's CancerNet Cancer Information: www.cancernet.nci.nih.gov

Medicare—The Official U.S. Government Site for Medicare Information: www.medicare.gov

Mental Health Net—About MHN: www.mentalhelp.net

The Health Resource, Inc.: www.thehealthresource.com

Society, the American Kidney Fund, the Cystic Fibrosis Foundation, and the American Heart Association. If clients are unaware of these resources, it is the nurse's responsibility to make them aware of these associations and the services they offer. Many of these associations provide magazines that contain the most recent information concerning research in the disease area. There is also print material that can provide the client and family with knowledge about the disease and its treatment.

The more resources the nurse can provide to the client and family, the more they will be able to manage their disease and the more in control they will feel over their own lives. Chronically ill individuals often feel that the disease has taken over their lives, and the more that the nurse can do to give them back some control, the more likely they will cooperate. With any information given to the individual, the nurse must make sure that it is readable, easy to understand, and accurate. To do this, the nurse must review the material, know the client who will use the material and his or her educational level, and provide material appropriate to that client.

Explore resources for chronic illness by completing Box 11–4.

Box 11-4	Student Learning Activity

Resources for Chronic Illness

Choose a chronic disease, such as diabetes, asthma, or depression; get on the Internet and put in the disease name. See how many web sites you find on that topic. Go into several sites and see how much information and what type of information is available. Describe what you have found.

Call or write a foundation for that disease and see what information they have available. Describe what you find, the cost of information, and how easy it was to obtain.

To help clients obtain information about their diseases, you may need to help them learn how to navigate the health-care system. The nurse may need to discuss with the client such information as where to call to get assistance and what questions to ask to get the needed information. They may need to help the client by calling the physician and describing symptoms so that the client can get information and help. The nurse may need to support the client and family in realizing what they are entitled to and how to access that information and help them to not become discouraged while working with the bureaucracy of health care. A personal experience that happened to me exemplifies this:

A year ago my 88-year-old mother fell and broke her hip. It required surgery and a period of rehabilitation. She needed assistance with her self-care activities and I worked full-time, which made it impossible to bring her home with me immediately after the surgery. She went to a long-term care facility where physical therapy and occupational therapy were ordered. She recovered from the fractured hip but 6 weeks after she returned home she fell again and fractured her pelvis. After the second fall she seemed to lose her will to live and became a total care. As her daughter, I was having to deal with my feelings of having a mother hospitalized, guilt that I had not been there to prevent the fall, and concern about how to handle her once she was discharged from the hospital. My work situation had not changed and she again went to a nursing home for physical therapy, which was covered under Medicare. Her time of being covered by Medicare was ending because the second fall had occurred so close to the first. I was faced with making some decisions regarding her long-term care, issues such as could I bring her home and get a home health aide to live in and help take care of her, or should I put her in a nursing home? There was nowhere to turn to get information regarding all the alternatives available to her and myself. I kept thinking, I am a nurse and have worked in the health-care system for years, yet I had no idea where to turn. She did not have the financial resources to pay for nursing home care, and I was forced to apply for Medicaid to cover the cost of nursing home placement. I have never felt more frustrated than during the process of obtaining the clearance for Medicaid—the amount of forms that needed to be completed, the information that was required, and the feeling that I was a criminal or trying to gain something for my mother that she was not entitled to. You

would fill out forms, then go to the office to submit the forms, and they would tell you they were not complete and you needed more information. You couldn't make an appointment for a specific time to turn in the forms, but went, signed in, and sat until they called you. You would get the new form, complete it, and then go back and sit and wait again. I know when the process was complete how much information I had learned, and I questioned how anyone who didn't have the health-care knowledge I had could ever accomplish that objective. I could see how a spouse trying to accomplish that for a loved one could get frustrated and give up, especially because all of this occurred and does occur while coping with a crisis within the family.

Families trying to get access to appropriate health care and answers to their questions can become frustrated. This may result in their giving up and not seeking further medical assistance, stopping treatment or using only home remedies, and picking and choosing things that fit their lifestyle and are more available. It becomes the nurse's role to advocate for clients and teach them how to become their own advocate. The worst feeling the client can have is that of being alone in coping with problems that seem overwhelming. Stresses can exacerbate diseases, and trying to cope with the health-care system certainly can become a stressor.

A final area of need that must be addressed is helping the client diminish feelings of social isolation. As the client's disease progresses, the ability to get out and attend normal functions may be lost. As this occurs, support systems are lost to the individual, and this loss can add to isolation and feelings of loss of independence. Individuals see themselves losing their normal roles and may experience this as a loss of personal identity. All of these changes can add to the stress of living with a chronic disease and increase frustration. The mother who can no longer care for her children and attend their functions or the older individual who can't get to the grocery store or drugstore or visit with friends can become depressed, be overwhelmed, and give up. The nurse must be aware that there may be many services available in the community for the elderly, such as a "phone friend" who will call housebound adults and talk to them; Meals-On-Wheels, which delivers meals to the housebound; and van transportation to adult day-care centers. Some of

these services are free and some have minimal charges based on the individual's income. There are also home-health aides who can do some housework as well as help with the client's self-care activities. The nurse must know the community and the resources available to assist clients in helping themselves to maintain some social contact outside the home. Cameron (1996) reported that Porter (1969) found that social isolation, such as living alone, was the major factor in nonadherence among patients on medication for chronic illness. Cameron also reported that Baekeland and Lundwall (1975) reviewed 19 studies that investigated social support and clients who dropped out of treatment. The literature revealed that those individuals who dropped out had low social support. The same article also reported that Becker and Green (1975) reviewed the literature and found that family support was strongly correlated with patient compliance. Support from family or significant friends can encourage the individual to maintain the treatment program and to have a positive outlook. The nurse can maximize this by including family and those individuals close to the client in the education process, as long as the client agrees.

Needs of the Family

Caregivers' needs also must be assessed when making a home visit to the family. Frequently, the burden of the care for the client falls on the parents, children, or spouse of the individual who is sick. The needs of these individuals can become as great as the need of the client who is chronically ill. The first area that the nurse should assess is the ability of the caregiver to manage the care of the client. The nurse must assess caregivers for their understanding and knowledge concerning the disease, drugs, and treatment regimen. The nurse must make sure that all the information the caregiver has provided is consistent and then must assist the caregiver in clarifying any misinformation. In a study of daughters caring for their mothers, Bull and Jervis (1997) found that home care was impeded when daughters had lack of access to information and resources. The nurse must be prepared to help the caregiver and the family find services to assist them in caring for their relative.

The nurse must be aware of difficulties caregivers may be having in making adjustments to the lifestyle changes that are required in their new role. Gravelle (1997) conducted a study on parents caring for children with a progressive life-threatening illness. She found that nurses should determine how parents define and manage their adversity, as well as be alert to the changing needs of the family. The changing needs usually occur as the health state of the child worsens. It is important to detect early signs that changes are occurring and to begin intervention immediately to help the family. Many of the areas discussed earlier in the chapter concerning assessment of the individual with a chronic illness also apply to the caregiver and family.

There are many support groups for the family of individuals with medical problems such as Alzheimer's, cancer, cystic fibrosis, asthma, and head injuries. These support groups can help the family members to better understand the needs of the individual who has the disease, as well as to understand their own feelings and frustrations. The more the nurse can help the client and family connect with support groups, the more he or she can help them both maintain some independence and deal with the emotional aspects of chronic disease. Support groups may not only provide an arena to vent feelings and frustrations, but also may serve as a good source of gaining information. Families who have dealt with the system or who have become aware of new treatments share that knowledge with one another. It becomes another type of chat room, only in this instance the individuals talk face-to-face, rather than over the Internet.

The nurse must be aware that other aspects of the caregiver's life do not disappear. This means that the caregiver is combining all normal roles with the new aspects of the care being provided to the chronically ill family member. The nurse may have to help guide caregivers through these changes and become a sounding board for caregivers as they struggle with new responsibilities. Rose (1998) discusses how the nurse must give appropriate help and support and not increase the demands on the caregiver. One individual in her study stated: "They come and I know they mean well, but it's just another thing to do. You know, you've got to make them a cup of tea, talk to them and it just wears you out." The caregivers in Rose's study also talked about how they need help in managing their time to accomplish all the tasks needed in a 24-hour period. The ability to manage time also involves helping all individuals involved in the care to be

coordinated in the care they are providing. The nurse must realize that giving care is not only physically demanding for the caregiver, but also emotionally demanding. The more the nurse can assist the individual in expressing concerns and frustrations, the more information that may be available to guide the caregiver. Caregivers need to have their confidence reinforced and they need to feel valued and supported, and the nurse is in a position to meet those needs.

The following is my personal experience:

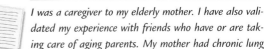

I was a caregiver to my elderly mother. I have also validated my experience with friends who have or are taking care of aging parents. My mother had chronic lung disease, a typical tuberculosis, hypertension, osteoporosis, and poor cerebral circulation resulting in [transient ischemic attacks] TIAs. As her condition began to deteriorate, it became harder and harder to leave her alone for any length of time. During the day when my husband and I were at work, I worried about her having an accident or falling and lying there until I would get home. I did not like going out in the evening without making sure that she was settled in bed. The first year that she started to become more disabled, my youngest child was a senior in high school and it wasn't as difficult. The next two years after that he was away from home in college and it became more difficult. The year he left for college my husband had to take him to school while I stayed home with my mother. It was very frustrating trying to meet all of my professional obligations and still be available for my mother. As she became less able to care for herself, she became more dependent on me for taking care of things. She would wait until I got home from work to ask me to do things for her when my husband had been there for several hours and she had not asked him for help. I had feelings of guilt because I was gone at work and frustration because I felt like I was not being a good daughter.

If it had not been for nursing friends, I would have had no idea where to turn to get assistance with her care. It gave me insight into the lack of knowledge I had and made me question how someone without medical knowledge could get the support they needed. I also found that the support of other friends who had experienced similar situations with their parents gave me additional knowledge in finding resources. Also it was the reassurance that I was not being a bad daughter that gave me the strength to cope with my mother's changes and the frustration of caring for her while fulfilling my other roles and responsibilities.

An area of concern that Gravelle (1997) discussed in her study of parents coping with children in the chronic stage of illness was trying to control services. Many parents encountered fragmentation of care, duplication of services, and gaps in services, all of which added to their frustration. The nurse became the one that helped family members work through the system, coordinated services, and directed them to resources to help them cope with the illness. This is important when the health situation is changing and the needs of the ill individual and family are changing. The nurse is the caregiver who should direct the family to resources and then help to coordinate them so that care is provided.

Sometimes the family can be a source of tension to the chronically ill client. Levine and Zuckerman (1999) report that few families are perfect in their functioning. Many families have overt or hidden tensions, and under the stress of the family member's illness those tensions can erupt. She states that long-standing but suppressed differences may emerge and new alliances may be forged. The nurse working with the family cannot ignore these situations, but must take them into consideration when assessing the family and client needs. The nurse must keep lines of communication open with families by being direct and honest with them. In addition, the nurse must be aware that differing religious, cultural, or ethnic backgrounds between clients, families, caregivers, or nurses can amplify conflicts.

As a nurse working in the community, you have a unique opportunity to approach the care of chronically ill clients from a new and different perspective. You are not restricted by the hospital and the demands the medical treatment requires. You go into the home to assess chronically ill clients and determine how they are handling their treatment plan. Your role is that of a nurse, but how you carry that role out is different than when you are in the hospital setting. You are in the client's home not only to perform procedures but also to assess the situation, the disease, and how your client is living with that disease. You enter the home with the knowledge of the health-care system, the disease, and the medical treatment. The role you play is that of helping clients blend the treatment plan into their lifestyle. There is no set clinical pathway for you to measure the client's progression. You determine success and failure of the care plan based on how well clients are handling the illness and integrating the treatment plan into their lifestyle. That means, when you enter the home, you must learn about the lifestyle of clients, their knowledge needs, and their goals and concerns and then guide them as they gain control over their lives and their illness. You need to learn what is important to the client and how the client fits into the family structure. What important role do they play in the family? You need to understand what is important to clients, what motivates them and how the disease is affecting their lives. Then, having that knowledge, use all the resources available to maximize the clients' ability to maintain a normal lifestyle and maximize their abilities. Communication is probably the most important tool you will need working in the community. You will need to be an active listener and realize that it takes time and patience to work in this environment. The reward comes in not seeing clients discharged from the hospital, but in having them stay out of the hospital and live a full productive life.

Research on Chronic Illness in the Community

Because many chronic illnesses are treated successfully outside of the hospital, nurses are encouraged to continually update their knowledge by reviewing current research regarding the care of clients with chronic illness in the community. Koch, Kralik, and Taylor (2000) studied type two diabetes in men using a Participatory Action Research (PAR) approach. The report of this research was the second of four group research projects related to type two diabetes. This study sought to understand men's

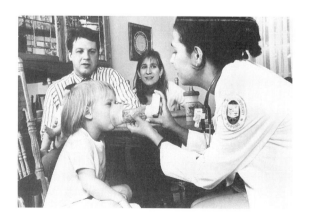

transition after diagnosis with type two diabetes and what it was like to live with diabetes.

The men with type two diabetes met with a researcher and two clinical nurse consultants for 2 hours once a week for 4 weeks in a community center. The results of the study indicated that the men felt that diabetes had a positive affect on their lifestyle. They felt they were taking better care of themselves, were confident in their knowledge about diabetes, and saw their diabetes as a part of their life, rather than as a disease. Men who had partners felt that those partners were helpful in managing their disease. These men were able to incorporate diabetes into their lives with minimal intrusion.

In another study, Williams, Freedman, and Deci (1998) sought to determine if clients with diabetes would feel more competent if they were autonomously motivated and thus would improve their glucose control. The 128 clients who formed the sample were between 18 and 80 years old, had no other major medical illnesses, and were responsible for managing their disease. The results of this investigation showed that when clients had choice, knowledge, and minimal external pressure applied to produce compliance with their treatment regime, they improved their control over their disease. The research demonstrated that the nurse needed to be a partner with the client in facilitating the client's control of his or her diabetes. The nurse needed an open, nonjudgmental attitude, and the clients needed to make the choice to control their blood sugar and their disease.

Cudney and Weinert (2000) investigated the impact of a telecommunication technology on middle-aged women with chronic illness living in rural areas who were unable to participate in a more traditional face-to-face support group. The Women to Women (WTW) Project was created to use a computer-based outreach tool to offer professional and group support and foster self-care to these women in isolated areas of Montana. Four cohorts of 30 women each participated in the project. The project consisted of four components: conversation, mailbox, HealthChat, and Resource Rack. A nurse monitor who was a certified advanced practice nurse provided oversight for the project. Women agreed to log on at least twice a week, but most women participated much more often. For example, the mean in one cohort group was 7.96 times per week. The project had a positive impact on the health of the participating women. The presence of the nurse monitor helped make participants secure in the quality of the information they provided.

With the increasing number of clients living with chronic illness in the community, more research is needed to better understand their needs. Further research must identify nursing interventions that are effective for meeting those needs.

SUMMARY

Information in this chapter should assist you in understanding the needs of chronically ill clients living in the community. It is important to arrive at a definition of chronic illness that is meaningful to you. Careful assessment of clients will help you to understand their perspective of the illness experience so that you can identify effective approaches to managing their care. You can help clients and families access important community resources and can be instrumental in identifying effective approaches to meet the unique needs of caregivers of the chronically ill client.

Active Learning Strategies

1. Write a story about a chronically ill client to whom you are assigned this semester. What is his or her perspective on the illness? What are the challenges you faced in helping this client to integrate the medical regimen into his or her lifestyle? What resources did you make available? How has the illness affected the family system?

2. You are assigned to visit Mr. Arthur, age 35. He is married and has four school-age children. Mr. Arthur has multiple sclerosis, which has been in remission. However, he is experiencing progressive deterioration in his ability to walk and has vision problems. After a recent hospitalization he has been unable to return to work. Develop a list of initial assessment questions to use on your first visit.

3. Visit your local multiple sclerosis association. Collect all available information on services they provide. Set up an interview with the executive director after you have reviewed the material so that you may ask specific questions about accessing services, cost, and so on.

4. Contact a local church. Explore all services that they provide to members of their congregation who are homebound.

References

Baekeland, F., & Lundwall, L. (1975). Dropping out of treatment: A critical review. Psychological Bulletin, 82(5), 738–783.

Becker, M. H., & Green, L. W. (1975). A family approach to compliance with medical treatment: A selective review of the literature. International Journal of Health Education, 18(3), 173–182.

Bull, N. J., & Jervis, L. L. (1997). Strategies used by chronically ill older women and their caregiving daughters in managing posthospital care. Journal of Advanced Nursing, 25(3), 541–547.

Burkhardt, M.A., & Nathaniel A. K. (1998). Ethics and issues in contemporary nursing. Albany, NY: Delmar.

Cameron, C. (1996). Patient compliance: Recognition of factors involved and suggestions for promoting compliance with therapeutic regimens. Journal of Advanced Nursing, 24(2), 244–250.

Cudney, S., & Weinert, C. (2000). Computer based support groups: Nursing in cyberspace. Computers in Nursing, 18(1), 35–43.

Gravelle, A. M. (1997). Caring for a child with a progressive illness during the complex chronic phase: Parents' experience of facing adversity. Journal of Advanced Nursing, 25(4), 738–745.

Koch, T., Kralik, D., & Taylor, J. (2000). Men living with diabetes: Minimizing the intrusiveness of the disease. Journal of Clinical Nursing, 9(2), 247–354.

Leidy, N. K., & Traver, G. A. (1996). Adjustment and social behaviour in older adults with chronic obstructive pulmonary disease: The family's perspective. Journal of Advanced Nursing, 32(2), 252–259.

Levine, C., & Zuckerman, C. (1999). The trouble with families: Toward an ethic of accommodation. Annals of Internal Medicine, 130(2), 148–152.

McWilliams, C. L., Stewart, M., Brown, J. B., Desai, K., & Coderre, P. (1996). Creating health with chronic illness. Advances in Nursing Science, 18(3), 1–15.

O'Neill, D. P., & Kenny, E. K. (1998). Spirituality and chronic illness. Image. The Journal of Nursing Scholarship, 30(3), 275–280.

Porter, A. M. W. (1969). Illness careers: The chronic illness experience. Journal of Advanced Nursing, 24(2), 275–279.

Prince, B. (1996). Illness careers: The chronic illness experience. Journal of Advanced Nursing, 24(2), 275–279.

Rose, K. (1998). Perceptions related to time in a qualitative study of informal carers of terminally ill cancer patients. Journal of Clinical Nursing, 17(4), 343–350.

Stuifbergen, A. K., & Rogers, S. (1997). Health promotion: An essential component of rehabilitation for persons with chronic disabling conditions. Advances in Nursing Science, 19(4), 1–20.

Turton, J. (1998). Importance of information following myocardial infarction: A study of the self-perceived information needs of patients and their spouse/partner compared with the perceptions of nursing staff. Journal of Advanced Nursing, 27(4), 770–778.

Williams, G. C., Freedman, Z. R., & Deci, E. L. (1998). Supporting autonomy to motivate patients with diabetes for glucose control. Diabetes Care, 21(10), 1644–1651.

Primary Care Skills for Community-based Practice

12 Health Assessment Concerns in the Community

Janet Schwab Merritt

LEARNING OBJECTIVES

1) Apply critical thinking in making complete client assessments in a community setting.

2) Understand the client's expectation and acceptance of health status.

3) Assess functional activities of daily living (ADLs), resources, adaptive strategies.

4) Understand assessment parameters that are indicative of urgent or emergency situations.

5) Apply assessment strategies in unexpected or out of the ordinary situations using problem-solving skills

6) Understand the need for continued supervision of care and assessment delivered in the community setting.

THE ART OF HEALTH ASSESSMENT

This chapter focuses on health assessment in the community. The lessons of mastering the techniques of observation, auscultation, palpation, and percussion of body systems are left to texts devoted to health and physical assessment. I see that as the *science* of health assessment. The goal of this chapter is to help the student gain insight into the *art* of physical and health assessment and how this is applied in community settings. The draft of the "Scope and Standards of Public Health Nursing Practice," proposed by the American Nurses Association (ANA) in early 1999, lists the assessment activities of a community-based nurse as including the client's environment, lifestyle, coping strategies, relationships, neighborhood, economic status, health status, and access to care, as well as other factors that might impact a client's health outcomes. Much of this *art* depends on the therapeutic use of self. Authors define and describe this in different ways. However, the essence remains the same: care occurs within and because of the relationship between nurse and patient (Peplau, 1952; Carson & Arnold, 1996; SmithBattle, Drake, & Diekemper, 1997; Deering, 1999). This is not a relationship of friendship, but a professional relationship that engenders trust by the client. It allows the nurse to become a partner in care with the client. The nurse can then become a credible and trusted advocate, teacher, coach, sounding board, and resource broker. The nurse's education, experience, and personality are all used to benefit the client's well-being. This chapter helps the student or novice nurse who has a community-based practice to hone assessment techniques. It suggests questions to ask to enhance knowledge of clients and their health status. Well-thought-out, organized questions with sensitive, perceptive listening helps each nurse develop a more complete picture of each client.

Taylor (1997) researched problem solving in clinical nursing practice. Her results point out differences between the novice and the expert nurse. She found that the novice tends to focus on one cue, whereas the expert is able to grasp many cues or signs and symptoms at once and organize them into a whole picture of the client. She found the expert is less distracted by internal cues of concern for doing a procedure correctly and is able to focus on many assessments concurrently. Taylor (1997) relates a story of a "subject" in her study who shared her thoughts after taking a client's blood pressure. She was focused on the fact that his arm wouldn't twist as she needed it to in order to take the BP. She recognized that there was something wrong with his arm, but was unable to realize that the arm was "bent and spastic" secondary to a cerebrovascular accident. Reading this chapter will assist the novice nurse in the ability to look beyond the one puzzle piece of client data to see more of the interlocking puzzle pieces of the client as a whole. Nurses must be excellent problem solvers. This requires strong clinical reasoning processes. The novice can move toward expertise by copying a role model who is more expert in recognizing all presenting cues (Taylor, 1997). Clinical instructors can serve the student well in this role.

The student nurse begins to get a view of this puzzle even prior to meeting the client or family from the client's chart or referral source. Try to get only as much information as necessary. Data are important. However, data often get interspersed with opinion. This increases the incidence of both positive and negative preconceived ideas. Try to view each client as a clean slate. Ignore statements that someone is rude or difficult. One never knows what the client was responding to when the previous *judgment* was made. If a clinician anticipates an angry client, for instance, he or she puts up a particular type of guard that may in and of itself promote anger in the client. I have recommended this strategy with my students. They have consistently met with clients prior to ever reading the chart or getting information about them. This allows them to interact without being harnessed by possible prejudices that have crept into previous assessments. The assessments and wisdom of others is valuable. Just try to use it *after* you have done your own initial assessment.

The relationship begins when the client first meets the student nurse. The nurse and the client's initial impression of this interaction sets the stage for the nurse-client relationship that will develop. It is the *nurse* who is responsible for maintaining this relationship, setting the relationship parameters, and clarifying expectations. The parameters of the relationship include when the student will be available to the client. I encourage students to make a contract with clients. This involves setting an appointment and time limit for the visit. Many students get snagged into staying longer than they have planned with clients who are lonely or seeking attention. They go to the door to leave, and the client remembers to mention a significant health concern. The student gets drawn in. Setting realistic limits on the time to be spent with a client lets both the student and the client know how long the visit will be. For the student nurse, this makes it imperative that an appointment not be missed. If an appointment is forgotten, or the nurse is late, the client may feel that the nurse does not value the visit. If there is a need to cancel, change, or arrive late to an appointment, the client must be made aware of this as soon as possible. An ill student may want to send in a colleague to see the client in his or her absence. This contract also adds responsibility to the clients. They are responsible for being present for the visit and can also be encouraged to plan for the visit with questions or concerns.

Another parameter involves what the client can expect from the nurse. It must be made clear that the relationship between the nurse and client is a professional one. The student nurse should not leave the client her home phone number. Nor should the student contact the client outside of the scheduled visit time unless this is specifically part of the care plan. (An exception is to confirm an appointment). The nurse may also need to verbalize that the relationship is confidential, but that it is not a friendship. Over time, genuine feelings of concern and compassion can develop between nurse and client; however, the student nurse must always be mindful of the nurse's role in the client's life.

These parameters help to build trust. The relationship is also benefited when the student has a nonjudgmental, positive regard for the client. Nurses need not condone lifestyle choices or health-care patterns, but the person is always to be respected. Novice nurses must avoid focusing on the failures and deficits seen in clients and concentrate on instilling hope (SmithBattle et al., 1997). The development of a rapport with the client mustn't be overlooked. It is via this avenue that the client will begin to trust the nurse and share problems and concerns regarding health problems.

THE CLIENT'S PERSPECTIVE

Clients' Expectation of Health

One important assessment parameter that is frequently overlooked is the client's expectation of health. Often the nurse enters a client's sphere of health with very different expectations of good health. For instance, a 63-year-old insulin-dependent diabetic may not be willing to do without sweets and may consistently have cookies as an afternoon or evening snack or candy when it is available. All of our nursing knowledge tells us this is not acceptable practice. However, if we assess that this client is not willing to change snacking patterns, we need to help with insulin adjustment and very thoroughly teach the client to know the signs and symptoms of hypo- and hyperglycemia. If the nurse "preaches" that the client can't have these "treats," then the client is likely to continue the behaviors and just not tell the nurse about them. It is far better for the client to admit "noncompliance" than to try to cover it up. This is what is meant by assessing and accepting the client's expectation

of health. This shows respect for what the client values in life. Using the same example, some clients live to eat, others eat to live. An understanding of the client's perspective aids assessment and the planning of appropriate interventions.

Without a doubt, for the client to be able to have a valid, reasoned perspective, the client must have a full understanding of the consequences of behaviors. Knowledge of risks does not always yield a health behavior change. Knowledge of risks doesn't keep a daredevil from escapades. Nor will knowledge of health risks always keep a diabetic from sweet treats. The client has the right to make personal health-care decisions. These decisions must be respected even if the nurse doesn't agree with them. The nurse must focus on assessing the adaptation to the illness and the effects of the illness on the client's life.

Adaptation is made to all illnesses or stress. Using the Adaptation model of nursing practice developed by Sr. Roy aids the understanding of what the nurse can do in assessment of this adaptation. Roy's premises describe man as an adaptive being whose adaptation level is a function of the interaction between adaptation mechanisms and the environment. Nursing interventions are focused on manipulation of the environment (Roy, 1981). In the previous example, the nurse can't change the illness. The important thing to assess is how the client is *adapting* to the illness. What resources are being used? What coping mechanisms are being used? Is the adaptation to the illness effective or ineffective? A thorough assessment based on this type of question leads to interventions to enhance the level of adaptive response.

Another example is of a client with chronic obstructive pulmonary disease (COPD). This client may arrange activities to maximize benefits of energy expenditure. If this client only shaves every other day, this is adaptive, not indicative of a lack of personal hygiene. We all make choices about what is important to us as individuals and live accordingly. The nurse must assess the client's expectation of his or her health and intervene to help the client achieve maximum adaptation. The nurse must also assess the client's wishes in regard to care. This includes end-of-life decisions, aggressive or palliative care measures, and whom the client chooses to make these decisions if or when the client is unable.

Box 12–1 will help you focus further on this area.

Box 12-1   Student Learning Activity

Client Situations

On assessment, a carotid bruit is heard in an elderly, frail client who wants no invasive treatments, is happy and content with her life, and seems to be integrating her life experiences adequately. Would you seek a referral to a physician who would recommend an ultrasound to be followed by a recommendation for an endarterectomy?

Why or why not?

Is it sufficient to express your findings and all alternative options to the client?

(Explain the reasons for your answer)

Does the nurse have an obligation to inform the adult daughter who cares for the client (prn) about the findings and recommendations?

---

full range of services be made available if this is what the client wants. This must be done in spite of the fact that some in the medical community may believe that aggressive intervention is futile.

For the nurse to be unbiased in his or her care in this type of a situation, she or he must be fully aware of personal values and beliefs regarding the end of life and the desirability of treatment regardless of its futility. This may be less of an issue in jurisdictions that are part of a nationalized Health Care Delivery System (HCDS). Currently, there are many diverse systems in different countries and even between different states within countries. These differences exist because of differing perspectives of who should pay for what health care. The problems of what care for whom may be more pronounced in a fee-for-service type of system. Regardless of what type of HCDS you practice in, the clients and their wishes are primary. As the character Patch Adams said in the movie by the same name, "If you treat an illness, you win or you lose. When you treat a person, I guarantee it, you always win" (Williams, 1998).

Ethical Principle of Autonomy and the Right of Self-Determination

The expectation and acceptance of what is "normal" for a particular client is also an ethical issue of autonomy and the right of self-determination. One of the most difficult lessons to learn, especially for the novice nurse in a community situation, is to respect the client's autonomy or the right to make independent choices. Many times the nurse's code of ethics that requires her or him to help in all situations (to apply beneficence) causes the nurse to help when help isn't wanted or needed. The nurse's perception of health is not necessarily the same as the client's. In a hospital, the nurse and other hospital staff are "in charge" in many aspects. The patient often feels powerless as a recipient of care. In the community, the client is more in control of the care received. The client can choose to partner with a nurse to learn healthy behaviors and to have health status assessed. However, the client controls his or her own care. This can be difficult for the student nurse in particular to accept. When one *knows* that there is a better, healthier way to live, it is hard not to try to *make* someone comply with the prescribed regimen. We can never *make* someone take our advice or

For some clients, the only expectation of life is to be loved and free from pain. Nurses must uphold the right of the client not to have numerous treatments or interventions that are not wanted. The medical community, which often focuses on treating an illness or problem rather than the person, may see interventions as necessary. On the opposite end of the spectrum, some clients have difficulty even talking about death and end-of-life decisions. For this client, the nurse must advocate that the suggestions. This is why the development of a trusting relationship is so important. If the client views the nurse as a trusted *partner* in care, then assessment information comes freely. Recommendations moving toward health are more respected. This respect for persons and their integrity is respect for autonomy or the right to self-govern. This issue becomes more complex if the client is not competent for one reason or another. This is addressed in the section on mental status assessment later in this chapter.

THE NURSE'S PERSPECTIVE

The Client at First Glance

Health assessment begins when the nurse first meets the client. The nurse must continually assess the client throughout the entire visit. It is important to move to some specific areas that need to be evaluated.

Box 12–2 presents a series of questions to help you practice assessment.

Mental Status Assessment

A Mini-Mental Status Exam (MMSE) is recommended for each visit. The formal exam should be conducted on initial interview. However, the assessment parameters should be addressed regularly. To assess orientation, the nurse can ask the client the current date and time and/or the scheduled date of the next appointment. In general conversation, the nurse must assess ability to comprehend and follow directions. These skills should not be taken for granted. Many clients who become demented are very socially skillful. They can learn and are even reinforced for the ability to hide or cover up their forgetfulness or poor judgment. Some clients may answer with rote phrases or frequently use clichés. One of my students worked with a very charming woman who she believed to be very cognitively intact until she conducted the formal MMSE. Even during the exam, the client tried to excuse her memory loss with statements such as, "Oh, you know I haven't had my coffee yet, let's just do this later!" and abruptly changed the subject. This can be difficult for the student who wants to show respect for the client and his or her need to appear as competent; however, the data collection that the MMSE affords is essential. I recommend that

---

Box 12-2   Student Learning Activity

Client Assessment

First glance assessments:

- How does the client greet the nurse?

- Is she or he able to come to the door?

- How are the client's gait, coordination, and general mobility?

- Is the client oriented to who you are?

- How is the pattern of speech? Skin color, respiratory pattern? Mood, affect?

- If the client is not able to come to the door, who is assisting her or him in the home?

- Does the home seem clean, safe, and free of hazards?

- What do you hear? Smell? Feel? See?

---

students make the basic elements of the MMSE part of every assessment. If the client asks why such questions are being asked, the student can truthfully say it is routine. The student must learn the complex task of respecting the client's right to make personal decisions and at the same time recognizing when the client is incapable of making informed choices. Allowing a cognitively or emotionally impaired client to muddle through complex health decisions is just as unethical as denying someone their right to decide.

Box 12–3 helps you to further examine ethical decisions.

Mental Health Assessment

In addition to an MMSE, each client should be assessed for signs and symptoms of mental illness. Many clients suffer from depression, anxiety disorders, and even suicidal ideations. Medications and medical conditions can mimic mental illness. What appears to be depression may be a side effect of antihypertensive medication or result from uncontrolled diabetes. In many situations, a full mental health assessment must be conducted. In each visit, however, a brief assessment of appearance, behavior, mood, communication, and thought content provides information needed to assess changes from the client's normal state.

When assessing appearance, the student must consider the appropriateness of dress, hygiene, and neatness. Also determine if the client's affect is appropriate for the situation. What does the client's behavior reflect? Is the client's response to you as it usually is or is there a change? Is their any evidence of hypervigilence, suspiciousness, paranoia, or response to hallucinations? Is the mood animated or flat and depressed? Can the client sit still for a discussion with you or is he or she moving around the room, pacing and restless?

Appearance is easiest to assess. Decide if the client is appropriately dressed for the weather. A client with bipolar disorder in a manic state may be in shorts and bare feet in the snow. A client with an exacerbation of schizophrenia may have on many layers of clothing and a hat to help hold himself or herself together or have aluminum foil wrapped around the head to deflect signals that are being "transmitted." Also note general hygiene practices and know that these become diminished with many mental illnesses such as depression, severe anxiety, and psychotic states. Behavior is closely associated with appearance. Is the client acting in a peculiar manner? This includes behaviors that indicate that the client is listening to voices or responding to hallucinations. Also pay attention to ritualistic behaviors such as checking or washing rituals that can be seen in conjunction with psychotic states and also with obsessive-compulsive disorders.

Communication assessment can follow. Does the flow of the conversation make sense, or does the client carry the conversation in illogical, loosely associated ways? Do the client's words fit with the emotional tone presented? Is the conversation coherent? Does speech seem pressured or is the rate and rhythm smooth and natural?

As part of the natural progression, thought content can be assessed next. The nurse must be alert to delusional content, somatic preoccupation, and most significantly, suicidal ideation. Table 12-1 presents some demographic information related to suicide. The U.S. Surgeon General, David Satcher, presented a call to action to prevent suicide on July 28, 1999. His report notes that suicide is the eighth leading cause of death in the United States. He also states that "the most promising way to prevent suicide and suicidal behavior is through the early recognition and treatment

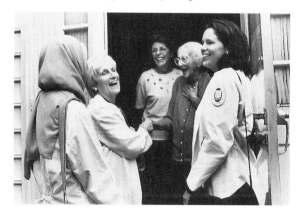

Table 12-1

Demographics of Suicide

The Problem

- Suicide took the lives of 30,535 Americans in 1997 (11.4 per 100,000 population).

- More people die from suicide than from homicide. In 1997, there were 1.5 times as many suicides as homicides.

- Overall, suicide is the eighth leading cause of death for all Americans and is the third leading cause of death for young people aged 15–24.

- Males are four times more likely to die from suicide than are females. However, females are more likely to attempt suicide than are males.

- White males account for 72% of all suicides.

- Together, white males and white females accounted for more than 90% of all suicides. However, during the period from 1979 to 1992, suicide rates for Native Americans (a category that includes American Indians and Alaska Natives) were about 1.5 times the national rates.

- Suicide rates are generally higher than the national average in the western states and lower in the eastern and midwestern states.

- Nearly 3 of every 5 suicides in 1997 (58%) were committed with a firearm

Suicide among the Elderly

- Suicide rates increase with age and are highest among Americans aged 65 years and older. The 10-year period, 1980 to 1990, was the first decade since the 1940s that the suicide rate for older residents rose instead of declined.

- Men accounted for 83% of suicides among persons aged 65 years and older in 1997.

- From 1980 to 1997, the largest relative increases in suicide rates occurred among those 80 to 84 years of age. The rate for men in this age group increased 8% (from 43.5 per 100,000 to 47.0).

- Firearms were the most common method of suicide by both males and females, 65 years and older in 1997, accounting for 77.1% of male and 32.7% of female suicides in that age group.

- Suicide rates among the elderly are highest for those who are divorced or widowed. In 1992, the rate for divorced or widowed men in this age group was 2.7 times that for married men, 1.4 times that for never-married men, and more than 17 times that for married women. The rate for divorced or widowed women was 1.8 times that for married women and 1.4 times that for never-married women.

- Risk factors for suicide among older persons differ from those among the young. Older persons have a higher prevalence of depression, a greater use of highly lethal methods and social isolation. They also make fewer attempts per completed suicide, have a higher-male-to-female ratio than other groups, have often visited a health-care provider before their suicide, and have more physical illnesses.

(Continued)

of depression and other psychiatric illnesses" (Satcher, 1999). Nurses in community settings are in a key position to recognize evidence of suicidal thinking or intent. A depressed, hopeless demeanor is frequently seen in suicidal clients. They feel as if there is nothing they can do to feel better and/or that there is nothing that can help them at all. Alternatively, people who seem to suddenly rise out of a sig-

nificant depression may be feeling relieved because they have made the decision to kill themselves and thus feel a release from the desperation of the illness. Often it is when the deepest depression begins to lift and the client has more energy that suicide is of the greatest concern. Consequently, these behaviors and cognitive changes need to be investigated thoroughly. It is okay, even recommended, that the

Table 12-1

Demographics of Suicide—cont'd

Suicide among the Young

- Persons under age 25 accounted for 15% of all suicides in 1997. From 1952 to 1995, the incidence of suicide among adolescents and young adults nearly tripled.

- From 1980 to 1997, the rate of suicide among persons aged 15 to 19 years increased by 11% and among persons aged 10 to 14 years by 109%. From 1980 to 1996, the rate increased 105% for African-American males aged 15 to 19.

- In 1997, more teenagers and young adults died from suicide than from cancer, heart disease, AIDS, birth defects, stroke, pneumonia and influenza, and chronic lung disease combined.

- Among persons aged 15 to 19 years, firearm-related suicides accounted for 62% of the increase in the overall rate of suicide from 1980 to 1997.

- The risk for suicide among young people is greatest among young white males; however, from 1980 through 1996 suicide rates increased most rapidly among young black males. Although suicide among young children is a rare event, the dramatic increase in the rate among persons aged 10 to 14 years underscores the urgent need for intensifying efforts to prevent suicide among persons in this age group.

(Satcher, 1999)

client be asked directly if she or he is considering suicide. Usually the client will answer honestly, especially if a relationship has been established. If the client answers in the affirmative, ask if a plan has been made and what has been done to facilitate that plan. The more concrete and completed the plan, the more imminent the danger. Some clients have suicidal thoughts but do not intend to act on those thoughts. Others keep suicide as a long-term, chronic option.

The second question to ask if the client does have suicidal thoughts is if he or she can contract for safety. Asking the client to make a verbal contract with you, the nurse, is an effective tool to postpone a suicide attempt, assess the client's ability to postpone a plan, and get the additional help that the client requires. For example, if a client states that he has purchased a gun with ammunition, has plans to drive to a remote national park, and his family and friends think he is out of town on a business trip for a few days, one can assess that his intent is very serious and imminent. This type of situation requires immediate intervention. Emergency mental health services must be initiated. This client must not be left alone.

If suicide is not an issue for a client, move to assess other maladaptive thought patterns. Those of a delusional nature must be assessed to determine if the cause is an illness itself (e.g., schizophrenia) or if it is a symptom of another problem. Possible medication side effects should be considered, as should electrolyte disturbances. It is difficult to assess whether a client is somatically preoccupied. Someone who is ill naturally focuses on the illness. However, a client who has significant complaints of illness without evidence of physical symptoms should cause the student to investigate if components of a mental illness are present. For somatic preoccupation beyond what seems normal, especially when the client is getting the needed emotional attention, the student is referred to psychiatric and mental health texts that discuss somatic disorders. Remember that a client with a severe depression may have mood-congruent delusions and hallucinations. An example is the client who believes that his or her internal organs are dead or crawling with worms, causing inability to eat. The depressed client in reality may be suffering from psychomotor retardation to the point that even the bowels are slowed and constipated, thus accounting for the uncomfortable feeling of the abdomen.

If a client is exhibiting a change in mental health status, a referral needs to be made so that additional treatment can be initiated. Use of the decision tree (see Box 12–4) for expected findings works well for this type of illness too.

Box 12-4   Student Learning Activity

Decision Tree Exercise

A change in health status has been noted in a client. Identify the change.

Assess and record the following:

Has the change been a gradual or rapid change? (small differences you have seen over time, vs. major change since the last visit)

Gradual/minor: Are these changes attributable to a specific, expected cause?

Yes: continue to observe and report

No: refer, advise client to see physician within the next few days

Rapid/major: If the client continues on the same path, how soon will serious consequences likely appear/occur?

Days: Advise the client to see a physician as soon as possible or call the physician and discuss concerns and schedule an appointment

Hours: Have the client immediately transported to the doctor's office or if this is not possible, transport via ambulance to local ER.

Emergent: The client is changing rapidly, steadily worsening, serious or life-threatening consequences seem inevitable: call 911 for emergency intervention.

NURSE-CLIENT PARTNERSHIPS

Assessing the Clients' Understanding of Illness and Medications

A 100-pound woman was routinely taking Bentyl and Valium to treat acid reflux, which had caused esophageal scarring and constriction. She fell and was treated in the local emergency department (ED). She was spared any fractures but suffered numerous contusions. She was prescribed Tylenol #3 with codeine. Her neighbors found her to be confused and unsteady on her feet the next morning. After sleeping for more than 3 hours, she was back to her normal mental status. Clearly she had reacted to an unintentional overdose. Had she informed the ED staff of her medicine regimen? Had they weighed her? Luckily the woman slept off what could have been a potentially serious overdose or a situation that could have caused another, more serious fall. This story illustrates the importance of the client knowing the medicines he or she takes and the illnesses for which the medicines are prescribed. Many rescue squads are now making packets available for people to place in their freezers that delineate the medications and medical conditions of the household's residents. This standard placement was enacted so that responses by rescue personnel would not be slowed, but could be improved based on a better knowledge of the client's health status. Other aids include medical-alert tags that can be worn. All clients on medications should be taught to keep a current list of their medications/illnesses in their wallet or purse. Identify if the client has this information readily available and if it is up to date.

In the early stages of the nurse-client relationship, the student nurse begins to assess the client's understanding of his or her illnesses and medications. Does the client have an understanding of both? Does he or she have a concept of the course of such an illness? When my father was to have an endarterectomy, my mother was rather unconcerned. My sister and I, both nurses, were very anxious about the risks involved. My father was well aware of the risks, but the three of us agreed not to tell my mother to spare her some anxiety. The surgery went well, but I often think back and wonder if we did the right thing by "protecting" her. Had my father not survived the surgery, she may have felt robbed of the opportunity of saying her good-byes. It is a difficult call. The client has the right to know, and the decision to tell others rests with him or her. My father was clear about the risks involved and was able to make a rational decision based on the facts. Each client needs to know in clear and understandable terms about illnesses, procedures, and medications that they have been or will be taking. Overwhelming or frightening the client are the risks of such interventions. Understanding this, the presentation of the information is critical. The nurse needs to clearly explain health information in a way that can be understood with the risks balanced appropriately with the benefits; however, it is important to respect the client's approach. Research has demonstrated that when people are acutely ill, they often wish for more direction from the health-care team. We need to be sensitive to the needs of

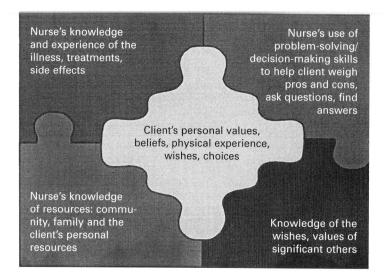

FIGURE 12–1

The complete puzzle represents a partnership between the client and nurse resulting in excellent care. It is the nurse who works to gather all of the pieces and work with the client to put them into place.

our clients in this regard and not expect them, especially elderly clients, to be comfortable with "partnerships." It must be a slowly introduced concept. It is important to recognize that this is a change in what has been a paternalistic medical model. Older clients may not be used to being partners in care. They may have relied on a physician to make all health-care decisions. It is the student, the newest generation of nurses, who must help all clients move to a standard of partnership in care. If a client is reticent to be involved in decision making, it is important to determine who will be making decisions for the client.

Before any visit is concluded, assessment of the client's understanding of what was said and done during the interaction is required. Providing a summary at the end of the visit helps identify that the visit is concluding and gives the client and the nurse an opportunity to ensure information was understood by both parties; for example, "So for today, Mrs. Smith, we talked a bit about your diabetes and how you have some questions about controlling your sugars better. We also discussed how you are concerned about your blood pressure in that you have some dizzy spells when you get up quickly." Asking the client to repeat back instructions is a way to assess if the information was understood. The student may also ask if the client has questions about the information. Encouraging questions is a very good strategy. The quality of questions gives the nurse a good indication if the information was understood. It also helps the student nurse know what

part of the information the client primarily focused on. In all situations, regardless of the educational level of the client, assess that the information is understood.

Mary S. was an obstetrical client that I was following in the community. She had experienced a miscarriage in her first pregnancy. Her husband, Bob, and she were elated that she was pregnant again, and they were anxious to do all that was necessary for Mary to retain this pregnancy.

Mary developed severe hypertension beginning in her fifth month. She was still working, and her midwife told the couple that she could continue to work, but that she would need to be on bed rest for all nonworking hours. Later, when Mary's blood pressure continued to escalate and her legs become more edematous, the midwife ordered complete bed rest.

The next evening I visited the couple to see how they were doing. They both were extremely concerned about the news they had heard. Only when Bob asked me if Mary would have to leave her job, did I realize how anxious they had been the previous day. I explained that Mary would have to be on bed rest continuously. We talked about how this would affect them financially and the kinds of support resources that they would need until the birth of the baby. I also notified their midwife so that she would be aware that the information she had communicated had not been understood. She thanked me and said she would be careful to assess their comprehension in the future.

Assessing the Client's Baseline

One of the most important assessment tasks is the ability to assess change. An observant nurse can note differences from one visit to the next. This is true of both positive and negative changes. In a child, the biggest clue of illness may be behavioral changes. A normally rambunctious, active child who is suddenly sitting quietly in the mother's lap for long periods may not feel well. Children have difficulty expressing pain and vague feelings of illness. Often, the caregivers know that the child "isn't acting right" without knowing why. This requires an assessment to rule out ear infection, flu, gastrointestinal upset, or other ailments common to this age group. This is also a time to evaluate the caregiver's ability to make assessments as well. It is good to observe the techniques used to take a temperature and how questions about illness are asked. With a little information, the parent or other caregiver can be taught to enhance the ability to assess signs of illness in the child or in themselves and give health-care providers the data needed to determine if the a visit to the primary health-care provider is needed.

In the geriatric client, both physical and behavioral changes may be subtle and may be the only indicators of change in health status. Walton and Miller (1998) reviewed this phenomenon and agree that "it is easy to attribute subtle or even dramatic change to the patient's age. Often even unintentional ageism can delay treatment and waste valuable time in assessment, data gathering, and problem identification" (pp. 85–86). Symptoms may be nonspecific and vague, but very important to observe and assess further. In the early stages of an infection, an elderly client may only complain of being tired or just of not feeling "right." This information should be treated as a symptom in itself and the classic seven characteristics of a symptom should be investigated. For example, while working with a particularly frail, elderly woman, I noted that she would occasionally have a fierce, dry cough. She described it as a tickle in her throat and told me that it frequently occurred at night and would waken her. She tried to treat it (unsuccessfully) with hard candies. These coughing spasms were quite severe and would frequently result in shortness of breath (SOB). These episodes concerned me because of her congestive heart failure (CHF), hypertension, and history of abdominal aneurysm repair. The client

had tried to adapt to these coughs, but they persisted and had lately gotten worse. It was when she told me that they had recently gotten worse that I made a connection. She had just seen her doctor who had increased her captopril, an angiotensin-converting enzyme (ACE) inhibitor. Knowledge of the side effects of this drug made me realize that this was the likely culprit for the cough. The physician changed the prescribed medication and the annoying, sleep-depriving cough was gone.

I would also like to emphasize that the client often knows when something is wrong or different without being able to express exactly what the problem is. Always listen to the clients. They know their own bodies better than anyone! It can be quicker and easier to attribute headaches to stress, heat, or family conflict. But if the client says "I really don't think that is the problem" be sure to follow the client's cue. This is when good, thoughtful open-ended questions come in handy. I believe that clients do have the information we need to make an accurate assessment, but it requires that we ask the right questions to draw out the information!

Box 12–5 provides additional open-ended health assessment questions.

Assessment of Functional ADLs

Many clients who are cared for in the community are very adaptive, as has been discussed. However, sometimes a client may not be as adaptive as he or she appears initially. Decreasing functional capacity generally occurs gradually. Appearances can be deceptive to family and friends as well. This is why the nurse must carefully assess the client's ability to manage his or her instrumental activities of daily living. Rarely will the individual recognize his or her own problem with ADLs. It is usually only when the electricity gets cut off or there is suddenly no money left in a checking account that significant others recognize a problem. The nurse can be more objective in this assessment.

The nurse can assess the client's ability to maintain functional ADLs in a number of ways. A quick look around the kitchen can give an indication if needed groceries are being obtained. Is the area clean? Ask if you can look in the refrigerator. Observe for signs of meal preparation. Is the stove consistently turned off? Do you see any signs of unsafe kitchen habits such as burned pots or

Box 12-5	Student Learning Activity

Health Assessment Questions

Practice using the following open-ended questions when doing a health assessment with one of your community clients. Record their responses.

- Tell me more about how you are feeling [about the particular concern].

- When does this occur?

- What makes it better/worse?

- Have you ever had anything like this before?

- Why do you think this happens?

- What have you done to try to take care of this?

- Point to where it hurts/feels funny.

- Does changing your position make it better or worse?

(Note that all of these questions with the exceptions of the last two can be asked not only for physical concerns/problems but for emotional ones as well.)

Assessment of Psychological, Emotional, Spiritual, and Cultural Health

To ensure the best quality of life for any client, a holistic approach is essential. Assessing physical needs is only one part of the assessment process. Psychological, emotional, spiritual, social, and cultural needs must also be assessed. When I think of this holistic perspective, an analogy of a small plant seems to fit. To *survive* it needs only minimal amounts of water, sun, and soil nutrients. To *thrive* it must have far more than the bare necessities. The plant must have good rich soil with the proper pH for it to produce flowers. It needs just the right amount of sunshine so that it won't be burnt by too much or whither without enough. It needs to have weeds pulled that encroach on its space and compete for the resources. The plant must be properly watered, the amount adjusted for the particular needs of the plant and soil conditions. The good gardener considers all of these parameters just as the nurse must consider emotional, spiritual, social, and cultural needs of each client. Box 12–6 helps you to think of one of your current clients.

Box 12-6	Student Learning Activity

Client Example

Using this analogy, think of a particular client.

What might be sunshine for him or her?

What is water?

What are the weeds that get in the way of growth?

How can the client's "soil" be enriched?

potholders? Do you see signs that the mail and newspapers are being read, sorted? Feel free to ask clients how they take care of their finances. The nurse has no need to know of specific financial information, but general information about whether the client is self-sufficient is important. Ask clients if they pay their own bills or if there is a system in place for this activity? Security measures such as direct deposit can be recommended.

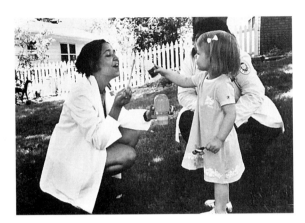

The gardening nurse must assess what the client's best growing conditions are. This requires attentive listening when interacting with the client. When your client Emily, age 8, tells her stories, what situations seem to make her content, happy? What activities, beliefs, or organizations are meaningful to her? These are the types of assessments that focus on activities that enhance personal development. Use of Erikson's developmental model (1963) aids the nurse's understanding of the developmental stage and tasks that the client is currently facing. For this school-age child to successfully develop a positive sense of self, Emily must accomplish the task of industry encompassing cooperation and personal competence. A sick child who is kept out of school or is consistently emotionally guarded because of a serious illness may lack opportunity to learn and practice the interpersonal skills needed at this age. Box 12–7 contains a client example for you to complete.

The nurse working in the community must be or become aware of the many resources available to clients and their families. Many communities have resources that are often underused. If the student is unaware of available resources, the local health department is a good place to start to become familiar with community resources. Churches, community groups, and schools are also valuable sources of assistance. Those resources used depend on the client's interests and needs. The most important task in recommending a resource goes beyond handing the client a pamphlet or just a phone number. It involves actively engaging the client in identifying needs that the resource can meet. If possible, it is often helpful to ac-

company the client on the initial visit or give the client the name of a specific person as a contact within the community resource service.

Assessment of Adaptive Strategies

Most clients, regardless of their age, have a need for some independence. This need should be supported. Even young children who have just learned to tie their shoes should be supported in this time-consuming endeavor. Many clients are very creative in adapting to decreased functional ability. There are many helpful strategies that clients develop to manage day to day at home, within

---

Box 12-7	Student Learning Activity

Client Example

Emily is home bound for at least a year because of a severe accident that occurred during a Girl Scout hiking trip. She suffered no cognitive damage. She had a complete fracture of her right femur requiring traction with absolutely no weight bearing.

What are the developmental tasks for this 8-year-old girl?

How can you as the nurse assist the client and her family to successfully manage the developmental milestones necessary at this age?

If Emily's mom is a single parent, solely responsible for her care, what resources could you suggest to help the mom meet her own developmental needs?

What support systems might be called on?

their own limitations. Seeing what one client does is information for the student to share with others. The nurse can add to the client's coping strategies by suggesting resources. These can range from tools to help reach things on top shelves (without dangerously getting on a chair!), to getting information about financial support for home modifications such as bathroom rails and ramps to replace stairs. Communities vary widely in the availability of resources. Many have child and adult day-care centers, Meals-on-Wheels, a local agency on aging, parenting classes, and play groups. Some have transportation assistance that can be used for things such as shopping, doctor appointments, or even to play cards at a community center.

Other examples of adaptive strategies include recommending that a client with loss of hand strength ask for medication in bottles that do not have childproof caps. Medication reminders that hold one day or one week of medications are also useful. Clients who take insulin and are unable to see well enough to draw it up themselves can have their regular dose drawn up by a nurse or family member ahead of time. For example, one client I know of has his daughter draw up a week's worth of insulin for him. He takes neutral protamine Hagedorn insulin (NPH) in the morning and again at 4 p.m. The daughter found a 1-inch thick rectangle of packing Styrofoam. She poked two rows of holes in two lines on the Styrofoam. One row held syringes for the a.m. doses and the other held the p.m. doses. The second Styrofoam "tray" held 2, 4, 6, 8, and 10 units of regular insulin that the client used for coverage. The Styrofoam was easily marked with a pen to avoid confusion. The client was taught to gently roll the syringe to appropriately mix the NPH insulin. He was proficient in checking his own blood sugar and injecting the insulin. He just lacked the dexterity and visual acuity to draw up the insulin. The client's independence was supported by a weekly visit by someone who could draw up his insulin, a task that took less than an hour.

This example shows how some creativity can enhance independence. The purchase of a cordless phone that can be carried in an apron pocket can give assurance to someone living alone that they have access to help if needed. This type of phone also prevents those with movement limitations from trying to dangerously rush to the phone when it rings.

Special Considerations of the Physical Examination in the Home or Non-acute-care Setting

As discussed previously, the client is in charge in a home environment. The nurse must ask where the client would be the most comfortable doing a physical exam. The nurse can request a bedlike surface with good lighting and privacy. Some clients may be very glad to have this done on the living room sofa whereas others may want you to do it in a reclining chair. The nurse must insist, with all due respect, that the client be in a position in which he or she can be adequately assessed. This may entail the nurse assuring the client that she or he will help the client to get dressed again or that the nurse will aid the client up and down stairs to a bedroom, or help the client into a different position. It is also important to convey that you really can't assess a decubitus ulcer of the coccyx when a large client is in a reclining chair! You must insist that the client allow you to look at the wound if this is part of the client's problem list. Remember that the client may not feel pain or may be modest about not having been able to adequately cleanse themselves. The nurse must often teach the client about the importance of a thorough exam.

Assessments That Warrant Attention

Urgent and emergency situations sometimes become apparent on assessment. There are times when a referral is necessary. A difficult task for the novice or student nurse is deciding when a client needs to be seen by a primary-care provider. This decision-making ability becomes easier as the nurse is more familiar with the clients in his or her care. It also helps to get to know the physicians that are caring for the clients.

In all of these situations, the student should call the nursing instructor for advice and counsel. The teacher or the student might also want to call the doctor or primary-care physician to discuss the case. More frequent visits can be scheduled with the client if this is appropriate in the particular clinical setting.

One example of assessing a potentially emergent situation is described in Table 12-2.

Table 12-2

A Client with Congestive Heart Failure

A client with CHF who has been stable for three months begins to have edema in her legs with eleven pitting edema and some increased SOB.

Plan: Assess life style changes: Change in diet? Increased salt intake? Change in activity level? Change in med compliance?

Assess physical changes: Change in vital signs? Has the client had pitting edema previously? Caused by what? What helped to decrease the edema? Any other symptoms such as evidence of a transient ischemic attack (TIA), insomnia, moist cough, chest pain, indigestion? Change in level of consciousness (LOC)? When assessing the client in the morning, ask how swollen her legs were the previous evening. In a bedridden client, assess for edema in the small of the back.

Assess med changes: Review with the client if there have been any medication changes that you were unaware of. Be sure that the client has not run out of medication.

If there are no known changes or causes that can be identified, it can be presumed that the change is in the client's physiology. If the client is becoming increasingly short of breath (SOB) while you are with her, this falls into the rapid/major change category and needs the intervention as mentioned. If these changes have occurred over the past week and the client confides that she has had more canned soup than usual because of the current cold weather, this is a more gradual change with an apparent cause (increased sodium from the prepared soup). This more gradual onset requires patient education and a follow up by the nurse in a few days to be sure the problem is resolving. Any time a student nurse is meeting with a client, the student nurse must assess what arrangements have been set up for the client to initiate if the client experiences a problem or emergency.

Know that many clients tend to downplay their symptoms. Clients may not want to draw attention to themselves or their physical problems. They may want to delay action. This is when the nurse *must* use the best assessments and intervene with the best nursing judgment and not be swayed by the client's reluctance to "make a fuss."

It is the nurse who knows when the client is in or moving toward an emergency situation.

Problem Solving

Handling Unexpected Situations Flexibly

When unexpected situations arise, try to be flexible. Lockstep routine can become tedious both for the client and the nurse. Enhance your repertoire of funny stories to tell. Take clients outside on beautiful sunny days. Don't be afraid to take them out in the snow as well. Being unpredictable and unconventional causes one to look forward to the next meeting. It also gives the client an opportunity to think of fun things to share with the nurse. Humor can bridge generational, racial, cultural, and socioeconomic barriers. A collection of outrageous hats purchased at second-hand stores can brighten many a dreary day. Share one with the client and make a dramatic entrance with yours on! Bubbles are also a delight. Carry some in your bag. Showing a child that you can blow gigantic bubbles with your gum can go a long way to decrease the intimidation often felt by kids. These activities aid in the relationship with the client, which always enhances assessment. Doing an exam with Grocho Marx glasses, nose, and mustache will lighten the routine. A side effect is that the clients can think of something other than what ails them for a while.

Many clients with serious or chronic illness and their families feel very socially and geographically isolated by the illness. The nurse can help to "normalize" the client with some creativity. Some parents with children in wheel chairs feel that they can never go to the beach. In reality, many beaches have special sand wheelchairs for those in need. Playing freely in the sand or even sitting in low surf can be renewing. It often takes the nurse to help the client get past the fears involved in such an adventure. "What if" problems can be explored and solutions thought out in advance to aid the client and family in planning. Another option is to bring the activity to the homebound person. If someone loves the church choir, invite the choir over to sing. If the child misses playgroup, have them all come over. If the spread of illness is a concern, it may even add more fun if all of the children that visit get to wear masks and gloves! The point is that many

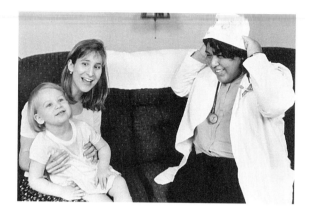

situations that are tremendously difficult can be brightened with humor. It doesn't make light of the illness, but rather reinforces that the illness is not all there is in the person's life. Illness is hard enough on families and clients without being additionally confined by the fear of living.

Writing this section caused me to think of the movie *Patch Adams* starring Robin Williams. I remember a "clinical intervention" that occurred late in the movie. An elderly client, who was not eating and seemingly had lost her will to live, was allowed to fulfill a fantasy she had since childhood. Early in the film she had told Williams' character that one thing she loved to do when she was young was to run her fingers through cooked spaghetti that her mother had made for dinner. Her fantasy was to be in a pool *full* of cooked spaghetti! Sure enough, "Patch" made it happen! She was joyous, renewed. Although the film shows nothing of the eventual outcome of this "intervention," one imagines that she is revitalized because of it. I relate this story because it is so unconventional. It was an intervention that met the objectives. Many times, unconventional approaches may have surprising effects. Often it is just because it *is* unconventional. It causes the client, the family, and the nurse to think "outside of the box." Table 12–3 presents some guidelines for you to consider when selecting interventions.

Children who have acquired a label of being "trouble maker" or having difficulties in schools, or adults who live in group homes can be marginalized. Our society seems to want to look past these individuals. Assessments can only be valid if these clients are made to believe that they are of value. Nurses and student nurses in particular can give new life perspectives to these clients. In one clinical setting, my

students sponsored a dance for indigent clients living in a large group home. Many had a history of mental illness. Most had little or no contact with family or friends outside of the group home. But when the students asked them to dance, treated them to special refreshments, and genuinely thanked them for coming, many clients were given something priceless: the knowledge that they were of value. This can open the door to helping clients become more active and interested in their own health. The relationships that develop enhance the ability to assess the client like nothing else will. A dance is not the answer for relationship building in every setting, but in this one, it was because of the fun we had that relationships were developed and trust emerged. Better health assessment and subsequent interventions were the result.

Assessing a Client with Dementia

The student may consider working with a client who has dementia as a task beyond the abilities of a novice nurse. This is not the case. It does require excellent assessment skills, good observations, and much patience. Noting changes in the client's behavior is an essential ingredient. Most people with dementia are unable to stay by themselves. Consequently, the primary caregivers are also key players when obtaining needed information. Parts of our society still hold onto prejudice of the elderly. What may be signs and symptoms of depression or physical illness are sometimes attributed to dementia.

If a client who is new to you has a diagnosis of dementia, be sure to ascertain who made the diagnosis. Family members or even some health-care workers may use the label. There are diagnostic criteria that must be met for someone to have the diagnosis of dementia. There are many types of dementia including Alzheimer's, Pick's, and Creutzfeldt-Jakob disease; all primary dementias and vascular dementia; AIDS dementia complex; depression; and dementia caused by brain lesions, which are secondary dementias (Carson & Arnold 1996). Appropriate physician diagnosis is essential because treatment can differ. For instance, if a senior citizen is depressed, treatment is available and effective. Medication or chemical imbalances that can mimic dementia are also treatable. Most true dementias are not curable, although in some cases progression of the disease can be halted or slowed. The student is referred to a comprehensive psychiatric/mental health text for a better understanding of the disease and appropriate nursing interventions.

Communication strategies to use with clients with dementia include using the five senses. For example, using pictures along with words may assist the client's understanding. You can show the client all of the equipment you will be using as you tell him or her that you will be assessing blood pressure. You may collect pictures of patients lying in different positions to aid your positioning of a client for examination. If successful, this type of communication assistance can also be taught to family members. If a client is reluctant to go with a caretaker to bathe, a picture of someone showering may be helpful to get the idea across. The use of touch in communication is also important with this type of client in that it helps to direct attention.

Another communication technique is validation of thought content. Previously, it was believed that reality orientation was the appropriate response any time a client was confused. Using reality orientation with clients who are demented can be ill advised. A client who begins to request to see her (long deceased) mother may grieve anew if told that her mother has died. Instead the nurse can reflect (validate) that the client is thinking of her mother and inquire more about the relationship the client had with her. This addresses the content of thought without reintroducing the facts that have been forgotten. You are caring for a client who has advanced dementia in the community. You wish to include pictures to facilitate communication. Con-

tent of speech that includes illness, pain, or the need to see a physician may be markers that the client is not feeling well. Observing facial expression when palpating any part of the body can be very significant because verbalizations are less trustworthy for this client. Agitation can also be an indication that the client is not feeling well. Working with family members, caregivers, or roommates of this client is crucial. It is they who can often assist the student nurse in establishing an understanding of the client's baseline.

Family Problems

All illnesses are family matters. One person's sickness affects the entire family constellation. Consequently, the nurse must assess not only the well-being of the identified client but also of the family as well. Assessments should include identifying what roles family members play. Are caregiving roles shared? How are decisions made? Who controls the finances? Are the voices of each family member respected? Does one member seem to carry the "family illness"? An example of this is seen in a family that had difficulty conceiving a child. After years of assessment and in vitro fertilization attempts, a child was conceived and delivered. The mother, so focused on the child, became suffocating in her care and protection. Interestingly, the child developed severe and chronic asthma—the overprotective parenting smothered her. Needless to say, other situations are less dramatic.

Family members adopt roles. Some of these roles are adaptive, but some are maladaptive. Appraisal of interaction patterns can assist the nurse in assessing the functionality of these interactions. Family systems theory assumes that the sum of the whole is different than the sum of its parts. As noted by Goodwin (1997), "The perceptions of each family member are interactional and co-construct a unit experience different than individual perceptions. The family system self-regulates through interactional patterns that constantly reshape its reality" (pp. 138–139). One student described her experiences:

I was assigned to a parish setting for my community-based clinical semester. Our instructor worked with the parish minister to identify families with specific health problems that could benefit from weekly home visits. An elderly woman asked for the student nurses to visit because

of her hypertension and anxiety. I was assigned to Mrs. T. Her middle-aged son, John, was living with her. As I began to develop a rapport with her she told me that John was an alcoholic and had many bad breaks since adolescence. She acknowledged that she "enabled" this behavior, but could not bring herself to change. For example, John had a serious fall and head trauma while he was intoxicated. The sequela was a seizure disorder. She would call 911 each time he had a seizure at home. My client was Mrs. T. However, I worked to intervene with John through her, as his illness was at the heart of the family problem.

Evidence of Abuse, Neglect, Potential for Violence

One observation that the nurse may be reluctant to acknowledge is evidence of abuse. This issue is very emotionally and value laden. The nurse's perspective is affected by his or her own experience with abuse. If a nurse has been threatened or beaten by a spouse, there may be a blurring of what is seen as abuse in clients. Children, women, and the elderly are the most vulnerable to abuse, but there have certainly been cases of men being both physically and emotionally abused.

During any assessment it is necessary to be alert to signs and symptoms of abuse and neglect. Some signs include bruises and cuts that are inconsistent with the described causative occurrence. When a person accidentally falls, the arms and hands automatically reach out to break the fall. If someone has small bilateral bruises on both upper arms, this can be from someone grabbing and shaking them. Also, when someone falls, it is usually "hard parts" that get bruised. It is normal for a young child to have bruised elbows and skinned knees from falls. However, bruises on the upper thighs are unusual in an accidental fall. Be sure to observe interactions between the client and significant others. Do they seem to cower from the stronger or more dominant person? Does there seem to be a reluctance to discuss the cause of trauma in the presence of this person? In all suspected cases of abuse and neglect, ask the client directly about your concerns or suspicions. Provide a private place to talk, if the suspected abuser is present. The client will most likely fear retaliation if an accusatory statement is made. Assure clients that you believe them

and that you will assist them in remaining safe. Abusers often tell their victims that it is the victims' fault, that they deserve the abuse. We, as nurses, must tell our clients that *no one* deserves to be abused and that it is *not* their fault. Also convey the message that the only way to stop abuse or neglect is to get it out in the open. Abusers generally don't or can't stop the abuse without education or other intervention. Always acknowledge how frightening it is to discuss the abuse. As awful as it can be, once abuse is recognized, it often means drastic changes in the living situation. Knowing this, clients may be reluctant to seek protection for themselves. In addition, threats are often made by the abuser to ensure that the person being abused does not disclose the activity. The nurse has to be able to ensure that the client will be safe once disclosures are made.

Most jurisdictions have laws that mandate nurses to report findings (or even suspicions) of abuse. Many localities have Child Protective Services and Adult Protective Services, which are agencies that investigate allegations of abuse and can remove vulnerable family members from dangerous situations if needed. Nurses working in the community must be aware of these services. Most communities have confidential women's shelters where an abused woman and her children can find housing and support for breaking away from the abuse. We are obligated ethically and legally to report all evidence of abuse. Table 12-4 offers examples of signs and questions you may use clinically if you suspect abuse or neglect.

Table 12-4

Questions to Ask a Client for Whom Abuse or Neglect is Suspected

- How did this injury occur?

- Has any one ever hurt you on purpose?

- Does anyone hurt you to make you do as they want?

- Has anyone told you not to tell about this situation?

- Has anyone ever touched you in a way that was uncomfortable to you?

HEALTH ASSESSMENT RESEARCH IN THE COMMUNITY

Research to assess client risk in the community setting has been done. This is congruent with a home and community focus on health promotion and disease prevention. If clients can maintain or improve functional status in the areas of basic and instrumental activities of daily living, they will be able to hold onto a better quality of life. Maintaining a client's functional level promotes independence, health, and mental health. When considering the entire health-care delivery system, this maintenance of functioning is also a cost-saving measure. It potentially allows a client to remain at home, receiving less illness/disability/dependent health care. This section reviews four current research articles, each of which concludes by recommending an assessment that I believe will be helpful for you in your nursing practice.

Beginning with the pediatric client and the family, Wimbush and Peters (2000) researched the benefit of obtaining a cardiovascular specific genogram (CVSG) to identify children and families at increased risk of cardiovascular disease. This specific area of assessment is becoming more urgent because of the statistical rise in cardiovascular disease and risk factors, even in young children. The authors developed the CVSG to gather information about three generations of a family's cardiovascular history. They found this assessment tool to be both valid and reliable. In this study, the tool was used on schoolchildren. The data generated provided evidence that "a preponderance of risk factors found in this research were those that were amenable to primary and secondary intervention strategies" (Wimbush & Peters, 2000, pp. 152–153). Even clients who consider themselves in good cardiovascular health can be aided by an assessment tool that assists the nurse in family health promotion, specifically, as an aid in planning intervention strategies to avoid cardiovascular disease.

There have been more studies that assess the decreasing functional ability and medical disability for the geriatric population. Two that are of interest focus are an assessment of modifiable risk factors (Sarkisian et al., 2000) and the association between chronic illness and functional change (Cho et al., 1998). Both of these articles support why nurses should be in the home promoting health.

In one study (Sarkisian et al., 2000) the researchers found that factors such as a slow gait, short-acting benzodiazepine use, depression, low exercise level, and obesity were significant predictors of functional decline for clients in daily activities. Additional factors such as loss of visual acuity, weak grip, and long-acting benzodiazepines affected basic functioning ability. Being able to recognize that these assessed changes can actually predict functional decline gives hope that these markers can be identified early and preventive interventions can be initiated. The old saying "an ounce of prevention is worth a pound of cure" is particularly valid with the geriatric client who has slower rehabilitation after injury or illness.

The Cho et al. (1998) study adds to this understanding by researching the association between chronic illness and functional change in a comprehensive assessment program. Researchers found that persons with gait and balance disorders and depression experienced a decline in both instrumental and basic ADLs. Hypertension and urinary incontinence led to declines in basic ADLs. Persons with coronary artery disease and an unsafe home environment also experienced declines in instrumental ADLs. Findings from this research suggest that active and early interventions help to avoid or decrease the rate of functional decline. Accurate assessment can identify those clients most at risk for functional change, once again supporting health promotion activities.

Specific mental health assessments for the geriatric population can also be enhanced to decrease morbidity. A study by Rabins et al. (2000) found more successful interventions for reducing psychiatric symptoms when using the Psychogeriatric Assessment and Treatment in City Housing (PATCH) program in a randomized trial of elders living in urban public housing. This study is important for those working toward health promotion who may not be comfortable with mental health assessment and intervention. There is a reluctance to diagnose and even discuss mental health problems by clients and health-care providers alike. This is an area, as noted by the authors of the study (Rabins et al., 2000), in which there is underrecognition by care providers.

Keeping abreast of assessment research done with community clients will always be important for your nursing practice. Staying current with research findings across disciplines aids assessment for all clients. It is similar to studying new puzzle designs and watching how others put them together. When I first encountered a two-sided puzzle, I wanted to quit before I ever started! However, once I talked to someone else who had found an effective strategy, I had the determination to give it a try. This "research" by a friend added to my practice skills of puzzle construction! Read the research! Even if you never face the same type of "puzzle" that the research addresses, the strategies are frequently helpful in many areas of practice.

CONCLUSION

As difficult as this may seem to a novice nurse, all of these assessments can be and are done during the general conversation and physical assessment of the client. You will be collecting volumes of data from many sources. You can think of it as collecting puzzle pieces for a puzzle that has more than one way to be constructed. You will be able to use and process the information in many different ways. This is the art of nursing. If a client had to answer a full battery of assessment questionnaires each time a nurse visited, the client would most likely decline the visit. The nurse is constantly assessing and making observations. The trick is to gain as much information from each interaction as possible. This requires the nurse to be very aware of all of the parameters to be assessed. With experience, differences or responses out of the range of normal will begin to leap out at the nurse just like an expert puzzler can quickly spot the needed puzzle piece. This work demands an attentive listener and the ability to arrange the puzzle pieces of a client's life in a meaningful and accurate fashion. The novice nurse in a community setting is in a challenging and ever-changing environment. This requires the nurse to have astute assessment skills, innovative interventions, holistic plans, and above all, excellent listening skills. With this challenge comes the reward of an exciting, changing, never-ending quest for health in an adventure that is pursued in partnership with clients.

Active Learning Strategies

1. Mr. S. is your 75-year-old client. When you arrive at your client's home you note that he is slow to come to the door to let you in. When questioning him about his health since your visit last week to follow up on postabdominal surgery he states he is "fine." However, he eventually reveals that he fell from a ladder yesterday evening. What questions would you ask about this fall?

   1. _____

   2. _____

   3. _____

   4. _____

   5. _____

   On physical exam you note the following: P: 102 and weak, BP: 98/54, R: 28. The client guards his abdomen, which is firm, almost hard on palpation. The client is pale, diaphoretic and lies on the sofa in a stiff, uncomfortable manner with his knees drawn up. What is your next action?

2. What pictures could you include in a binder to assist your communication with a client who has an advanced dementia?

   How would you use these pictures?

3. Check your assessment skills. Invite a student colleague to join you on a home visit to one of your community clients. Using Box 12-2 first glance assessments, complete your observations independently. Compare your assessments with your student colleague. How did you do?

4. Contact your local Mental Health Association. Check the suicide rates among the elderly persons, persons under age 25, and rates by gender in your community. Check them against rates cited in this chapter. Did you gain any new perspectives on your community?

References

American Nurses Association (ANA). (1999). Scope and standards of public health nursing practice. (Draft).

Carson, V. B., & Arnold, E. N. (1996). Mental health nursing: The nurse-patient journey. Philadelphia: W. B. Saunders Company.

Cho, C., Alessi, C. A., Cho, M., Aronow, H. U., Stuck, A. E. Rubenstein, L. Z., Beck, J. C. (1998). The association between chronic illness and functional change among participants in a comprehensive geriatric assessment program. The Journal of American Geriatrics Society, 46(6), 677–682.

Deering, C. G. (1999). To speak or not to speak, self disclosure with patients. American Journal of Nursing, 99(1), 34.

Erikson, E. H. (1963). Childhood and society (2nd ed.). New York: W. W. Norton & Co.

Goodwin, S. S. (1997). The marital relationship and health in women with chronic fatigue and immune dysfunction syndrome: View of wives and husbands. Nursing Research, 46(3), 138–146.

Peplau, H. E. (1952). Interpersonal relations in nursing. New York: G. P. Putman's Sons.

Rabins, P. V., Black, B. S., Roca, R., German, P., McGuire, M., Robbins, B., Rye, R., Brant, L. (2000). Effectiveness of a nurse-based outreach program for indentifying and treating psychiatric illness in the elderly. Journal of the American Medical Association, 283(21), 2802-2809.

Roy, C. (1981). Theory construction in nursing: An adaptation model. Englewood Cliffs, NJ: Prentice-Hall.

Sarkisian, C. A., Liu, H., Gutierrez, P. R., Selley, D. G., Cummings, S. R., Mangione, C. M. (2000). Modifiable risk factors predict functional decline among older women: A prospectively validated clinical prediction tool. The Journal of American Geriatrics Society, 48(2), 170–178.

Satcher, D. (1999). The surgeon general's call to action to prevent suicide, 1999. (On line) http://www.surgeongeneral.gov/osg/calltoaction.

SmithBattle, L., Drake, M. A., Diekemper, M. (1997). The responsive use of self in community health nursing practice. Advances in Nursing Science, 20(2), 75–89.

Taylor, C. (1997). Problem solving in clinical nursing practice. Journal of Advanced Nursing, 26 (2), pp 329-336.

Walton, J. C., & Miller, J. M. (1998). Evaluating physical and behavioral changes in older adults. MedSurg Nursing, 7(2), 85–90.

Williams, R. (1998). Patch Adams. Directed by Tom Shadyac. Universal Studios.

Wimbush, F. B., & Peters, R. M. (2000). Identification of cardiovascular risk: Use of a cardiovascular-specific genogram. Public Health Nursing, 17(3), 148–154.

13 Teaching Clients in Community-based Sites

Margaret J. Cofer

LEARNING OBJECTIVES

1) Describe the community settings in which nurse educators teach.

2) Discuss the use of the nursing process to promote teaching and learning.

3) Describe the characteristics of a good learning environment.

4) Describe ways to adapt teaching for different clientele.

5) Identify learning resources for teaching clients in the community.

6) Identify the implications of the use of alternative therapies for nurse educators.

7) Discuss the advocacy role of the nurse in client teaching in community-based practice.

8) Discuss current research in teaching and learning.

Client education within the community setting is changing. Many may view certain community sites as unlikely places for health education to occur, but now more than ever, students and registered nurses (RNs) are identifying new opportunities for teaching clients. Nurse educators have begun to respond to the increased need for community-based nurses, and as a result, students are finding themselves in innovative places in which teaching can benefit clients.

The following story, written by a nursing student, illustrates the sometimes surprising challenges you may encounter in planning teaching programs in community-based settings:

SKIPPY

Placement for my community clinical is in an elementary school. Attending to runny noses, bellyaches, and the dreaded head lice are my daily tasks. The acuteness of children is not high. However, regardless of whether we work with a sick or a well population, nursing requires teaching skills. This is reinforced by my experience with a special third grader named Grant. Although not exactly health related, Grant has an unusual problem. He desperately wants to learn how to skip.

Grant is very frustrated. All the other kids know how to skip, and he doesn't understand why he can't get the hang of it. As hard as he tries, his arms and legs will not cooperate. Grant is a determined and dramatic little boy. Every Tuesday and Thursday he wanders into the clinic tearful and anxiety stricken, with scraped knees and elbows. Concerned and curious, I continue to question him about his being accident-prone. Lying on the cot with his hand to his forehead, he moans, "Can I just have an ice pack, please?" Suppressing my giggle, I fulfill his request. He reminds me of a little Woody Allen. After some coaxing, Grant reveals that he needs to learn how to skip before he reaches middle school. Although his problem is not life threatening (except to him), I offer to teach him how to skip. I reassure him, tell him that middle school is still a few years away, and that I am confident we will have him skipping in no time. His big brown eyes widen and for the first time, he smiles. Grant is eager to start learning.

Well, easier said than done! The nursing diagnosis is acute anxiety related to the inability to skip, manifested by scraped knees and elbows. As suspected, none of my nursing texts have a readily available care plan for this particular problem. Some research and investigation is in order! I try skipping myself, watch my husband skip (a six-foot Marine and a good sport), and observe Grant as he gives it his best effort. I now have a better feel for the mechanics of skipping. I devise a care plan, which divides the art of skipping into smaller achievable goals. Grant relentlessly works on each of these, one by one, during recess and at home. We work on his arm and leg coordination and use dance for his rhythm. Slowly, Grant begins to get the

hang of it. Within a month he is skipping everywhere. I nickname him "Skippy."

Grant reminds me that nursing isn't always working with sick people. Although I didn't eradicate head lice from the school, I did teach a little boy how to skip. Seeing Grant constantly smile and watching his anxiety level plummet as he learned how to skip was a thrill for me. Sometimes, stuck in traffic, Grant skips through my mind. I smile and traffic seems to move a little quicker.

As suggested in the preceding story, you will encounter teaching needs in many different areas of the community and for many different topics. Community-health organizations are employing more nurses as a result of decreased length of stay in the hospital and sub-acute-care settings, and these nurses are responding to opportunities for client teaching. Client education is going beyond the traditional view of teaching, that is, teaching that takes place primarily in health-care institutions. In fact, the American Nurses Association formally recognized this notion in 1991 when it suggested that nurses must provide and clients must receive self-care information in more client- and family-oriented sites.

EDUCATIONAL SETTINGS IN THE COMMUNITY

The community-based focus in today's health care has led to an increase in the number of settings where teaching can occur. These settings, as shown in Table 13–1, are

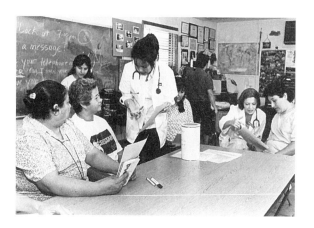

Table 13-1

Educational Setting by Category

HEALTH-CARE SETTING	HEALTH-CARE-RELATED SETTING	NON-HEALTH-CARE SETTING
Hospitals	Alzheimer's Association	Businesses
Health Maintenance Organizations (HMOs)	American Cancer Society	Industry
Visiting Nurse Associations (VNAs)	American Heart Association	Church-related associations
Physician offices	American Lung Association	Civic associations
Community health centers	Muscular Dystrophy Association	Parent-teachers associations
Diagnostic centers	Diabetic Club	Community service clubs
Wellness centers	Head Injury Support Group	Senior centers
Nurse-managed centers		Sheltered workshops
		Shelters for specific populations
		YMCA and YWCA

O'Halloran, V. (1997). Defining education settings to improve client teaching. MedSurg Nursing, 6 (3), 131. Reprinted by permission of the publisher, Jannetti Publications, Inc., East Holly Avenue Box 56, Pitman, NJ.08071-0056; Phone (609) 256-2300; FAX (609) 589-7463.

classified according to the primary purpose of the organization or agency that sponsors client health education. All of these educational settings serve to benefit the health-care consumer in communities. The key function of the nurse educator can range from teaching in an organization in which the importance of service is first and teaching is secondary to the overall care delivered, as in hospitals. Health education, disease prevention, and programs to improve the quality of lives are offered in health-care-related settings. Teaching by nurse educators can also be conducted in noncare settings. In these facilities health care is an incidental or supportive function of an organization. For example, a business can offer screening and make available instruction in job-related health and safety issues to meet the Occupational Safety and Health Administration (OSHA) regulations or provide opportunities for health education through wellness programs to reduce absenteeism or improve employee morale (O'Halloran, 1997).

NURSE EDUCATORS IN THE COMMUNITY

The organization in which nurse educators have an opportunity to provide teaching creates a framework of reference by defining or categorizing educational settings by their primary purpose. The role of the educator is clarified using the framework for reference (Murray, 1998). There is greater understanding of the target audience and the resources within the environment influencing the educational task to be accomplished. Each of these factors affects the nurse's ability to meet specific learning needs.

The variety of settings illustrate the many changes that have occurred in health care and also enables nurses to recognize the many opportunities for teaching that exist in today's health-care environment. As a result, nurse educators can more accurately determine who the potential learner is and then consider the circumstances under which learning is to take place. An additional benefit from categorizing settings is that doing so assists teachers in learning about available resources that can limit or dictate specific teaching strategies (O'Halloran, 1997)

The primary purpose of many organizations has remained constant; however, many have undergone change. Many have assumed greater shares of responsibility, whereas others have only begun to evolve. Health care is moving from a technology-based to a consumer-oriented focus. Home health, for example, has expanded responsibilities and church-related roles in health promotion are evolving. The influences leading to the shifting of responsibilities are secondary to the decreased length of stay in the hospital setting. Although economic reasons are usually cited as the major reason for this shifting, other influences have played a major role. If the influences are viewed on the macro level, demographics, health-care legislation, changes in society, and health-care reform have contributed to the impact. Significantly, these changes have affected the micro level—individual nurses and their need to meet the challenges and opportunities brought by the macro influences. For example, trends such as the aging population and changes in the leading cause of death from infections, such as pneumonia, have been reduced. These trends have led to an increase in the number of persons with chronic diseases, and the aging population has led to an increase in the need for long-term care. An important role for the nurse educator in community-based education is to move the clients in health-care settings toward health.

Mrs. R., 63, was diagnosed with rheumatoid arthritis at age 17. Because of an inability to tolerate pain associated with walking, she successfully underwent a right total hip replacement and was discharged from acute care to long-term care on the fourth postoperative day. On postop day seven, Mrs. R. experienced pain, redness, and an elevated temperature. Because of long-term steroid therapy for arthritis, Mrs. R.'s wound failed to heal. On return to the hospital, the orthopedic surgeon ordered an infectious disease consult, and a decision was made to treat the client with 6 weeks of antibiotics twice daily. A surgeon was consulted to provide central venous access for long-term antibiotics. A Groschong catheter was inserted, and four days later, the patient was discharged to the home of her daughter. A home-health consult was processed with the goal of teaching the client and daughter administration of intravenous (IV) antibiotics and care of the Groschong catheter. Prior to discharge, the orthopedic nurse administered the first dose of the antibiotics. Mrs. R. was discharged home with instructions that the home-health nurse would administer the second dose that day.

Developing a plan in which Mrs. R. can be taught these specific behaviors is crucial. The nurse educator's first priority is defining objectives in behavioral terms, for example, "the client will be able to administer IV antibiotics through a Groschong catheter by the third home visit." Defining measurable outcomes is necessary for cost reimbursements. Health-care settings do not separate out the cost of patient teaching activities, because many third-party payers at present do not reimburse organizations for inpatient or outpatient teaching. The value placed by the organization on health education determines the percentage of financial support provided to such programs as well as the time given for nurses to prepare teaching plans and teaching (O'Halloran, 1997). Another consideration nurse educators must determine is the extent to which health teaching activities are rewarded. Although the responsibility to teach self-care is spelled out in the majority of Nurse Practice Acts and the American Hospital Association's (1974) Patient's Bill of Rights, teaching efforts may not be as highly valued as other roles of the nurse. Administrative support is a major factor in how teaching is viewed. Box 13–1 provides a student activity for teaching clients with IV catheters.

Box 13-1	Student Learning Activity

IV Catheters

What types of intravenous (IV) catheters have you encountered in your community-based sites? List behavioral objectives for clients who have IVs. Would behavioral objectives be similar for clients with different types of IVs?

Table 13-2

Coping with Alterations in Health Status

REHABILITATION	PREVENTION OF COMPLICATIONS	PSYCHOLOGICAL SUPPORT
Physical activities	Knowledge of risk factors	Sharing
Adaptive equipment	Environmental hazards	Promote well-being
Safety in the home		

Health-care-related Setting

Lifestyle modification programs have been devised, implemented, and evaluated by volunteer organizations such as the American Lung Association and the American Cancer Society. Private organizations may offer these classes too. Many hospitals offer these classes as part of their community organizations. Often, hospitals offer classrooms and auditoriums in support of the organization.

Health-care-related settings offer disease-specific education. The American Lung Association is an example. The association provides educational programs on lung disease, air quality, tobacco use, and smoking. Publications are provided for the purpose of teaching and supporting healthy habits for clients. Programs for participants vary from teaching the disease process to promoting a greater sense of quality of life as these clients participate in physical activities determined by the participants' capacities.

Many of the larger, well-supported organizations have professional nurses on staff as paid employees or as volunteer members to develop health education materials and to plan and participate in programs such as conferences, health screenings, or to lead support groups. Teaching is a major responsibility of nurses functioning within these organizations that operate in the health-care-related setting. A major goal of health-care-related settings is teaching coping with alterations in health status. Table 13–2 presents some important aspects to consider in your teaching. Box 13–2 provides space for you to write about applying some of these ideas to some of your clients.

These organizations receive funds from donations, planned giving, and local community support. A signifi-

Box 13-2   Student Learning Activity

Client Teaching

Have you met clients coping with alterations in health status? Describe how you would teach a client coping through rehabilitation. What needs to be considered when teaching clients about environmental hazards? How would you promote sharing and a sense of well-being in your client?

cant focus for these organizations is research, which helps to inform the public about healthy living. Many of these organizations have national headquarters; however, they offer local services that are community-based.

Non-health-care Setting

Generally termed as "wellness programs," these organizations have gained momentum over the past decade. Because chronic disease, such as heart disease, stroke, and cancer, are caused by smoking, poor diet, stress, inactivity, and misuse of alcohol and drugs, it is recognized that changes in lifestyle practices can prevent the occurrence of disease and improve health. To promote health in non-health-care-related settings, nurse educators are teaching stress reduction, smoking cessation, and physical fitness (O'Halloran, 1997).

On the macro level, the soaring cost of health insurance has spurred these programs. Health insurance costs impact private health insurance carriers like Blue Cross, and government-sponsored health insurance facilitated through private insurance like Medicare. Insurance premiums associated with rising health-care costs impact employers and employees. Currently, there is a great deal of concern that employer-paid health insurance costs have inflated to the degree that this insurance option is a risk (Brown & Wyn, 1996). This inflation is a result of the increased cost of health care. In an attempt to deal with the rising costs, employers realize a reduction in the dollar amounts paid for sick care by investing in keeping their employees well. In non-health-care settings, nurses teach self-care measures. Table 13–3 lists some potential topics.

NURSING PROCESS TO PROMOTE TEACHING/LEARNING

Teaching clients in community-based settings requires nurses to plan for the multiple and varied opportunities for teaching. The teaching process assists the nurse in planning purposeful activities. Applying the teaching process increases the likelihood that individuals will learn (Boyd, 1992). The five phases are assessment, nursing diagnosis, planning, implementation, and evaluation.

Assessment

The assessment phase of the teaching process is perhaps the most crucial element because what the nurse accomplishes in this stage influences the following stages. The systematic and thorough collection of data relevant to the teaching process is the basis from which learning needs are identified, objectives are developed, and a workable plan is designed. Data collection assists the nurse educator to determine several factors (Table 13–4).

Assessment of Learning Needs

The nurse's data-collection techniques directly influence the determination of learning needs. A learning need is "something a person ought to learn for his [or her] own good, for the good of the organization, or for society" (Knowles, 1980, p. 88). Although this step is often overlooked (Lancaster, 1992), it is crucial for the client to learn. The PRECEDE model (Green, Kreuter, Deeds, & Partridge, 1980) is a seven-phase framework that offers nurse educators a guide to conducting assessments (See Table 13–5). The PRECEDE model is beneficial to nurse educators in other ways. This model facilitates identification of an educational diagnosis (Phases four and five). Clearly defining an educational diagnosis prevents oversight of determining learning needs.

Application of the PRECEDE Model

The PRECEDE model was used in a 1997 study by Schneider and colleagues to teach children in community-based schools self-care measures to manage asthma. As a result of teaching, the children experienced fewer hospitalizations and emergency room visits related to acute attacks. Although the researchers demonstrated the benefits of learning self-care measures, this

---

Table 13-3

Topics Related to Self-Care

Exercise

Nutrition

Stress reduction

Avoiding injuries (e.g., back safety)

Screening

Smoking and tobacco use

Table 13-4

Factors Determined in Assessment

Learning needs

Level of motivation

Ability to learn

Resources for learning

Table 13-5

PRECEDE Model

Phase One:	Social diagnosis with quality of life defined by the individual and indicators such as absenteeism, unemployment, and discrimination.
Phase Two:	Social diagnosis: demographic and health problems resulting from phase one.
Phase Three:	Behavioral diagnosis: Identify specific health-related behavior linked to the selected health problem.
Phases Four and Five:	Educational diagnoses
Four:	Categorize into predisposing factors (knowledge, values), enabling factors (resources, skills), reinforcing factors (attitudes and behaviors of other personnel, peers, parents, employers)
Five:	Decide which factors make up the three classes on which the intervention will focus.
Phase Six:	Administrative diagnosis: develop and implement the program
Phase Seven:	Evaluate the program

From *Health Promotion Planning: An Educational and Environmental Approach*, Second Edition by Lawrence W. Green and Marshall W. Kreuler. Copyright © 1991 by Mayfield Publishing Company. Reprinted with permission of the publisher.

project was supported by a time-limited grant project, and the project was ended when financial support expired. However, the study demonstrates how teaching self-care management benefits clients. It also demonstrates that teaching and learning based in the community decreases the need for acute-care medicine and the costs associated with acute care. See Table 13–6 for a teaching plan using behavioral objectives in the cognitive, affective, and psychomotor domains and Table 13–7 for assessment of learning needs as determined by the PRECEDE model.

Assessing Learning Needs of the Family

The goal of the community-based nurse educator is to manage acute and chronic conditions while promoting self-care measures among individuals and families (Zotti, Brown, & Stotts, 1996). Because of the emphasis on self-care measures for individuals and families, the goal differs from past goals of health care. Past goals were based on treating episodes of illness with teaching sessions in

acute-care facilitates with discharge instructions to support self-care. Box 13–3 provides space for you to list specific learning needs for a client.

Box 13-3	Student Learning Activity

Learning Needs

Consider clients you have met in your community-based experience. List learning needs that address positive and negative predisposing factors, enabling factors, and reinforcing factors. You can do this exercise with the child who needs dental care.

Nurse educators in community-based settings must recognize the need for learning and incorporate teaching into their contact with families. The sources for determining learning needs come from assessment data as the nurse

Table 13-6

Teaching Plan

A. Objectives

  1. Establish an asthma education program that teaches:

    a. The importance of early and consistent compliance with medication

    b. The implications of pollutants, and preventive measures to avoid development of acute episodes.

  2. Implement the program in one inner-city school

  3. After 6 months, evaluate, revise, and offer the program at two additional schools.

  4. After 1 year, evaluate, revise, and offer the program in two more additional schools.

B. Client Objectives

Cognitive: Following an asthma health education program, 90% of clients will demonstrate knowledge about importance of asthma care and implications for preventive acute attacks, and the effects of pollutants.

Affective: Asthma clients will share their attitudes, values, and perceptions regarding their current disease process.

Psychomotor: 90% will attend all classes.
        70% will attend all scheduled appointments at community clinic.
        50% will report self-reports compliance with prescribed medication, coping with stress, and avoiding pollutants.

C. Teaching Content

  1. Handouts with presentations. One handout per session for six sessions. Handouts will be in English.

  2. Sessions will cover welcoming and explanation of meetings, what to do when asthma attack occurs, how to keep attacks from occurring, medications, making choices about asthma, and exercise and sports.

D. Implementation

  1. Select school for initial presentation

  2. Assign and orient nurse educator

  3. Design and test appropriateness of handouts

  4. Determine clarity and accuracy

  5. Revise handouts as needed

From Health Education Planning: A Diagnostic Approach by Lawrence W. Green, Marshall W. Kreuter, Sigrid Deeds, and Kay Partridge. Copyright 1980 by Mayfield Publishing Company. Reprinted by the permission of the publisher.

Table 13-7

Learning Needs

PREDISPOSING FACTORS: DEMOGRAPHIC VARIABLES, KNOWLEDGE, ATTITUDES, VALUES, AND NORMS	ENABLING FACTORS: AVAILABILITY OF RESOURCES, ACCESSIBILITY, AND REFERRALS	REINFORCING FACTORS: ATTITUDES, AND ACTIONS OF HEALTH PERSONNEL, FAMILY, AND OTHERS
Positive attitudes, beliefs and values to build on: The child with asthma knows how to administer medications. Negative attitudes, beliefs, and values to address: The child with asthma does not understand the need for consistent dosing of medications.	Positive skills and resources to address: Parents believe in the importance of regular visits for health care Negative skills and resources to address: Transportation is difficult to arrange	Positive support to build on: School nurse expresses to the health department concern about inadequate health services. Negative support Inconsistent care on visits to health-care practitioner.

From Health Education Planning: A Diagnostic Approach by Lawrence W. Green, Marshall W. Kreuter, Sigrid Deeds, and Kay Partridge. Copyright 1980 by Mayfield Publishing Company. Reprinted by the permission of the publisher.

Table 13-8

Family Health Related Topics

Nutrition

Physical activity

Stress control and management

Health responsibility

Family resilience and resources

Family support

comes into contact with families in the community. There are several sources for data collection (Friedman, 1998). For example, client interviews are a source in which the client relates to past and present experiences with health concerns and problems. Objective findings, such as the observation of the home and its facilities, help determine needs. Subjective appraisals of experiences from family members can guide the nurse educator. The last, and perhaps the most frequently used method, is written and oral information from referrals, various agencies working with the family, and health team members. Pender's (1996) assessment guide for family strengths and weaknesses can serve as a reference for determining learning needs. Table 13–8 details family health-related topics.

With the increase in volume of home-health referrals from hospitals, the home-health nurse needs to identify the main caregivers and involve them in all phases of the teaching plan. Including the main caregivers and the family in client education is vitally important. Educating the client without the family members frequently results in poor self-care and poor outcomes (Rankin & Stallings, 1996). First in the sequence of teaching is identification of the nursing diagnoses, and together with the client and family, decisions are made regarding the priority of needs. The teaching plan includes behaviors in the three learning domains.

Nurses who are teaching a client and the family in the home must be informed about resources in the community. Providing access to financial resources for families can be a priority before learning a caregiver role (Graham & Gleit, 1992). Here, the nurse educator may work in a team approach with social workers. In today's health-care market, financial resources are not only for poor citizens. Often, clients have an income above the limits set for Medicaid, yet are unable to afford health insurance or are locked out for any number of reasons. For example, many clients are unable to enter health maintenance organization (HMO) plans because of preexisting diseases. In these cases, clients benefit from knowing how to access other resources. Families in rural areas may experience lack of health-care services, in addition to lack of resources.

Nursing education has identified the need for students in community settings to focus on available resources that are supportive to the family as well as individuals. In their curricula, students are asked to identify resources that focus on services for women and children, access to clinic services, schooling, financial resources, child abuse, gang violence, and services for the older adult (DeNatale & Lantz, 1998). Once teaching and learning begin, students and nurses in home-health care can promote the role of the family in maintaining health, identifying stressors, and teaching coping strategies. Client and family education is the foundation for home-care services (Graham & Gleit, 1992).

Learning Needs and Alternative Therapies

Traditional health care emphasizes the treatment of disease in a body rather than restoring balance to the mind, body, and spirit (Schuster, 1997). This gap is being recognized. Within a few years, health education programs will incorporate holistic perspectives and therapies into health-care professional curricula (Scott & Riedlinger, 1998).

Today, the need for an integrated approach to health care is highlighted by the increasingly large numbers of clients using traditional and holistic therapies at the same time. In 1997, in a follow-up to a 1993 pioneering study, David Eisenberg and colleagues (1997) found that 83 million people, or 42 percent of the population, had used at least one of 16 alternative therapies during the previous year, up from 60 million, or 34 percent, in 1990.

The survey findings of the U.S. population suggest that between 1990 and 1997, the total number of visits to alternative medicine practitioners rose by 47.3 percent, from $427 million to $629 million, and expenditures for alternative medicine professional services increased by 45.2 percent, from $14.6 billion to $21.2 billion in 1997. Out-of-pocket payments to alternative medicine practitioners amounted to $12.2 billion in 1997, and total out-of-pocket expenditures on alternative therapies reached $27 billion.

What are the implications for the nurse who is teaching in the community? Nurses must constantly expand their knowledge base to keep current with the ever-growing body of information on therapies and disease management. However, trends in patient interests and demand are important driving forces. In the United States a critical mass of clients are demanding a personalized, thorough, and preventive approach to health care. These demands for a more holistic approach, coupled with greater interest in self-care, natural products, and an integration of spirituality and health, have resulted in a public acceptance of alternative therapies (Scott & Riedlinger, 1998). These facts are well documented in the Eisenberg study (1997).

These statistics have implications for nurse educators. Many clients who benefit from alternative therapies, including herbal medicine and alternative therapies such as acupuncture, and who also rely on traditional medicine, often do not give a complete history during health-care visits to traditional practitioners. As a result, several dissimilar practitioners provide fragmented care. Clients should be taught the importance of giving a complete history of therapies during practitioner/client interviews.

Assessing Learning Needs of Culturally Diverse Clientele

As nursing care moves to a community-based setting, the impact of culture on nurse educators-family relationships will become more pronounced. Culture can influence how patients interpret their diseases and how they relate to their health-care providers. Conversely, culture may influence how nurse educators interpret their clients or the clients' diseases. Because nurse educators are expected to conduct assessments for clients and families from diverse cultures, he or she must be skilled in accessing a client's values, beliefs, and practices. This allows data collection without depending on a written fact about that specific culture or formulating stereotypes about such a group. By conducting a cultural assessment, the nurse educator learns the client's perceptions of his or her health and illness, as well as the client's perception of what needs to be learned (Camphina-Bacote, 1995). Three assessments guides are identified.

Cultural Assessment Tools

The nurse educator must integrate the cultural assessment into existing nursing history and assessment forms to reflect culturally relevant questions. By integrating the two approaches, questions about cultural beliefs and background are embedded in the existing nursing assessment form. Therefore, culture is not "singled-out," but rather appropriately integrated into the client's history. Tables 13–9, 13–10, and 13–11 are all examples of such assessment forms.

Matching culturally diverse nurse educators to client populations of the same background is helpful. This is necessary for language barriers. Teaching and learning can be complicated when clients speak languages that are different from that of the nurse. In addition, these nurses can act as teachers for their colleagues. Because there is a shortage of nurses from diverse backgrounds, all nurses must support existing nurses to care for patients of different cultures.

MOTIVATION TO LEARN

Motivation is a prerequisite to learning (Lancaster, 1992). Often people are willing to learn about health-related topics because they see a benefit for themselves. For example, an 80-year-old in stable health is told of an elevated blood sugar on routine physical examination. The client is taught control measures based on proper diet management. Blood sugar values on a return visit 1 month later reveal a level within normal limits.

Motivation can either be internal or external (Rankin & Stallings, 1996). If a client, discovered to have an elevated blood sugar on routine physical exam, understands that diet management must be learned, the learner will have sufficient internal motivation to comprehend appropriate diets. External motivation requires that others generate feelings of expectancy in the learner that rewards will result from learning. If a client seems unmotivated to change habits, the nurse educator must look for environmental issues, lack of knowledge and skills, or social stimuli that may inhibit the person's readiness to learn (Wells-Federman & Edwards, 1994).

The nurse educator can provide external motivation by helping the client to define attainable goals (Rankin & Stallings, 1996). Motivation can also be generated by

---

Table 13-9

Berlin and Fowkes' Learn Model (1982)

Listen to the client's perception of the problem.

Explain your perception of the problem.

Acknowledge the similarities and differences.

Recommend interventions that involve the client.

Negotiate a teaching plan with the client.

Table 13-10

Kleinman, Eisenberg, and Good (1978) Patient's Explanatory Model

What do you think has caused your problems?

Why do you think they started when they did?

What do you think your sickness does to you?

What kind of treatment do you think you should receive?

What are the most important results you hope to achieve from these treatments?

What are the chief problems your sickness has caused?

What do you fear the most about your sickness?

Table 13-11

Fong's "Confher" Guide (Fong, 1985)

CULTURAL COMPONENT	VARIABLE
Communication	Language and dialect preferences
	Nonverbal behavior
	Social status
Orientation	Ethnicity identity
	Acculturation
	Value orientation
Nutrition	Symbolism of food
	Preferences and taboos
Family Relationships	Family structure and roles
	Family dynamics/decision making
Health Beliefs	Alternative health care
	Health, crisis, and illness beliefs
	Response to death
	Disease disposition and resistance
Education	Learning style
	Informal and formal education
	Occupation and socioeconomic level
Religion	Preference
	Beliefs, rituals, and taboos

helping the client reach a learning goal and by encouraging a sense of commitment toward a caregiver (Redman, 1997).

In an on-line dialogue between Canadian and American nursing students discussing challenging aspects of teaching clients, one student from George Mason University wrote the following comment:

I think we motivate people by taking their individual situation into account. For example, one of my clients has a horrible time with edema and pain in her left leg, related to her hypertension. It is in her interest to be rid of the edema and pain. Although this may not be achieved solely by hypertension prevention/control teaching, the steps taken will eventually assist her with her leg. This motivates this client. Another

client may be motivated by being able to control her diet. It may give her a sense of authority and control in her life, in a setting where there is very little autonomous control. Some clients are motivated to learn simply for approval by the health-care provider—this could be a good or bad thing, for we do not want our clients to stop caring for themselves once the professional relationship ends. . . . It is not effective to simply give a client information without knowing what "makes them tick" (so to speak!!!).

A University of Windsor student added the following important comment that relates to motivation for learning:

I think the nurse being a partner is excellent. It leaves the client more open to control his or her own care. . . . Feeling more of an equal is a form of empowerment to the client, to give them control.

Ability to Learn

The nurse educator must assess the client's ability to learn. Many factors affect this determination. Sensory deficits, such as poor vision and hearing impairment, affect learning. Attention span deficits and cognitive levels must be determined. The demographics of people with poor education and reading abilities suggest that they represent a significant proportion of health-care consumers who have serious difficulty reading and comprehending written patient education materials and information routinely given to them (Wilson, 1996).

The on-line dialogue between American and Canadian students demonstrated that students in both countries shared similar challenges in teaching of clients. One George Mason University student wrote about a real-world experience with teaching:

I can comment on the challenges faced when trying to implement a simple teaching plan on hypertension. The population at this home is very diverse: we have mentally retarded clients, clients diagnosed with schizophrenia, depression, Alzheimer's, etc. I carefully prepared my teaching materials and set up the time and date, only to discover that most of the clients had "forgotten" about it, or simply had no

interest. The two individuals I was able to teach (both had severe hypertensive conditions), had a very short attention span, and yet, to my amazement, knew their medications' side effects better than any nurse! So, the lesson here is flexibility in adapting nursing care to suit the individual's needs! Teaching materials were kept short and simple, verbiage was kept in laymen's terms . . . yet, these two clients still had a fairly complex knowledge of their meds.

Matching teaching strategies to the client's developmental stage enhances learning. For example, school-age children need repeated practice for psychomotor skills, as in proper use of an insulin syringe; adolescents learn best when immediate benefit is gained; and learning in adults occurs when the client values the information being taught (Potter & Perry, 1995). Most children and adults are responsive to teaching strategies that employ stimulation of several senses and participatory learning exercises whenever possible (Rankin & Stallings, 1996).

RESOURCES

Resources for learning depend on the organization supporting the teaching. Standardized topic-specific teaching materials, such as pamphlets and films, are often provided by vendors who service health-care settings. Closed-circuit TV and mobile TV/VCR units can be easily provided to any client-occupied area. Posters are an excellent means of conveying information. Computer-assisted learning modules are available in certain agencies. These strategies reduce the time the nurse educator spends teaching, allowing for diverse learner needs and providing the pace and repetition for learning (O'Halloran, 1997).

Nurse educators, with no resources, may resort to very basic needs. For example, creatively using newspaper in lieu of poster board may help convey the same lesson. The nurse must determine the minimal requirements in resources. This may mean determining that a chair to sit on is the least, but most essential, requirement for learning.

Planning for Teaching and Learning

Planning begins with prioritizing clients' learning needs. Learning needs can be prioritized by taking into account the degree of the client's needs and the amount of time the nurse has available to teach. Setting priorities helps separate the "must know" from the "ought to know." By assessing each person's learning needs, the nurse can better allocate time and ensure that the primary learning needs are met. The three learning needs developed by George (1982) are:

- Immediate need (urgent) versus a long-range need (can be met at a later time)
- Specific need (related specifically to the learner's condition or treatment plan) versus a general need (something done for all learners)
- Survival need (the learner's life may depend on it) versus a well-being need that is helpful, but not essential

Realistically, teaching may involve only one session (Rankin & Stallings, 1996). These decisions are often made by determining the cost/benefit ratio, while establishing priorities among competing needs (Egan, 2001). Managers in the organization offering the client services can be made aware of conflicts about competing needs and costs of teaching by nurse educators.

Next, the nursing diagnosis is determined. Among the nursing diagnoses for learning needs are knowledge deficit, impaired coping, altered health maintenance, and self-care deficit. Coping may have to be taught after more urgent needs are met. For example, the client must learn about medications for emphysema before learning how to cope with the limits imposed by the disease.

The nurse must take into consideration the individual's needs and readiness to learn and the amount of time available for teaching (Boyd, 1992). Nurses must meet immediate and specific needs and plan to meet more

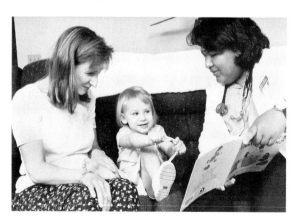

general needs in the future. It is important to remember, too, that teaching does not have to entail blocking out an hour of time. Teaching can be integrated into the overall plan of care for clients (Graham & Gleit 1992)

Team-Oriented Teaching

Teaching in community-based settings requires prioritizing and planning with other disciplines. Many clients need a multidisciplinary approach to regaining self-care abilities. Remember Mrs. R. and her total hip replacement? She must have a teaching plan that considers information from other health-care providers. Based on documented need for the service, Medicare reimbursements are provided to occupational therapists to conduct an assessment of bathroom safety in homebound clients following hip replacement surgery. Occupational and physical therapists also teach clients how to use durable medical equipment (e.g., elevated toilet seat), and activities of daily living (ADLs) for the home environment, for example, use of a sock aid (facilitates putting on socks without extreme flexion and internal rotation of the operative leg). Physical therapists teach clients with hip replacements postoperative leg and hip exercises, crutch walking, how to descend and ascend stairs, and transfers in and out of the bed, chair, and car (preparation for travel home). Often, nurses conduct these duties. Regardless, time spent teaching the client depends on coordination of time and overlapping responsibilities with other disciplines. Although limited in the number of visits into the home, physical therapists' and occupational therapists' home visits are covered under Medicare.

Planning a Teaching Episode

The first step in developing a teaching plan is to generate reachable goals and outcomes for the client(s) based on the assessment data and in collaboration with the client, family, and significant other. Outcomes should be developed to reflect three learning domains:

- The cognitive domain reflects the learner's ability to recall information, apply previously learned information to new situations, and break larger pieces of information into smaller parts.

- The psychomotor domain refers to the types of physical skills required of the learner during the educational process. For example, a psychomotor skill for clients with hip replacements may be the goal of ambulating 100 feet with two crutches, using partial weight-bearing only, to the operative leg.
- The affective domain deals with attitudes, values, feelings and self-expression, such as the ability to value progress from ambulating 50 feet to 100 feet, and self-reporting pride in the advanced progress.

In the teaching plan, outcomes must be appropriate for the learner, clear, concise, measurable, and attainable. Outcomes must be attainable in a short period of time because they serve as a gauge toward longer-range goals. Farquharson (1995) offers an alternative way to state and measure outcomes. He suggests using the formula A + B = C, in which "A" is what you want your learners to know, "B" is what you want your learners to feel, and "C" is what you want your learners to be able to do following the lesson. Table 13–12 applies this model.

Thus, an outcome statement for a homebound, postop client having undergone total hip replacement that is on Coumadin therapy would read as follows: The client, currently taking Coumadin for the prevention of deep vein thrombosis, will self-administer medication correctly and with confidence.

Teaching episodes are interventions that can vary in length from 10 minutes to an hour or more. In long-term teaching interventions, several teaching episodes are linked together. One model that can be used to guide the process of designing such a teaching intervention is known by the acronym EDICT (Farquharson, 1995). The advantage of this model is that it avoids the teacher-centered approach and involves and invites the participation of clients. It is particularly important to understand that the five elements do not need to follow the sequence suggested by the letters in the EDICT acronym:

E = Explain (Main ideas, sequencing of issues, and outcome.)

D = Demonstrate (Hands-on demo by nurse educator or provide an example in a story.)

I = Involve (Nurse involves the learner by providing an exercise that requires him or her to use or apply the ideas of information presented.)

C = Coach (Based on observations made during the "involve" stage, the teacher then coaches the learner by providing feedback.)

T = Test/Transfer/Terminate (If outcomes have been accomplished, the nurse educator designs a mechanism for checking to see if the learner transfers the new behavior or knowledge to the real world, and then terminates the learning activity.)

Planning Related to the Environment

When possible, the physical environment is assessed in advance of the teaching session. The home can be ideal for client, family, and caregiver teaching. This setting offers the client a sense of familiarity with surroundings that can be amenable to learning. Community-based education can be varied and numerous; however, basic principles apply to all settings. Plans must consider the number of persons to be taught, need for privacy, noise, room temperature, ventilation, furniture, lighting, and equipment needed for the teaching session (Potter & Perry, 1995). The time of day at which the teaching is to occur must be considered in concert with the age of the population. Consider the senior citizen who would appreciate entering a course to learn the importance of controlling blood pressure but who stays at home because of a fear of driving during hours of heavy traffic.

The psychosocial environment affects a client's ability to learn. Anxiety levels can be high because of chronic illness or social issues such as poverty, homelessness, and stress associated with living in areas of crime. Symptoms of distress such as fatigue, along with the client and family's

---

Table 13-12

Farquharson (1995) A + B = C Model: An Application

A: Client knows Coumadin dose.

B: Client feels confident administering Coumadin to self.

C: Client appropriately self-administers correct dose of Coumadin.

perceptions of the illness and support systems available, may adversely affect the person's ability to learn. Regardless of the psychosocial readiness factors, the health-care system and nursing profession mandates self-care teaching and appropriate referrals for all clients (O'Halloran, 1997). Clients with multiple health problems should be identified immediately as requiring more intense teaching.

Implementation

Implementation involves believing that each interaction with a client is an opportunity to teach (Fetter, 1997). The nurse educator acts on these opportunities for effective learning and uses a variety of approaches to create an active learning environment. Throughout the implementation phase of teaching and learning, the nurse educator must continue the phases of assessment, planning, and evaluation to keep abreast of evolving needs (Boyd, 1992).

A teaching plan serves as a guide to assist clients toward a goal. During the implementation phase, the teaching strategy chosen may fail to meet the client's learning needs. This may occur for a number of various reasons. For example, the client may be tired. It is during this phase that the nurse educator must continue to assess, plan, and evaluate to stay tuned to the learner's abilities.

A student from the University of Windsor wrote the following to her American colleagues in the on-line international dialogue, reflecting on the difficulties often experienced in implementing teaching in the home and having to structure it around many uncontrollable variables:

I worked with a couple in the community. The mom was due in about 3 months and had developed hypertension, possibly pregnancy induced. My barriers mostly fell into two categories. One is that her husband worked 10-hour shifts so I was never able to meet or talk with him. The other category is that the visits had to fit into her schedule and then mine. Although I was able to visit once a week for 3 weeks, I feel it would have been very beneficial to visit twice a week during a time that included her husband and for a span of time longer than 3 weeks. I felt that a total of 3 to 4 hours (over the three visits) was inadequate to ensure that the client understood all of what was taught and would be able to carry this over into her daily cooking and other activities. . . . Overall, time is a barrier.

CASE STUDY—IMPLEMENTATION AND EVALUATION

The nurse educator has developed a teaching plan based on learning needs of the residents in an assisted-living setting. These residents are independent and maintain their own apartments. It has been determined that the clients have a knowledge deficit related to chronic, nonmalignant pain. The plan is to teach two 1-hour classes. The goal of the program is teach self-management of pain.

The nurse educator begins the first session by lecturing on the pharmacological management of pain. The content includes medication actions, possible side effects, and the most effective time to take certain medicines. Written information is distributed with the clients knowing that the written material supports the information imparted by the nurse. A dialogue is held. The participants and nurse discuss aspects that are general to everyone and to each individual's needs. The last part of the session is devoted to evaluating the learner's knowledge. The nurse asks the residents to briefly explain the action of the medication and possible side effects. The residents are encouraged to bring written questions to the second session. Feedback during the second session enables the nurse to determine the other outcomes of this pain management education program.

One week later the nurse begins the second session by inviting the participants to describe and discuss how pain has affected the ability to perform activities of daily living. Each participant is encouraged to participate in the dialogue. Participants encourage each other. The nurse asks questions to promote clients' use of the information for their own problem solving. The nurse educator is alert to cues suggesting confusion. The nurse clarifies by restating.

The nurse then has the physical therapist and the occupational therapist demonstrate the appropriate use of devices to assist with activities of daily living such as walkers, zipper pulls, and long-handled shoe horns. A question-and-answer session follows. Time is allotted for individual problem solving. This allows application of new knowledge for each individual's health concern. Although coping strategies that require cognitive skills are not used often with older adults, this may be more related to their lack of exposure to these methods than to ability or willingness to perform them (Davis, 1997). Nurse educators must document the effectiveness of the strategies they used and report the success or must reevaluate.

COMMUNICATION AND TEACHING

The most important element in the relationship between nurse and client is open and honest dialogue. For instance, there is anecdotal evidence of clients with emphysema that suggests that some clients remove nasal oxygen, and continue to smoke, but say they do not, even stating fictitious outcomes in the smoking cessation classes. The apparent reason for this is to keep the educator happy; the patient feels unable to say that he or she is not carrying out the suggested steps to quit smoking, perhaps for fear of disapproval by the nurse. Any exchange in which the patient feels unable to be honest can be considered a waste of time for both parties. If a problem is identified rather than hidden, then the issues that might contribute to the problem can be explored and addressed (Brown, 1997).

Individuals with chronic diseases, such as emphysema, are living with a condition that affects most aspects of their lives. Unless nurse educators have personal experience with chronic illness, they cannot know what it's like to live with the condition. Use of open questions helps reveal what it is like living with a chronic illness. For example, the nurse might ask, "What does having emphysema mean to you? How do you feel about having emphysema?" These questions can be asked at the beginning of a program and again in subsequent sessions to help place the patient in an appropriate context. Questions subsequently directed to patients, based on eliciting this type of information, encourage them to share the problems they encounter in dealing with the day-to-day management of emphysema. Open questioning is a skill that can be used to promote equality in the communication between the nurse and the patient, as well as to enable clients to speak of their own experience. Closed questions are most commonly used for assessment (Brown, 1997). These can be answered using one word, and there is no way of understanding how relevant they are to the patient's situation. The conscious use of open questions can minimize this tendency.

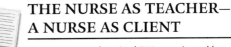

THE NURSE AS TEACHER— A NURSE AS CLIENT

Ms. C., a recently retired RN, experienced burning and itching on the top of the left foot. This symptom occurred during a class at the Learning Resource Center (LRC) for senior citizens during an afternoon session devoted to learning computer technology. A momentary scratch alleviated the itching. No further thought was given to the symptom—the scratch did the trick.

On the following Saturday morning, the symptoms once again appeared. The itching and burning returned. This occurrence was accompanied by an increased amount of redness that extended up the left leg to midthigh. Ms. C. applied 1 percent hydrocortisone cream from her own medicine cabinet to the affected area. By Saturday evening, symptoms were worsening. The itching and redness were extending to the right ankle and foot. Ms. C.'s husband drove to the local pharmacy and purchased an oatmeal bath. Ms. C. felt these self-help measures would be beneficial. The treatments had worked for her clients during her nursing practice.

On Sunday, Ms. C. discovered more extension of the problem. The itching was extending up both legs and the areas on the left foot and ankle had begun to ooze clear fluid. She was further alarmed when she noticed redness higher up both legs and the itch intensified. On Monday morning, the dermatologist was called and an appointment was made for an office visit. Ms. C. felt anxious.

Once the physician examined the client, a diagnosis was made of a classical allergic reaction. The history was reviewed and a tentative diagnosis of an allergic reaction to poison ivy was proposed. Ms. C. had worked in her garden for many years without any problems with allergic responses. This response was assumed to be the onset of an allergy to poison ivy.

The physician gave an explanation of the treatment, but there was no time for discussion or answering Ms. C.'s questions. The physician was on his way to the next client. After all, Ms. C. had been squeezed in on a very busy day in the office. However, Ms. C. did not understand the information hastily given to her by the physician. After a few moments Ms. D., the nurse, entered the room.

The office nurse had a calm reassuring voice. She began the session by asking Ms. C. to repeat the physician's instructions. She immediately recognized Ms. C.'s knowledge deficit and began explaining the rationale for each treatment verbally. First, she explained the need for a short-acting and long-acting cortisone injection to be given intramuscularly and described possible side effects. Next, Ms. D. explained the need for oral cortisone and listed dates, dosages, and times the medication was to be taken. On the first and second days she instructed Ms. C. to take 2 tablets 3 times per day. On the third and fourth day she was instructed to decrease the dose by 1 tablet. On the subsequent days, weaning doses of the cortisone were to be taken until all medication was taken. Instructions were given to call the office for problems or concerns.

Ms. D. stayed with Ms. C. and listened to her concerns. She responded in a knowledgeable, caring, and supportive manner. Ms. C.'s anxiety was completely gone.

Nurse as Advocate for Client Teaching: From Illness to Wellness Care

Professional nurses possess the expertise and special skill needed to provide information on managing illness and promoting health. Although many clients may prefer to depend on nurses and medical care to meet their needs, starting at this point, teaching can move a client forward, to grow toward the responsibility for maintaining or improving health. Community-based nurses are in a strong position to promote such behaviors. Providing clients and families with facts and resources is a function that today's nurse must value.

Use of Health-Care Facilities and Services

As part of the nurse educator's assessment of clients in the community-based locations, the nurse must determine if the clients need to be taught how to use health-care facilities (Brown & Wyn, 1996). For instance, a child with asthma may be brought to the emergency room by the parents who are using this service as primary care. In many instances, individuals must be told who to call for appointments they need. Advocating for clients without health-care insurance requires referrals to social services. Nurses must document events when clients are not covered by Medicaid's historic guarantee of health coverage for the poor, seniors, children, and citizens with disabilities (Shalala, 1997). Box 13–4 contains an activity on client advocacy for you to complete.

Box 13-4	Student Learning Activity

Advocacy

Have you been an advocate for your clients in the community-based sites? Have you observed an RN advocate for a client? Have you witnessed a need for client advocacy?

Write objectives in behavioral terms that consider advocating for the client.

Research in Teaching and Learning

Four recent research studies are presented here that have significant implications for nurse educators. Remember the discussion of teaching in non-health-care-related sites? Thompson, Edelsberg, Kinsey, and Oster (1998) report that obesity was estimated to cost U.S. businesses $7.7 billion in health care in 1994. Women ages 25 to 34 lost 9 workdays per year as a result of obesity whereas women ages 35 to 44 lost 10 workdays per year. These statistics support the importance of teaching by nurse educators. Businesses offering self-care instruction can gain the benefits of health promotions programs.

The next research article examined patient education material. Wilson (1996) conducted a study to examine the readability of patient education information material used by nurses in three community-based sites. Results showed that a ninth-grade reading level was required for the patient education material. Culturally sensitive information was found in only four (8.5 percent) of the education materials. These materials showed African Americans, but no other minority group was represented. The author suggests, "[I]f written materials are the method of choice for communicating with and educating patients, then using materials that exceed clients' ability to read and comprehend is clearly not an option, especially given the fact that an informed patient is mandated by the Patient's Bill of Rights" (p. 203).

The next two articles reflect the need for cultural considerations in client education. Corkery and colleagues

(1997) conducted a study to determine the effect of a bicultural community health worker (CHW) on completion of diabetes education in an inner-city Hispanic patient population and to evaluate the impact of completion of the education program on patient knowledge, self-care behaviors, and glycemic control. All clients received instruction from a certified diabetes nurse educator. Participants were randomly assigned to one of two groups. One group received intervention by a bicultural CHW. The second group did not receive intervention by a CHW. The findings of the study suggest that intervention by a bicultural community health worker improved rates of completion of the diabetes education program, and knowledge, self-care behaviors, and glycemic control improved after completion of the program.

Goeppinger and Lorig (1997) reviewed community-based arthritis patient education studies conducted between 1980 and 1995. The authors found that arthritis patient education programs in the United States have not reached racial and ethnic minorities, those with less than high school education, and inner-city residents. The review found community-based arthritis patient education has provided convincing evidence that relatively well educated, Caucasian, rural and urban adults and elders benefit.

The last two research articles address current trends in health care. First, Baker and colleagues (1996) interviewed 467 native-Spanish-speaking and 63 English-speaking Latino patients after admission to a Los Angeles area emergency department with nonurgent medical conditions. Although 26 percent of the Spanish-speaking patients had an interpreter, another 22 percent said that one was needed. When the patient's English and the clinician's Spanish were both poor, an interpreter was absent 34 percent of the time, and 87 percent of the patients in this situation said one was needed.

Another article that reflects current trends in health care is a seven-year review of use of alternative therapies. Morgan (1998) reported between 1991 and 1997 the number of visits to alternative medicine practitioners rose 47.3 percent. As a result, employers are more willing to offer coverage. The number of larger organizations, those with more than 500 employees, offering insurance coverage for alternative therapies rose 24 percent in 1997.

This chapter has addressed client teaching in community-based sites. Changes in health care and community-based sites in which education occurs were discussed. Facilitating a good learning environment for clients and adapting teaching to the individual client were described. Types and methods of teaching and learning resources for teaching clients in the community were explored. Finally, recent research in teaching and learning was reviewed.

Active Learning Strategies

1. Write a teaching plan for a client or family with whom you are working in the community. What learning needs have you identified within the cognitive, affective, and psychomotor domains? Identify expected outcomes and interventions. Then evaluate the effectiveness of the interventions and planning.

2. You have volunteered to participate in a nutritional screening in a homeless shelter. Assessment data are gathered by the survey method. Develop a plan including implementation and evaluation for participants that are found to be malnourished.

3. List characteristics that enhance your ability to be an effective nurse educator. Start with the strengths you possess. Then reflect on possible areas that will improve the ability to affect learning for the client.

4. Search the following Internet addresses to familiarize yourself with the organizations that offer alternative therapies.
   American Chiropractic Institute
   www.amerchiro.org
   American Association of Oriental Medicine
   aaom.org
   American Message Therapy Association
   www.amtamassage.org
   American Yoga Association
   alignment.org/default.asp

References

American Nurses Association. (1991). Nursing's Agenda for Health Care Reform: Executive Summary. Retrieved January 5, 1999 from www://nursing world.org/readroom/magenda.htm.

American Hospital Association. (1974). A patient's bill of rights. Chicago: The American Hospital Association.

Baker, D., Parker, R., Williams, M., Coates, W., & Pitkin, K. (1996). Use and effectiveness of interpreters in an emergency department. The Journal of the American Medical Association, 275 (10), 783–789.

Berlin, E., & Fowkes, W. (1982). A teaching framework for cross-cultural health care. Western Journal of Medicine, 139, 934–938.

Boyd, M. (1992). The teaching process. In N. Whitman, B. Graham, C. Gleit, & M. Boyd (Eds.), Teaching in nursing practice (2nd ed., pp.155–170). Stamford, CT: Appleton & Lange.

Brown, E., & Wyn, R. (1996). Public policies to extend health care coverage. In R. Anderson, T. Rice, & G. Kominski (Eds.). Changing the U.S. health care system: Key issues in health services, policy, and management (pp. 41–51). San Francisco: Jossey-Bass.

Brown, F. (1997). Patient empowerment through education. Professional Nurse Study Supplement, 13(3), S4–S6.

Camphina-Bacote, J. (1995). The quest for cultural competence in nursing care. Nursing Forum 30(4), 19–25.

Corkery, E., Palmer, C., Foley, M., Schechter, C. Frisher, L., & Roman, S. (1997). Effect of a bicultural community health worker on completion of diabetes education in a Hispanic population. Diabetes Care, 20 (3), 254–257.

Davis, G. (1997). Chronic pain management of adults in residential settings. Journal of Gerontological Nursing, 23 (4), 16–22.

DeNatale, M., & Lantz, J. (1998). Community health strategies. Nurse Educator, 23(4), 11–12.

Egan, G. (2001). The skilled helper (7th ed.). Pacific Grove, CA: Brooks/Cole.

Eisenberg, D., Davis, R., Ettner, S., Appel, S., Wilkey, S., Van Rampay, M., & Kessler, R. (1997). Trends in alternative medicine use in the United States, 1990–1997, The Journal of the American Medical Association, 280(18), 1517–1572.

Farquharson, A. (1995). Teaching in practice. San Francisco: Jossey-Bass.

Fetter, M. (1997). Patient-family-community education: No longer frills. MedSurg Nursing, 6(3), 119–120.

Fong, C. (1985). Ethnicity and nursing practice. Topics in Clinical Nursing, 7(3), 1–10.

Friedman, M. (1998). Family nursing: Research, theory, & practice (4 ed.). Stamford, CT: Appleton & Lange.

George, G. (1982, May). If your patient tries your patience, try this plan. Nursing '82, 50–55.

Goeppinger, J., & Lorig, K. (1997). Interventions to reduce the impact of chronic disease: Community-based arthritis patient education. In J. Fitzpatrick & J. Norbeck (Eds.), Annual Review of Nursing Research, 1997 (pp. 101–122). New York: Springer Publishing.

Graham, B., & Gleit, C. (1992). Teaching in selected settings. In N. Whitman, B. Graham, C. Gleit, & M. Boyd (Eds.), Teaching in Nursing Practice (2nd. ed., pp. 31–47). Stamford, CT: Appleton & Lange.

Green, L., Kreuter, M., Deeds, S., & Partridge, K. (1980). Health education planning: A diagnostic approach. Palo Alto, CA: Mayfield.

Kleinman, A., Eisenberg, L., & Good, B. (1978). Culture, illness and child care: Clinical lessons from anthropological and cross-cultural research. Annals of Internal Medicine, 88, 251-258

Knowles, M. (1980). The modern practice of adult education: Androgogy versus pedagogy (2nd ed.). Chicago: Follett Publishing.

Lancaster, J. (1992). Education models and principles applied to community health nursing. In M. Stanhope & J. Lancaster (Eds.), Community Health Nursing. St. Louis: Mosby.

McCarthy, N. (1994). Health promotion in the community. In C. Edelman & C. Mandle (Eds.), Health promotion throughout the lifespan (pp. 202–219). St. Louis: Mosby.

Morgan, S. (1998). The stampede to alternative medicine. Healthcare Trends Report, 12(12), 1–2. Bethesda, MD: Health Tends, Inc.

Murrary, T. (1998). Using role theory concepts to understand transitions from hospital-based nursing practice to home health nursing. The Journal of Continuing Education in Nursing, 29 (3), 105–111.

O'Halloran, V. (1997). Defining education settings to improve client teaching. MedSurg Nursing, 6(3), 130–136.

Pender, M. (1996). Health promotion in nursing practice (3rd.ed.). Stamford, CT: Appleton & Lange

Potter, P., & Perry, A. (1995). Basic nursing: Theory and practice (3rd ed.). St. Louis: Mosby.

Rankin, S., & Stallings, K. (1996). Patient education: Issues, principles, practices. (3rd ed.). New York: Lippincott.

Redman, B. (1997). The practice of patient education (8th ed.). St. Louis: Mosby.

Shalala, D. (1997). Recognizing community outreach nurses. Nursing Management 28(8), 64–65.

Schneider, S., Richard, M., Huss, K., Huss, R., Thompson, L., Butz, Eggleston, P., Kolodner, K., Rand, C., & Malveaux, F. (1997). Moving health care education into the community. Nursing Management, 28(9), 40–43.

Schuster, J. (1997). Wholistic care: Healing a sick system. Nursing Management, 28(6), 56–61.

Scott, C., & Riedlinger, J. (1998). Promotion education about complementary or alternative therapies. American Journal of Health-System Pharmacy, 55(23), 2525–2527.

Thompson, D., Edelsberg, J., Kinsey, K., & Oster, G. (1998). Estimated economic costs of obesity to U.S. business. American Journal of Health Promotion, 13(2), 120–127.

Wells-Federman, C., & Edwards, L. (1994). Health education. In C. Edelman & C. Mandle (Eds.). Health promotion throughout the lifespan (3rd ed., pp. 243–264). St. Louis: Mosby.

Wilson, F. (1996). Patient education materials nurses use in community health. Western Journal of Nursing Research, 18(2), 196–205.

Zotti, M., Brown, P., & Stotts, R. (1996). Community-based nursing versus community health nursing: What does it all mean? Nursing Outlook, 44(5), 211– 217.

CHAPTER

14

Communication as the Fabric of Community-based Nursing Practice

Rosemarie C. Brenkus
and
Mary Narayan

LEARNING OBJECTIVES

1) Describe nine factors that influence communication.

2) Discuss the importance of self-disclosure in therapeutic communication.

3) Describe important factors in nonverbal communication.

4) Differentiate between personal and professional communication.

5) Identify therapeutic communication techniques for different age groups.

6) Discuss important considerations in cross-cultural communication.

We all communicate one way or another every day. Some people are excellent communicators whereas others are poor communicators. What makes a good communicator? There is no "best" way of communicating effectively. We encounter people from very diverse backgrounds and values every day. This precludes any hope we may have of finding one specific way to communicate with people in general. This chapter focuses on ways to communicate effectively with different groups, specifically, children, the elderly, and various cross-cultural groups, in community health settings. The content in this chapter, although basic, is the cornerstone of all effective communication.

Almost all communication falls under "interpersonal communication." The word *interpersonal* is often used to modify the word *communication*. When it is used in this way, interpersonal means more than just two persons communicating face to face. It refers to a type of human contact that can be a telephone conversation, a heated argument, a large committee meeting, or a public speech. One definition of interpersonal communication states that interpersonal communication is characterized by the way each person talks and listens to maximize one's humanness (Stewart, 1986). Keep in mind that communication is something that happens between people, not something one person does to someone else.

One of the most difficult, yet essential, things we struggle to do as human to human is to develop the ability to fully communicate. No one can really know us unless we are able and willing to tell about ourselves through our words and our actions. Buscaglia (1978) believes that we all have the right to make our statement and have it heard and understood. However, unless we are content to talk to ourselves, only we will know who we are. Others will only know who we are when we are able to say what we mean.

VARIABLES THAT INFLUENCE COMMUNICATION

According to Potter and Perry (1995), there are nine variables that influence communication: perceptions, values, development, space and territoriality, emotions, sociocultural background, knowledge, roles and relationships, and environmental setting. The following is a short explanation of each of the factors.

Perceptions

Each person senses, interprets, and understands events differently. Perceptions are a person's personal view of events occurring in the environment and are formed by goals and expectations; differences can be obstacles to effective communication. Perceptions shaped from years of similar experiences are difficult to change.

Values

Values reflect the things a person considers important in life. Different experiences and expectations lead to the formation of different values; they influence the way a person expresses ideas and the way the ideas of others are interpreted.

Development

The rate that speech development varies among children is related to neurological competence and intellectual development. Environment also affects speech and language development.

Space and Territoriality

During social interaction, people consciously maintain a distance between themselves. When personal space is threatened, persons may respond defensively and communicate less effectively. Nurses often work very closely with clients, so it is important to consider the influence that personal space may have on your communication with them.

Emotions

Emotions are subjective feelings about events; these influence the way a person communicates and relates to others. The nurse attempts to ensure that emotions do not interfere with providing optimal care. However, the nurse must be empathetic. Emotions can cause a person to misinterpret or not hear a message.

Sociocultural Background

Culture affects a person's generalizations and perceptions about the world. Language, gestures, and attitudes reflect

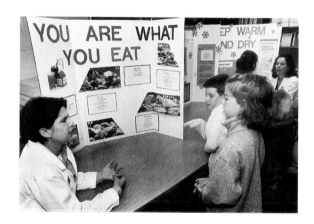

cultural origins. A nurse must accept a client's cultural background and frame of reference.

Knowledge

Different levels of knowledge make communication more difficult. A common language is essential. Knowledge is a product of development, education, environment, and sociocultural factors.

Roles and Relationships

Persons communicate with others in a style they assume is appropriate for various roles and relationships. The formality or informality of communication depends on the roles and kinds of relationship one has with others. Effective communication is possible if the participants are aware of their roles. We feel more comfortable expressing ideas to individuals with whom we have developed a positive relationship.

Environmental Setting

Communication is more effective in a comfortable environment. Noise or lack of privacy or space may cause confusion, tension, or discomfort. Environmental distractions can distort communication.

Self-Disclosure

One of the most important aspects of effective communication is establishing and maintaining trust and self-disclosure. Self-disclosure is the deliberate communication of information about yourself to others. Self-disclosure needs to be well timed to suit the occasion and the expectations of the people involved. Revealing too much too soon can make the other person feel uncomfortable and anxious to terminate the relationship early. Thus, when we first meet someone, we disclose information that is not too revealing or personal. As we feel more trusting in our relationship, we reveal more personal information.

The Johari Window is an excellent model for demonstrating how willingness to self-disclose affects our relationships with others (Beebe & Masterson, 1986). The Johari Window describes four types of information about you. The model, as shown in Figure 14-1, identifies four quadrants. Imagine that this *window* has panes that are movable and move from side to side and up and down.

	Open	Blind
Known to others	Known to self	Known to self
Unknown to others	Hidden	Unknown

FIGURE 14–1 The Johari window

Quadrant one is called the *open area*. It refers to information that others know about you and that you are also aware of. The more information you reveal about yourself, the bigger this pane or quadrant becomes. Therefore the more risks you are willing to take by self-disclosing, the larger your open area will be. Typically, when we first meet people we self-disclose information that is very basic such as age, occupation, the area where we live, and other things that anyone can know about us. As we become more familiar and comfortable with someone, we begin to reveal more about ourselves, thereby allowing our open area to get larger and larger.

The second quadrant is known as the *blind area*. This area consists of information about you that is known to others but not known to yourself. For example, you may think you are a rising opera star, but others think your voice is terrible. It is not until you allow people to get to know you better that they feel free to tell you that your chances of making it as an opera singer are not very good. As you learn how others see you, this second pane becomes smaller. Usually, the more we know about ourselves and about how others see us the smaller the blind area becomes.

The *hidden area,* the third quadrant in the Johari window, contains information that you know about yourself but that others do not know about you, nor do you want them to know. We all can think of many things about ourselves that we do not want other people to know. Perhaps we failed college in our earlier years or had our driver's license suspended for speeding—all embarrassing things that we want no one to know. Many counselors believe that we never need to reveal all things about ourselves to anyone—not even our closest friends. Self-disclosure can enrich a trusting relationship. However, the person you disclose this information to must be able to accept it. Otherwise, you have decreased communication, rather than increased it.

The last quadrant is called the *unknown area.* Information that is unknown to both you and others is found in this pane. We do not know how we will react in certain situations or what side we might take in an argument. Others may not know this either. We assume that this area exists because eventually some of these things become known to ourselves, to others, or to both.

The Johari Window demonstrates that people trust us only when they see us as trustworthy. The objective in any trustworthy relationship is to have our open area as big as possible and our blind, hidden, and unknown areas as small as possible. The more we trust someone, the more we self-disclose and vice versa. Think of this in a community setting when working with families as a small group. This family self-discloses things you need to know to provide proper care only when family members feel they can trust you. This is a challenge to all of us in health care.

Each of us is a unique individual; we interpret verbal and nonverbal communication differently. Take for example the phrase *picture window.* We all know what a picture window is but we all have a different way of defining it. In an exercise called "I am more like this than that" students are given words such as *summer* or *winter, screened porch* or *picture window, fly swatter* or *fly paper.* They are then asked to write down the phrase of each pair that best describes them. Through discussion, students are asked to explain why they chose the particular word and what the word meant to them. Some students feel that a picture window is very open and panoramic whereas others see it as very confining and restricting. The point of this exercise is to show that although we all hear the same word and know objectively what the word means, we all have different interpretations of the word. This is a very important factor to remember when communicating with clients. As health professionals, we must remember that the way we define a word may not be the same way our client is defining it. Therefore, clarification is very important. We all have different experiences in our life that generate different definitions of words. In health care we should never assume that the client interprets things as we do.

Nonverbal Communication

To communicate effectively we must be able to communicate both verbally and nonverbally. Many experts in the field of communication believe that 80 to 100 percent of all communication is nonverbal. It is important to remember that our body language and intonation should be sending the same message as our spoken words. Even if we say nothing, we are communicating. Our nonverbal cues affect the delivery of our message and many times are more powerful than the words we say. For example, a person who screams at you in a very angry voice telling you that "nothing is wrong" is sending two different messages—a verbal message and a nonverbal message. The receiver then needs to interpret it the way he or she sees fit—and it may not be the correct way. Becoming an accurate observer of nonverbal behavior takes time and practice. The following are some areas we should be concerned about when considering nonverbal communication:

Body Posture and Movement

The way a person moves, walks, stands, and sits can reflect emotions, self-concept, and either wellness or illness. Leaning backward can imply withdrawal, whereas leaning forward can imply being involved. An "at attention" kind of posture can demonstrate attentiveness or a feeling of wellness, whereas a slumping position can mean boredom or illness. Observing posture and movement can allow the nurse to collect valuable information.

Eye Contact

Eye contact usually indicates interest in a conversation or person. A lack of eye contact indicates anxiety, defensiveness, and a discomfort and lack of confidence in communicating. Movement of the eyes communicates feelings and emotions. The level at which eye contact occurs significantly influences communication. (Potter & Perry, 1995)

Facial Expression

The face is the most expressive part of our body. According to Knapp (1978), the face reveals six primary emotions: surprise, fear, anger, disgust, happiness, and sadness. When a patient tells us something, our reaction to it is revealed in our facial expression. Even the slightest movement of our forehead or lip can reveal our reaction to the client's statement. Take, for example, the client who just revealed to you that she had an abortion several years ago. A grimace or pursing of your lips can say that you do not approve.

Touch

Touch can facilitate a sense of trust and empathy. From our experiences as young children we began to learn how much we could trust people by the way they touched us. We tend to trust those people whose touching has satisfied

us or brings us pleasure. The greater the satisfaction received, the greater the interest we have in maintaining the relationship. We choose our physicians, dentists, or nurse-practitioners by the gentleness of their touch. It is important to remember that although touch is very important it must be used with discrimination. Touch must always be used in a professional, ethical manner and must be clearly accepted by the patient. Touch in other cultures will be discussed further in this chapter.

Personal Appearance

Personal appearance affects the way people perceive us. It influences our abilities to persuade others and is one of the first things noticed when others first see us. A nurse who is not clean and tidy can send a message to the client and family that this nurse is not going to give good care. "Someone who does not take the time to be tidy cannot possibly take time to give good care" is the impression the nurse may give. In other words, physical appearance is key in "first impressions." Fortunately or unfortunately, we live in a society today in which the "ideal body" is the standard for us to live by.

Territoriality and Personal Space

Clients generally respond better and feel more comfortable at a personal distance. This is discussed in detail later in the chapter. There are times when intimate space is necessary, especially when certain treatments are being given to the client. The sooner the client is comfortable with this, the better for both parties involved.

Listening

Box 14–1 contains an activity to help you think about your nonverbal behavior. The most important tool of all communication is listening. Listening is an active process through which we select, attend, understand, and remember. Understanding is probably the most important of all of these elements. All too often we "hear" someone say something, but we do not understand what was said. To listen effectively we must actively work at understanding the other person. Listening implies the message "You are important to me" and "I am interested in talking to you."

Box 14-1	Student Learning Activity

Non-verbal Communication

Think about how you structured communication with one of your patients. How do you think the following behaviors affected your nonverbal communication?

- Body posture

- Eye contact

- Facial expression

The following story illustrates one student's growing awareness of the importance of listening:

When we look around us in today's hectic society almost every one of us is striving to achieve a better standard of living to include a bigger house, better cars, more vacations, and more things for our kids. I never had such things growing up but never felt shortchanged because of it. On the contrary, I reveled in our vacations being in a tent and my Grandmother and Grandfather always going for walks with me, our picnics consisting of jelly sandwiches and a bottle of water, and stopping by a stream while out driving to get our feet wet. Never was an appreciation of the simple things in life brought home to me more than when having to deal with the youngsters of today during my latest clinical rotation, which took place in a local school system.

The area of my clinical rotation is an economically booming part of the state with a particularly highly educated and upwardly mobile population. There is particular affluence with the influence of the well-paid highly technical jobs that are abundant in this location. However, with this high-demand stress field there seems to be a price being paid by a largely forgotten population here, and that is the children of those in this field.

I was particularly perturbed by a specific incident with a teenager with whom I came into contact at one of my sites. It was early in the morning and she was already in a school setting that is more or less a last chance at high school graduation before the county gives up on a student and they fend for themselves. It was my first day at the school and I was in a very cramped little clinic with no privacy at all when I noticed her hanging around the door of the clinic. After questioning her as to what she was there for, she told me that she had a headache. The look on her face and body language strongly suggested that a headache was the least of her problems, but how to find out what was really going on was my next task. The nurse I was assigned with that day had other kids coming and going from the clinic so I took it upon myself to investigate further. I did not know quite how to approach it to begin with so I went right in there with questions and after a clumsy start was able to ascertain the problem and uncover one of the saddest situations I have ever come across.

This young woman had just had her sixteenth birthday the previous day and on that birthday she had no celebration of any kind. Instead, she found out that one of her best friends was in a coma in a local hospital after a suicide attempt and his chances for recovery were slim at best. If this was not bad enough, this friend was the younger brother of her previous best friend who had successfully attempted suicide almost a year prior to the day. This followed the suicide of both of the boys' father a year prior to that. The family who had once consisted of six was now down to three with one whose life was hanging in the balance. This teenager stated that he had been the "happy one" but nobody seemed to listen. She went on to describe what both of the boys had conveyed to her from their experiences at the mental health services, which were that they do not listen to you, take you seriously, or they are just there for a sham. All of which indicates that, justified or not, their interpretation was that of abandonment and having nobody to turn to, least of all their parents.

To be honest I made a few suggestions to this young lady that seemed to temporarily help her through what she was dealing with immediately but I was going from that location so I was not able to follow up on the outcomes of the situation. However, I must confess to feeling shocked at the grief bestowed on one family and woefully inadequate in how I was supposed to respond to one so young carrying such a heavy burden. As a new parent and soon to be new nurse I think that my most valuable lesson comes from acknowledging the importance of time. Time needed to guide and nurture our children of today who undoubtedly face *challenges that were previously unknown. Time for our patients who have lives and issues that reach far beyond whatever specific ailment they may be coming to see us with. And, the time to always remember that the clients, students, or patients are more than people with whom physical or mental problems are separate entities to be addressed without consideration to all other aspects of what makes up their life. I have never really faced the problem of not being able to communicate with anyone but the more I find out about nursing from experience, the key is not only being able to talk to someone, but being able to listen. This is what makes the difference between being a nurse who treats conditions and a nurse who makes a long lasting difference to a person's life. Hopefully, I will never forget to leave my ears open.*

Glatthorn and Adams (1983) suggest that there are three types of listening: hearing, analyzing, and empathizing.

Hearing is receiving the message as sent. Glatthorn and Adams (1983) say that to achieve this, you must:

- Receive the sounds as transmitted
- Translate these sounds into the words and meanings that were intended
- Understand the relationship of those words in the sentences spoken
- Note the relevant nonverbal cues that reinforce the message
- Comprehend the entire message as intended

Analyzing is using critical or creative judgment to discern the speaker's purpose. Analyzing involves the following steps:

- Hearing the message accurately
- Identifying the stated purpose
- Inferring the stated purpose
- Determining if a critical decision or judgment is required
- Responding accordingly

Empathizing requires concentration, a sensitivity to the emotional content of messages, an ability to see the world from the point of view of the speaker, and a willingness to suspend judgment. It involves these steps:

- Hearing the message accurately
- Listening to the unstated purpose
- Withholding judgment
- Seeing the world from the perspective of the speaker

- Sensing the unspoken words
- Responding with acceptance (Beebe & Masterson, 1986)

To listen effectively, you must work at understanding the other person. To be an effective communicator, it is your responsibility to listen attentively. O'Brien (1974) has identified common listening problems. Ask yourself these questions and evaluate your own listening ability.

- Are you able to listen to another without being distracted into thinking of someone or something else?
- Do you engage in an activity while someone is speaking—writing, doodling, watching another situation such as television, listening to the radio or stereo, reading the newspaper or a report, signing papers, and so on?
- Are you so concerned with having an answer to the situation or question that you do not hear the problem?
- Are you committed to your ideas to such a degree you do not listen to the responses of another?
- Are you negative about viewpoints that differ from yours and therefore reject new ideas or trends?
- Do you feel that most people are valuable and that communication with them is important?
- Are you abrupt with people, interrupting them to tell your story?
- Do you strive to accent the positive attributes of the speaker or do you look for flaws in his presentation?
- Can you summarize the ideas of others without asking them to repeat the dialogue again?
- Do you break in to complete the thoughts of others, either because you feel they are too slow in getting to the point or because you feel more capable? (O'Brien, 1974).

THERAPEUTIC COMMUNICATION

One student's story illustrates the importance of developing skills and confidence in therapeutic communication:

VISITS WITH MRS. V.

I've chosen to talk about my partner's client who is in the end stages of multiple sclerosis. She is 55, has been married for more than 20 years to a loving husband, and has an adopted son who is now 20. She has lost complete function of her extremities with the exception of movement in her neck. It causes her great pain to speak so she answers most questions with a nod of yes or no. She can eat but her main source of nutrition comes from a gastric tube (g-tube).

Our first visit caused a wide variety of emotions. I felt many emotions—pity, anger, fear, terror, and love. Ms. N., the day nurse, said that Mrs. V. had talked more with us than anyone else in months. She even said to me, "It's your turn to talk," because I wasn't saying much throughout the conversation. I felt fortunate that she allowed us to see a part of her that has been lost in the disease. When we left her home, I felt intense rage. How could such a beautiful young woman have such a terrible, debilitating disease? Why did this happen to her? How could God have allowed such a terrible disease to exist? I felt feelings of terror and fear because MS strikes people when they are in the prime of their life. What is stopping any of our classmates from having the disease? I wanted so much to stop her pain and my first thoughts were "Where is the cure, the pill, the magic potion?"

Visits to her house have taught me lessons that will impact me the rest of my life. . . . I believe she has taught me the importance of therapeutic human interaction. She has exhausted all means of treatment and has been poked and prodded to the point of no return. All that is left is human interaction and pain management. This scares me because I am a student who is not skilled in the area of therapeutic communication. I don't want to say the wrong thing or retrieve uncomfortable memories. Since the first visit there have been times when she doesn't respond to our questions and I wonder if we are making a difference in her life. When I question myself, I think of the first visit when she was energetic and talked throughout the entire interaction. During this interaction she seemed to forget that she was dying and she focused on our conversation. I believe that these moments, however small, have brought some joy during our visits.

Therapeutic communication requires planning so that the nurse consciously influences less-able persons into directions and actions beneficial to their welfare. Various authors who have defined therapeutic communication have in common the key words of *planning* and *consciously influencing*. Keep in mind that there is a difference between personal and professional communication. In contrast to social or personal conversation, therapeutic conversation should have a direction related to the health and well-being of the client. It should focus on helping the client learn about his or her illness and how to cope with it. It should also be goal directed and time limited. This type of communication is client centered and considers (1) the client's perspective and strengths, (2) readiness to learn, (3) ways of relating to others, (4) physical and emotional condition, and (4) sociocultural norms as relevant factors in planning and implementing communication strategies. Table 14–1 provides examples for using therapeutic communication.

COMMUNICATING WITH CHILDREN

We must remember that we cannot communicate with all people the same way. We need to communicate differently with children than we do with the elderly. Children do not have the same experiences to draw on that adults do. To communicate effectively with children at different age levels, we must understand the child's cognitive, developmental, and functional level. To have an effective relationship with the child client, the nurse must understand feelings and thought processes from the child's perspective. Seeing the world as the child perceives it is crucial in developing rapport with the young person. To determine what is appropriate communication, we first need to determine the developmental stage of the child. Each stage (infants, toddlers, preschoolers, school-age, or early adolescence) requires different types of communication.

In infancy, nonverbal communication is a key factor. Because touch is one of the prime sources of communication, we need to be very aware of how we approach this child. We must be gentle and avoid fast, abrupt movements. Gently patting the infants on their backs while holding them gives them reassurance and a sense of feeling secure. Many infants respond to low, comforting tones, regardless of the words. We must also be cognizant of our voice tone and facial expressions because we want the infant to see us as a comforter. It is also wise to keep the parent in view while caring for the infant.

The toddler and preschooler communicate both verbally and nonverbally. During this developmental phase the child is egocentric and focuses primarily on the self. Children in this stage are not in a sharing orientation because they feel the world revolves around them. Communication must be concrete and direct. It is a good idea to allow the child to explore things that may be used in their care, such as the stethoscope or thermometer.

Table 14-1

Techniques of Therapeutic Communication

TECHNIQUE	DEFINITION	EXAMPLE
Using broad opening statements	Initiating the discussion by allowing the client to determine what will be discussed	"Is there something you would like to tell me?"
Using general leads	Indicating that the nurse is listening and is interested in what the client is saying	Yes," "Oh?" "And then . . .," "Go on."
Reflecting	Repeating all or part of the client's words	Client: "I am terribly worried." Nurse: "Terribly worried?"
Sharing observations or perceptions	Stating to the client your perceptions or observations	"You're grimacing when you turn," "You seem to be in pain."
Acknowledging the client's feelings	Verbalizing acceptance and understanding of clients feelings or thoughts	"It must be extremely upsetting to you to be confined."
Selective reflecting	Directing back to the client what the nurse believes to be main idea client has stated	Client: "It's too much! I will never be able to go home!" Nurse: "Too much?"
Using silence	Maintaining an attentive, expectant silence to promote reflection	Silence conveys sadness, distress, anger, contemplation.
Giving information	Providing client with information to answer questions or dispel misinformation	"When you wake up, you will be in the recovery room, where the nurse will. . . ."
Clarifying	Requesting that the client make his or her meaning clear	"I'm not sure that I understand. . . ."
Verbalizing implied thoughts and feelings "	Verbalizing implied thoughts and feelings to verify nurse's impression of the client	Client: "I think this is going to do the trick." Nurse: "You are eager to get discharged aren't you?"
Validating	Requesting the client to validate that need has been met	"Are you feeling better now?"

Adapted from Leddy & Pepper (1993), p. 355.

The school-age child is a verbal person who is very curious about everything and wants to know "why" and "how." These children are eager to learn and want information. They need information that is easy to understand, for even though they may be thirsting for knowledge, they do not have the ability to process complex information. If the information is too overwhelming, the child may process the information inaccurately.

The adolescent or teenager is not yet an adult, but does not want to be seen as a child. They also may see adults (especially parents) as "old-fashioned" and "out of touch." Friends are of prime importance and the use of teenage language or slang is the way communication takes place. Imposing our values and judgments on this age group is a sure way to shut off all communication. The use of slang is controversial, but if you do not understand a word that is being used, you must ask the teen to help you understand it. Allowing the teen time to talk and listening attentively helps immensely in allowing for a successful communication process.

A Canadian nursing student participating in an international dialogue with nursing students at George Mason University showed how she met the challenge of teaching a child living with two blind adults through creative communication techniques:

LEARNING THROUGH COMMUNICATING

I worked with a very special family in the fall. The mother and her live-in boyfriend were both blind. The mother had a very active, fully sighted 3-year-old daughter. They requested information on healthy eating for their daughter because she was being "picky" and they were worried about her. The mother was also feeling really badly that she couldn't see to teach her child psychomotor skills such as colouring in between the lines. . . . Overcoming the visual barrier made this an extremely exciting family to work with. How did I overcome it? Every time I met with them, I spoke right away to tell them of my presence and gently touched a shoulder or a hand to tell them I was close by. I enlarged every handout I made so that they could use them in their special reading machine. I also taught the mother how to colour in the lines by making stencils for her. The mother could colour inside the stencils and then show her daughter how it was done. . . . The mother was afraid that her child would be behind developmentally if she was raised in her home. I eased her anxiety by completing a Denver II assessment and assuring her that she was actually above normal for her age. This was a wonderful family to work with and I learned so much from them.

Table 14–2 provides information to help you communicate successfully with children in the age ranges just discussed.

COMMUNICATING WITH THE ELDERLY

The term "older adult" refers to people who are 65 years of age or older. By the year 2030, it is projected that 22 percent of the U.S. population will be older adults (U.S. Department of Health and Human Services, 1991). The older adult represents the most diverse of the age groups. Effective use of the principles of communication as they relate to relationships with older adults requires a clear understanding of the uniqueness of older persons. Unfortunately, the stereotypical image of the older adult is that of a frail, not very competent person. Older adults vary greatly in capabilities, interests, and capacities of relationships. Some elderly are frail and have reduced intellectual function as a result of disease, and some retain a high level of physical and intellectual function until their death (Arnold & Boggs, 1999).

Years ago, the elderly were held in high esteem and recognized for their wisdom. They passed their wisdom from generation to generation by word of mouth and were seen as valuable teachers to the younger generation. Because the elderly died at much younger ages than the elderly today, there were fewer of them, and their contributions to society were considered special. Then came the advent of inventions like the microwave, computers, and technology. Too often in today's fast-paced society, we do not take the necessary time to communicate carefully with the elderly.

Almost all elderly experience diminished sensory communication. (Arnold & Boggs, 1999). One important problem of communication faced by the elderly is decreased processing of information resulting from age-related sensory loss (Carmichael, 1985). The developmental life cycle is sometimes considered unfair by many

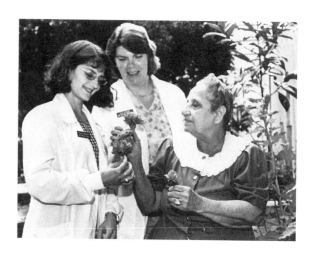

Table 14-2

Communicating with Children

AGE GROUP	CHARACTERISTICS	COMMUNICATION TECHNIQUES
Infants	Nonverbal is primary mode	Use stroking, soft touching, holding; soothe with crooning voice tone.
	Kinesthetic	Use motion (rocking, for example) to reassure. Allow freedom of movement, avoid restraining when possible.
	Bonded to primary caregivers only, infants more than 8 months may display anxiety when approached by strangers.	Use parents to give care. Arrange for one or both parents to remain nearby. Establish rapport with caregiver (parent) and keep at least 2 feet between nurse and infant at first. Talk to and touch infant and smile often initially. Learn some specific aspects of how primary caregiver provides care in term of sleeping, bathing, feeding, and attempting to mimic. Allow mother to always be within sight of child and vice versa.
	Vision—20/200–20/300 at birth	Encourage infant's caregiver (parents) to use a lot of intimate space interaction (8–18 inches). Mimic same when trust is established.
	Minimal receptive language skills	Use soft, slow voice tone; smile often, sit down as often as possible or stoop down so as to appear less imposing. Talk out loud in an active listening manner. Say such things as "Mommy is here and she loves you," "Mommy will keep you safe."
	Separation anxiety when primary caregiver is absent.	Provide for kinesthetic approaches; offer self while infant is protesting (examples: stay with the child; pick the child up and rock or walk; talk to the child about mommy and daddy and how much the child cares for mommy and daddy).
	Short stature	Sit down on chair, stool, or carpet to decrease posture superiority.
Toddlers	Limited vocabulary and verbal skills	Make explanations brief and clear. Use child's own vocabulary words for basic care activities. Assess (for example, use the child's word for defecate—"poop, gooies," urinate—"pee-pee, tinkle"); learn and use self-name of child.
	Speak in phrases	Rephrase child's message in a simple, complete sentence; avoid baby talk.
	Limited vocabulary	Use vocabulary skills to get to know primary caregiver first before approaching child. For example, allow the child to see that the nurse can be a friend with mommy.
	Kinesthetic	Allow ambulation when possible (toddler, chairs, walkers). Pull child in wagon often if child cannot achieve mobility.
	Struggling with issues of autonomy and control	Allow child some control. (For example, say, "Do you want half a glass or a whole glass of milk?" Reassure child if he or she displays some regressive behavior (example: if child wets his pants, say "We will get a dry pair of pants and let you find something fun to do"). Allow child to express anger and to protest about his or her care (example: Say "It's OK to cry when you are angry or hurt").

(Continued)

Table 14-2

Communicating with Children—cont'd

AGE GROUP	CHARACTERISTICS	COMMUNICATION TECHNIQUES
		Allow the child to sit up or walk as often as possible after intrusive or hurtful procedures. Say, "It's all over and we can do something more fun." Use nondirective modes, such as reflecting an aspect of appearance or temperament (example "You smile so often") or playing with a toy and slowly coming closer to and including the child in play.
	Fear of bodily injury	Show hands (free of hurtful items) and say "There is nothing to hurt you. I came to play/talk."
	Egocentrism	Allow child to be self-oriented and accepted. Use distraction if another child wants the same item or toy rather than expecting the child share.
	Direct questions	Use nondirective approach. Sit down and join the parallel play of child. Reflect messages sent by toddler (nonverbally) in a verbal and nonverbal manner. For example, say "Yes, that toy does lots of interesting and fun things."
	Separation anxiety	Accept protesting when parent(s) leave. Hug, rock the child, and say, "You miss mommy and daddy! They miss you too." Play peek-a-boo games with child. Make a big deal about saying "Now I am here." Show an interest in one of child's favorite toys. Say "I wonder what it does," or the like. If child responds with actions, reflect them back.
Preschoolers	Speaks in sentences but unable to comprehend abstract ideas	Use simple vocabulary; avoid lengthy explanations. Focus on the present, not the distant future; use concrete meaningful references. For example, say "Mommy will be back after you eat lunch" (instead of saying "at 1:00"). Use play therapy, drawings.
	Unable to tolerate direct eye-to-eye contact (some preschoolers)	Use some eye contact and attending posture. Sit or stoop and use a slow, soft tone of voice.
	May react negatively and with increased anxiety if long explanation is given regarding a painful procedure	Complete procedure as quickly as possible, give explanations about its purpose afterwards. For example, say "Jimmy, I'm going to give you a shot" (quickly administer the injection). "There, all done." It's OK to cry when you hurt. I'd complain, too. This medicine will make your tummy feel better."
	Short attention span and imaginative stage	Explain, using imagination (puppetry, drama with dress ups): use music. Use play therapy; allow child to play with safe equipment used in treatment. Talk about needed procedure happening to a doll or teddy bear, and state simply how it will occur and be experienced. Use sensory data: Say, for example, "The teddy bear will hear a buzzing sound."
	Concrete sense of humor beginning	

elderly because as sensory losses diminish, there is a simultaneous loss of friends through death, retirement, or relocation. In many instances, there is the loss of a spouse as well. It is difficult to understand the loss the elderly person is feeling because we have not experienced this. Frustration exists when family members are trying to deal with this person who once guided them and now is seeking guidance from them. The family must learn new coping skills and ways to increase tolerance.

As we age, physical changes occur that can alter our self-esteem and communication ability. Hearing and vision loss are two of the more significant losses we experience in addition to change of body shape and image. Many people choose to exercise to keep their bodies in as good a shape as possible, but working with hearing and visual impairment is not always as easy.

By the age of 50, we all begin having hearing loss. To what extent we lose our hearing is never predictable. Because hearing is an essential part of the communication process, we must learn strategies for working with the elderly who are hearing impaired. Arnold and Boggs (1999) suggests 12 strategies:

1. Determine whether hearing is better in one ear, and then direct speech to that side.
2. Help elderly clients adjust hearing aids. Lacking fine motor dexterity, the elderly client may not be able to insert aids to amplify hearing. Check batteries.
3. Speak distinctly but in a normal voice.
4. Address the person by name before beginning to speak. It focuses attention.
5. Do not speak rapidly; about 125 words a minute is best.
6. If your voice is high pitched, lower it.
7. If the older adult does not understand, use different words when repeating the message.
8. Face the older adult so he or she can use facial expression and/or lipreading to enhance comprehension. For example, humor is often communicated by subtle expressions.
9. Use gestures and facial expression to expand the meaning of the message.
10. Do not talk with your hands in front of your mouth or with food or gum in your mouth.
11. Keep background noises to a minimum (e.g., turn down the radio or television when talking).
12. Obtain feedback periodically to monitor what the person hears.

Vision decreases as we get older. What we once were able to distinguish is not as easy anymore. This impairment leads to problems involving dressing, preparing meals, driving, taking medication, using the telephone, and other daily functions that we all take for granted. This impairment almost always affects the person's ability to function autonomously. Some important things to remember: have eyeglasses available as needed, always keep the room arranged in the same way so the elderly person will not have to continually learn where things are placed, and be sure the room is well lighted.

Dealing with the psychosocial needs is not always as concrete as dealing with hearing and visual losses. Many times the elderly suffer from isolation and loneliness caused by loss of contact with friends and relatives because of death or perhaps relocation to an aging facility. Many younger people get impatient talking to an older person because the older person repeats things over and over. It is very important to know that the elderly person is experiencing changes that are uncontrollable and in many instances frustrating. Think for a moment how you would feel if people did not want to hear what you had to say and saw you as a burden. This is how the elderly may think that other people see them. When elderly clients are in a nursing home or in a community setting, a smile and a hello can change their whole day. We must become a society in which we are able to relate more to the elderly than we do today. Less than 5 percent of all the elderly are in nursing homes. Most are functioning people who do not want to be seen as incapable, but rather want to be seen as capable, contributing members of society.

Box 14–2 helps you apply the concept of age-appropriate communication.

CROSS-CULTURAL COMMUNICATION

No discussion about communication in community health is complete without considering the diversity of communication patterns that nurses find in today's communities. Throughout the world, but particularly in North America, communities are becoming more culturally diverse.

Immigration and travel patterns are changing the faces of many communities. The community-health nurse increasingly cares for people from many different cultures; cultural diversity in health care is becoming the norm instead of the exception.

Cultural diversity is accompanied by diversity in communication patterns, which present special challenges to the community-health nurse. Different cultures have different values, beliefs, and practices, including *communication* values, beliefs, and practices. Because of these differences, nurses and patients frequently *miscommunicate*, each taking the wrong message from a communication encounter. Consider the following nurse-patient encounters:

- While teaching a non-English-speaking Pakistani man how to perform self-urinary catheterization, the nurse uses the "thumbs up" gesture to indicate the patient performed the technique correctly. However, the patient becomes quite upset because in his culture, "thumbs up" is an obscene gesture.

- A Navaho patient avoids eye contact while the nurse is teaching her about diabetes management. The nurse perceives the lack of eye contact as disinterest and nonunderstanding and gives up on the teaching. However, in the patient's culture, lowered eyes are a sign of respect for the nurse, her expertise, and her knowledge.

- The nurse makes a home visit to a patient from India. The nurse has many visits that day and is trying to be very efficient with her time. On entering the home, the nurse refuses the offer of tea saying she needs to hurry. The family is offended, perceiving the nurse to be very rude and disrespectful. As the nurse attempts to instruct the family in the care of the patient, she finds she does not have the rapport necessary for teaching. The nurse did not realize that, from the family's cultural perspective, before "business" it is very important to establish a social bond through sharing refreshment.

- A refugee family from the Sudan has an appointment at the clinic at 10:00 A.M. They arrive at 12 noon as the nurse is eating her lunch. The nurse is very frustrated with the family. From the nurse's culturally developed perspective on time, being late for appointments communicates a lack of interest. The nurse feels the parents are irresponsible to show so little interest in their children's health. However, to the Sudanese family, who do not share the same time orientation as the nurse, the children's health is of utmost importance.

Each of these situations shows how easy it is to mis-communicate when providing cross-cultural health care. In each of the scenarios, the nurse misinterpreted what the patient meant to convey or the patient misunderstood the message the nurse was trying to give.

Obstacles to Effective Cross-Cultural Communication

Communication is a complex phenomenon, difficult in the best of circumstances. However, when the patient and the nurse come from very different cultural backgrounds, effective communication becomes more challenging. There are four main obstacles to effective cross-cultural communication:

- First, people from different cultures frequently communicate in different languages. When there is a language barrier between the nurse and the patient, communication is obviously impeded.
- Second, communication consists not only of words and sentences but also of nonverbal messages. It is estimated that we communicate more with our nonverbal communication messages than with our verbal messages. However, the same nonverbal communication patterns can mean different things in different cultures. For instance, making eye contact carries different meanings in different cultures.
- Third, communication occurs within a social interaction, and different cultures demand different social conventions in social interactions. For example, one culture may require a preliminary period of socializing before "business" whereas another culture values "getting down to business" in the most efficient and forthright way.
- Fourth, as we begin communicating with another, we make a number of assumptions on which we base our communication. We tend to assume that the person with whom we are attempting to communicate holds the same basic values and beliefs that we do. It is from here that we begin to communicate. However, the values, beliefs, and practices that we assume because they are so widely held in our own culture can be very different in the culture of our patient. For instance, many Americans assume that punctuality is an indicator of how important a person thinks an appointment is. However, the assumptions and values given to time vary from one culture to another.

The role of community-health nurses is to facilitate optimal health and well-being for their clients. Nurses do this by establishing mutually agreeable health goals with their community-health clients. Before nurses can reach these goals, nurses must communicate effectively with their clients. One of the first steps in assisting clients reach "well-being" is to determine how the client defines well-being. What "well-being" is differs from culture to culture and person to person. It is the clients who define what well-being is for them. Therefore, effective communication must be established for nurses to accomplish their role.

Strategies for Dealing with a Language Barrier

When the patient does not speak English and the nurse does not speak the patient's language, the ideal way to meet the patient's communication needs is with the help of a medical interpreter. Medical interpreters are professional interpreters who have special training in facilitating cross-cultural communication concerning health problems. Patients have the right to translation services that ensure they are able to make informed decisions regarding their care. Translation is a complex skill and it has been found that there are many dangers in using nonprofessionals as translators, such as in the following situations:

- When the translator is from the patient's family or community, the patient may be reluctant to relate the details of the illness and its symptoms out of embarrassment or fear. The patient may fear the illness will stigmatize the patient or the patient may downplay symptoms so as not to worry family or friends. Conversely, the translator may be embarrassed for the family member or friend or may be unable to accept what the patient reports out of fear or disbelief and may omit or downplay the symptoms in the translation.
- When the translator is from a rival region or state, which frequently happens between ethnic groups that share the same language, the patient may feel intimidated by the translator and the patient's vulnerable position in relation to the translator. The patient may not accurately divulge embarrassing parts of their medical history to the translator.

- In many cultures, particularly among Middle Eastern, Arab, North African, and Asian cultures, it is unacceptable to discuss certain body parts or processes with members of the opposite sex. If the translator is from the opposite sex, the patient may feel that discussing symptoms violates the culture's norms of modesty.

As can be seen from these concerns, many considerations must be taken into account when choosing an appropriate translator. Although medical translators are the "translator of choice" to ensure quality translation, community-health nurses frequently must cope with less-than-ideal translators because of time and financial constraints. There are several ways the nurse can enhance the quality of the translator's interpretation of the health interview:

- Explain the purpose of the interview to the interpreter.
- Explain to the interpreter the need to translate exactly the patient's own words; the interpreter should not "interpret" the patient's problem.
- Look and speak directly to the patient instead of to the interpreter during the interview.
- Look for the patient's nonverbal communication.
- Check the adequacy of the interpreter's translation by asking the patient to verbalize understanding of the conversation. Instruct the interpreter to repeat the patient's words exactly.
- Plan extra time for an interpreted interview. When an interpreter is required, the interview takes twice as long as normally expected when the nurse and the patient communicate in the same language.

Although many culturally diverse patients in our communities have learned to speak and understand English, their understanding and abilities in English fall along a continuum. Some can understand but can't speak English, some can speak but cannot read English, and some understand most of the time, but sometimes become confused. The nurse must assess the patient's knowledge and skill in the language before providing teaching. There are a several techniques the nurse can use to enhance communication when interviewing or teaching in a patient's second language:

- Use short simple sentences.
- Choose the most common or simple words in explanations.

- Do not use negatives in questions. Example:
  Wrong: "You don't take the medications together, do you?"
  Right: "Do you take the medications together?"
- Do not use contractions.
- Avoid metaphors, idioms, and colloquialisms.
- Pantomime words and actions while verbalizing them.
- When giving time-sequenced instructions, give steps in order. Example:
  Wrong: "*Before* you inject the medication, pull the plunger up to check for blood."
  Right: "*First,* pull the plunger up to check for blood, then inject the medication."

NONVERBAL COMMUNICATION VARIABLES

We have all heard the expression, "Your actions speak louder than your words." All people tend to "hear" very strong messages from another's body language. When we are talking with others, we pay as much attention, if not more, to what they are saying with their eyes, their facial expressions, their gestures, their use of pauses, their use of touch, and their tone of voice. From early childhood, multiple experiences with others teach us what a head nod, raised eyebrows, or a particular hand gesture means. However, the same nonverbal pattern can mean one thing in my culture and carry a different meaning in yours.

Eye Contact

American children learn that it is important to make eye contact when talking with others. They learn to see eye contact as a sign of respect, paying attention, and honesty. By the time Americans reach adulthood, they tend to interpret a lack of eye contact as a sign of disrespect, disinterest, or dishonesty. However, in many cultures, making eye contact is a sign of arrogance, intimidation, or sexual overture. An American child is told "Look at me when I talk to you!" But a Navaho child may be told, "Look down when I talk to you."

Even though Americans value eye contact, they do not like too much eye contact. Americans maintain eye contact, but the eye contact is not sustained for a long period. We briefly break our eye contact a couple of times within a minute while talking with others. Too much eye contact is perceived as a "stare" or as "invasive." The French tend to maintain eye contact longer than Americans do. Many Americans perceive the French as arrogant. Could part of this feeling about the French come from the length of their eye contact? The point here is that the meaning of eye contact varies from one culture to another; the message we tend to take from another's eye contact is the message it means in our own cultural perspective.

Facial Expressions and Head Gestures

There is a saying, "Everyone understands a smile." In one sense this is true: a smile is a positive expression toward another. However, different cultures assign other meanings to a smile in addition to the positive feeling towards another. For instance, consider this case:

The nurse instructed the Cambodian mother of a toddler how to use a shampoo preparation to treat her daughter's head lice infestation. The mother spoke limited English but seemed to understand the instructions. During the instruction, the mother frequently smiled at the nurse, nodding her head up and down, which the nurse perceived as understanding and agreement. However, to the Cambodian mother, her smile and head nodding were not indicators of agreement and understanding. Instead, they were indicators of the mother's respect for the nurse and her appreciation that the nurse was trying to help her child. The mother gave the shampoo to the child as an oral preparation.

How people from different cultures indicate agreement varies widely from culture to culture. In America, we tend to nod our heads up and down. The Yupik Eskimo indicates agreement by raising the eyebrows, a very subtle facial expression, which is missed by most Americans. The Eastern Indian frequently expresses agreement by rolling the head back and forth, which is perceived by most Americans as "I don't know," but in the Eastern Indian culture means "yes."

Gestures

The meaning of hand gestures also varies from culture to culture. In America, the "thumbs up," "OK" sign made by making a circle with the thumb and index finger, and the "V" for victory or peace sign are all very positive gestures.

However, in some other cultures these same gestures are obscene gestures. In many cultures, especially in those found in the Middle and Far East, one must be careful of the placement of one's feet. To cross one's legs so that the sole of the foot points towards another is an insulting gesture.

Use of Space

People are acculturated into different perceptions about personal space. In American culture, most people tend to distance themselves about 18 inches to 36 inches from the person with whom they are conversing. To move closer is to invade another's personal space and is perceived as an aggressive, intrusive behavior. To distance one self farther than 36 inches is perceived as "distant" or "aloof" behavior. However, personal and conversational space are defined differently in other cultures. An appropriate conversational space in some cultures is 9 to 24 inches and in other cultures the appropriate space is further than 36 inches. The feelings we get from the movement in and out of our comfortable social space can be quite strong and are frequently misinterpreted between people of different cultures, as can be seen by the following example:

The visiting nurse was attempting to teach a Saudi Arabian gentleman about his elderly father's diabetes management plan. As they sat down together on the couch, the Saudi gentleman sat very close to the nurse. The nurse felt very uncomfortable, and pulled herself as far into the corner of the couch as she could. The Saudi man drew closer to her. The nurse's discomfort exacerbated. Although she did not put her feeling into words, her discomfort reflected her feeling that the patient's son was in her intimate space. She felt as though her were making a sexual advance and she cut the teaching short. The gentleman, however, was just trying to get into the socially acceptable space that meant appropriate interest within his culture.

Use of Touch

The way touch is perceived varies from culture to culture. In American culture, touching a person's arm or shoulder is usually interpreted as a sign of caring, but in some cultures it may be perceived as rude behavior. Touching of children or patting them on the head in some Asian and South American cultures is considered to be dangerous to the child.

STRATEGIES FOR MANAGING NONVERBAL COMMUNICATION PATTERNS IN DIVERSE CLIENTS

Nurses in community-based sites must be very cautious about how they perceive the nonverbal behaviors of clients who come from different cultures. Usually, we tend to perceive the messages from nonverbal behaviors subconsciously from our own cultural perspective. One strategy for decreasing the miscommunication that can occur is to make conscious our subconscious interpretations of these behaviors. For instance, when the nurse who was teaching the Saudi Arabian man about his father's diabetes felt uncomfortable, she could bring into her consciousness that she feels uncomfortable because the man is moving into her personal, intimate space, which from her experience in her own culture, usually means a sexual advance. She needed to remind herself that the way she interprets the behavior may be an erroneous interpretation from the man's cultural perspective. She then needs to ask herself what the gentleman means by this nonverbal behavior. In addition, nurses must be sensitive to the variety of interpretations that may be given their own nonverbal behaviors.

Kavanagh and Kennedy (1992) make several recommendations about ways to avoid miscommunication with nonverbal behavior patterns:

- Mirror the client's nonverbal patterns. How much and when does this client and family make eye contact? What facial expressions do they use to express agreement? Disagreement? How much space do they place between one another during conversations? How fast do they talk? How loud?
- When the nurse gets a feeling that the patient has become defensive or that "things are not going well," the nurse can stop, apologize for any offense given by her behavior, and express her desire to assist the client meet his or her health goals.

Box 14–3 will allow you to apply your knowledge about culturally competent communication.

Social Etiquette

Communication occurs within a social interaction, and different cultures demand different social conventions in

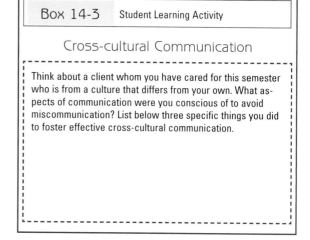

Box 14-3   Student Learning Activity

Cross-cultural Communication

Think about a client whom you have cared for this semester who is from a culture that differs from your own. What aspects of communication were you conscious of to avoid miscommunication? List below three specific things you did to foster effective cross-cultural communication.

social interactions. We do not jump into effective communication until we have adhered to the socially acceptable conventions. Before a meaningful conversation can take place, the social conventions for communication must be observed or communication will be hindered. In general, we do not realize that we follow these conventions, because, within our own culture, they are so "second nature" to us. Depending on the situation, in American culture, we open a conversation by greeting the other person, shaking hands, offering a seat, and in a number of other socially acceptable ways let the person with whom we are beginning a conversation know that we are ready to communicate. Even before initiating the conversation, we make sure we are addressing the right topic, to the right person, at the right time, and in the right place. These communication "rights" are frequently culturally determined.

Greetings

How we open a conversation differs greatly between cultures. Some cultures shake hands, others kiss on the cheek, others require asking about one another's families, others necessitate the sharing of refreshment, and still others require a prolonged period of "chit-chat" before "business" can begin. Some cultures are very formal, requiring formal greetings and formal forms of address whereas others value a casual approach and a familiar form of greeting. In some cultures, it is very important to greet the elders before greeting the younger members in a group.

During the Communication Encounter

Within American culture, we show interest in the conversation by nodding, interjecting comments like, "and then what happened" and "yes, I see." Other cultures may show interest by maintaining a thoughtful silence or by smiling and nodding even if they don't agree.

The Right Topic, Person, Time, and Place

Each culture determines what topics should be discussed with whom at what time and place. Very often, this differs from the American norm. Nurses are socialized into a Western Biomedical approach to the four communication "rights" early in their career. Nurses learn that the patients have the right to know about their illness and their options for treatment. We believe that patients should be the decision makers about their care. This belief grows out of the Western Biomedical ethical concepts concerning patient autonomy and truth telling. Table 14–3 illustrates how these concepts differ in other cultures.

Within the different value systems found in different cultures, the patient may not be the decision maker about

his or her care. Another family member may be the appropriate person to whom to address the health interview and the care instructions. This is sometimes hard for American nurses to accept because of our deeply held values of equality, independence, and self-reliance. However, if our patients do not share these values but instead value hierarchy and family interdependence, we do not enhance their sense of well-being by violating their deeply held culturally determined values. Table 14–4 presents some common differences in values between Americans and other cultures.

Strategies for Effective Communication Despite Diversity in Social Values and Etiquette

There are hundreds of different ethnic cultures and different cultural variables. It is beyond the scope of this chapter on communication to describe the different cultural variables for all the different cultures we find in our communities. Here we address some general strategies that will help you communicate effectively across cultures.

Table 14-3

Diversity in Beliefs about Health

WESTERN BIOMEDICAL CULTURE	VARIOUS OTHER CULTURES
Disease has physical cause	Imbalance causes disease
Mind-body separation	Mind-body-spirit unity
Truth telling	Hope
Autonomy	Decisions by family head; family interdependence
Self-care	Family meets patient's needs
Reliance on biomedicine	Reliance on traditional, home, folk practitioners/remedies
Pain borne stoically	Pain expressed openly
Western Bioethical principles	Ethical principles from different perspectives

Table 14-4

Diversity in Social Values

TYPICAL AMERICAN VALUES	VALUES FROM VARIOUS OTHER CULTURES
Self-reliance	Interdependence of family
Independence, autonomy	Family decision making
Competition, achievement	Cooperation, relationship
"The things money can buy"	Spirituality, nature, people
Technology—bigger, better	Tradition
Internal locus of control	External locus of control
Equality	Honor, hierarchy
Youth	Elderly
Physical beauty	Wisdom
Punctuality	Presence to person
The future	The present or past

Cultivate Attitudes Associated with Excellent Transcultural Nursing Care

According to Emerson (1995), there are six attitudes that characterize nurses who excel at cross-cultural nursing care: empathy, caring, openness, flexibility, a positive response to cultural differences, and a willingness to learn. To communicate effectively across cultures, you need to communicate these attitudes to your culturally diverse clients.

Be Sensitive to the Impact of Culture on the Health and Communication Values and Practices of the Client—and the Nurse

Most health, communication, and social values and practices are culturally determined. They have been passed down from generation to generation. Because these values are deeply embedded in us, they are very difficult to change. Each culture has developed values and practices over centuries of tradition, and it is not the task of the nurse to say that these are not valid. In providing cross-cultural health care, it is important to be open-minded and nonjudgmental about the cultural beliefs and practices of others. Respect for our patients involves respect for their cultural beliefs, values, and practices.

Obtain Background Information about the Patient's Culture

When our patients come from cultures different from our own, it is helpful to obtain information about these cultures before we attempt to provide care for these patients. There are a number of resources that provide information about specific cultures, the rules for polite behavior within the culture, and the norms for verbal and nonverbal communication, as well as information on health and dietary patterns (Giger & Davidhizar, 1995; Lipson, Dibble, & Minarik, 1996; Purnell & Paulanka, 1998; Spector, 1996). With awareness of these cultural norms, the nurse's efforts to establish rapport, start a therapeutic relationship, and open the lines of communication are enhanced. However, the nurse must be aware that any particular client may or may not follow the norms of his or her culture of origin. No one is a stereotype of his or her own culture.

Discover the Client's Views and Practices for the Health Problem by Performing a Cultural Assessment

Because communication is most effective when both parties begin with the same understanding of the problem, a cultural assessment of the health problem can facilitate the rest of the communication and nursing process. There are a number of cultural assessment tools available in the nursing literature (Andrews & Boyle, 1998; Giger & Davidhizar, 1995; Leininger, 1991; Narayan, 1997; Spector, 1996). Through a cultural assessment, the nurse seeks first to understand the health problem from the client's point of view. The Explanatory Model Interview (Klienman, Eisenberg, & Good, 1978) is among the quickest ways to get to the cultural overlay of a health problem in the shortest amount of time. These questions are included in the cultural assessment checklist found in Table 14–5. Box 14–4 will help you practice your cultural assessment skills.

Box 14-4   Student Learning Activity

Cultural Assessment

Use the cultural assessment checklist in Table 14–5 to assess one of your clients from a culture different from yours. Were you surprised at some of the information that did not fit your preconceived idea of a client from this culture? Briefly summarize the findings from your assessment.

CURRENT RESEARCH

As more nurses assume roles in community-based practice, there is a need for research related to the specific types of communication problems these nurses might encounter. One area for study is that of interdisciplinary communication in health care. Russell and Hymans (1999) explored outcomes related to collaboration and communication between undergraduate nursing and social work students. In partnership with a neighborhood organization, these two groups of students worked together to identify and meet needs of the community. Communication between the groups helped students from each discipline identify similarities and differences between their professions that could be used to design effective interventions in the community. Results suggest the benefits of pairing nursing students with students from other health professions to gain experience in professional communication and collaboration.

There is very little research that addresses how clients signal their needs for health care information. A study by Levinson, Gorawara-Bhat, and Lamb (2000) addressed this problem through looking at clues that clients present in conversations with their physicians. Their findings also appear relevant to nurses. The researchers recorded 116 physician/client interactions and found that clients present important clues that are opportunities for health-care professionals to implement therapeutic communication strategies. Some of these clues appeared to be a "cry for help." In the majority of cases, physicians failed to respond to opportunities to adequately acknowledge clients' feelings. It is interesting that visits characterized by these missed opportunities tended to be longer than visits when physicians did respond positively. Results of the study suggest that healthcare professionals need to be alert to clues presented by clients to demonstrate understanding and empathy and, thus, to enhance the therapeutic relationship.

Another study looked at physicians' perceptions of how well they communicated with clients when explaining things versus the clients' perception of the same. Although physicians thought they communicated well, especially when efforts were made not to use unfamiliar terminology, the clients felt they were not familiar with the terms and things were unclear (Bourhis, Roth, & MacQueen, 1989). This study has important implications for nurses and other health-care personnel. We must never take for granted that the client understands what we are explaining and need to identify ways to complement the client's need for information, whether through audiovisual materials, one-on-one discussions, pictures, or various other resources.

Table 14-5

Cultural Assessment Checklist

PATIENT IDENTIFIED CULTURAL/ETHNIC GROUP RELIGION	CLIENT'S EXPLANATION OF PROBLEM	NUTRITION ASSESSMENT	PAIN ASSESSMENT	MEDICATION ASSESSMENT	PSYCHOSOCIAL ASSESSMENT
Social Customs	*Diagnosis.* What do you call this illness? How would you describe this problem?	Pattern of meals: What is eaten? When are meals eaten?	Cultural patterns/patient's perception of pain response	Patient's perception of "Western" medications	Decision maker
Typical greeting. Form of address? Handshake appropriate? Shoes worn in home?	*Onset.* When did the problem start? Why then? What started the problem?			Possible pharmacogenetic variations	Sick role
Social customs before "business." Social exchanges? Refreshment?	*Cause.* What caused the problem? What might other people think is wrong with you?	Sick foods			Language barriers, translators
Direct or indirect communication patterns	*Course.* How does the illness work? What does it do to you?	Food intolerance and taboos			Cultural/ethnic community resources
Nonverbal Patterns of Communication	What do you fear most about this problem?				
Eye contact. Is eye contact considered polite or rude?	*Treatment.* How have you treated the illness? What treatment should you receive? Who in your family or community can help you? Traditional practitioners?				
Tone of voice. What does a soft voice or a loud voice mean in this culture?	*Prognosis.* How long will the problem last? Is it serious?				
Personal space. Is personal space wider or closer than in the American culture?	*Expectations.* What are you hoping the nurses will do for you when we come?				
Facial expressions, gestures. What do smiles, nods, and hand gestures mean?					
Touch. When, where, and by whom can a patient be touched?					

CONCLUSION

Communication is one of the most important skills for health professionals to master. It is also one of the most difficult because we work with people from all age groups and all cultures. The United States is becoming more culturally diverse. In 1990, one out of every five Americans was classified as a minority. The Census Bureau estimates that by 2050, "minorities" will account for more than one-half of the population. Caring for patients from different cultures is, and will increasingly be, the norm. Because communication is so significantly impacted by the patient's and the nurse's cultural backgrounds, nurses must be sensitive to the patient's cultural communication needs and adjust their communication techniques to meet those needs.

Knowing how to communicate effectively takes practice, understanding, patience, and acceptance. Value neutrality is one of the most difficult things a healthcare worker must acquire. Communication never stops and can be the most important element to aid the well-being of the client. We must work at accepting the client at face value, even though at times we may find this difficult.

References

Andrews, M., & Boyle, J. (1998). Transcultural concepts in nursing care. Philadelphia: Lippincott.

Andrews, M., & Boyle, J. (1998). Transcultural concepts in nursing care. Philadelphia: Lippincott.

Arnold, E., & Boggs, K. (1999). Interpersonal relationships: Professional communication skills for nurses. Philadelphia: WB Saunders.

Beebe, S., & Masterson, J. (1986). Communicating in small groups: Principles and practices. Glenview, IL: Scott, Foresman and Co.

Bourhis, R., Roth, S., & MacQueen, G. (1989). Communication in the hospital setting: A survey of medical and everyday language use amongst patients, nurses and doctors. Social Science Medicine, 28, 339–346.

Buscaglia, L. (1978). Personhood: The art of being fully human. New York: Ballantine.

Carmichael, C. (1985). Cultural patterns of the elderly. In L. Samovar & K. Porter (Eds.), Intercultural communication: A reader. Belmont, CA: Wadsworth.

Emerson, J. (1995). Intercultural communication between community health nurses and ethnic-minority clients. (Doctoral Dissertation). Fairfax, VA: George Mason University.

Active Learning Strategies

1. Discuss with a classmate your experiences trying to communicate effectively with a child, an adolescent, and an elderly person.

2. Make a list of five of the most common forms of nonverbal communication you observed in your last clinical experience. Ask a classmate to do the same and compare lists.

3. Interview a nurse from a culture different than yours regarding ways you both communicate. Make a list comparing and contrasting your similarities and differences.

4. Using the Johari Window, determine which "pane" is largest for you, as an individual in your class, in your clinical group, in your family.

Giger, J. N., & Davidhizar, R. E. (1995). Transcultural nursing: Assessment and intervention (2nd ed.). St. Louis: Mosby.

Glatthorn, A., & Adams, H. (1983). Listening your way to management success. Glenview, IL: Scott, Foresman and Co.

Kavanagh, K. H., & Kennedy, P. H. (1992). Promoting cultural diversity: Strategies for health care professions. Newbury Park, CA: Sage.

Kleinman, A., Eisenberg, L., & Good, B. (1978). Culture, illness and care: Clinical lessons from anthropologic and cross-cultural research. Annals of Internal Medicine, 88, 251–258.

Knapp, M. L. (1978). Non-verbal communication in human interaction. New York: Holt Rinehart & Winston.

Leddy, S., & Pepper, J. M. (1993). Conceptual bases of professional nursing. Philadelphia: JB Lippincott.

Leininger, M. (1991). Leininger's acculturation health care assessment tool for cultural patterns in traditional and non-traditional lifeways. Journal of Transcultural Nursing, 2(2), 40–42.

Levinson, W., Gorawara-Bhat, R., & Lamb, J. (2000). A study of patient clues and physician responses in primary care and surgical settings. Journal of the American Medical Association, 284(8), 1021–1027.

Lipson, J. G., Dibble, S. L., & Minarik, P. A. (Eds.). (1996). Culture & nursing care: A pocket guide. San Francisco: UCSF Nursing Press.

Narayan, M. C. (1997) Cultural assessment in home care. Home Healthcare Nurse, 15(10), 663–672.

O'Brien, M. (1974). Communications and relationships in nursing. St. Louis: C. V. Mosby.

Potter, P., & Perry, A. (1995). Basic nursing: Theory and practice (3rd ed.). St. Louis: Mosby.

Purnell, L. D., & Paulanka, B. J. (1998). Transcultural health care: A culturally competent approach. Philadelphia: Davis.

Russell, K., & Hymans, D. (1999). Interprofessional education for undergraduate students. Public Health Nursing, 16(4), 254–262.

Spector, R. E. (1996). Cultural diversity in health and illness. Stamford, CT: Appleton & Lange.

Stewart, J. (Ed.). (1986). Bridges not walls. New York: Harper and Row.

U.S. Department of Health and Human Services. (1991) HEALTHY People 2000. Washington DC. Public Health Service.

CHAPTER 15 Working with Families in the Community

Georgine M. Redmond

LEARNING OBJECTIVES

1) Define the family in broad terms and as a health-care unit.

2) Describe various family forms.

3) Describe the structural, functional, and developmental aspects of the family.

4) Describe crisis within a family and identify examples of developmental and situational crises.

5) Differentiate family resilience from crisis.

6) Identify a model for family crisis intervention.

7) Explore the nurse's role in family health promotion.

8) Describe the components of family assessment and diagnosis.

9) Evaluate current family research in community-based settings.

10) Describe the nurse's role in comprehensive care of the family.

This chapter focuses on your care of families in community-based settings. You will work with families at various points along the health-illness continuum—from healthy families caring for the birth of a baby in a "Home Tomorrow" program in which you follow up on an early discharge to an elderly family with a dying member with whom you work in a church community. After performing a family assessment, you may provide any number of direct or indirect services like teaching and supporting breast-feeding efforts to vital signs monitoring. Communication, counseling, and case management skills are especially needed in these settings as you work with your families. This chapter provides some background information on families, giving some specific examples of types of family issues that you may confront in a variety of community-based settings.

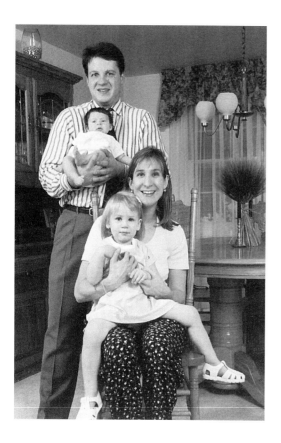

FAMILY

The term *family* conjures up many images for us. Our perspective on family arises from our experiences within our own families and the "ideal" families portrayed on TV and in movies as we grew up, as well as broader definitions of family that we see in the media and society today.

The families that you meet in community-based settings should be asked to self-define their family for you; it is their definition and perspective that you will use to collaboratively conduct assessments, identify needs, and plan interventions. Box 15–1 will give you an opportunity to formulate your definition of family.

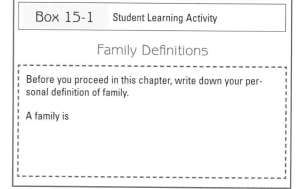

> **Box 15-1**   Student Learning Activity
>
> ## Family Definitions
>
> Before you proceed in this chapter, write down your personal definition of family.
>
> A family is

Definition of Family

Common definitions of families are:

"Two or more persons who are joined together by bonds of sharing and emotional closeness and who identify themselves as being part of a family" (Friedman, 1998, p. 9), or more broadly, a "group of individuals closely related by blood, marriage or friendship ties (nuclear family, cohabiting couple, single parent, blended families, etc.) that may be characterized by commitment, mutual decision making and shared goals" (Bomar, 1989, p. 120).

Essential elements that exist in any definition of family include two or more persons and the emotional attachments that are present. Geographical proximity has been deleted from most definitions of family, because situational factors like divorce or military assignments may alter this.

You will identify each family's definition of itself as you collaborate with them to provide the necessary nursing care. Asking questions directly about who their family is, observing their living circumstances, and observing with whom they spend time and share confidences will help you to get at this personal definition. A nurse who wishes to provide family-centered care must have this information.

Family Forms

Contemporary family life takes on many forms. Common terms used in discussing family forms are family of origin and family of procreation. Each person has a *family of origin,* the family into which an individual is born or adopted and socialized; many have a *family of procreation,* the family created by marriage, childbearing, or adoption.

In addition, other terms used to describe family are nuclear and extended family. The *nuclear family* is usually considered the traditional family form composed of mother, father, and children by birth or adoption. A more contemporary view of the nuclear family today includes married or unmarried couples living together with or without children, single-parent households, blended families (second marriages), homosexual families, and communal families.

The *extended family* usually refers to a group of individuals beyond the nuclear family, often related by blood, such as grandparents, aunts, uncles, cousins, and other kinfolk who may or may not live with the family. Today, because of the distance that exists within the extended family, many families seek to expand their kinship ties to include friends and neighbors in their current environments who become part of their extended families. Table 15–1 depicts types of family forms.

Based on this information, take a few minutes to apply your knowledge of current family forms to the experiences you are having in your community-based site.

There are three predominant perspectives through which you can understand the families with whom you work in the community. These are the structural-functional, developmental, and system approaches. The *structural-functional* approach looks at the arrangement of the parts that compose the family as a whole and the functions that the family carries out in the larger society and on behalf of its members. The *developmental approach* views the family and its progress through normal developmental periods from the time it is established through marriage to the death of one or both spouses. The *systems approach* views

Table 15-1

Types of Family Forms

Nuclear Family: Husband, wife, and children by birth or adoption

Couples: Married or unmarried individuals living together without children

Single-parent Family: One parent of either sex and a child or children

Blended Family: Husband, wife, and children of either or both by previous marriages, plus children they produce

Homosexual Family: Two adults of the same sex with or without children

Communal Family: Group of unrelated adults and children committed to living as a family

Plural Family: Husband, wives, and their collective children by birth or adoption

Extended Family: Close relatives of a nuclear family, such as grandparents, uncles, aunts, and cousins

Adopted Extended Families: Friends and neighbors in current environments adopted by the nuclear family

---

Box 15-2   Student Learning Activity

Exploring Family Forms

What types of families have you encountered in your community-based experience? List them and discuss any particular issues you have dealt with that arise from their family forms.

---

the family as a complex social system and as a unity from which an individual family member's behavior flows. The family as a system constantly exchanges energy, information, and material with the environment.

Family structure refers to how the family is organized and the relationships among its members. The elements involved in family structure include roles, value systems, communications patterns, and power structure (Friedman, 1998).

Roles

Individuals within the family may occupy many roles. A role is a set of behaviors, attitudes, beliefs, principles, and values that characterize the occupant of a given social position or status (Friedman, 1998). For example, "father" is a role in a contemporary family that carries expectations of shared child care and child socialization, a partner in providing for the financial needs in the family, as well as home management and maintenance. It is important to remember as you work with families in the community that roles are developed through a sociocultural lens. Recognition of this is important to provide culturally competent care to your families. Therefore, a contemporary definition of "father" in the American society may not fit that of immigrant families.

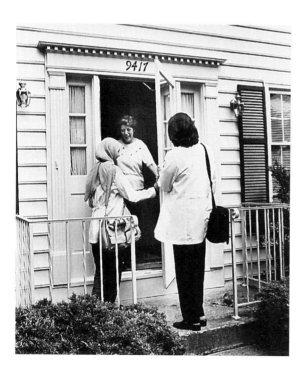

The following story describes a student's home visit to an international family and illustrates the impact of culture on role:

My first home visit was to a family from Pakistan. I was really nervous but my instructor assured me that everything would go just fine. The family moved here because the father wanted his children to receive a good education. The father was a professor of French in their home country. The family lives in a subsidized housing apartment. It is furnished with beautiful furniture and collectibles from their country. The sofas were arranged around the walls so that everyone could see each other while speaking. There were many classic novels on the bookshelves and a set of encyclopedias. It was a very beautiful home.

Talking with the father and sister of the little boy we were there to discuss went very well. The family was so thankful that we were there to help the boy with his asthma and to inform the family of his condition and treatment options. The father spoke through his daughter because he did not speak English very well. They were both very nice. We wanted to speak with the mother but she stayed in the kitchen. I figured that it was the custom in their country to let the male handle any business that needed to be conducted.

As we went to leave the father came out of the kitchen with two very large vacuum packed bags of dates. He wanted us to have them as a way of saying thank you for our help. As our instructor told us many times, we were not supposed to accept gifts for our services. We tried to decline very politely but it was apparent that the father would be extremely insulted if we did not accept his gift. We took them with a smile on our face and a thank you and left to go back to our school. I thought about the family that night and realized that the visit went well and that we were able to help them even if it was such a small way.

Roles in contemporary society are more interactive then specifically prescribed by tradition as in the past. In general, if role behaviors are clearly defined and communicated, a family functions very well. That is when the performance of one member matches the expectations of other members, and vice versa. When *role complementarity* exists, family balance is maintained. The following story illustrates role conflicts that can occur in families.

Jim and Megan Maguire were in their 30s. They had been married 4 years before they decided to begin their family. Both had consuming professional careers, Megan as a teacher and Jim as sales manager in a large computer networking company. They had many friends and an active social life. Both realized that a baby would limit their current lifestyle but they finally felt ready. Before the birth of the baby, both had decided that Megan would stay home for at least a year to care for the baby since Jim's career was going so well.

Megan had a difficult labor, which ended in delivering Marie, who weighed 5 pounds and 13 ounces, by Caesarian section. At first everything went well as Jim realized that Megan needed additional help and support postpartum. Megan's parents, sister, and brother lived close by and they too provided a lot of help and support to the family.

After the postpartum period, Megan and Jim began to argue about their respective roles in the family. Jim seemed to expect that Megan would take total control of Marie as well as the housework. Megan felt that Jim still should do his share as she now had a 24-hour-a-day job caring for Marie.

Box 15–3 will help you to think through interventions for the Maguires.

Box 15-3   Student Learning Activity

Role Expectations

What issue are the Maguires dealing with now that their family has expanded?

How would you as the nursing student making a follow-up 3-month home visit help them to resolve this conflict? What resources might assist them?

Value System

A family's value system is the conscious and unconscious ideas, attitudes, and beliefs by which a family is joined together in a common culture. Values influence the way roles are allocated and the way members perform their roles. For example, if families value closeness, they eat together and plan outings and vacations together.

Family values also determine how families view health and illness. In families that value primary prevention, parents are likely to attend to children's immunizations, provide dental and physical checkups, and provide adequate nutrition. All families value health for their members. Some families that you meet in the community may not demonstrate this value because of lack of knowledge or resources regarding preventive health behaviors. It then becomes your responsibility to provide educational information and sources of needed resources for the family. Box 15–4 will help you develop these ideas further.

Box 15-4   Student Learning Activity

Valuing Primary Prevention

List two resources in your community that provide food to low-income families.

List two resources in your community that provide low-income children with free dental care.

Communication Patterns

Effective communication within a family is critical if it is to achieve its purpose as the primary socializing agent. Clear communication exists when family members work to accurately reflect their feelings. Communication involves sending and receiving messages, expressing feelings, expressing power, and resolving conflicts.

> For example, families from Caribbean countries communicate their likes and dislikes for others' behavior directly. Within the culture and family this type of communication is understood, but in North American society it may be viewed as rude or insensitive. Families whose members come from different cultural backgrounds are more common in today's society. This situation can complicate communication within the family itself, as well as influence the way individual members communicate with others. There may be a blending of cultural communication styles with a resulting pattern that is unique. Nurses must be sensitive to a family's cultural orientation to avoid potential misinterpretation of communication patterns, but must also avoid assuming that communication will be determined solely by culture. (Redmond, 1992, p. 195)

Value systems, socioeconomic situations, and ethnicity significantly affect communication. It is important not to stereotype the communication of various cultures. For example, I grew up in an Irish-American family. A stereotype of the Irish might lead one to believe that Irish-American communication was predominantly negative in relation to building children's sense of self. This type of family communication is designed in this culture to keep children humble and to prevent them from having an exalted opinion of themselves. My family experience was totally different. I received extensive positive communication regarding my personal abilities. I was led to believe that I could do anything I wanted to do, and family support for personal growth was high.

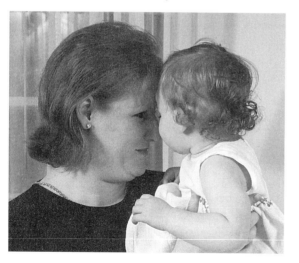

Power Structure

Power is one dimension of the family system. The family power structure is the ability of one family member to influence the behavior of another.

Power influences decision making in families. For example, if the mother is the most influential member of the family, the children's career choices may be shaped by her expectations. In assessing a family, it is important for you to determine with whom the power resides concerning particular issues, because this has implications for the health decisions that the family makes. For example, among Hispanic families, men generally are the decision makers. Therefore, a male family member would probably make choices regarding types of health-care providers and health-care facilities. As with communication, it is important for you to consider that culture is not the sole determinant of family power structure. Exposure to other cultures and other values concerning relationships may alter traditional power relationships in families. Moreover, power in families may be issue related, rather than universal. For example, one family member may have the strongest decision-making power regarding finances, whereas another is influential regarding health-care decisions. Box 15–5 allows you to expand your thinking on family structure.

Box 15-5   Student Learning Activity

Family Structure

As you assess the families with whom you work in the community, give some examples of structural elements that were particularly noteworthy.

How have you modified your interventions with the families based on your assessment of these particular structural elements?

Table 15-2

Family Functions

FUNCTION	DEFINITION	BEHAVIORAL EXAMPLE
Affective	Stabilizing adult personalities and meeting the psychological needs of the family.	Actively listening to a teenager's concerns.
Socialization and social placement	Preparing children for their expected roles in society and helping them to become productive societal members. Instilling family's value system.	Involving children in community projects that assist the poor or homeless.
Reproductive	Continuing family lines and providing future citizens.	Pregnancy and childbearing.
Economic	Providing financial resources to meet the family needs and allocating them wisely.	Budgeting for effective use of finances.
Health Care	Providing health care and physical necessities such as food and housing.	Providing nutritional meals for the family.

Redmond, G. (1992). Family health. In K. Berger & M. B. Williams (Eds.), Fundamentals of nursing (pp. 190–207). East Norwalk, CT: Appleton & Lange.

Family Function

Family function refers to what the family does, for example, how the family protects its members from stresses of modern day life. What the family does is based on structural elements, roles, values, communication patterns, and power (Friedman, 1998). Family functions are outcomes of the family structure or how the family organizes itself. You might ask yourself, "For what purpose does the family exist?" Family may be said to have five functions, which serve various purposes for the family members, the family unit, and the society. Table 15–2 depicts these functions.

Affective Function

The affective function is focused on meeting the needs of family members for affection and understanding. It is central both to the establishment of the family through the marital union as well as for the continuation of the family unit (Friedman, 1998). The family must meet the need for affection of its members to maintain family integrity. The socioemotional needs include building self-esteem and morale, as well as creating a loving environment in which members are nurtured and feel secure. The affective function is often influenced by the family's economic conditions. For example, more affluent families have the luxury of placing greater emphasis on companionship and love, whereas poorer families must place greater emphasis on working to acquire the physical necessities of life. It is important that societal support allows all families this opportunity by providing excellent, nurturing schools and child-care facilities because of the increasingly common need for both parents to work to meet the family's economic function.

Socialization and Social Placement Function

The socialization and social placement function of the family is the process by which the child learns attitudes, behavioral skills, and the interpretation of social norms from significant others. Social placement refers to the conferring of status, that is, the socialization of the child into the family social class and the instillation of relevant aspirations and values (Friedman, 1998). The family provides learning experiences for its members so that they can function effectively both within the family and in the larger society. In the family, children learn language, roles, and understanding of right and wrong. The individual's sexual role patterning and development of initiative and creativity are also part of the socialization process (Friedman, 1998). In today's society, the socialization function is shared more and more.

Reproductive Function

The reproductive function is the process by which the family perpetuates itself (Friedman, 1998). Reproduction is a basic function of the family, although it is no longer limited to nuclear families in our society. There are many single-parent families in our society and many pregnancies outside of marriage, especially among teenagers. Couples whose reproductive ability is complicated by physical and social barriers may seek solutions to accomplish this function through other means such as adoption, artificial insemination, in vitro fertilization, and the use of surrogate parents. Teaching about safe, effective contraception including natural, chemical, and mechanical means to assist couples to determine the time of family expansion is one way nurses may facilitate this function as a basic responsibility. It is becoming more common for couples to delay or permanently defer reproduction.

The following student story illustrates the importance of maintaining a nonjudgmental attitude as you work with family members on issues related to their reproductive function.

I was introduced to the walk-in clinic by the public health nurse on duty. She stated that today would be "pretty routine." The clinic was responsible for administering immunizations, pregnancy tests, doing purified protein derivative (PPD) checks, and caring for ill babies. The afternoon seemed like "the usual." People of all ages came in for immunizations for school health requirements and for foreign travel. All the pregnancy tests were for teenagers. These girls seemed to be uninformed, practicing regular unprotected sex, influenced by the needs of their partners, or overcome by a sense of invincibility. I was unable to grasp where their minds were wandering, why protection was so difficult to remember, why taking care of themselves seemed too tedious, and why having children was their lifelong answer to happiness. I found that I was applying my

standards of living; that I had to take a step back and understand the life they were struggling with. Perhaps our backgrounds were diverse or our education was varied. Perhaps our parents had alternative ways of caring and relationships simply meant providing food on the table. Differences set aside, there was one aspect I knew we had in common . . . the need for love, especially for self-love. Probably one of the most difficult lessons to learn.

The clinic seemed less busy than I had thought. I imagined long lines, more nurses, and a diverse clientele. As the afternoon came to an end, the last client walked in. The client was a Caucasian teenage girl of 18. She was accompanied by her mother. Ms. K. requested an HIV test for her daughter. The nurse had hoped to locate a file but to no avail. She was a new client. As the nurse asked Ms. K. whether I could remain in the room for the appointment, my mind flashed with questions. I wondered why she was here. Had she had unprotected sex with someone who had HIV? Had she shared needles? Had she tried to gain some self-worth by hoping to win over the awe of some foolish boy? Had she given in to her feeling of invincibility to engage in risky behavior? What exactly was it that she did to bring her here today, worried enough to be tested?

As all of us were about to enter the room, the nurse asked Ms. K. whether she wanted her mother to join us. Ms. K. was informed that it was solely her decision. Her mother's presence was not a requirement. Ms. K. stood silent for a moment, then she motioned for her mother to come in. We closed the door and proceeded with the exchange of information. Questions were swapped. Answers were given. It soon became obvious that Ms. K. was familiar with HIV. She had done some reading on her own. As the interview unfolded, her history was slowly pieced together. She was here for an HIV test because her rapist's HIV status was unknown. One had already been administered to him in prison but remained confidential to his victims. The rapist was her step-grandfather. He molested her at age 9. She was one of 17 victims for which he was now imprisoned. As the mother revealed her daughter's story, my mind raced with shock. I had been unfair in my thoughts and allowed unnecessary questions to clutter my judgment. Nonetheless, I was still unable to fully comprehend their experience, their anger, their pain, or the trauma it had caused throughout the years. However, I did understand that this client, like all clients, deserved respect, support, and the best possible care. Her path to healing would be a long and arduous one, self-love being a most crucial step.

Economic Function

The economic function refers to the provision and allocation of sufficient material resources to meet the family's needs for food, clothing, shelter, and health care (Friedman, 1998). Nurses are often involved in helping families to find resources for healthful living when they are poor or unemployed, such as by assisting families to apply for food stamps or make contact with community resources for other types of financial assistance. The following story illustrates one student's attempt to assist an international family deal with a problem with their finances.

Although I have lived within Northern Virginia all my life, I never realized what or who makes up the community around me. At the beginning of this clinical I had no set expectations, but quickly came to learn that this was a whole new realm of nursing. I was unclear as to how I felt about my role. What could I do?

Patients were assigned to me including a 36-year-old Hispanic female who has six other children in El Salvador and one newborn in the States. M.A. has never raised any of her children alone. Her mother would always do most of the job. M.A. speaks no English and is illiterate in both languages. Also, she is somewhat intellectually delayed. The health department has helped her throughout her pregnancy and now she needs to be educated about the infant.

As the semester comes to an end she is very accepting of my advice and teachings. M.A. follows my directions but fails to complete all instructions. Tasks must be given one or two at a time. Throughout my visits, M.A. keeps all appointments, including WIC and doctor visits, for the baby and herself. She keeps all important papers and bills in a plastic bag and asks for help whenever she has a question.

On Tuesday, November 3, M.A. handed me a bag I had never seen before and asked if Medicaid would cover these. To my surprise, there were almost 50 bills and late notices within this bag. Shocked by the amount and the time that had passed before I learned of these, I slowly began to read through each letter. The majority were from the hospital and pediatric center. Many were dated as far back as August. The bills covered all medical procedures and hospital stays from April 1998. The hospital bills were all past due and now being paid by a medical credit company including interest.

The hospital and all affiliated companies are aware that M.A. does not understand English, yet all her bills are written in English. None had Spanish translation. Although frustrated with the situation, I helped M.A. sort her bills and find Medicaid cards for both herself and the baby.

One phone call giving the hospital billing company M.A.'s Medicaid number took care of the bills. I cannot understand why a facility that is dedicated to caring for individuals could not foresee this situation. I was very glad to be an advocate for M.A. and take at least one burden away from many others.

Completing Box 15–6 will assist you to identify financial resources in your community.

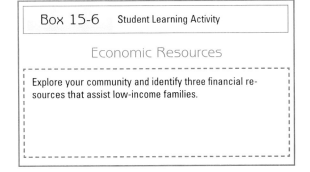

Box 15-6	Student Learning Activity

Economic Resources

Explore your community and identify three financial resources that assist low-income families.

Health-care Function

The health-care function refers to the ways the family protects the health of its members. The health care of the family is significantly related to family structure and function. For example, the health beliefs and values are related to the family's level of knowledge about health and illness and what is considered normal or usual within the socioeconomic or cultural group. In low-income groups, many people do not consider themselves ill unless they can no longer work. In high-income groups, people are more aware of symptoms as indicators of illness.

Family deterioration is often related to poor health of family members. When a family member becomes ill, nurses may be able to help other family members clarify their values and roles or work with them on improving their communication skills and power balances to prevent deterioration of family functioning. The following story describes how one student sought to assist an international family in protecting the health of one of its members.

I have found home visits to be eye-opening and rewarding. My experiences have really taught me how important our social and physical environment is to our health.

Our client, Sharon (I have changed her name), her husband, and daughters immigrated from Africa. They came for a better life and, although I do not understand the exact story, to leave political unrest and fear of violence behind. Like many immigrants, they have few material goods, but they have more resources for success than my other clients.

They both speak English, so language is not a barrier. The husband is college educated and works as a substitute teacher. Sharon has a part-time job in a restaurant. Their oldest daughter is in kindergarten and the youngest is 3. Sharon came to the health department because of an unplanned pregnancy. It is easy to like Sharon because of her lovely smile and gentle personality.

On my first home visit the primary concern was for her nutrition, because the clinic assessment revealed that she was not gaining weight. Sharon looked tired and uncomfortable, but was attentive to my advice to eat small meals and information on how to improve her diet. As the visit progressed, I learned that housing was her primary concern. Sharon and her family were staying in an apartment with acquaintances, but the situation was far from ideal. They had very little money and needed to move as soon as possible. That day I modified my plans about nutrition to include information on how to find affordable housing in Fairfax County.

I researched county housing resources, talked to housing counselors at Northern Virginia Family, and called United Way for referrals to other organizations that might help. I learned about Section 8 and the long waiting list.

On my next visit I gave this information to Sharon along with a recipe for rice pudding in the hope of increasing the foods with calcium using WIC allowances. Sharon said she liked the pudding, but couldn't fix it. It was on this visit that I finally came to understand that she had very little access to the kitchen! Her slow weight gain resulted from the stress of her living environment and lack of access to a kitchen!

As a student, I felt that the only thing I could really do was to encourage her and her husband in their search for an apartment. I called often to support their efforts and to let Sharon know that I cared about her and her situation.

Sharon and her family did find a home on their own. I don't really know if my information and caring made a difference, but I like to think that it did. I believe that with her own kitchen, her diet will improve along with the chances of having a healthy baby. But I like best what I saw in her face on my last home visit—hope!

FAMILY LIFE CYCLE AND DEVELOPMENTAL STAGES

Another approach to viewing the family unit is the developmental approach. This approach studies the family and its normal developmental crises from its establishment in marriage through the death of one or both spouses. The successive stages of growth and development that families go through as a unit are referred to as the *family life cycle* (Friedman, 1998). Knowledge of the family life cycle prepares nurses to be aware of the developmental crises a family may face. Although each family is unique, there are universal characteristics of each developmental period. Involved in each stage is both negotiating some change and the accomplishment of some developmental tasks to transition from one stage to the next.

Table 15–3 illustrates the six stages of the family life cycle and the associated tasks.

Danielson et al. (1993) note that stage six—added to the discussion of the family life cycle because people are living longer and having fewer children—is the least understood and, for most families, has the longest duration

Family events like divorce and subsequent remarriage of one or both spouses alters family development. Danielson et al. propose additional stages that these families must negotiate. Table 15–4 outlines the alterations to the family life cycle with the associated task that must be addressed.

Table 15–5 describes stages and tasks when parents remarry and form reconstituted or blended families.

FAMILY SYSTEMS THEORY

Family systems theory has gained broad acceptance in health care during the past decade. Of all the perspectives used in viewing families, it has the most relevance to understanding family stress and the impact of illness on the family (Danielson et al., 1993). As mentioned earlier, the family system is a holistic unit from which individual family behaviors flow. The family has great power in facilitating or repressing the growth of its members. Family interactions are complex, influenced by both family

Table 15-3

Six Stages of the Family Life Cycle

STAGE	MAJOR TASK
1. Unattached young adult who is between families	1. Parent and young adult successfully separating from one another
2. New marriage	2. Committing to a new family system
3. Family with young children	3. Accepting new members into the system
4. Family with adolescents	4. Remolding the boundaries of the family to allow the children independence
5. Launching the children and moving on	5. Accepting many exits and entrances into the family
6. Later Life	6. Accepting shifting generation roles and death

Danielson, C., Hamel-Bissell, B., & Winstead-Fry, P. (1993). Families, health and illness: Perspectives on coping and intervention. St. Louis: Mosby, p. 6. (Based on the work of Carter, E. A., & McGoldrich, M. (Eds.). (1980). The family life cycle: A framework for family therapy. New York: Gardner Press.)

Table 15-4

Stages of the Family Life Cycle during Divorce

STAGE	MAJOR TASK
1. The decision to divorce	Accepting the mobility to resolve marital discord
2. Planning the breakup in the system	Creating viable arrangements for all members of the system
3. Separation	Resolve attachment to spouse; develop cooperative coparenting relationship
4. Divorce	Resolve emotional divorce

members and the larger society. The following story illustrates the systems perspective.

Jean and Bob Gold have been married for 7 years. They have two children, Barbara, 2, and John, 4. They all have relationships with each other.

In addition to the relationship they have with each other, each one has a relationship with the outside world. Bob plays golf and is an associate in a law firm; Jean attends exercise classes and works as a case manager for children with disabilities 20 hours a week. The children are in play groups, day care, tumbling, and swimming. They have just bought their first house and are preparing to move, which places increased stress on both parents. At the same time Bob is preparing for a trial and is away a great deal, including weekends. Jean is experiencing abdominal pain to the point of being unable to care for her children. She is undergoing a series of tests to identify the source of her pain. The whole family feels tension until the stressful situations are resolved and a state of balance is restored.

Table 15-5

Stages of the Family Life Cycle for the Reconstituted Family

STAGE	MAJOR TASK
1. Entering a new relationship	Recovery from the loss of the first marriage
2. Planning a new marriage	Accepting peers of all system members; accepting complexities with patience
3. Remarriage and reconstitution of family	Final resolution of attachment to former spouse; acceptance of a different type of family with permeable boundaries

Danielson, C.B., Hamel-Bissell, B., & Winstead-Fry, P. (1993). Families, health and illness: Perspectives on coping and intervention. St. Louis: Mosby, p. 7. Used with permission.

Each of the three perspectives for understanding families—structural-functional, developmental, and systems—provide essential information as you assess the families with whom you work in the community.

Family Crisis

A crisis occurs when a family encounters problems and obstacles that cannot be resolved through their usual coping behaviors. Usually a period of disorganization follows as the family makes abortive attempts at solving the problem or overcoming the obstacle. Crisis always involves change and loss. Crisis is different from transition in that "transition refers to passage or movement from one state or place to another that occurs over time, involving changes that can be managed." (Murray & Zentner 1997, p. 243).

Family Crisis Intervention

The goal of crisis intervention is to restore the family to its precrisis state or to raise it to a higher level of coping. Nurses need to be sensitive to family members' needs for reassurance about their ability to manage crisis. At the same time, nurses may need to provide concrete assistance to help families meet their everyday needs for food, transportation, and child care. Crisis disorganizes families and depletes members of the energy needed to resolve the problem. Energy is lost through high anxiety levels caused by feelings of lack of control and abortive

attempts to resolve the crisis. Blaming should be discouraged; it is frequently a way of avoiding the truth and decreases the likelihood of a healthy adaptation.

Types of Family Crises

There are two types of family crises: situational (or accidental) and maturational (or developmental). Situational crisis occurs suddenly in response to an external event or conflict involving a specific event (for example, destruction of the family home in a disaster, birth of a handicapped child, or divorce). Maturational crisis relates to the change involved in the developmental stages and the accomplishment of developmental tasks discussed in the previous section. This type of crisis occurs when the family is unable to complete the developmental task of one stage, creating a deficit that interferes with completing the tasks of the next stage. For example, a family in which a teenager is chronically mentally ill may be unable to assist the teenager to balance freedom and responsibility, later preventing "launching" from occurring smoothly. Family crisis can be understood by looking at the crisis-producing situation, the family's perception of the situation, the family resources that can be used to deal with the situation, and the degree of disorganization the family is experiencing (Redmond, 1992). Some families are destroyed by crisis and persistent stress, whereas others emerge stronger and more resilient than ever.

The following story illustrates a family experiencing a situational crisis. Divorce is a stressful event that can easily become a crisis if the individuals do not have adequate coping behaviors or situation support. (Edelman & Mandle, 1994).

> Barbara, 33, and Frank, 35, have been married 11 years. They met and married in college during Barbara's freshman year. Both left college, and Frank got a job because Barbara became pregnant shortly after their marriage. They had three children, Scott, 12, Laura, 10, and Carl, 8. Frank eventually returned to school earning a baccalaureate and masters degree while continuing to work. Barbara made few trips outside the home except to accomplish things like shopping and activities related to the children. She had no friends except casual acquaintances among her neighbors. The children all did well in school and were involved in activities after school and in sports in the local community. Frank was absorbed in his work and school. Later, after he was employed by a large computer company in a responsible management position, he frequently went to work-related social events but discouraged Barbara from coming with him because, as he said "she had little in common with his friends or their wives." One evening after the children were in bed Frank announced that he wanted a divorce. He left the house that night.
>
> Barbara went to one of her elderly neighbor's homes the next morning. She was distraught and feeling overwhelmed. She was questioning over and over again, asking, "What did I do wrong? Why did this happen to me? What am I going to do? How will I manage?" She expressed extreme feelings of loss and inadequacy for not preserving her marriage.
>
> Barbara's neighbor attends Blessed Sacrament Church and she invited her to attend Mass with her at noon that day. Barbara's neighbor introduces her to the Parish Minister who interviews Barbara. It is later decided that a nursing student will work with Barbara and her children in that setting twice a week.

Table 15–6 illustrates an example of crisis intervention that can be used with Barbara.

Table 15-6

Steps in Crisis Intervention

FAMILY OBJECTIVE	NURSING INTERVENTION
1. Confront crisis in manageable increments and identify facts to clarify the crisis event.	• Allow Barbara to ventilate feelings about her husband and pending divorce.
	• Encourage Barbara to allow children to ventilate their feelings individually and as a group.
	• Consistently reflect your belief in their ability to manage.
	• Help them to identify strengths.
2. Find and accept help.	• Refer to local mental health center for couple, children, and family intervention.
	• Refer to attorney through Legal Aid or other community resource.
	• Assist in identifying employment resources like want ads and State Employment Agencies.
	• Assist Barbara to find local support groups for separated and divorced persons.
	• Encourage her to accept help from neighbors and expand her network of friends.
	• Encourage low-/no-cost family outings.

Crisis resolution occurs when a family perceives the stressful event realistically and, by means of appropriate support services and adequate coping mechanism, solves its problems. However, crisis resolution is a complex phenomenon; resolution of long-standing individual and personal problems that sometimes contribute to crisis may require extended psychotherapy.

FAMILY RESILIENCE

Another relatively new construct related to crisis is family resilience. Family resilience refers to how families withstand and rebound from crisis and adversity (Walsh, 1996). Family processes like cohesion, flexibility, open communication, problem solving, and an affirming belief system help the family manage crisis, buffer stress, and move on. A family resilience lens helps you to view the families in crisis in the community as capable of repair. The following student story is illustrative of family resilience. Though this family experienced repeated crises and adversity, their ability to trust illustrates the concept of resilience.

I had spent a rather routine morning in the multiservices clinic at Springfield Health Department. We had done school immunizations, PPDs, and follow-ups on tuberculosis (TB) clients on isoniazid (INH) therapy. As I was standing in an examination room with a patient, a bright little face peeked around the corner and waved excitedly at me. What a wonderful surprise! The little girl was one of the children from the Headstart class I had worked with during my junior clinical. I waved back, suppressing a whoop of glee and whispered that I would come out to see her in a few minutes. After we finished with the immunizations, I walked out to the waiting room to say hello. I bent down to greet her, held open my arms and was instantly knocked back as 40 pounds of preschool joy hurtled into my waiting arms. It was so good to see her! I carefully unclasped the fingers clenched around my neck and pulled her back gently to look at her. How she had grown! I felt tears well up in my eyes and I realized again how much I had learned from the children and how much I missed them. As we chatted, I felt someone's eyes on me and glanced up to see a middle-aged woman with intensely blue eyes watching me. She, too, had tears in her eyes and seemed incredibly moved by the sight of us. I was somewhat puzzled but was pulled back by an incessant tug on my lab coat and an incredible torrent of words. After spending a few minutes with the child, I hugged her again and stood up to re-

turn to the examining room. After a few minutes, the nurse called out, "Number eight?" The middle-aged woman stood up and followed us back to the room. "Immunization?" the nurse asked the woman as we walked back. "Yes" she responded in a thick foreign accent. I was struck by her quiet dignity and her intense blue eyes. As she sat down, the nurse asked which arm she would like to have her shots in. "Is this one OK?" he asked, patting her left arm. She smiled, misunderstanding his question somewhat, and answered that it was almost completely healed. The nurse inquired if it had been injured and she nodded and replied that it had been broken but was doing better. He asked her how she had broken her arm. She hesitated briefly, looking from him to me and then said in halting English, "I am Albanian. You cannot understand how terrible things are in my country. You can trust no one, not even your neighbors. Neighbors kill neighbors and, if they find out you are trying to leave, they soap you when you flee.

"Soap," she repeated and looked around as though trying to come up with a way to explain it. "Soap—like you use for your hands," she explained as she made a washing motion with her own. "Oh, soap!" the nurse and I exclaimed in unison. I volunteered, "We know what soap is, but I'm afraid we don't understand what you mean." She explained, "If they find out you are leaving the country, they soap your stairs. They put soap on them to make you fall," she explained as she made a scrubbing motion with one hand. "The morning that I left, the taxi was waiting in front of my house to take me to the airport. I only had 12 stairs to go from my house to the car. They soaped the last two stairs. As I ran down the stairs, I slipped on the soap and fell. I got up quickly and I rushed to the car. I was so afraid. The taxi took me to the airport to Tirane. I flew from the airport in Tirane to Zurich and then to the United States. I did not notice that my arm was broken until I reached Zurich. I had been so afraid, I hadn't felt the pain. I could not trust the doctors in Zurich even. Not like I can trust you." She smiled at each of us and continued, "I didn't get help for my arm until I reached the United States." Both the nurse and I had been shocked by the story she told us. She continued with tears in her eyes, "Coming from my country to the United States was like coming from Hell to Paradise. You do not know how wonderful it is here." I swallowed a huge lump in my throat and choked back the tears. The nurse said, "Well, now you are here and you are safe. I just have to get a few things and I'll be back to give you your shots." After he left the room, the woman turned to me and whispered, "Every morning when I wake up I am full of terror and I think they are coming to kill me. Then I realize that I am in the United States and I am safe." As she described this feeling on awakening, I realized that

she most certainly must be suffering from posttraumatic stress syndrome as a result of living through a war and watching so much horror. "That must be very frightening for you," I responded. "Yes," she replied, "you cannot imagine the things I have seen." "No, you're right . . . I cannot. I have been very fortunate to live here all of my life," I replied, realizing as I said it how incredibly true it was. "The dreams that you have and the terror that you feel are not unusual for someone who has gone through what you've been through. But you made it here and now you are safe and, gradually, the dreams will go away and you will feel safe. And if you need to talk to someone about those dreams, we can give you the number of someone who can help you." She sobbed softly and looked at me. "In my country, even the doctors cannot be trusted. They may betray you or turn you in. But I can trust you—you will not hurt me." It came to me as she spoke that perhaps her emotion on watching me hug the little child from Headstart somehow had to do with this very issue. Tears welled up in my own eyes yet again and I smiled, "Yes. You can trust me. You can trust us." She sighed and said, "Thank you." After the nurse came back and gave her the needed immunizations, I walked her back to the waiting area. She took my hand in hers and said, "Goodbye. Thank you." I said goodbye and realized that my life had been forever changed. I realized that the trust the Albanian refugee had placed in me was a very precious gift. I vowed to myself that I would uphold her trust and the trust of the countless patients that would follow during my upcoming career. I vowed that each time I cared for a patient, I would be thankful for the trust they placed in me. I vowed that each time I cared for a patient, I would endeavor to earn that trust, to cherish it, to nurture it—to value the precious gift I had been given and guard it wisely.

FAMILY HEALTH PROMOTION

According to Petze (1991), "families are a primary target for health promotion in community health nursing" (p 355). Definitions of health promotion vary, and most address the individual. For example, O'Donnell (1987) defines health promotion as "the science and art of helping people change their lifestyle to move toward a state of optimum health" (p. 5). Therefore, building on their definitions, family health promotion involves assessing the family's current health status, risks, and health goals while at the same time helping them to make decisions about needed lifestyle changes.

Gordon (1993) developed an assessment of functional health patterns that will help you identify cur-

rent health status, risk factors, and lifestyle for your families. These functional health patterns include assessment of health-perception–health-management patterns, nutritional-metabolic patterns, elimination patterns, activity-exercise patterns, sleep-rest patterns, cognitive-perceptual patterns, self-perception–self-concept patterns, role-relationship patterns, sexuality-reproductive patterns, coping/stress tolerance patterns, and value-belief patterns. (See Appendix A for Functional Health Patterns Assessment Guidelines for Family.)

Problems in functional health patterns are seen as dysfunctional problems and not disease, for instance, speech and vision problems. Potential dysfunctions are predicted on the basis of risk factors, for example, smoking with heart disease. According to Edelman and Mandle (1994) family-related risks can be inferred from such factors as lifestyle, biological dimensions, environmental attributes and sociopsychologic factors. The objective of doing a family risk analysis is to provide the family with knowledge about realistic health threats before they have signs and symptoms.

As you work with families in the community, you will be involved in many health-promotion activities such as vital signs measurement, hearing testing, and teaching self-care for minor illnesses like abrasions and colds. Other categories of health-promotion activities include assisting with environmental changes like safety-proofing a home for a toddler and helping families to manage diabetes through diet and exercise teaching. According to Edelman and Mandle, health promotion involves more than education; it must involve the family changing its behavior. As you work with families, it is important to gear interventions toward helping them to accept responsibility for their own health and for the health and safety of the whole family.

You are also a vital link to appropriate community resources for your families. Not only do they need to know about available resources but they also need to learn to use them appropriately. Frequently, families need specific help and support to use complex community systems. At first you may need to accompany them to access the services that they need. At times, you must advocate for needed services, because families may not understand their entitlements. When I was a graduate student at a large metropolitan university, I worked in an outpatient facility in a low-income community. One of the families on my caseload was a Puerto Rican immigrant family with eight children. The

Table 15-7

Nurses' Role in Family Health Promotion

- Collaboratively assess health status and goals with the family.

- Review family lifestyle and with the family identify strengths and unhealthy patterns needing change.

- Act as a family advocate and assist family to negotiate complex community systems and ensure that the family gets needed services available.

- Help family to identify needed community resources appropriately.

- Health education role—teach appropriate information to make lifestyle changes, e.g., nutrition, exercise, positive parenting behaviors.

- Assist families to plan for lifestyle modification.

- Researcher role—read and critically analyze research and incorporate into practice.

- Care manager role—coordinate and prevent duplication of services.

- Work for social and policy change to promote family health

family was labeled "noncompliant" because family members had not followed through on securing diagnostic testing for the youngest, 5-year-old Maria. After a lengthy family assessment and a period of trust and rapport building, I found out that diagnostic tests were to be completed 10 city blocks across town from where the family lived. Mrs. R. had made several abortive attempts at keeping her appointments. However, Maria constantly vomited on the bus because of the noise, people, and closeness of the situation.

Once I was able to secure money for a taxi and accompany the family, we at least got there. I was then able to go through the admission procedures with Mrs. R. and explain the logistics of the large city hospital, the clinic, and their procedures. We drew a map, with landmarks she would recognize, when bringing Maria alone. After several visits the testing was completed.

As you provide the necessary education for your families it is important that you incorporate the needed

lifestyle change into the mutually developed implementation plan. For example, if a family member's goal is weight reduction, but he or she has a sedentary lifestyle, exercise must be incorporated into activities of daily living. Initially, this might be done by taking the stairs instead of the elevator and parking the car at a distance from the workplace and the mall.

You also may be involved in care coordination of the family's health-promotion activities. This ensures that needs are met but services are not duplicated.

Looking for research opportunities as you work with your families, perhaps comparing the outcomes of two different health education approaches, is part of your role as well. Minimally, you must continue to read and analyze family health-promotion research and incorporate it into your interventions. Many of the changes that are needed for optimum family health come from political and social change. Part of your role in family health promotion is to be involved politically at the grassroots level, working for that change.

Table 15–7 summarizes the nursing role in family health promotion. Box 15–7 will help expand your understanding and skill in facilitating health promotion.

Box 15-7   Student Learning Activity

Health-Promotion Application

- Give a brief description of a family with whom you are working in the community and their health- promotion needs.

- List three family health-promotion activities that will meet these needs and help them change unhealthy behavior.

- What lifestyle changes must be made to maintain changed behavior?

FAMILY ASSESSMENT

Family assessment in nursing is the collection and analysis of data relative to family health. Family assessment is concerned with family structure, function, and environment, particularly as these factors influence the health of individual members and the family as a whole. In community-based settings where nurses care for clients, family assessment is one of the most important functions that nurses carry out because of the relationship of the individual to the family's health. An understanding of how family assessment is performed is therefore important knowledge for the nurse to have. Two family assessment tools are included in Appendix A and B.

Purpose of Family Assessment

Nurses carry out family assessment for several important reasons. These include: (1) promoting awareness of family health practices; (2) raising the family's consciousness regarding its structure and functioning and their impact on health of the family; (3) providing an opportunity to collaborate with the family by listening to its concerns about health; (4) identifying the families' needs for referral to other resources; (5) individualizing care to be given by the health-care professions in community-based settings; and (6) promoting a sense of family responsibility for improving health.

CHARACTERISTICS OF HEALTHY FAMILIES

In assessing families, nurses must identify the healthy aspects of each family and capitalize on these family strengths when planning care. Family theory literature concurs on the following five characteristics of healthy families (Friedman, 1998; Danielson et al., 1993):

- Mutual respect and support. Mutual respect and support is the basis for healthy family dynamics. All characteristics of healthy families depend on mutual respect. Respect implies valuing other family members for who they are and recognizing the unique contribution that each family member provides to the integrity of the family as a whole. An atmosphere of acceptance prevails. When there is mutual respect, support flows naturally. To families that respect each other, relying on one another for

assistance or encouragement demonstrates a healthy mutual dependency.

- Open communication. Open communication in a family is the ability and willingness to honestly discuss all issues of concern to the family. Open communication can involve routine family decisions or matters of greater significance; for example, a child talking about school problems, a teenager sharing thoughts about experimenting with drugs, or a couple speaking with one another about sexual concerns. Open communication involves self-disclosure, sharing aspects of self that may be personal or private. This kind of openness involves risk of rejection or punishment. Therefore, it requires self-confidence and trust in other family members. Not all families that function well operate under conditions of complete openness, but it is generally agreed that the fewer the areas of closed communication, the healthier the family.

- Shared problem solving. Shared problem solving implies that family decisions are made with input from all appropriate family members. Mutual trust and open communication make shared problem solving more effective. Families may address day-to-day problems, such as allocation of responsibility for household chores, or more serious problems that threaten family structure or functioning, such as serious illness of a family member.

- Flexibility. Flexibility implies willingness among family members to adjust family process or roles to accommodate changes in the needs of individual members. For example, children may agree to switch household chores with each other so one of them can attend team practices that conflict with chores.

- Enhancement of personal growth. Healthy families recognize the need of individual members to develop their full potential. This may require temporary or long-term adjustments in family process to accommodate the needs of a particular member. For example, the husband/father may desire a career change that requires returning to school, which in turn may create a financial burden that necessitates family lifestyle changes such as omitting a family vacation or limiting the number of family outings; or one parent may take on an extra part-time job to help with a child's college expenses. Enhancement of personal growth of individual family members also incorporates maintaining a balance between shared activities and separate activities. Each member is recognized as an individual, as well as a family member (Redmond, 1992).

Nurses in community-based practice may encounter families through health screening activities or when a family member is ill. Nurses can help families recognize their family strengths to cope with ongoing decisions or a family member's health problem. The same approach is effective when collaborating with families facing maturational stressors, such as dealing with a teenager learning to balance freedom and responsibility with the family automobile.

Components of Family Assessment

To assess the family, nurses collect data related to three different categories: environment, family structure, and family function. The data collected helps nurses make appropriate nursing diagnoses with the family's input. Table 15–8 contains commonly used family nursing diagnoses.

CURRENT FAMILY RESEARCH

Vanderwater and Lunford (1998) investigated the relationship among family structure, parental conflict, and child well-being in 618 children from ages 10 to 17 and their parents. Structure defined as "married—never divorced" versus "divorced—not remarried" showed no influence on children's well-being. However, findings showed that parental conflict (high versus low) influenced children's well-being. Well-being was defined as internalizing and externalizing behavior and trouble with peers. In addition, analysis of the data by gender indicated that parental warmth toward the child mediated the

---

Table 15-8

Examples of Family Nursing Diagnoses

NURSING DIAGNOSIS	EXPLANATION
Ineffective Family Coping: Compromised	A usually supportive family member provides insufficient, ineffective, or compromised support, comfort, or assistance to another family member experiencing a health challenge when support, comfort, or assistance is needed to master the challenge. For example, a client is facing a difficult decision about treatment alternatives at the same time that his partner, who usually supports him in a shared decision-making process, is experiencing an intense emotional response to the situation and is unable to participate in shared decision making.
Alteration in Family Processes	A family that has been functioning well experiences a stressor and has difficulty functioning. For example, a family experiences a death of one of its members and is temporarily unable to carry on the activities of daily living.
Impaired Home Maintenance Management	A family is unable to maintain a safe home environment because of illness in a family member, poor hygienic practices, an impaired caregiver, or lack of support from family and friends. For example, alcoholic parents are unable to maintain a physically safe environment for their children.
Alterations in Parenting	A real or potential inability of one or more adult members of the family to provide a positive environment that facilitates the growth and development of children. For example, an emotionally disturbed adult caregiver in a family is unable to meet the children's needs for affection.
Family Coping: Potential for Growth	Family member(s) has (have) effectively adapted to a health challenge of one family member and is (are) exhibiting desire and readiness for enhanced health and growth for self and affected family member. For example, the family of a handicapped child who exhibits readiness to use community and health resources to promote optimal social, emotional, and physical development of the child.

Redmond, G. (1992). Family health. In K. Berger & M. B. Williams (Eds.), Fundamentals of nursing (pp. 190–207). East Norwalk, CT: Appleton & Lange, p. 206.

relationship between conflict and well-being for girls. However, in boys, conflict and parental warmth impacted well-being independently. Based on the results of this research, health-promotion programs to assist parents to change unhealthy interactions should be developed to improve child well-being.

Another study (Rogers & White, 1998) developed a model of parenting satisfaction and tested it on a national panel of 1200 parents interviewed between 1988 and 1992. The model focused on the effects of three factors—marital satisfaction, family structure, and parents' gender—on parenting satisfaction. A cross-sectional analysis, panel analysis, and structural equation analysis were used. Findings indicated that parenting satisfaction depends mostly on the three factors studied. These factors have both independent and interactive effects on parental satisfaction. Parental satisfaction was insensitive to other variables like number and ages of children, social class, and parental employment patterns. Fathers reported low parental satisfaction and their evaluation was more related to their assessment of marital satisfaction than was that of the mothers. Parental satisfaction was also high in those parenting their biological children. There was a strong two-way relationship between marital and parental satisfaction for both mothers and fathers. It seems clear that education for parenting and family change during pregnancies strengthens both marital and parental satisfaction.

In another study related to families of mentally ill adults, Doornbos (1996) investigated the characteristics of families with a mentally ill relative. Families of the seriously and persistently mentally ill historically have been directly or indirectly blamed for the mental illness of their family member. As biological research into the cause of serious mental illness has progressed, it has become clear that serious mental illness is like multiple sclerosis or any other chronic illness. Dysfunctional coping patterns may result from the impact of the illness on the family, but dysfunctional coping does not cause the illness. This study sought to document the health and strength of families with a seriously mentally ill member.

Using two different scales to measure family stress and coping and four different instruments to operationalize family health in terms of subconcepts of adaptability, cohesion, satisfaction, and conflict, Doornbos studied 85 families with serious mental illness from community mental health agencies, public and private psychiatric hospitals, and support groups. These families were compared with a normative group of families on the same variables.

As expected, families of the mentally ill reported significantly more stressors than the normative sample. Also statistically significant was the fact that the families of the mentally ill relied more heavily on the coping strategies identified in the instrument than did the normative families. They used specific coping strategies such as passive appraisal, reframing, seeking social support, seeking spiritual support, and using community resources.

In relation to family health, they experienced statistically significant less cohesion, significantly greater adaptability, less conflict, and a lesser level of satisfaction with the functioning of their family unit than did the normative sample. The ability of families of the mentally ill to adapt and be flexible to various situational and developmental stressors and to manage conflict within their families are acknowledged as strengths and characteristics of healthy families. It appears that the impact of mental illness on the family does not affect the functional abilities of the family, but their affective evaluation of the family, that is, their feeling of being less bonded with the family and less satisfied with family functioning.

The results of this study provide validation of family strengths and health in coping with serious mental illness. Nurses in community-based practice should reinforce family coping strategies in working with families who have mentally ill members.

The self-perceived informational needs of caregivers were explored in a qualitative study conducted by Conley and Burman (1997), a purposive sample of 14 individuals who had been the primary caregivers for family members who had died within the preceding 12 months. Understanding the context of care as described by the informants in this study is important to understanding their informational needs. Every caregiver studied described the all-consuming nature of the caregiving process. Within the context of exhaustion and constant care, the caregivers had difficulty conceptualizing and articulating their informational needs.

However, two distinct categories of informational needs emerged from the data: (1) the need for information related to the patient's disease and course of the disease, and (2) information related to available supportive services through health-care and community agencies.

The researchers make the following recommendations for home-care nursing practice: (1) coordinate sources of support and care for the family to reduce caregiver stress, and (2) counsel caregivers about the usual course of their family member's disease, expected symptoms, treatments, expected side effects, and what to expect during the dying process.

Because half of the caregivers in their study preferred oral information, the researcher recommended both continuing to use printed information in addition to using verbal reinforcement to ensure comprehension of information.

This chapter has focused on information to assist you in meeting the needs of families in the community. Components of family assessment, that is, family definitions, forms, family structure and function, and family development, characteristics of healthy families, and family nursing diagnoses are included. Family crisis and health promotion are discussed as opportunities for nursing intervention in the community. Current family research is reviewed.

Active Learning Strategies

1. Write a story about a family with whom you are working in the community. What family needs have you identified collaboratively with the family? Have family dynamics affected its ability to meet its needs? In what way?

2. You are assigned to Mrs. Braden to make a follow-up postpartum visit after discharge from the hospital. You find out that her baby was stillborn. Mr. and Mrs. Braden have two other children, Barbara, 4, and Mary, 2. Develop a list of assessment questions to use on your first visit.

3. Explore services for the Braden family in your community and on the Internet. Visit one or two agencies helpful to families who have experienced a neonatal loss.

4. Set up an appointment ahead of your visit if possible to find out the specifics of eligibility, referral, and cost. Gather as much material and information as possible.

5. Contact local churches in your community. Explore outreach services that they provide to both parishioners and nonparishioners.

References

Bomar, P. J. (1989). Nurses and family health promotion concepts, assessment and intervention. Baltimore: Williams & Wilkins.

Conley, V. M., & Burman, M. E. (1997). Informational needs of caregivers of terminal patients in a rural state. Home Healthcare Nurse, 15(13), 808–817.

Danielson, C. B., Hamel-Bissell, B., & Winstead-Fry, P. (1993). Families, health and illness: Perspectives on coping and intervention. St. Louis: Mosby.

Doornbos, M. M. (1996). The strengths of families coping with serious mental illness. Archives of Psychiatric Nursing, 4, 214–220.

Edelman, C. L., & Mandle, C. L. (1994). Health promotion throughout the lifespan (3rd ed). St. Louis: Mosby.

Friedman, M. M. (1998). Family nursing: Theory and assessment (4th ed.). East Norwalk, CT: Appleton & Lange.

Gordon, M. (1993). Manual of nursing diagnosis: 1993-1994. St. Louis: Mosby.

Gordon, M. E. (1987). Nursing diagnosis: Process and application (2nd ed.). New York: McGraw-Hill.

Murray, R. B., & Zenter, J. P. (1997). Health assessment and promotion strategies through the lifespan (6th ed.). Stamford: CT: Appleton & Lange.

O'Donnell, M. (1987). Definition of health promotion. Journal of Health Promotion, 1(4), 5–9.

Petze, C. F. (1991). Health promotion for the well family, In B.W. Spradley (Ed.), Readings in community health nursing (pp. 355-364). Philadelphia: J. B. Lippincott Company.

Redmond, G. (1992). Family Health. In K. Berger & M. B. Williams (Eds.), Fundamentals of nursing (pp. 190–207). East Norwalk, CT: Appleton & Lange.

Rogers, S. J., & White, L. K. (1998). Satisfaction with parenting: The role of marital happiness, family structure, and parents' gender. Journal of Marriage and the Family, 60, 293–308.

Vanderwater, E. A., & Landsford, J. E. (1998). Influences of family structure and parental conflict on children's well-being. Family Relations, 47, 323–330.

Walsh, F. (1996). The concept of family resilience: crisis and challenge. Family Process, 35(3), 261–281.

Appendix A

Eleven Functional Health Patterns Assessment Guidelines for Family Assessment

The 11 functional health pattern areas are applicable to the assessment of families. Families are the primary clients in community-health nursing. In some cases, a family assessment may be indicated (1) in the care of an infant or child whose development is influenced by family health patterns or (2) when an adult has certain health problems that can be influenced by family patterns. The following guidelines provide information on family functioning:

1. Health-perception–health-management pattern

History:

a. How has family's general health been (in last few years)?

b. Colds in past year? Absence from work/school?

c. Most important things family does to keep healthy? Think these make a difference to health? (Include family folk remedies, if appropriate.)

d. Members' use of cigarettes, alcohol, drugs?

e. Immunizations? Health-care provider? Frequency of checkups? Accidents (home, work, school, driving)? (If appropriate: Storage of drugs, cleaning products, scatter rugs, etc.)

f. In past, ease of finding ways to follow suggestions of doctors, nurses, social workers (if appropriate)?

g. Things important in family's health that I could help with?

Examination:

a. General appearance of family members and home.

b. If appropriate: Storage of medicines, cribs, playpens, stove, scatter rugs, hazards, etc.

2. Nutritional-metabolic pattern

History:

a. Typical family meal pattern/food intake (describe)? Supplements (vitamins, types of snacks, etc.)?

b. Typical family fluid intake (describe)? Supplements: type available (fruit juices, soft drinks, coffee, etc.)?

c. Appetites?

d. Dental problems? Dental care (frequency)?

e. Skin problems? Healing problems?

Examination:

a. If opportunity available, examine: refrigerator contents, meal preparation, contents of meal, etc.

3. Elimination pattern

History:

a. Family use of laxatives, other aids?

b. Problems in waste/garbage disposal?

c. Pet, animals waste disposal (indoor/outdoor)?

d. If indicated: problems with flies, roaches, rodents?

Examination:

a. If opportunity available, examine: toilet facilities, garbage disposal, pet waste disposal; indicators of risk for flies, roaches, rodents.

4. Activity/exercise pattern

History:

a. In general, does family get a lot of/little exercise? Type? Regularity?

b. Family leisure activities? Active/passive?

c. Problems in shopping (transportation), cooking, keeping up the house, budgeting for food, clothes, housekeeping, house costs?

Examination:

a. Pattern of general home maintenance, personal maintenance.

5. Sleep-rest pattern

History:

a. Generally, family members seem to be well rested and ready for school/work?

b. Sufficient sleeping space and quiet?

c. Family finds time to relax?

Examination:

a. If opportunity available, observe: sleeping space, sleeping arrangements.

6. Cognitive-perceptual pattern

History:

a. Visual or hearing problems? How managed?

b. Any big decisions family has had to make? How made?

Examination:

a. If indicated: language spoken at home?

b. Grasp of ideas and questions (abstract/concrete)?

c. Vocabulary level?

7. Self-perception–self-concept pattern

History:

a. Most of time family feels good (not so good) about themselves as a family?

b. General mood of family? Happy? Anxious? Depressed? What helps family mood?

Examination:

a. General mood state: nervous (5) or relaxed (1)? (Rate from 1 to 5.)

b. Members generally assertive (5) or passive (1)? (Rate from 1 to 5.)

8. Role-relationship pattern

History:

a. Family (or household) members? Members ages and family structure (diagram)?

b. Any family problems that are difficult to handle (nuclear/extended)? Child rearing? If appropriate: spouse ever get rough with you? The children?

c. Relationships good (not so good) among family members? Siblings? Support each other?

d. If appropriate: income sufficient for needs?

e. Feel part of (or isolated from) community? Neighbors?

Examination:

a. Interaction among family members (if present).

b. Observed family leadership roles.

9. Sexuality-reproduction pattern

History:

a. If appropriate (sexual partner with household or situation): sexual relations satisfying? Changes? Problems?

b. Use of family planning? Contraceptives? Problems?

c. If appropriate (to age of children): feel comfortable in explaining/discussing sexual subjects?

Examination:

None

10. Coping-stress tolerance pattern

History:

a. Any big changes within family in last few years?

b. Family tense or relaxed most of time? When tense, what helps? Anyone use medicines, drugs, alcohol to decrease tension?

c. When (if) family problems, how handled?

d. Most of the time is this method of coping successful?

Examination:

None

11. Value-belief pattern

History:

a. Generally, family gets things they want out of life?

b. Important things for the future?

c. Any "rules" in the family that everyone believes are important?

d. Religion important in family? Does this help when difficulties arise?

Examination:

None

From Gordon, M. (1993). Manual of nursing diagnosis: 1993–1994. St. Louis: Mosby.

Appendix B

The Friedman Family Assessment Model (Short Form)

The following form is shortened for ease in assessing families. Two words of caution are called for before using the following guidelines in completing family assessments. First, not all areas included are germane for each of the families visited. The guidelines are comprehensive and allow depth when probing is necessary. The student should not feel that every subarea needs be covered when the broad area of inquiry poses no problems to the family or concern to the health worker. Second, by virtue of the interdependence of the family system, unavoidable redundancy exists. For the sake of efficiency, the assessor should try not to repeat data, but to refer the reader back to sections where this information has already been described.

Identifying Data

1. **Family name**
2. **Address and phone**
3. **Family composition**
4. **Type of family form**
5. **Cultural (ethnic) background**
6. **Religious identification**
7. **Social class status**
8. **Family's recreational or leisure-time activities**

Developmental Stage and History of Family

9. **Family's present developmental stage**
10. **Extent of developmental stage fulfillment**

11. **Nuclear family history**
12. **History of family of origin of both parents**

Environmental Data

13. **Home characteristics**
14. **Characteristics of neighborhood and larger community**
15. **Family's geographic mobility**
16. **Family's associations and transactions with community**
17. **Family's social support network**

Family Structure

18. **Communication Patterns**
    - Extent of functional and dysfunctional communication (types of recurring patterns)
    - Extent of affective messages and how expressed
    - Characteristics of communication within family subsystems
    - Types of dysfunctional communication processes
    - Areas of closed communication
    - Familial and external variables affecting communication

19. **Power Structure**
    - Power outcomes
    - Decision-making process
    - Power bases
    - Variables affecting power
    - Overall family power

20. Role Structure

- Formal role structure

- Informal role structure

- Analysis of role models (optional)

- Variables affecting role structure

21. Family Values

- Compare the family with American or family reference group values and/or identify important family values and their importance (priority) in the family.

- Congruence between family's values and values of family's subsystems as well as family's reference group and/or wider community

- Variables influencing family values

- Does the family consciously or unconsciously hold these values?

- Presence of value conflicts in family

- Effect of the preceding values and value conflicts on health status of family

Family Functions

22. Affective Function

- Family's need/response patterns

- Mutual nurturance, closeness, and identification

- Separateness and connectedness

23. Socialization Function

- Family child-rearing practices

- Adaptability of child-rearing practices for family form and family's situation

- Who is (are) socializing agent(s) for child(ren)?

- Value of children in family

- Cultural beliefs that influence family's child-rearing patterns

- Social class influence on child-rearing patterns

- Estimation of whether family is at risk for child-rearing problems and, if so, indication of high risk factors

- Adequacy of home environment for children's needs to play

24. Health-care Function

- Family's health beliefs, values, and behavior

- Family's definitions of health-illness and their level of knowledge

- Family's perceived health status and illness susceptibility

- Family's dietary practices

- Adequacy of family diet (recommend 24-hour food history record)

- Function of mealtimes and attitudes toward food and mealtimes

- Shopping (and its planning) practices

- Person(s) responsible for planning, shopping, and preparation of meals

- Sleeping and resting habits

- Exercise and recreation practices (not covered earlier)

- Family's drug habits

- Family's role in self-care practices

- Family's environmental practices

- Medically based preventive measures (physicals, eye and hearing tests, and immunizations)

- Dental health practices

- Family health history (both general and specific diseases—environmentally and genetically related)

- Health-care services received

- Feelings and perceptions regarding health services

- Emergency health-care services

- Dental health services

- Source of medical and dental payments

- Logistics of receiving care

Family Coping

25. **Short- and long-term familial stressors**

26. **Family's ability to respond, based on objective appraisal of stress-producing situations**

27. **Coping strategies used (present/past)**

   • Differences in family members' ways of coping

   • Family's inner coping strategies

   • Family's external coping strategies

28. **Areas/situations where family has achieved mastery**

29. **Dysfunctional adaptive strategies used (past and present)**

From Friedman, M. M. (1998) Family Nursing: Research, Theory & Practice. pp. 579–581. Reprinted with permission of Prentice Hall, Inc., Upper Saddle River, NJ.

CHAPTER 16

Working with Groups in the Community

Ann H. Cary

LEARNING OBJECTIVES

1) Describe the general concepts of group work essential to community-based nursing practice.

2) Differentiate the kinds of group work appropriate to the community-based nurse.

3) Articulate the leadership and coleadership dimensions for managing groups commonly experienced in community-based nursing practice.

4) Describe community-based nursing practices that facilitate group improvement of outcomes for the health of the individual and the family.

Nurses functioning in community-based practice have many opportunities to work with groups. The evolution of hospitals to health-care systems requires that health professionals be knowledgeable about patients and population needs that exist where people live, recreate, and work. Use of community resources to manage the acute or chronic conditions of people in their natural venue requires knowledge of group and organizational functions as well as knowledge of the needs of patients experiencing similar demands and diagnoses. For nurses working on interdisciplinary teams, group and team dynamics, functions, and interventions are critical competencies in community-based practice. Interdisciplinary practice groups are the mainstay of success to achieve coordination of care and integration of services (Erkel, Nivens, & Kennedy, 1995).

This chapter describes the general concepts of groups in the context of "client" or "provider" of health care. Discussion focuses on the nurse's roles in leading groups and advocating for group constituents as partners in health-care delivery. Finally, the chapter envelopes the tenets contained in the systems perspective of the human ecological model, which serves as the philosophy for community-based nursing. (Bronfenbrenner, 1979; Chamberlin, 1988). Both the nurse and the clients interact with multiple social networks during the provision of care in community settings.

You have had many experiences with groups. Your family is your first and most enduring example of a group. In primary and secondary education, groups are formed to organize the teaching and learning of knowledge, skills, and attitudes. Extracurricular activities revolve around the formation of groups, for example, team sports, bands, or clubs. You may be a member of a community group striving to fund civic projects, keep neighborhoods safe, or influence policymakers to be sensitive to your issues. Some of you may even participate in a health-related group designed to facilitate new knowledge of health behaviors, adhere to weight-control programs, change personal actions or attitudes, or provide personal awareness and growth. In fact, you have experienced a large part of your own growth and development personally and professionally through group experiences.

As a community-based nurse, you are responsible for forming, leading, and evaluating groups with a common goal related to health and the ecological systems, which support or destroy the health of individuals, families, and communities. When you are not in the leadership role, you may find yourself serving as an advocate for group efforts or a coalition partner for groups wishing to work toward a unified goal. In the advocacy role, you are a promoter of a group's autonomy and self-determination (Cary, 2000). Clearly, whether you fulfill the leadership or advocacy role in working with groups, you will implement your role based on knowledge and experiences of group behaviors.

WHAT ARE GROUPS?

Groups are a collection of people who interact and are interdependent in achieving a goal. Although most groups function face-to-face in the same environment, this method of meeting as a group is giving way to electronic methods. Research with groups has yet to conclude that one method is superior to the other. However, as electronic methods increase in frequency, data to support which method works best for a particular instance provides specific guidance for groups and leaders.

Groups function effectively and efficiently when they stimulate interaction in a coordinated and (typically) structured manner. A group is effective when it achieves its goals. It is efficient when it uses discussion and interaction to conduct the activities necessary to achieve the goal in a prescribed time frame. Effective and efficient

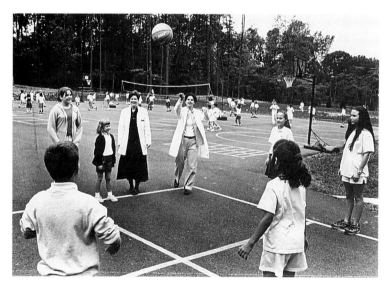

group functioning benefits from clarity of goals; member support for goals; leadership actions among members to facilitate interaction, learning, and achievement of the goals; and mutual satisfaction among members.

As you improve your skills in leading groups in the health-care environment, it is notable to recognize the importance of these four core activities of leaders.

Core Group Activities of Members and Leaders

Clarify Goals

The intent of using a group format to meet health-care needs necessitates a clear statement of one or more goals for the group. The discussion and clarification of goals occur when recruiting members and at the first meeting or during the initial portion of the meeting. As a leader, you may find that members will seek reclarification throughout the process. Alternatively, you may find that members' behaviors (questions, interactions) indirectly beg for clarification of goals during the process. Be liberal in taking the time necessary to clarify the goals—this is an essential process to achieving the subsequent group activities.

Examples

- At the conclusion of our group, you will be able to identify solutions to the cause of our children being inadequately immunized.
- The goal of this meeting is to determine how physical therapy referrals can be initiated within the first 24 hours of admission to home care.
- We are meeting as a group to understand your concerns about the hazardous waste landfill scheduled to be built in the county.

Seeking Member Support for the Goals

Clarifying and supporting a group's goals are "two sides of the same coin." Group members must understand the goal and see it as relevant to their unique and collective needs. Members need to verbalize their commitment to the goal and support behaviors that work toward it. It is likely that members may have other ambitions for the group of which they may be aware or unaware. For example, some may attend to meet high social needs (to be liked, to conform, or to vent frustration). Others may wish to learn or contribute to additional dimensions of the goal outside of the intent of the group (to be seen as an expert, to broaden the group's mission, to bring the group to premature closure). Still others may be misinformed about the group's goals and activities and view the experience as not meeting their needs. However, it is essential that members whose needs are met by the goal support the group goals. Two-way communication (listening and talking) is a critical element in members' decisions to support the goals. Encourage each member to actively participate in effective communication so that their feelings and performance are apparent. When members are ambivalent, the leader must take time to clarify the goal and the thinking behind the ambivalence so that understanding is achieved. Group members who can support the goal stimulate cooperation, collaboration, and a high level of commitment to the group and the goal. Support for alternative goals should be discussed and either incorporated or resolved by agreement to plan for additional venues of action at the appropriate time.

For example, the leader may summarize using the following statements:

- Now that the goals of the group have been stated, what are your thoughts about them?
- Does anyone in the group have other goals in mind? If so, please share them now.
- How can the group's goals support any of the goals you may have?

Leadership Actions—Yours and Theirs Together

Generally speaking, participation and leadership is shared and distributed among members in the group. Participation by both leaders and members is key to effective learning. The formal leadership provided by the leader may be augmented by informal leaders in the group. Informal leaders are recognizable by the expertise they share, the authority they represent, or the impact their actions create in facilitating or antagonizing the group process. Remember that leadership facilitates the group to achieve its goals. The facilitative skills of informal leaders must be recognized and viewed as collaborative. The leader must reinforce attempts to participate and empower members to bring knowledge and experiences that further group goals. The leader is responsible for providing enough structure for members to meet the goals by identifying starting and ending times and number of meetings, recognizing and validating group norms, clarifying levels of confidentiality, summarizing progress, clarifying decision-making procedures that match the situations, providing problem-solving guidance and strategies for groups experiencing stagnation or impasse toward the goal, and bringing closure to the group.

For example, the leader may summarize using the following statements:

- During the last 15 minutes we have discussed the barriers to immunization. Now let's spend the remaining time designing strategies to meet our immunization goals of 95 percent.

- To get a complete picture of our referral pattern, could the members of the physical therapy department share with us their procedures for intake?

- There is clearly a difference of opinion about the siting of a hazardous waste landfill in the county. What additional data should this group provide to solidify our recommendations to the zoning committee?

Promoting Mutual Satisfaction among Members

When individuals are members of a group, they bring individual needs even while participating in the achievement of group goals. Satisfaction derives from various motivations of group members: altruism, inclusion, team membership, caring, learning, empowerment, similarities with others, connectedness, solving problems of importance to the members, values clarification, better health, additional resources, and so forth. Meeting the needs of group members and promoting mutual satisfaction for member needs as well as with group goals are keys to successful group experiences. The leader can gather clues about member needs from verbal and nonverbal behaviors. Words and statements from members tell others the direct message about needs, for instance, "Yes, I believe you understand how isolated I feel." Nonverbal behaviors including body language and tone of voice often reveal the real feelings behind the verbal message (e.g., "Yes, I believe you understand how I feel," said with sarcasm, averted eyes, and a frown). Clear communication in groups entails congruence between a verbal and a nonverbal message. A group leader must assess the degree of mutual satisfaction with the group process and outcomes by being attentive to both verbal and nonverbal messages.

Incongruence in communication may be addressed as an invitation to the group members to clarify their needs within the group. Facilitating mutual support among group members often suffices to meet member needs outside the goal. Attentiveness to human behaviors as well as to group processes that must be completed as the group works toward its goal is an arduous but beneficial skill of facilitators and leaders.

The leader may use the following statements:

- Aside from generating three innovative approaches to immunization success, what else have you learned about your ability to work with this team?

- Physical therapy has just provided critical information for our referral process. How can we show them how important their service is to the referral success?

- It appears that there are two commonalties between the environmentalist and the industrialist on the siting situation of the hazardous waste landfill. Can our group support these two principles as a basis for further discussion?

These four core activities of leaders are applicable to all groups involved with community-based nursing. Whether meeting with church groups to identify high-risk members in need of health promotion or home care, a group of newly diagnosed diabetics, or health-care providers on an intake team, your ability to work effectively to facilitate group goals is enforced by the application of the nursing process, knowledge of individuals, group behavior, and systems thinking. Box 16–1 provides an opportunity for you to identify some important leadership strategies for a group.

Box 16-1	Student Learning Activity

Leadership Strategies

List some leadership strategies you could use to facilitate the four core functions of a group you plan to lead in your community practicum.

TYPES OF GROUPS

There are a variety of groups to which nurses deliver care. For purposes of this chapter, several categories are reviewed with respect to the emphasis of the group. The practice, knowledge, and skill of the nurse are as critical to success in a group as are the facilitation process skills. For specialized groups, leaders must have practice and process skills to facilitate the group safely and effectively.

A junior student described her feelings on leading a support group for her clinical practicum:

I learned from my instructor that the members of the faith community in which we were having our community-based clinical requested a "Living with Cancer" support group and that I would be asked to facilitate the group. I was apprehensive, yet excited. I had all of the theory on groups and had participated in some support groups myself. My mother was a cancer survivor so I had some insight into the issues she had dealt with during and after treatment. When I met the group for the first time, there were six clients within four months of diagnosis of their disease. During that first meeting, all members shared a little information about themselves, their disease, treatment, and their reason for wanting to participate in a group. Joanne had recent surgery for metastasis from the breast to the pelvic cavity. As she shared her story, the tears came as she expressed her fears of future treatment, nausea, and alopecia. I realized that she'd been there before and knew what might be in her future. The group discussed each fear and shared their experiences (good and bad). Some even shared funny stories, which served as tension relievers. Joanne stated that it had helped to share her fears with the group, and I was relieved that our first session was over but also eagerly awaited the next group session.

Therapeutic groups may be characterized as essentially healthy members who are experiencing a crisis. Examples of therapeutic groups are disaster victims and bereavement groups.

Self-help groups are typically organized and facilitated by patients who work to solve problems as group members define them. Examples include Alcoholics Anonymous (AA), AlAnon (for family members of substance abusers), cancer support groups, parenting groups, and Students Against Driving Drunk (SADD). These groups are formed to assimilate certain values among their members as well as to serve as a social reference for meeting and learning from others attempting to incorporate or maintain these values. Although the community-based nurse may be unlikely to lead these groups, the nurse's knowledge of these support resources and attention to referral options is important.

Support groups often have an educative function that is useful for members to incorporate new behaviors and effectiveness. Self-improvement through a support group is characterized by the provision of emotional support and health-related information (McCloskey & Bulachek, 2000). Typically, cognitive awareness of one's own behaviors is achieved in these groups, although no attempt to alter personality is made. Encounter groups and sensitivity groups were common in the 1970s and 1980s. Contemporary examples include assertiveness groups, relaxation groups, weight management groups, and caregiver support groups. Because many of the group interventions used by the community-based nurse incorporate support functions, the Nursing Intervention Classifications (NIC) offer a useful guide for implementation strategies with support groups (McCloskey & Bulachek, 2000).

Cooperative learning groups involve the use of small groups so that members work together to maximize their learning (Johnson, Johnson, & Smith, 1991). Through cooperative learning there is an opportunity for active engagement by members, growth of social skills, increased retention, and joy in learning. The five elements of cooperative learning include: positive interdependence, individual accountability, face-to-face interaction, interpersonal and small-group skills, and group processing (Cinelli, Symons, Bechtel, & Rose-Colley, 1994). In contrast, traditional learning groups are not reflective of these specific characteristics. Traditional learning groups tend to be more homogeneous, have one appointed leader, emphasize one task, and have less of a focus on group processing (Black, 1994) Cooperative learning groups are ideal for health-education activities and instructional strategies of these groups require members to participate to reinforce learning.

Psychotherapy groups are used to treat the psychiatric conditions of members in the group. Personality reconstruction is a hallmark of these groups as well as strengthening of interpersonal relationships by virtue of the group. This type of group is outside the community-based generalist nurse's scope of practice.

Focus groups comprise carefully selected participants who are asked to reveal as much as possible about their experiences and feelings on a specific topic. They have historically been used by market researchers to elicit consumer feedback, by social scientists to develop questionnaires, and by program evaluators (Frey & Fontana, 1993). In health-care systems and communities, focus groups are rapidly increasing as a method of choice for understanding consumer-provider needs (Crosby, Ogden, Kerr, & Heady, 1996). As an employee, you may be asked to conduct or participate in these groups to better understand consumer or colleague views or to assist others to understand your views. It is likely that new health-care services have been developed based on the results of focus groups. Likewise, new organizational schemes are often predicated on employee and customer focus group data. With consumerism in health care remaining a strong value in today's systems, your involvement with focus groups is likely to be evident.

As a focus group leader, one might elicit opinions using the following statements:
- How much are consumers willing to pay out of pocket for community-based nursing care?
- Which community-based nursing services are necessary in small rural communities?
- What are the experiences of the patients for access to primary and specialist care in your community?

In Box 16–2 write your ideas about how to effectively influence a focus group.

These typologies of groups are not all inclusive but are meant to illustrate the differential characteristics of groups with inference to possible general goals, purposes, and requirements for leaders and facilitators. Perhaps this will stimulate the reader's thinking about the nature of groups and nursing intervention possibilities in the community.

Functions in Groups— The Leadership Challenge

To meet both goal achievement and maintenance of the group as an entity, task and maintenance functions need to be balanced. Bales' (1953) classic research notes that roles emerge in a group to ensure that group goals and member needs are met. When group commitment to the goal is high, task behaviors result in high productivity. When group commitment is mixed or low, leaders and members must exhibit both task and maintenance behaviors.

As a group member and a leader, you must possess both task and maintenance skills, but you may not have known the skills by these names the last time you were in a group. Observe your behavior and the behaviors of others and note the impact of both task and maintenance interventions. Table 16–1 provides nine administrative behaviors useful in a group (Bales, 1953).

The group leader often assumes several roles to enhance group relations, such as encourager, diplomat, communication facilitator, trust builder, standard setter,

---

Box 16-2	Student Learning Activity

Focus Groups

Think about what you would do if you were in a focus group in which the leader asks too many questions and members become fatigued. What specific changes would you make if you were the leader?

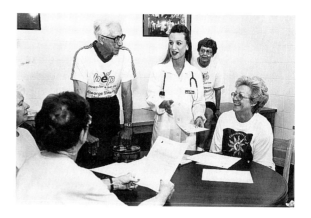

Table 16-1

Task Functions: The Nine Administrative Behaviors

1. Initiation: Define goals and problems and begin to work toward problem solving.

2. Elaboration: Expand on ideas and plans.

3. Information and opinion giver: Offer helpful information for problem solving.

4. Information and opinion seeker: Request data and feedback from members.

5. Coordinator: Clarify information presented and coordinate input of group members.

6. Evaluator: Evaluate group decisions in relation to identified goals.

7. Energizer: Stimulate group to operate at highest potential.

8. Orienter: Raise questions about direction of the group process.

9. Liaison: Communicate and bridge needs and concerns of group with external world. (Bales, 1953)

Table 16-2

Counterproductive Functions: Typical Behaviors

• Aggressor: Exhibits behavior that meets his or her needs, but that reduces others' status and contributions. May attack the task of the group.

• Blocker: Returns to issues that have previously been discarded or rejected. Uses resistance and negative behaviors.

• Playmate: Displays a lack of concern and involvement through irrelevant behavior or "horseplay." Remains detached or aloof.

• Monopolizer: Dominates group communication and creates group hostility.

• Recognition Seeker: Boasts of accomplishments, acts flamboyantly, arrives late, and leaves early.

• Victim: Encourages rescue by group members then rejects support and assistance. "Yes . . . but" language used.

• Rescuer: Oversupportive of group balance, fears conflict, and attempts to "smooth over" contradictory views and ideas.

• Truster: Uses excessive or premature self-disclosure, which threatens other members.

• Mistruster: Rejects trust and elicits hostility from others. Accusatory.

• Isolator: Becomes passive, dependent, and fearful of sharing thoughts, feelings.

• Dominator: Acts as an expert and perfectionist who tries to undermine the leader and questions the competency of the group and its abilities to meet the goal.

(Benne & Sheats, 1948; Bodganoff & Elbaum, 1978; Yalom, 1975)

follower, evaluator of emotional climate, and tension reliever (Bales, 1953; Johnson & Johnson, 1975).

Task and maintenance behaviors assist the group to achieve goals and help to meet the needs of the group. However, you have probably participated in groups in which other behaviors have been observed that meet the needs of individuals at the expense of the group goals. These behaviors meet the intrapsychic needs of members and are counterproductive to the group. The behaviors identified by classic group theorists and practitioners related to counterproductive functions are identified in Table 16–2.

Leaders usually address counterproductive behaviors that interfere with the progress of the group in one of two ways. The leader can share observations about the behavior with the individual(s) outside the group and jointly collaborate with the individual(s) to increase

functional behaviors while replacing the counterproductive behaviors. Likewise, the leader can increase the group's awareness of allowing members of the group to behave in a counterproductive manner. For example, the leader may say, "The group is allowing Tim to do all its work solving the issues of time management" or "Why does the group allow the aggressive behavior to continue?" These statements by the leader can serve to do the following:

1. Bring awareness to the group of the group's reaction to the counterproductive behaviors.
2. Identify the issues or reasons for the group's responses.
3. Support all group members to replace the counterproductive behaviors.

Clearly intervening with counterproductive behaviors in groups is challenging for the leader and requires technical and critical thinking to determine improved outcomes for the group. The leadership role for this behavior requires recognition of interpersonal needs and conflicts and mechanisms to reduce the impact of counterproductive behaviors for the success of the group.

Stages of Groups

All groups operate in stages as they progress toward their goals. The leader's view of the unfolding of these stages may differ among colleagues in much the same manner as the variety of models described by earlier theorists. For perspective, several classic models are described to help the reader recognize stages of development in groups.

Tuckman's early research (1965) revealed that groups generally undergo four stages or changes. According to Tuckman's view of stages, the group progresses from being nonproductive to achieving outcomes, as illustrated in the following:

- Forming: Members come together, exhibiting dependency on the leader, and test their individual values in the group. "Tell us what to do."
- Storming: Members engage in sharing personal needs and disparate values, often rich in emotional expression. Conflict may emerge among members as well as with group goals.
- Norming: Members seek to identify rules and guidelines of acceptable behaviors. Interdependency with one another may develop, and cohesion or attractiveness among members occurs.

- Performing: Members work to focus on and accomplish the task or goal.

Marram (1978) views group development as occurring in the following three phases:

- Introductory phase: Members meet one another and establish a climate of self-expression, trust, and interpersonal safety. Norms or ground rules are discussed.
- Working phase: Members begin to take responsibility for making change. The leader and other members reinforce members' initiatives to change behaviors or to become active learners.
- Termination phase: Members summarize experiences, view the group from the perspective of goal achievement, and recognize the loss of separation from the group.

Marram's model is applicable today to nontherapeutic groups, especially groups in which education of group members is the goal. Groups are generally not bound by a specific schedule of progression in stages. Rather, stages should be viewed as the unfolding of process events guided by leader facilitation and member behaviors. The goal of recognizing group stages is to plan for both a linear and cyclical pattern of group activities as the group attempts to achieve its mission, goals, and purposes. In some groups, there may be a clear and sequential movement of group activities from the unproductive to productive phases. Yet in other groups, the movements progress, stagnate, recycle, and proceed in a cyclical manner until the goal is reached. During a one-episode group meeting, the stages maybe compressed or invisible. However, in multiple group meetings the stages may unfold quite clearly. The function of the leader is to recognize stages, encourage full participation during each stage, confirm members' ability to progress, and assist members to accomplish the goals throughout the staging process.

EVALUATING GROUP OUTCOMES AND PROCESSES

Working within groups constitutes a nursing intervention strategy. You can use multiple evaluation methods of data from the audiences or stakeholders who have a commitment to the group or its outcomes.

Your evaluation can be collected verbally or in writing. You can ask group members, consultants, faculty, peers, and employers to provide evaluation data. It is useful to include your own views on the group as a part of the evaluation. Multiple methods of input comprehensively inform the evaluation outcomes. Evaluation data can be summarized and examined to determine the effectiveness and efficiency of the group. Five evaluation areas

outlined by Looney and Muir (1997) can guide the leader's understanding of group goals, communication, norms, leader and member roles, decision-making, and problem-solving procedures. These are illustrated in Table 16–3.

Looney and Muir (1997) developed a helpful Postmeeting Reaction Form (Table 16–4) that can be adapted to meet specific evaluation needs of various types of groups. It provides a quick scanning mechanism useful to quantifying processes and outcomes.

Table 16-3

Evaluating Group Work

- Are there clear and accepted group goals?

- How well does the group understand its charge?

- Does the group know and accept limits on its area of freedom?

- Do members understand what they are supposed to produce?

Communication Skills and Interaction Patterns

- How clearly do members express their ideas and opinions?

- How well do members listen to each other?

- Do members complete one topic before they switch to another?

- Is verbal participation equally balanced among all members?

Leadership and Member Roles

- Is the leadership appropriate for the group's needs?

- Are the roles performed by members appropriate both for their skills and the needs of the group?

- Are there any needed functions not being provided?

Decision-Making and Problem-Solving Procedures

- Are members adequately prepared?

- Is the group using an agenda? If so, how well is it being followed? Does it serve the group's needs?

- Is anyone providing periodic, internal summaries so members can keep track of major points of discussion?

- How are decisions being made?

- Has the group defined and analyzed the problem before members begin developing solutions?

- Do members understand and agree on criteria in making decisions?

- How creative is the group in presenting the information, or deriving a solution?

- Are information and ideas being evaluated critically or accepted at face value?

- Do you see any tendency toward *groupthink* (group members become closed minded and pressure others to conform).

(Looney & Muir, 1997)

Table 16-4

Members Postmeeting Reaction Form

Instructions: Circle the number that best indicates your reactions to the following questions about the discussion in which you participated:

1. *Adequacy of Communication.* To what extent do you feel members were understanding of each others' statements and positions?

| 0 | 1 | 2 | 3 | 4 | 5 | 6 | 7 | 8 | 9 | 10 |

Talked past each other;   Communicated directly with
misunderstanding   each other; understanding well

2. *Opportunity to Speak.* To what extent did you feel free to speak?

| 0 | 1 | 2 | 3 | 4 | 5 | 6 | 7 | 8 | 9 | 10 |

Never had a   Had all the opportunity to
chance to speak   talk that I wanted

3. *Climate of Acceptance.* How well did members support each other, show acceptance of individuals?

| 0 | 1 | 2 | 3 | 4 | 5 | 6 | 7 | 8 | 9 | 10 |

Highly critical   Supportive and receptive

4. *Interpersonal Relations.* How pleasant and concerned were group members with interpersonal relations?

| 0 | 1 | 2 | 3 | 4 | 5 | 6 | 7 | 8 | 9 | 10 |

Quarrelsome, status   Pleasant, empathic,
differences emphasized   concerned about group members

5. *Leadership.* How adequate was the leader (or leadership) of the group?

| 0 | 1 | 2 | 3 | 4 | 5 | 6 | 7 | 8 | 9 | 10 |

Too weak or   Shared, group-centered
dominating   and sufficient

6. *Satisfaction with role.* How satisfied are you with your personal participation in the discussion?

| 0 | 1 | 2 | 3 | 4 | 5 | 6 | 7 | 8 | 9 | 10 |

Very dissatisfied   Very satisfied

7. *Quality of Product.* How satisfied are you with the discussions, solutions, or learning that came out of this discussion?

| 0 | 1 | 2 | 3 | 4 | 5 | 6 | 7 | 8 | 9 | 10 |

Very dissatisfied   Very satisfied

(Continued)

Table 16-4

Members Postmeeting Reaction Form—cont'd

8. *Overall.* How do you rate the discussion as a whole apart from any specific aspect of it?

0	1	2	3	4	5	6	7	8	9	10

Awful; waste of time   Superb; time well spent

9. *Goal Attainment.* To what degree was the goal of the group met?

0	1	2	3	4	5	6	7	8	9	10

Unmet   Met fully

Add any other comments here:

(Adapted from Looney & Muir, 1997.)

Managing Conflict in Groups

You may have noted that as groups proceed through stages, diverse values, opinions, and facts emerge. This is healthy behavior because it expresses the "reality orientation" of the members. For the leader, it demands careful facilitation of the competing behaviors, so that members understand their differences, discover any commonalties, dedicate their work to building on those commonalties, and decide how to manage the contrasting behaviors. When group members' values are in conflict, the leadership role is more complex. This is because values emanate from a member's core reality of beliefs that are typically steadfast. Values clarification, in which values are communicated, explored, and evaluated, assists members to learn more about themselves and others. Discovery of the universality of values is essential to develop cohesion and trust in a group. In contrast, conflict in groups may emerge from competing "factual" information. This situation results when members provide facts or statements that contradict each other. The leadership role is to provide guidance to members to substantiate the facts as well as to provide knowledge that is accurate and contemporary.

Members in groups may react to conflict in a number of ways, including the following:

- Avoidance: Because no benefits of conflict exist, the member and group as a whole may deny it, refuse to continue the discussion, or change the topic.
- Reduction: Reducing the level of the conflict while suppressing some needs and issues to keep the conflict manageable.
- Proliferation: Spreading the conflict in terms of time or additional issues and persons. The emotional tone of communication during conflict may result in shouting, personal anger, and violence.

From classic research on the use of conflict behaviors, Thomas and Kilmann (1974) revealed that individuals engage in five orientations that vary in the degree of assertiveness on behalf of one's needs and cooperation with others' needs in a conflict situation. Individuals have a predominate orientation to use some of the five behaviors to the exclusion of others. Successful conflict management strategies occur when all five behaviors can be applied skillfully by matching the behavior to the situation at hand. For example, the use of accommodation as a conflict strategy may be effective when one person's needs can be delayed to move the group process forward. However, exclusive use of accommodation behaviors by a group member signals a risk that this individual's needs may be ignored and result in a dissatisfying group experience. Leaders in the group

Table 16-5

Five Orientations to Conflict

Accommodating: Neglects own concerns to satisfy the concerns of others.

Avoiding: Acknowledges no concerns.

Compromising: Attempts to find solutions that partially satisfy others.

Collaborating: Finds solutions that satisfy others so that mutual gains are recognized by all.

must be cognizant of conflict behaviors that facilitate and disrupt group process from goal attainment. Encouragement in the full array of conflict management behaviors for group members may be more productive to meeting group goals. Thomas and Kilmann (1974) identified five characteristic behaviors often seen in conflict management of groups. These five orientations to conflict are defined in the Table 16–5.

You will experience individual and group behaviors that meet each of these descriptions. The goal of conflict management is to direct the process of the group so that its goals are met. This may mean that individual conflict is acknowledged; yet, in the absence of immediate resolution, the members agree to work toward the goal while finding individual resolution through an external referral (mediation or arbitration) or meeting outside the group as individuals to resolve any differences desired.

Looney and Muir (1997) offer the following guidelines for facilitating the productive outcomes of conflict:
- Communicate with members about the issue: Avoid stereotypes and hidden agendas.
- Refute the position or idea rather than attacking the person.
- Construct reasonable arguments with facts rather than unsubstantiated claims.
- Work for a "win–win" solution by keeping an open mind toward the ideas of others.
- Be open to opportunities for compromise and collaboration.

- Encourage outside intervention through mediation and arbitration when the group dissolves because of conflict.
- Clearly specify in the group the acceptable rules and norms for managing conflict. Set the tone for these norms with the group initially.
- Use neutral rather than emotionally charged language.
- View disagreement in the spirit of inquiry, not defensiveness.
- Ask for criticism of ideas and opinions.
- Actively listen to others and hear the messages they convey.
- Clarify misunderstandings.

Managing conflict in a group will vary in intensity and leader energy. However, group members committed to working toward the goal will be able to find areas of consensus so that the group's work can be achieved. The leader's actions remain to assist the group to achieve its goals.

In Box 16–3, write some potential conflict resolution ideas for use in a support group.

Box 16-3	Student Learning Activity

Conflict Behaviors

You are assisting in leading a support group when you become aware that some sort of conflict is disrupting your planned approach to meeting the goals that you have identified. At one point, some of the members withdraw their participation. Identify three things that you would do to attempt to resolve the conflict:

1.

2.

3.

Leading Groups

Most of the groups conducted by community-based nurses have a formal leadership structure. Groups can be led by a single leader or facilitated by coleaders. Yet most groups succeed because the leadership functions are distributed among group members. Success results when all group members take responsibility for group productivity. Learning in groups occurs when members participate, interact, and perform leadership functions—whether they are task or maintenance activities.

Coleadership is a plausible leadership approach in groups. It requires clear, frequent communication and goal setting for coleader strategies to evolve to the point at which the group is enriched by this approach. Even as the group is experiencing stages of group development, coleaders are experiencing their own stages of coleadership as each attempts to recognize and manage their skills and limitations.

Dick, Lesseer, and Whiteside (1980) recognized four stages in the sequence of coleadership development. During *formulation,* leaders deal with issues of philosophies of groups, personality styles, identity, confidence, performance anxiety, and activity level. The *development* stage entails leaders collecting data about the strengths and limitations of self and the other. It is important that coleaders recognize the complementary skills they provide as a team as well as the gaps in skills that may exist. *Stabilization* constitutes a stage of establishing mutual trust and growing confidence in oneself and the other leaders. *Refreshment* is the final stage, comprising satisfaction, creativity, new perspectives, and seamless leadership.

Coleadership has both advantages and disadvantages. Advantages include augmented knowledge and emotional support, lower leader anxiety, expanded energy, and leadership behaviors as well as group continuity in the event of leader absence. Disadvantages are noted as well. Seamless coleadership develops as a process and is not instantaneous. It requires maturity, respect, temperamental compatibility, trust, and likeability. It also requires additional time commitment, increases the complexity of leadership, and costs more for additional salaries. Proper care in selecting a coleader may entail consideration of several factors: age, gender, ethnicity, leadership styles, affect, cognitive style, verbal and nonverbal activity, level of competitiveness, defensive patterns, and self-esteem (Janosik & Phipps, 1982). However, once coleadership unions are mutually established, the coleading approach in groups generally results in efficient and effective group processes and outcomes. Box 16–4 provides a space for you to list important activities you would want to consider in coleadership of a bereavement group.

Box 16-4	Student Learning Activity

Coleadership

You and another student have been assigned to be coleaders for a bereavement group session starting in 10 days. You meet together to plan leadership activities for the group. List six activities you would do to prepare for the group session:

1.

2.

3.

4.

5.

6.

Tips for Leading Groups

Special activities foster the productivity of members. Recruitment of members is an important initial step. Clear communication about the nature and goals of the group is critical. Members who self-select and whose needs mesh with group goals are more likely to experience success. Age, gender, and ethnic characteristics may also promote more success with either similar or different member characteristics, depending on the goals of the group. Costs may encourage or dissuade members from joining. Access to time and place must be planned for those who are employed or have other school and family responsibilities. Other characteristics may include diagnosis, functional status, mental status, provider status, and reimbursement status. Sliding scale fees encourage membership. Group size is important; 8 to 10 members are usually ideal.

Whether working with groups of providers and peers or with patients, general group facilitation skills are useful to achieve outcomes. Groups can be an economical method to provide service and general communication as well as to elicit data. The provision of an adequate amount of structure and guidance typically depends on the nature or goal of the group. A clear agenda or articulated goals and commitment by members all contribute to successful processes and outcomes. Experienced group leaders are flexible in their approach, focused on the present but with an eye toward the outcomes to be achieved in the future. They empower members to share knowledge and solve problems in a manner that meets the member's need to take as much control of his or her situation as is possible. General strategies for leading groups are noted in Table 16–6.

Groups are a uniquely effective care delivery strategy when the contributions of group members aid in learning and healing of both individuals as well as the group entity that emerges. You will find ample opportunities to initiate, lead, facilitate, and evaluate care services, patient outcomes, and community needs by working with groups. Group-oriented care delivery highlights both leadership skills and your role as a change agent for the improvement of individual health and the health status in a community (Zotti, Brown, & Stotts, 1996).

The 21st-Century Challenge: Teleconferencing Application to Group Work

The evaluation of technology enhances access to group work as an intervention strategy for community-based nursing practice. This can also apply to nursing education. A group of nursing students at the University of Windsor and at George Mason University used WEB CT to participate in an on-line information group to compare and contrast their community-based nursing experiences in the two different countries.

One student from the University of Windsor wrote:

I just finished reading for my community exam a couple days ago and the "first" community nurses had (difficult) situations on a regular basis—no soap, no electricity, no running water. Now that we are even more into the community, we come across this situation more often and have to become more creative and versatile than perhaps we thought we would ever need to be—especially today in what is supposed to be a very "advanced society."

A peer at George Mason University replied:

I feel that the changes have had a great impact on nursing. I believe like Kim that it's not where you practice nursing, but how you practice it. I believe that the impact it's had on my education is by the College of Nursing incorporating this into our curriculum. I believe that we as nursing students are getting a well-rounded education. We are learning the technical parts that are required in nursing, as well as the way nurses practice in the community. I know that this semester in community has opened my eyes to things that I had never thought of before. I don't believe that this could be learned in the hospital.

The on-line project revealed the busy life of students; they would post a message and then reappear after getting caught up with their responsibilities in school and elsewhere. An American student wrote:

Table 16-6

Tips for Leading Group Discussions

Initiating Discussion

- Help reduce primary tensions.

- Briefly review the purpose of the meeting, outcomes to be achieved, and limitations to be observed.

- Give members informational handouts as needed.

- Make sure special roles (such as recorder) are established.

- Suggest procedures to follow.

- Ask a clear question to help members focus on the discussion issue.

Structuring Discussions

- Keep the group goal oriented; watch for digressions and topic changes.

- Put the discussion or problem-solving procedure in writing on the chalkboard or in a handout.

- Summarize each major step or decision.

- Structure the group's time.

- Bring the discussion to a definite close.

Equalizing Opportunity to Participate

- Address comments to the group as a whole.

- Control compulsive, dominating, or long-winded speakers.

- Encourage less-talkative members to participate.

- Listen with genuine interest to infrequent participants.

- Do not comment after each member's remarks.

- Bounce questions of interpretation back to the group before you offer an opinion.

- Remain neutral during arguments.

Stimulating Creative Thinking

- Encourage members to search for other alternatives.

- Suggest techniques (such as brainstorming) designed to tap a group's creativity.

- Discuss components of a problem one at a time.

- Be alert to suggestions that open up a whole new line of thinking.

Stimulating Critical Thinking

- Encourage members to evaluate information and reasoning.

- Make sure all members accept the standards, criteria, or assumptions used in making judgments.

- Evaluate all solutions thoroughly before making them final.

(Adapted from Looney & Muir, 1997)

 It has been some time since I "checked in" but I will be better about it from this point forward. . . . Anyway, I wanted to take the opportunity to comment on questions posted. First of all, community-based nursing has forced many nurses and students to take a good look and to learn more about the "entire person." No longer is the "client" just a "sick patient" in a hospital bed in need of acute care. We now have to deal with their families, their "healthy" environment, and their different backgrounds. I hope that even should I move into the acute nursing field, that I will always remember that different patients have different situations and we, as professionals, should not judge or assume anything without a good background check.

Through the on-line information group, the two groups of students in two countries shared not only information about their clients in community-based experiences, but also about the stresses in their student lives. The group sometimes evolved into a support group, as well as an information group. This is only one example of how, as our society becomes more "high tech," we are offered many opportunities for new ways to conduct work in groups. Some of these approaches involve audio conferencing, video conferencing, desktop and multimedia teleconferencing, or hybrid meeting formats. Users of these group conferencing tools can select the mechanisms that best suit their group work needs, budget, and equipment compatibility.

Audio conferencing uses voice communications via standard telephone lines and new technologies such as integrated services digital networks (ISDNs) and the Internet. If several group members are in each location, speakerphone or audio-conference terminal equipment may be used. More than two locations optimizes audio capability through use of multiple network building equipment or Internet-based software.

Although introduction of voice allows for a fuller understanding of members' communication than e-mail or "chat room" dialogue in groups, audio conferencing may diminish the full communication potential of group members because nonverbal components of communication are absent. Leaders and members alike may need to implement the use of frequent intermittent summaries and validity checks—"Does anyone feel differently about . . . ?"—to incorporate those whose responses are less assertive, ambiguous, or ambivalent.

Audiographics technology can connect graphic display devices such as computer monitors located at distant sites. Some systems allow still-frame visuals, annotation, writing, or drawing on the screen. Audiographics are typically used to enhance both audio and videoconference capability, a feature useful for educative groups (International Multimedia Collaborative Communications Alliance [IMCCA], 2000).

Computer or asynchronous conferencing uses electronic file strategy and e-mail to provide an asynchronous conference in which group members can join the dialogue at any time, read, and add their comments. This vehicle can be adjuvant to the real-time conference mechanism by supplying advanced preparatory materials, assignments for an upcoming audio conference, or for continuing discussion that originated during a video or audio conference (IMCCA, 2000).

Video conferencing is used by groups to communicate to others in the group using real-time interaction with audio and video communications network technology. Desktop video conferencing mixes personal computing with audio, video, and real-time technology from a single personal computer. A point-to-point group conference incorporates video conferencing between two systems, whereas multipoint conferencing involves three or more videoconference systems. Some systems allow for a continuous presence of group members—a "Hollywood Squares" format in which each member is seen in a quadrant for the entire length of the meeting (IMCCA, 2000).

Hybrid group meeting formats allow for a mix of conference technology users, assuming compatibility of technology and requisite bandwidth capabilities (IMCCA, 2000).

Teleconferencing methods described offer electronic channels to facilitate communication within a group or between groups for purposes of meeting, education, training, collaboration, and commuting for work. Technology mechanisms include telephone, ISDN, Satellite, Internet local area network/wide area network (LAN/WAN), T1, and DS-3 lines.

Questions must be raised and answers provided for the technological application of group work to be effective. Table 16–7 lists several planning questions to consider when selecting a technological approach to implement in groups.

Should response to the questions in Table 16–7 focus favorably on the use of teleconferencing for group sessions, the actual conduct of the session must next be considered. This requires planning, choreography, and nuances for effective transmission, reception, and engagement of group members. Considerations include:

- Select time, date, participant list, and reserve lines.
- Connect to bridging site at beginning of setup period to test that all sites connect.
- Adjust volume on monitor to 60 percent and place microphone close.
- When not speaking, mute the microphone or all participants may see and hear you sneezing, mumbling, or shuffling papers (unless it is critical to group process).
- If the group is in progress and the audio changes, contact the operator for the meeting to make adjustments.

Table 16-7

Technology Applications: Considerations for Group Work

- Who is in charge? Is the leader also the technology person or can the leader focus on the group process?

- What is the goal of this group meeting? Do participants have a copy of the goal and agenda?

- What is the desired outcome? How can the group process best be facilitated?

- What alternatives from a technology standpoint are available to facilitate the group process?

- Who will be communicating with whom? What is context and form of communication? Where are participants located?

- What experience have group members had with groups, the technology, and subsequent outcomes? How do they feel about it?

- What training is required to facilitate effective group members' participation?

- What are the costs for equipment, transmission, and training?

- Is the production capability in house or would on outside vendor be more efficient and affordable?

- Where do the meetings occur? Have selections for lines or satellite times been made?

(Adapted from Earon, 2000)

- Often there is some noticeable audio delay, so try not to interrupt the speaker and provide sufficient time for participants to respond. Otherwise, a videotape and audio track can become fumbled and confusing.
- Camera angles for three or fewer participants at a site are usually stationary; however, for more than three people the camera may need to be moved to see the person speaking.
- If graphics are used, allow for vertical presentation and sufficient white space with large font sizes.
- Have clear meeting objectives.

- Prepare yourself and materials prior to the meeting—rehearsal is helpful.
- Dress with video in mind—solid colors work best.
- Introduce yourself and others when your site is the focus of the conference.
- Establish the leader to keep the group focused.
- Disallow non–group-member interruptions; silence beepers, phones, faxes.
- If someone has not spoken for a time, elicit that person's participation.
- Avoid facing, standing up, swiveling, or leaning too close to the camera. Try to stay seated in front of the camera (Earon, 2000).

The advent of technology application for group work provides the potential for more users to have access to group participation from remote areas (rural areas, prisons, international sites, and so on). However, until the technology is generally affordable and distributed, training is sufficient, refinements of conducting and outcomes of group work are achieved, and acceptability by group members is clear, the widespread use of teleconferencing will take time. Should you select teleconferencing as a method of conducting group work, incorporate evaluation activities from the provider and user perspectives, the economic perspective, the goal and outcome perspective, and the technology friendliness perspective to determine its usefulness compared with on-site face-to-face group work in the community. Community acceptability is essential to the outcomes possible with teleconferencing group interventions.

RESEARCH WITH GROUPS IN THE COMMUNITY

As nurses gain sophistication in leading and participating in groups, they can effectively use findings from the increasing number of research studies focused on groups. Three different studies are described here. A study by White and Dorman (2000) examined the results of an on-line support for caregivers of Alzheimer's patients. The researchers studied the content and themes of 532 messages posted on a public Alzheimer's mail group during 20 days. Members used the mail group to find and give information, to share ideas and experiences, and to provide encouragement. The researchers suggest that by becoming aware of the potential benefits of on-line support groups, nurses can

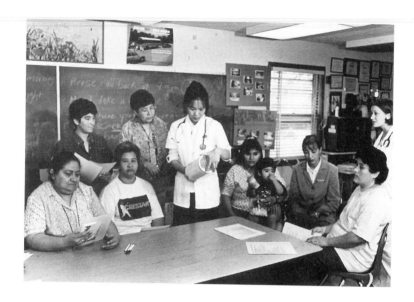

encourage Alzheimer's caregivers to use on-line groups as a practical alternative to traditional groups.

Another type of support group was evaluated by Kleffel (1998). This evaluation research was carried out to study a caregiver community-based support program. Caregivers reported that they sometimes felt overwhelmed, isolated, and lacked time for a personal life. They described their lives as being "on hold." Researchers concluded that the community-based support program was a powerful mechanism for helping the caregivers to socialize and to learn to care for themselves.

An exploratory, descriptive pilot study was undertaken to describe the Young Parents Project, a computer network offering health information and support to adolescent mothers (Hudson, Elek, Westfall, Grabau, & Fleck, 1999). Nine adolescent mothers were provided with computers so that they could participate in the Young Parents Project from their homes. Findings from the study indicated that participants accessed the computer network 834 times for a total of 7,046 minutes during the first year of the study. Themes that emerged from content analysis of the participants' electronic messages included infant sharing, finances and education, and postpartum problems. The researchers concluded that the project served as a helpful approach to providing health information and social support to the adolescent mothers.

Finally, Rodriguez (1999) used a participatory action research methodology to study the problem of domestic violence in migrant farmworker women in California. Data gathered over a 4-year period were analyzed, including observations, field notes, informal conversations, interviews, and written stories from the women. The "power of the collective" emerged as a critical base for battered migrant farmworker women to help them support and care for each other. Concepts of liberation, enlightenment, and "conscientizacion" were important aspects of the collective experience.

CONCLUSION

As nursing roles in community-based practice increase in both numbers and complexity, nurses will need to use groups for a variety of traditional and nontraditional purposes. With the increased sophistication of many in the community in the use of computers, it makes sense for nurses to become knowledgeable about the use of this technology for such purposes as group discussion, support, and teaching. Groups often offer unique advantages such as efficient use of time, opportunities for comparison of ideas, and peer support that make them important nursing interventions in community-based practice.

Active Learning Strategies

1. Discuss with a partner the importance of recruitment criteria when forming groups. Use three examples of different groups you might lead in the community and the recruitment criteria for each.

2. List and discuss the differences between task, maintenance, and counterproductive behaviors in a group.

3. Discuss the reasons to encourage the emergence of conflict in the group. What type of behaviors are you likely to see as group members respond to the conflict?

4. Observe a focus group session and an educational group session. Discuss the similarities and differences between these relative to the following:
   - Goals
   - Member behaviors
   - Task and maintenance functions observed by making a checklist
   - Leader behaviors
   - Composition of group

5. Participate in role playing exercises for the following scenarios:
   - A leader orienting the group to the goals of the group
   - Coleaders discussing their strengths and limitations
   - Intervening with a member who is monopolizing the group
   - Providing corrective information to a member who states "We all know that diabetes is caused by eating too much sugar"

6. You have just learned that a quarterly goal for your home-health agency is that all family caregivers become knowledgeable about respite services in their community. Debate the use of individual versus group methods to achieve this goal. What are the advantages and disadvantages of each method for the caregivers, staff, and agency resources? Outline a plan to achieve this goal.

References

Bales, R. F. (1953). A theoretical framework for interaction process analysis. In D. Cartwright & A. Zander (Eds.), Group dynamics, research and theory. Evanston, IL: Row, Peterson.

Benne, K. D., & Sheats, P. (1948). Functional roles of group members. Journal of Social Issues 4(2), 41–49.

Black, S. (1994). Group learning. The Executive Educator 14(9),18–20.

Bogdanoff, M. A., & Elbaum, P. L. (1978). Role lock: Dealing with monopolizers, mistrusters, isolates, helpful Hannahs, and other assorted characters in psychotherapy. International Journal of Group Psychotherapy 1(2), 247–262.

Bronfenbrenner, U. (1979). The ecology of human development, experiments by nature and design. Cambridge, MA: Harvard University Press.

Cary, A. H. (2000). Case management. In M. Stanhope & J. Lancastee (Eds.), Community and public health nursing: Process and practice for promoting health (5th ed.). St. Louis: Mosby.

Chamberlin, R. W. (1988). Beyond individual risk assessment: Community wide approaches to promoting the health and development of families and children. Washington, DC: National Center for Education in Maternal and Child Health.

Cinelli, B., Symons, C. W., Bechtel, L., & Rose-Colley, M. (1994). Applying cooperative learning in health education practice. Journal of School Health 64(3), 99–103.

Crosby, F. S., Ogden, A. B., Kerr, S. L., & Heady J. (1996). Focus groups describe rural nursing in New York State. Journal of the New York State Nurses Association 27(2), 4–8.

Dick, B., Lesseer, K., & Whiteside, J. (1980). A developmental framework for co-therapy. International Journal of Group Psychotherapy 30(3), 273–285.

Earon, A. (2000). Seven steps to successful video conferencing. Accessed at http://www.imcaa.org/cl-imcca/framesettest.htm/?whitepaper/videosteps/control

Erkel, E. A., Nivens, A. S., & Kennedy D. W. (1995). Intensive immersion of nursing students in rural interdisciplinary care. Journal of Nursing Education 34, 359.

Frey, J. H., & Fontana, A. (1993). The group interview in social research. In D. L. Morgan (Ed.) Successful focus groups (pp. 20–34). Newbury Park, CA: Sage Publications, Inc.

Hudson, D. B., Elek, S. M., Westfall, J. R., Grabau, A., & Fleck, M. O. (1999). Young Parents Project: A 21st-century nursing intervention. Issues in Comprehensive Pediatric Nursing, 22(4), 153–165.

International Multimedia Collaborate Communications Alliance. (2000, May 24). General glossary. Accessed at http://www.imcca.org-imcca/general101.htm/may.

Janosik, E., & Phipps, L. B. (1982). Life cycle group work in nursing. Belmont, CA: Wadsworth.

Johnson, D. W., & Johnson, F. P. (1975). Joining together. Upper Saddle River, NJ: Prentice Hall, Inc.

Johnson, D. W., Johnson, R. T., & Smith, K. (1991). Active learning in the college classroom. Edina, MN: Interaction Book Co.

Kleffel, D. (1998). Lives on hold: Evaluation of a caregiver's support program. Home Health Nurse, 16(7), 465–472.

Looney, S., & Muir, J. K. (1997). Working with small groups. Workshop presented at George Mason University, Fairfax, VA (available from authors at Department of Communication).

McCloskey, J., & Bulachek, M. (Eds.). (2000). Nursing interventions classification. St. Louis: Mosby.

Marram, G. D. (1978). The group approach in nursing practice. St. Louis: Mosby.

Muir, J. K. (1993). Introduction to interpersonal and small group communication. Dubuque, IA: Kendall/Hunt.

Rodriguez, R. (1999). The power of the collective: Battered migrant farmworker women creating safe spaces. Health Care for Women International, 20(4), 417–426.

Thomas, K. W., & Kilmann, R. H. (1974). Thomas-Kilmann conflict mode instrument. New York: Xicom Corp.

Tuckman, B. W. (1965). Developmental sequence in small groups. Psychological Bulletin 63, 384–399.

White, M. H., & Dorman, S. M. (2000). Online support for caregivers. Analysis of an Internet Alzheimer mailgroup. Computer Nursing, 18(4), 168–179.

Yalom, I. D. (1975). The theory and practice of group psychotherapy (2nd ed.). New York: Basic Books.

Zotti, M. E., Brown, P., & Stotts, R. C. (1996). Community-based nursing versus community health nursing: What does it all mean? Nursing Outlook 44, 211–217.

CHAPTER 17

The Nurse in the Community-based Child-care Center

Maureen Kirkpatrick McLaughlin

LEARNING OBJECTIVES

1) Discuss past, current, and future trends of child care.

2) Discuss how the nurse's professional values, competencies, and knowledge impact a child-care center.

3) Discuss the role of the nurse as provider, designer, manager, and coordinator of care in relation to the community-based child-care center.

4) Identify the key indicators and tools used to assess quality in a child-care center.

5) Discuss the advocacy role of the nurse to influence federal, state, and local governments to improve the quality of child care.

6) Explore the role of the nurse as child-care health consultant.

This chapter discusses how a national crisis in child care provides vast opportunities for nurses to practice and apply their values, competencies, knowledge, and technical skills in a community-based child-care center. The chapter explains how health-care issues of access, cost, and quality are concerns for care of children, as well as adults. It also discusses research studies and assessment tools that can help improve the quality of child care. In addition, the chapter discusses questions most frequently asked of nurses about child-care issues, the past and future trends of child care, and how you, as a nurse, can advocate to ensure that children will be in safe and healthy child-care environments in the future.

Consider the following three scenarios:

> *I was totally taken by surprise. One of our parents informed me her 18-month-old son was a carrier of Hepatitis B. It wasn't a problem, until he started biting other children and broke the skin of another child.*
>
> *One of my staff came to me and said, "We have a problem. The wrong baby was just given a bottle of breast milk."*
>
> *One of my teachers informed me she had a 4-year-old boy who upon awakening after a nap had a glazed look about him. When I questioned her further, she said the boy also had some mild facial twitching and that he started to "wet his bed" during naptime. Shortly thereafter he was in the Emergency Room having a grand mal seizure.*

Each of the preceding stories is true. They are examples of the wide array of health and safety issues that a child-care center director faces on a regular basis. Because most directors of community-based child-care programs are not health professionals, they can benefit from nurses' assessments at the center to ensure safe and healthy environments for young children. You, the nurse, can meet this community-based need. Box 17–1 provides a space for you to list health issues to consider in a child-care center.

Box 17-1   Student Learning Activity

Health Issues in Child-care Centers

Take a moment to reflect on what it would be like to work in a child-care center. What other examples of health issues do you think could occur in a child-care center?

PAST TRENDS IN CHILD CARE

Throughout history, child-care programs have been designed to meet societal goals as they arise. They have been needed to provide care and education for children while parents worked, to provide custodial care for children while parents learned new job skills to avoid public assistance, to provide compensatory education, and to extend the functions of the home. Early childhood education and care has a history of more than 200 years. Given the increase of mothers in the workforce, this history will extend well into the 21st century. In Box 17–2, write your ideas about child-care placement.

Box 17-2   Student Learning Activity

Child-care Placement

Think about the first time you heard about a child being placed in a child-care program. What do you remember thinking and feeling about it?

For years, there has been a controversy between mothers who work outside of the home and mothers who do not. Many mothers work, even without financial necessity, and the stigma once prevalent toward the "working mother" has dissipated.

When did children start leaving the home for educational purposes? In France, as early as the 1700s, children 2 years of age and older were grouped together in "knitting schools" where they gathered around "teachers" who knitted. In Colonial America, "dame schools" came into fashion for 4- to 7-year-old children. These schools were operated by widows and young, single women and later evolved into boarding schools (Decker & Decker, 1997).

In the 1780s, "common schools" delivered education to young boys, who were taught by men who focused the learning on morality. "Infant schools" were brought from Scotland to Indiana in 1825 by Robert Owen, a mill owner who believed in providing his workers a happy place for young children to learn good practical habits using "hands-on" activities. In the 1850s, "kindergartens," education programs that enrolled children ages 3 to 7, came to the United States via a German immigrant. A "nursery school" for children of poor women was created in 1854 in cooperation with the Child's Hospital of New York City to reduce infant mortality. At that time, these nurseries were considered necessary to counter children in the labor force, to discourage exploitation of women, and to help alleviate immigrants' cultural assimilation problems (Decker & Decker, 1997). "Montessori schools" began in 1906 when Maria Montessori, the first woman to graduate from an Italian medical school, began work with children with mental disabilities. This type of school emphasizes that children can teach themselves with minimal adult guidance (Decker & Decker, 1997).

For the next 40 years, most mothers stayed at home. When World War II broke out, many mothers reentered the workforce to support the war effort; the federal government provided financial support to pay for child-care services (the Lanham Act). Following the war, mothers returned to the home to care for their children, and funding to cover child-care needs decreased. In 1947, only 12 percent of mothers with children under the age of 5 were in the workforce. Over the next 30 years, the percentage of working mothers with children under the age of 18 more than doubled—from less than one third in 1960, to two-thirds in 1990 (Children's Defense Fund [CDF], 2000).

CURRENT TRENDS IN CHILD CARE

Since the late 1980s, there have been concerns throughout the United States that child care for working parents was too expensive, had too many waiting lists, and was of mediocre to poor quality. A national debate occurred over the nature and extent of our nation's child-care problems, and researchers began to study the problems. In response to this debate, federal support for child care was expanded by establishing the Child Care Development Block Grant and the At-Risk Child Care Program as part of the Omnibus Budget Reconciliation Act of 1990.

Child care is a daily necessity for millions of working parents, and although efforts are being made to improve child care, it remains in crisis. A child will spend more than 2000 hours per year in child care (Decker & Decker, 1997). In 1999 the National League of Cities produced "Ten Critical Threats to America's Children: Warning Signs for the Next Millennium: A Report to the Nation." Child care is listed as one of these threats.

Types and Definitions of Child Care

The National Association for the Education of Young Children (NAEYC) defines early childhood as birth through age 8 (NAEYC, 1998). Many names are associated with caring for young children, such as day care, child care, early care and education, preschool, and nursery school. Box 17–3 provides a space for you to write your definition of child care.

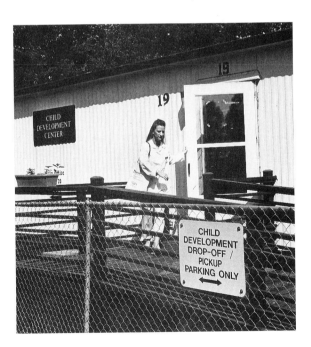

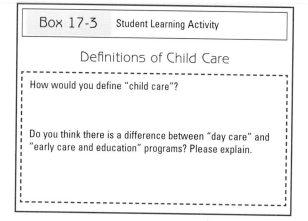

Box 17-3   Student Learning Activity

Definitions of Child Care

How would you define "child care"?

Do you think there is a difference between "day care" and "early care and education" programs? Please explain.

There are two basic kinds of child care: *center care* and *family child care*. A *child-care center* is defined as an out-of-home program and facility serving children who need care for part or most of the day while their parents work. These facilities are regulated by the state to meet minimum licensing requirements and may serve children ranging in age from 6 weeks to school age. Some child-care centers are not-for-profit and are sponsored by state and local governments, religious groups, or parent cooperatives. For-profit centers are usually owned and operated by individuals or family corporations (Decker & Decker, 1997).

Family child care is care provided in a home other than the child's own and in which the group size is relatively small. According to Willer (1990), most of these programs operate as independent businesses and approximately 60 percent are "unregulated."

Day care is a term frequently used to indicate that children are being cared for in a place other than their home. It has no correlation with quality, licensure, or accreditation. Early childhood professionals are working diligently to educate society to replace this word with *early care and education*. This phrase better defines that quality child care, from infancy to prekindergarten, contributes to early brain development and prepares children for school readiness.

Licensed or *regulated* child-care programs are programs that meet "Minimum Standards for Licensed Child Day Centers." These regulations, as defined by the state or local jurisdiction, are available from the state Department of Social Services, which usually administers these services and provides operating licenses for centers and homes. These standards include specific guidelines

for centers such as administration, staff qualifications and training, staffing and supervision, programs, special services, the physical plant, special care provisions, and emergencies. These guidelines are minimum requirements and many do not meet the National Health and Safety Standards for Out-of-Home Child Care Settings developed by the American Academy of Pediatricians and the American Association of Public Health.

Licensing specialists visit the home and the center for both formal announced visits and also unannounced visits to ensure that regulations are being followed. Many departments are understaffed, and mandatory visits have decreased. This further jeopardizes the health and safety of children.

Unlicensed or *unregulated* care is usually provided in a home and does not meet any state or local regulations; this type of child care is considered illegal. Many parents are unaware of this, and daily send their child into a neighborhood home that may be unhealthy and unsafe, but available and affordable. These providers usually ask for cash payment so that there are no records to document child-care transactions and no penalties for taxes.

Accredited means that a child-care center has voluntarily met the "seal of approval" established by the National Association for the Education for Young Children (NAEYC) through a self-study process that includes administrators, teaching staff, and parents. This team works together to evaluate and improve the quality of the program. These standards, established in 1985, represent the current consensus on what constitutes a high-quality child-care program. Although attaining this credential is a great achievement and is to be renewed every three years, it does not guarantee parents that the program will not change. *Nonaccredited* means that a center has not been accredited. It does not imply that the center has lesser quality, simply that it has not gone through the self-study process.

Demographics and Economics of Child Care

According to the National Center for Education Statistics, in 1995 there were approximately 21 million infants, toddlers, and preschool children under age 6 in the United States, and almost 13 million of them were in child care.

It is estimated that 75 percent of women with children under the age of 5 will be employed and in need of child care in the early part of the 21st century (U.S. Department of Health and Human Services, 1996). Children in licensed centers and homes are being cared for by 3 million child-care teachers, assistants, and family child-care providers. Females compose 97 percent of the teaching staff, 41 percent have children, and 10 percent are single parents. The average salary of a child-care provider is approximately $14,820 per year (CDF, 2000). Child care center teaching staff earn annual wages of less than one-half of wages earned by comparably educated women in other professions and less than one-third of those of comparably educated men (Willer, 1990).

Earnings are even lower for many home providers. According to data from Wheelock College, The Economics of Family Child Care Study, family child-care providers earn $9,528 per year. Unregulated child-care providers earn even less at $5,132 annually. Only 18 percent of child-care centers offer fully paid health-care benefits to teaching staff. One-third of all child-care teachers leave their centers each year. This high turnover of staff is a contributing factor to poor quality of care. The demand for child-care services keeps growing, yet the supply is not meeting this demand. This ever-growing number of children in out-of-home settings for early care and education has brought with it questions about quality, affordability, and access, the very same issues that are prevalent in health care. In Box 17–4, briefly describe an experience with a child-care program.

Quality, Affordability, and Access to Child Care

Quality

Research over the last 25 years shows that high-caliber early care and education programs can benefit children. Children need to be safe, healthy, and appropriately stimulated. Yet many parents are unfamiliar with what to look for in a quality program. Many parents' first question to directors is: "How much does it cost?" Dombro et al. (1996) point out that the quality of early care and education is linked to healthy development and well-being. Yet only 12 to 14 percent of young children are likely to be in child-care environments that prepare them to enter school ready to succeed, and between 35 and 45 percent of infants and toddlers are in settings that are potentially harmful to their growth (Dombro et al., 1996).

What are the other indicators for quality child care? Table 17–1 presents some of these indicators.

The Quality 2000 Initiative documents warn of a "quality" crisis in early care and education in the United States and suggest a plan for improvement (Kagan, 1997). What can parents do? Table 17–2 presents some important areas to consider in relation to childcare providers.

Box 17-4	Student Learning Activity

Use of Child-care Programs

What has your own experience, or that of a friend, been with child-care programs?

Table 17-1

Indicators of Quality Early Care and Education Programs

Children benefit in small group sizes

High staff-to-child ratios

Warm, caring staff who are well educated and who have specialized training

Higher compensation levels for staff

Low turnover of staff

Administrative stability

Table 17-2

Parent Checklist for Child-care Providers

A TOOL TO ASSIST PARENTS IN CHOOSING A CHILD-CARE PROGRAM.

DOES THE CHILD-CARE PROVIDER:

Have a license to operate a child-care center?

Have previous experience, training, and education in working with young children?

Have certification in first aid and CPR?

Understand the different ages and stages of childhood development?

Share the same philosophy of caring for your child as you do? (Including difficult behavior.)

Appear to enjoy his/her work?

Seem to be someone your child will enjoy being with?

Have additional help?

Provide a variety of developmental activities that will stimulate your child's learning?

Table 17-3

Questions to Ask about a Child-care Center

Is the center clean?

Is there enough space to play?

Are the teachers kind and caring?

Are sick children kept home so as not to infect the well children?

Are immunization records up to date?

Table 17–3 lists some questions to consider related to quality in a child-care center.

Recognizing that quality care depends on quality child-care providers, North Carolina is addressing this issue by improving caregiver compensation through the NC Cares program. This program provides health benefits and salary supplements to child-care providers who continue their education in the early childhood development and education field. In Box 17–5, describe how you think the education of health-care providers affects the quality of child care.

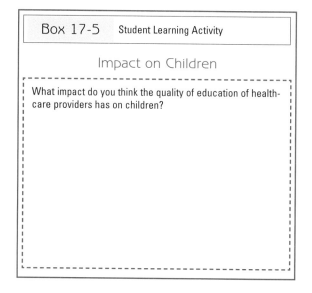

Box 17-5	Student Learning Activity

Impact on Children

What impact do you think the quality of education of health-care providers has on children?

Affordability

For those who can afford to put their children in a licensed child-care center, there are not always guarantees that these children will be safe. In many states, parents have no guarantees that even the minimum health and safety standards will be enforced.

Costs for full-day child-care services range from $4,000 to $10,000 per year. One-third of families with young children earn $25,000 per year or less; many do not receive any financial assistance to meet this expense (CDF, 2000). A 1999 U.S. Department of Health and Human Services report found that out of 15 million children eligible to receive financial assistance for child care, only 1 out of 10 actually received it (CDF, 2000).

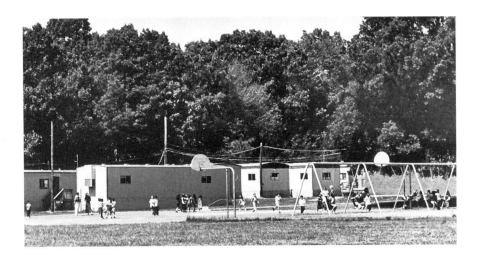

Access

Accessing child care is still a problem for low-income families even though Head Start was enacted in 1965 to provide comprehensive preschool to low-income 3- and 4-year-old children. It has been a model program for quality early childhood education offering physical and mental health care, nutrition, social services, and parent participation. Additional attention and assistance to low-income families was provided in 1976 by the Dependent Care Tax Credit created by Congress to partially offset child-care costs. Later, the Family Support Act of 1988 was enacted to help transition families off of welfare by helping to pay for child-care costs. The Child Care Development Block Grant (CCDBG) was passed in 1990 to assist low-income children (CDF, 2000).

Although child-care needs are evident, the low-income populations are still finding access difficult. High-quality programs are sometimes beyond the reach of parents because of unaffordable costs. Parents, out of necessity, sometimes turn to programs that they can afford, but that are poor in quality. According to The Study of Children in Family and Relative Care, 13 percent of regulated and 50 percent of nonregulated family child-care providers offer care rated as inadequate (Dombro, et al. 1996).

Parents cannot be productive on the job unless they have care for their child when and where they need it. Communities are not able to keep up with the increased demand for child-care services. The working poor and those who work nontraditional hours have an even more difficult time finding care for their children. Almost half of working poor parents work rotating schedules, so the Monday to Friday from 7 A.M. to 6 P.M. schedules at most child-care facilities may not be adequate. Many parents have to piece together child-care arrangements using a child-care program for one or two days, a neighbor the next, and an adolescent on another day. These factors can create problems for the child in terms of security and positive mental health.

Welfare reform has brought attention to this need for nontraditional hours for child-care services. Marriott International is an example of a corporation that has created a program that operates 24 hours a day, 365 days a year to meet the needs of employees in Atlanta. Other companies addressing the child-care need for nontraditional hours are Longaberger, America West Airlines, AT&T, Saturn, and Toyota.

THE NURSE IN THE CHILD-CARE CENTER

How does this background information relate to you? Nurses can play a critical role in improving the quality of child care in the community by using their core values, competencies, knowledge, and advocacy skills.

In Box 17–6, list some professional values that you think are important in a child-care center.

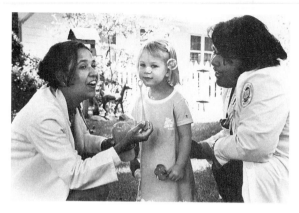

Box 17-6   Student Learning Activity

Professional Values

What professional values do you think you need to demonstrate in a community-based child-care center? Are they similar or different compared with those needed in acute-care settings?

Professional Values and Behavior

The values you need to work in a community-based child-care center are the same values you need to practice in any nursing role, namely: caring, altruism, autonomy, respect, integrity, and social justice (American Association of Colleges of Nursing, 1998). Concern for the well-being of children, a vulnerable population, means you have the opportunity to advocate for their needs and those of their families and providers. You can do this by demonstrating an empathetic and caring approach, taking time to better understand cultural similarities and differences that may impact the quality of care being provided, and advocating for healthy and safe environments.

The right to self-determination (autonomy) can be practiced when you provide health information and education to parents, families, and child-care providers on behalf of children. For instance, using a partnership approach, you can promote and teach healthy habits to parents and providers, which in turn can prevent injury and illness. Some examples of how you can do this include:

- Emphasizing the use of a properly secured infant car seat at all times
- Making sure an infant is put to rest on his or her back
- Ensuring that the crib being used has slats no more that 2 ⅜ inches apart
- Providing a smoke-free environment for the child
- Never leaving a baby unattended

It is through this information and education that parents and providers learn. It is by knowing what is right, safe, and healthy for their child that parents and providers then feel empowered to make their own right choices.

Respect is a core value in building and maintaining working relationships with children and their families. Without it, there can be no trust. Respect of the child, parents, and providers is demonstrated by the way you walk, talk, and act. Table 17–4 presents some ways to show respect for children and adults in a child-care center environment.

Think about how your body language conveys respect. Practice empathy. Stoop down to the level of the child's height to listen and to speak. Call him or her by name. Look directly at children and adults when you speak. Do

Table 17-4

Respect in the Child-care Center

- Look both children and adults in the eye. (Recognize this is not the norm for some cultures.)
- Call the child or adult by his/her name.
- Use a respectful tone of voice.
- Smile or frown as appropriate to the situation.
- Be nonjudgmental.
- Listen.
- Remember to keep information confidential.

you smile or do you frown? Do you use a diplomatic approach when confronting difficult situations, such as informing a mother that her daughter was biting one of her little friends today? Are you nonjudgmental when it comes to understanding each child and parent? Do you understand that parents may be afraid to ask you questions because they think you are the expert on children's issues and they don't want to be embarrassed?

You must be knowledgeable of, and open to, cultural similarities and differences. What is standard practice in one family is not in another. Do you inquire about these differences so you may better understand them, or do you remain a silent observer? Which approach would you want to have taken if you were the new parent in a different country?

Your integrity is critical. You must be open, honest, and sincere. It is important to be able to communicate when and how you can be of assistance, when you can provide that assistance, how you will provide it, and why. It is not always easy. The caring nurse, who is self-aware, also uses an "emotional intelligence" (Goleman, 1995) and an "intuitional intelligence" (Kaiser, 1999). These types of intelligences are additional skills, much like a sixth sense, that can assist you when "you just know" that something is not right. The nurse who hones in on these skills learns to listen, to accept, and to explore these feelings. In Box 17–7, write your ideas about how infection is related to interactions in child care.

Box 17-7   Student Learning Activity

Intuitional Intelligence

Reflect on a time when you "just knew" something was going to happen. Did you listen to your inner voice? What happened? For instance, maybe you noticed a change in the way a child was interacting with a parent. The child may have appeared afraid and reluctant to go home. Maybe you have observed a change in the child's disposition. You have a "feeling" something is wrong. What should you do? What did you do?

Upholding moral, legal, and humanistic principles (social justice) is another value that nurses need to demonstrate in nontraditional settings. Protecting the privacy and confidentiality of children and their families is an ethical obligation. You need to remember that information is treated confidentially in a child-care center, just as it would be in any other health-related environment. Box 17–8 provides a space for you to list types of confidential information you might find in a child-care center.

Box 17-8   Student Learning Activity

Social Justice

What are examples of confidential information that you might encounter in a community-based child-care center?

The following are examples of situations that must be treated confidentially:

- Information on children, such as who is doing the biting in a classroom setting
- Knowing a child is a carrier of hepatitis B
- Information on child-care providers, such as a teacher being fired for using inappropriate discipline methods with a child or a teacher who has informed you that he or she has the HIV virus
- Information on parents, such as knowing who is divorced, separated, or remarried; where they work; and what their family income may be

Social justice implies ethical, moral, and legal obligations, so it is important for the nurse to be familiar with current laws that impact a child-care program such as the Americans with Disabilities Act. Would you know what to do if a director of a child-care center told you that he or she was refusing to enroll a child with special needs into the center? A resource that defines questions and answers related to children with special needs and child care is the 1993 Child Care Law Center publication called

"Caring for Children with Special Needs: The Americans with Disabilities Act."

Another important way the nurse can be proactive in moral obligations in the child-care setting is by observing admission procedures. For instance, you may learn that the center's admission procedures do not even inquire whether children have access to health care. The nurse can be instrumental in promoting universal health care for children by informing and educating parents and providers of how uninsured children may be eligible for health-care insurance through the national Children's Health Insurance Program (CHIP). Child-care center enrollment practices can be easily revised to include the question of each and every parent, "Does your child have a primary-care physician?" This one question can make the difference as to whether children and their families receive the necessary health-promotion and injury-prevention care needed during the early years.

Your professional values are the foundation to practice and guide your interactions with clients, colleagues, and other health professionals. A resource that should prove valuable is "The Essentials of Baccalaureate Education for Professional Nursing Practice," which was originally developed in 1986 by the American Association of Colleges of Nursing and revised in 1998 (American Association of Colleges of Nursing [AACN], 1998). Although these guidelines were formalized for baccalaureate nursing programs, the content will benefit nurses at any stage of their education.

Competencies

Your basic function as a nurse in the community-based child-care center is to "first do no harm" and to promote optimal health for children, their families, and child-care providers. How do you do this? What core competencies and knowledge are needed? How does your role develop from being a student nurse to an experienced nurse? How do you transition from being a student of care to a provider of care? What experiences will help you develop further into a designer, a manager, a coordinator, or a consultant for health care? Competencies that are important to consider in relation to the nursing role in the child-care center include critical-thinking, communication, assessment, and technical skills.

Critical Thinking

Critical thinking is crucial to the nurse's work in the child-care setting. When the director of a child-care center calls the nurse with a problem, she or he must help. You must attentively listen and hear *all* of the facts. You must be adept at asking questions to get to the root of the problem without being judgmental. You must be clear and specific to gather more information. You may need to know how to analyze the data, synthesize it, interpret it, and recommend action to ensure the health and safety of children. The following is an example of how you might use your critical-thinking skills:

The director called and asked if I would help her with a problem. I immediately thought, "Now what?" I had heard this center was having problems, and quite frankly, I didn't want to get involved. After all, my child was safe. My curiosity took over and I found myself asking a lot of questions and finally agreed to meet with her. The director informed me she was having a lot of problems with children being injured on the playground. I immediately "put on my thinking hat" and started problem solving.

Working together, we identified the problem and a plan of action. The director later told me the plan had been effective in significantly reducing the number of injuries on the playground.

In Box 17–9, list questions you would want to ask the director in the situation just described.

Box 17-9	Student Learning Activity

Critical Thinking

Before you continue reading, think about what you would do if presented with the preceding problem. What type of questions would you be asking the director?

Look at the following list and see how you did using your critical-thinking skills.

- How many injuries were there in a day? A week? A month?
- What type of injuries?
- How did these numbers compare with the previous month?
- What has changed? New staff? New children? New equipment?
- Are younger children out on the playground at the same time as the older children?
- Are staff strategically located around the playground so that all children are within sight and sound?
- When was the last time the equipment was inspected? By whom?
- Are there written records that document the injuries and the staff involved?
- Are there playground rules? Do staff know and enforce these rules?
- How are parents informed of injuries? What action is taken with the staff?

Communication

You will need to communicate effectively using oral, nonverbal, and written communication skills. If you have never been in a community-based child-care center, you might have a misperception that "baby talk" should be used. On the contrary, as recent brain research indicates, it is during the first 3 years of life that the vast majority of brain "wiring" is produced (Shore, 1997). Verbal and nonverbal communication is stimulating to the children during these "prime times" and will most likely have a decisive and long-lasting impact on their future development (Shore, 1997).

The communication skills you demonstrate in the child-care center are important. You will need to be an active listener to decipher some of the new forming words of the toddler. You will quickly learn to tell children *what you want them to do,* instead of what you *don't* want them to do. For instance, instead of telling Johnny not to wipe his nose on his shirt, you would hand him a tissue and ask him to use it. After he tosses it into the trash and washes his hands, you would then praise him for using "healthy behavior." This communication style is a positive approach to learning and promotes children's mental health. When communicating with child-care providers and parents, be

Table 17-5

Child-care Center Jargon

DAP—Developmentally appropriate practice

Todds—Toddlers

DSS—Department of Social Services

IEPs—Individual education plans

NAEYC—National Association for the Education of Young Children

careful not to use "medical jargon." You will discover the early childhood education field has its own jargon (see Table 17-5) and "DAP," "Todds," " DSS," "IEPs," and "NAEYC" will become familiar to you as well!

Communication with parents requires diplomacy and a need to think carefully before you speak. Normal childhood growth and development can bring challenging behaviors such as biting, hitting, use of inappropriate language, and temper tantrums, all of which are painful to parents. How these incidents are communicated to the parent strengthens or weakens a relationship. Remember to use language that is supportive and and emphasizes that you want to work together to do what is best for the child. As in all other health-care environments, your written communication skills are important. Your documentation must be clear, accurate, and relevant.

Assessment

Assessment is gathering data about the health status of the client, analyzing and synthesizing the information, making judgments about interventions based on the findings, and evaluating the outcomes. It also includes understanding the child, family, or target populations and using the data from organizations and systems to plan and deliver services (AACN, 1998).

Examples of assessments that can be done in the child-care center are:

- Well-child assessments
- Risk-reduction assessments
- Environment and playground assessments

- Quality care assessments
- Developmental assessments
- Nutritional assessments
- Mental health assessments

Table 17-6

Assessment Tools

Caring for Our Children: The National Health and Safety Performance Standards for Out-of-Home Child Care Programs. Book and/or videos can be obtained by calling the National Child-care Information Center (NCCIC) at 800-616-2242.

Food for Thought: Nutrition and Children: Addresses children's dietary needs, food preparation, sanitation, and the social experiences of mealtime. Can be obtained by calling NAEYC Resources Sales at 800-424-2460.

Infant Toddler Environment Rating Scale (ITERS) and Early Childhood Environment Rating Scale (ECERS -R): Assessment tools used to measure quality in the child care environment. Authored by Harms & Cryder, they can be purchased through the Teachers College Press, New York.

Accreditation Guidelines for Early Childhood Education Programs: A self-study guide for programs seeking national accreditation. Contact National Association for the Education of Young Children (NAEYC) at 800-424-2460.

Table 17–6 presents examples of sources for some assessment tools.

Technical Skills

Acquisition and use of technical skills are required for the delivery of nursing care (AACN, 1998). Scientific principles underlie these skills, which are developed through course work and clinical experiences.

In Box 17–10, list important technical skills needed in a child-care center.

Following is a list of some technical skills that can be performed in a child-care setting:
- Vital signs
- Hand washing
- Teaching personal hygiene
- Immunizations
- Applying bandages

- Well-child assessments
- Medication administration
- Nebulizer treatments
- Applying heat and cold
- Administering cardiopulmonary resuscitation (CPR)
- Administering first aid
- Applying infection control measures
- Apnea monitors
- Teaching body mechanics to child-care providers
- Diaper changing
- Handling body fluids

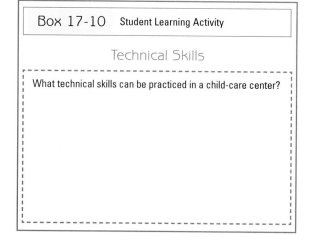

Box 17-10   Student Learning Activity

Technical Skills

What technical skills can be practiced in a child-care center?

Core Knowledge

Health Promotion, Risk Reduction, and Disease Prevention

Health promotion in the child-care environment requires knowledge about health risks and the methods to prevent or reduce those risks. To do this, it is essential to understand children's normal growth and development. Disease prevention knowledge includes methods for keeping an illness or injury from occurring, diagnosing and treating a disease early in its course, and preventing further deterioration (AACN, 1998). Health promotion and disease prevention in the child-care setting helps children, families, and child-care providers achieve an optimal level of wellness.

In Box 17–11, write your ideas about important core knowledge for child-care professionals.

Following is a list of health-education activities you

Box 17-11   Student Learning Activity

Core Knowledge

Write down some examples of health-promotion and disease-prevention activities you can provide in the child-care setting.

can provide in the child-care setting to promote health and reduce injury:

- Car seat safety
- Importance of dental care
- Poison control
- Infant sleeping positions to help prevent sudden infant death syndrome (SIDS)
- Importance of up-to-date immunizations
- Normal growth and development
- Positive discipline and behavior management

You may find that the Websites listed in Table 17–7 provide helpful information in implementing health-promotion, risk-reduction, and disease-prevention activities for children.

Table 17-7

Internet Resources

Healthy Child Care America: www.aap.org

National Resource Center for Health and Safety in Child Care: www.nrc.uchsc.edu

InsureKidsNow: www.insurekidsnow.gov

National Child Care Information Center: www.nccic.org

National Center for Education in Maternal and Child Health: www.ncemch.org

Illness and Disease Management

Illness and disease management require knowledge about pathophysiology of the disease, assessment and management of its symptoms, and the pharmacology used to treat the illness (AACN, 1998). Children who attend child-care programs are at increased risk for infectious disease, most commonly upper respiratory, diarrheal, and skin diseases (Dooling & Ulione, 2000). However, if current conditions persist, the major childhood diseases of the 21st century will be asthma and diabetes, and these illnesses will be seen at a much higher frequency in child-care centers.

Asthma rates are increasing worldwide. In the last 10 years, the rate has almost doubled in the United States. Asthma is the leading serious chronic illness among children and affects approximately 5 to 6 million children under age 18. Since 1979, asthma-related hospitalizations have increased 61 percent among children. According to a 1998 Centers for Disease Control and Prevention (CDC) report, asthma rates for children from birth to age 4, have increased 160 percent from 1980 to 1994 (Ruppenkamp, 1999). The nurse in the child-care center can play a vital role in preventing complications for these illnesses by providing health-education programs for the providers and the parents. Chapter 19 contains additional information about the problem of asthma for children in an elementary school.

In Box 17–12, list content you might teach about asthma.

Box 17-12   Student Learning Activity

Illness and Disease Management

Write down key elements you would teach providers and parents about the management of asthma.

It is also important for the nurse and the providers to have knowledge on the social, physical, psychological, and spiritual responses of the child and family with the illness so that they can serve as a support system. Using knowledge of illness and disease management, the nurse can do the following:

- Assess and manage symptoms
- Assess and manage pain
- Administer medications and therapies
- Anticipate and manage complications
- Anticipate and provide psychological support
- Link families with community services as needed

Ethics

The nurse in the community-based child-care program must be able to identify potential and actual ethical issues. As described in Chapter 7, ethics includes values, codes, and principles that govern decisions in nursing practice, conduct, and relationships. Read again a scenario used at the beginning of this chapter:

 I was totally taken by surprise. One of our parents informed me her 18-month-old son was a carrier of Hepatitis B. It wasn't a problem, until he started biting other children and broke the skin of another child.

List ethical considerations for this scenario in Box 17–13.

Box 17-13   Student Learning Activity

Ethics

Write down what you think are the ethical considerations in the preceding scenario.

How would you handle this situation, and why?

This situation is an example of what is actually happening in child-care centers. Cases like this present an ethical dilemma and an opportunity to use the critical-thinking skills as discussed earlier. Your knowledge and skills in the following areas should prove helpful to you as you encounter ethical dilemmas (AACN, 1998):

- High personal and professional values
- Application of the code of ethics
- Application of an ethical decision-making model
- Excellent communication and negotiation skills
- Personal accountability

Human Diversity

Your presence in the child-care center, as in any other environment, may present you with opportunities to experience cultures, races, religions, lifestyle variations, and socioeconomic levels different from your own (AACN, 1998). It will be important that you be open to understanding and learning about these differences. What you may discover is that we are all more alike than different. Remember to seek first to understand rather than to be understood, collaborate with others, be sensitive to cultural differences, and provide a holistic approach.

The Nurse as Advocate

Americans are voicing strong support for making quality child care, including early education and after-school care, a major national priority (CDF, 2000). In a poll conducted in August 1999, two-thirds of those surveyed agreed that providing access to early education programs and after-school programs was more important than cutting taxes (CDF, 2000). Faith Wohl, president of the Child Care Action Campaign, recommends four ways to bring higher-quality and more affordable child care to more children, namely speak out for better care, create new partnerships, work to influence public policy, and take part in a broader campaign (Wohl, 1999).

Furthermore, role development can take you to other opportunities to advocate for the needs of children and families in the policy arena either at a local, state, or federal level. These are opportunities to advocate for health care and child care for *all* of America's children.

Table 17-8

What Nurses Can Do to Advocate for
Healthy Child Care

1. Advocate for quality child-care programs!

2. Promote access for all children to have a medical and
   dental "home."

3. Advocate for improvement of local and state health and
   child-care regulations.

4. Offer expertise to provide health screenings.

5. Provide health-education programs for children, families,
   and staff.

6. Assist in the development of health policies and
   procedures.

7. Scan the environment, identify risk factors, and make
   recommendations for improvement.

8. Promote the integration of health and safety in daily lesson
   plans.

9. Be a positive role model of healthy behavior to others.

Nurses interested in advocating for children's child-care needs are obtaining training at the National Training Institute for Child Care Health Consultants at the University of North Carolina at Chapel Hill. The training program addresses health-care issues such as: inclusion of children with special needs, facilitation and consultation skills, injury prevention, nutrition, child abuse prevention, infectious diseases, mental health, and advocacy. This program is provided through federal funding from the Maternal Child Health Bureau, Health Resources and Services Administration, as part of the development of a systems approach to integrate health, child care, and social services.

RESEARCH STUDIES

Community-based studies have addressed the quality of child care. The executive summary of The National Child Care Staffing Study done in 1989 noted that serv-ices provided by most centers were rated as having barely adequate quality (National Center for the Early Childhood Workforce, 1989).

In other research, a four-state study of quality in child-care centers discovered that only one out of seven were rated as "good" quality (Cost, Quality and Outcomes Study Team, 1995). This same study reported that 1 out of 10 child-care centers provided inadequate care and jeopardized the health and safety of children. Another national survey identified that only four states met the standards recommended by experts for adult supervision in child care (Holcomb, 1999).

The author carried out a telephone survey to find out the most frequently asked questions to nurses from staff in child-care centers. Table 17–9 presents results from this survey.

Table 17-9

Top 10 Frequently Asked Questions of
Nurses by Child-care Providers

1. What child-care health policies do I need?

2. When should I exclude a child from the center?

3. How sick is too sick?

4. Do I have to take a child with special needs into my
   center?

5. How long do children with head lice need to stay home?

6. Should a child with thick nasal mucus see a doctor?

7. How high should I let a fever go before I call the parent?

8. What should I do with the child whose behavior is
   disruptive?

9. Can we expel a child who keeps biting?

10. What are the tricks for toilet training?

*Source: Author's telephone survey of Child Care Health
Consultant colleagues, 1999.*

FUTURE TRENDS

Air and water pollution, along with lead poisoning, will continue to be environmental hazards for children. The American Academy of Pediatrics (AAP) published the *Handbook of Pediatric Environmental Health*, which has more than 30 chapters on prevention and treatment of childhood environmental health problems (CDF, 2000).

Be prepared to see a paradigm shift as we move farther into the 21st century and the focus for child-care services shifts from "child-care centers" to "family centers." The

evolution to a family center model has already begun in some places where child-care centers now offer additional services, such as take-home dinners for busy working parents and dry cleaning services where parents can drop off their laundry with their child and pick both up at the end of the day. Programs will focus on the whole family and not just the child, recognizing that for the child to be successful, the needs of the entire family must also be met. Table 17–10 reflects the paradigm shift from child development centers to Family Centers (Greenman, 1999).

Table 17-10

Paradigm Shift from Child Development Center to Family Center

BASIC UNIT	THE CHILD	THE FAMILY
Primary Focus	Child's well-being and security	Whole family's well-being and security
	Comprehensive child development and education	Comprehensive child and family development and education
	Social development	Child and family social development
	Emotional development	Child and family emotional development
	Physical development	Family economic development
	Child-oriented values	Family-oriented values
Services	Primarily for children under age 6	Care/education for all ages
	Primarily 6 A.M.–6 P.M.	Hours to fit family's schedule
		Tailored services
		Back-up care
		Emergency care
		School-age/teen care
		Elder-care support
		Educational services
		Adult/family services

CONCLUSION

Societal needs are dictating that health services be provided in nontraditional locations such as child-care centers. Nurses can play a vital role in improving the health and safety of children using their values, competencies, skills, and knowledge. Nurses can act as advocates to promote and change health and child-care policies to advance national, state, and local health objectives, which can increase the span of healthy lives, reduce health disparities, and increase access to prevention services.

Active Learning Strategies

1. Interview a child-care center director to determine the daily health and safety issues that are encountered and ask how you can provide assistance.

2. Interview three parents who currently have their children enrolled in a child-care program. Ask them to rate the center, staff, and curriculum on its level of quality.

3. Interview one of your local legislators and ask what her or his views are on child care. Ask for examples of how the crisis is being addressed.

4. Identify one area in the early care and education field that you feel needs attention. Research your area of interest. Write an article to a newspaper or journal advocating for change.

References

American Association of Colleges of Nursing (AACN). (1998). The essentials of baccalaureate education for professional nursing practice. Washington, DC: Author.

Children's Defense Fund (CDF). (2000). Yearbook 2000: The state of America's children. Washington, DC: Author.

Cost, Quality, and Outcomes Study Team. (1995). Cost, quality and child outcomes in child care centers, technical report. University of Colorado at Denver.

Decker, C., & Decker, J. (1997). Planning and administering early childhood programs. Upper Saddle River, NJ: Prentice Hall.

Dooling, M., & Ulione, M. (2000). Health consultation in child care: A partnership that works. Young Children, 55(2), 23–26.

Dombro, A. L., O'Donnell, N. S., Galinsky, E., Melcher, S. G., & Farber A. (1996). Community mobilization: Strategies to support young children and their families. New York: Families and Work Institute.

Goleman, D. (1995). Emotional intelligence. NY: Bantam.

Greenman, J. (1999). The family center of the 21st century. Solutions. Spring/Summer. Cambridge, MA.

Kagan, S. (1997). Highlights of quality 2000. Young Children, 52, 54–62.

Kaiser, L. (1999). Intentional Intelligence. The Health Forum Journal, 42(50), 180–183.

National Association for the Education of Young Children (NAEYC). (1998). Guide to accreditation. Washington, DC: Author.

Ruppenkamp, J. (1999). 101 ways to reduce allergens in your home for people living with allergies or asthma. Merrifield, VA: Positive Publishing.

Shore, R. (1997). Rethinking the brain: New insights into early development. New York: Families and Work Institute.

U.S. Department of Health and Human Services. Healthy Child Care America: Blueprint for action. (1996). National Center for Education in Maternal and Child Health. Washington, DC: Author.

Willer, B. (Ed.). (1990). Reaching the full cost of quality in early childhood programs. Washington, DC: NAEYC.

Wohl, F. (1999). Making a difference in child care through advocacy. Solutions, 6–7.

Applying Primary Care Skills to Community-based Practice

CHAPTER 18

Community-based Nursing Practice in a Senior Center

Joanne C. Langan

LEARNING OBJECTIVES

1) Define primary health care, primary care, and primary prevention.

2) List selected primary-care skills that may be applied in a senior center.

3) Describe the demographic trends in growth of the population aged 65 years or greater.

4) Identify opportunities, challenges, and action plans to enhance the students' personal and professional development.

Some of the key tenets of our junior-level community-based clinical at George Mason University College of Nursing and Health Science are health promotion, disease prevention, and the application of primary-care skills in a community-based practice. We also seek to provide these primary-care skills to a vulnerable population. We chose the elderly as our population in the clinical section placed at a senior center. This chapter presents a definition of primary health care and describes specific skills that are used in the performance of primary care.

Student excerpts are presented to illustrate the application of primary-care skills, the strengths of the clinical site, and the challenges.

WHAT IS PRIMARY HEALTH CARE?

Primary health care is differentiated from early definitions of primary care. Primary health care is defined as an "approach to health care that focuses on promotion of health and prevention of disease across the continuum of care. In contrast to primary care, in which the principal focus has been on the professional-client dyad and a client's first contact with medical providers, primary health care is concerned with the health of communities or populations" (National Nursing Research Agenda, 1993, p. 2). The panel defines primary health care as including the following:

a. All members of a population having access to health services

b. Individual, family, and community involvement in the identification of health priorities and the planning and implementation of health-care services

c. Services that are preventive and health promotive rather than just curative

d. Integration of health development with economic and social development

e. Attention to clients' culturally acceptable health practices (p. 2).

PRIMARY CARE AS COMPLEMENT TO PRIMARY HEALTH CARE

The Institute of Medicine's definition of primary care has varied over time. Earlier definitions emphasized comprehensive and accessible provision of care by accountable personnel (Institute of Medicine, 1978); and provision of services "to a defined community, coupled with systematic efforts to identify and address the major health problems of that community." (Institute of Medicine, 1988, p. 2). The Institute of Medicine later redefined primary care to include concepts such as "integrated, accessible health care services, accountability of providers, attention to a wide range of individual needs, development of a long-term partnership with clients, and the broader family and community context of health care" (1994, p. 1). This definition of primary care complements the definition of primary health care, because primary health care focuses on the provision of care for individuals, families, and communities on a continuum. The notion of a continuum of care requires a great deal of communication and coordination among caregivers and providers. In both primary health care and the Institute of Medicine's redefinition of primary care, health promotion and education efforts are considered part of integrated, long-term health plans. These long-term health plans are to target individuals,

families, and communities and include attention to social and economic factors that may compromise health and well-being. The goal is to enable individuals and groups to choose a healthy lifestyle and to support them in assessing their lifestyle changes and caring for family members.

PRIMARY PREVENTION

Armentrout (1998) states that primary prevention measures are taken to prevent a problem before it occurs. Primary prevention measures include wearing seatbelts and bicycle helmets and obtaining health education and immunizations. Primary prevention is equated with health promotion because both attempt to increase health and prevent illness. Armentrout predicts that greater effort will be made to keep people healthy in a cost-effective way, and great value in the form of reimbursement will eventually be placed on health and wellness promotion and primary prevention. These concepts take on special meaning for specific populations. The elderly as a specific, vulnerable population are the focus of this discussion.

DEMOGRAPHIC TRENDS OF THE AGED

Demographic trends continue to show an increasing proportion of older adults in the population. In 1990, 12.6 percent of the U.S. population was 65 years old or older (U.S. Bureau of the Census, 1990). By the year 2020, persons over age 65 in the United States are expected to constitute 20 percent of the total population. Between 1980 and 1991, the population between 75 to 84 years of age grew by 33 percent to 10.3 million. The population 85 years and over grew by 41 percent to 3.2 million. The total number of persons exceeding age 65 has reached over 30 million (U.S. Department of Health and Human Services, 1994). Ninety-five percent of older adults live independently in the community or interdependently with support networks from family, friends, or neighbors (Arrington, 1997).

An increasing vulnerability and chronic illness that can threaten older adults' ability to live independently often accompany advancing age. Nursing care at home or

> *When health is absent*
> *Wisdom cannot reveal itself,*
> *Art cannot become manifest,*
> *Strength cannot be exerted,*
> *Wealth is useless and*
> *Reason is powerless.*
>
> Herophilus

in a senior center is part of an integrated approach to community-based, long-term care that can facilitate independence and manage health-care issues over time (Magilvy, Congdon, & Martinez, 1994).

Although disabilities such as arthritis, visual impairment, hearing impairments, high blood pressure, depression, and diabetes increase with age, there has been a trend toward better relative health among the aged in the last two decades. Improved health practices throughout the life span and a higher level of education have been found to contribute to the trend toward healthier aging (Fries, Williams, & Morfeld, 1992).

Greater numbers of elderly live independently in the community as a result of healthier aging. One form of independent living is found in retirement communities. These communities generally attract well elderly individuals (Arrington, 1997). Another client setting is the adult day-care center. In this setting, well elderly individuals with minor health deviations may socialize, enjoy nourishing meals, and be intellectually stimulated in a safe, protected environment. In either of these types of settings, nursing faculty and students can support healthy aging and learn valuable lessons about aging by encouraging health-promotion activities, providing health monitoring, and presenting health education information.

Nursing academicians realize that our future nurses must be prepared to provide care to this aging population in a variety of settings. Arrington (1997) stated, "The extraordinary number of elderly expected to live into the next century calls for creative inclusion of this population in learning experiences for students in baccalaureate nursing programs . . . [communities] offer a rich environment for interaction and learning with the well elderly that encourages students to consider the limitless possibilities for nursing interventions with our greatest national resource: the elderly" (p. 82). In this particular clinical course, we emphasized the practice of primary-care skills in a community-based setting, a combination of adult day care/assisted living senior center (senior center).

HOW PRIMARY-CARE SKILLS ARE APPLIED TO THE ELDERLY: THE GEORGE MASON UNIVERSITY SENIOR CENTER MODEL

The experiences that are shared in this chapter are largely the experiences of the first junior-level nursing section to experience a community-based clinical at this combination adult day care/assisted living senior center. The students and faculty members collaborated with the health-care team both within and outside of the senior center to achieve the application of primary-care skills in this setting.

The goal of the application of our primary-care skills was to teach individuals and their families how to choose a healthy way of living. We offered support to families in assessing their lifestyle changes and showed caring for family members, both the assigned clients and their caregivers. We needed to assess the readiness of the individuals, family members, and groups to participate in their own health care and the degree of their involvement in active decision making. Some of the elderly clients were mentally and intellectually intact and participated actively. They were able to listen attentively and apply the primary-care skills that were taught. Others were only partially or not capable of the application of health-promotion strategies independent of family members. However, through a variety of teaching methods, the students were able to "reach" all of the clients in the adult day-care program and most of the clients in assisted living in some way. The students made a difference. A humorous example of this is the level of competition that developed among the assisted living residents during seated daily exercises. One 80-year-old lady wanted to be the one to raise her extended leg or arm higher than anyone else in the group. That group's keen sense of competition did not diminish with advancing years!

Table 18-1

Sample List of Nursing Student Teaching Projects at Senior Center

Community resources for the elderly

Finger stick method and blood glucose values

Progressive phases of Alzheimer's disease

What is blood pressure and how is it measured?

Exercise for seniors

Hearing loss and practical tips on the use and care of hearing aids

Proper fit and care of dentures

The list of student teaching/learning projects (Table 18–1) shows the shift from an illness focus to one emphasizing disease prevention and health promotion. Proper fit and care of dentures aid in the promotion of appropriate nutrition. Proper fit and care of hearing aids promotes increased communication and participation in social activities, which promotes a sense of well-being. The seniors were very interested in the blood pressure screenings and the true meaning of the measures. This knowledge promoted compliance with healthy eating habits and medication administration. Though the nursing students' teaching could not cure any of the preexisting conditions of this population, they could impact the current state of wellness.

Although this junior-level clinical was concerned with the elderly as a vulnerable population, our focus was on individuals, families, and small groups. We offered the same access to services to all persons at the senior center. Some of the participants in the adult day-care program and some of the residents in the assisted living unit refused to participate, and we honored their choice. By recognizing the individual freedom to choose, we also involved the individual and family members in the identification of health priorities and the planning and implementation of health-care services. For instance, one individual's assessment revealed urinary incontinence. With the individual and family, a plan was developed to implement bladder training. The assigned student offered trips to the toilet on regular intervals and assessed for incontinence and skin breakdown. This was a very positive experience for all involved. The client enjoyed the attention and intact skin, the family appreciated the opportunity to provide input into the plan and evaluation, and the student learned the application of the nursing process and collaboration and was thrilled with the positive outcome of her preventive and health-promotive measures.

In the case of the incontinent client, the preventive and health-promotive interventions clearly proved to be cost effective. The client's family was able to avoid the purchase of additional units of incontinence briefs. There was no added expense of barrier creams, skin care treatment, or treatment for potential complicating infection processes. Interestingly, the client also agreed to the promotion of hydration because the problem of incontinence was being addressed.

Another important focus of this clinical was the attention to clients' culturally acceptable health practices. The students learned the "language" of some of the elderly, such as the use of "powders" for pain, and the measurement of "sugar" instead of blood glucose. Some of the clients were willing to divulge a great deal about their current health and health history whereas others chose to keep this information private. Certainly, in most cases, more information was forthcoming once rapport and familiarity with the students were developed. The students implemented additional culturally sensitive behaviors. They learned that they needed to escort the clients more slowly, speak in the front of the clients at eye level, and present less health information in shorter sessions. Those clients who wanted more specific information about selected topics were given supplemental teaching/learning opportunities on an individual basis. Complete Box 18–1 to further discuss the teaching needs of the elderly.

In keeping with the concept of primary health care, communication and coordination among caregivers and providers was evident at the senior center. The codirector shared much information with the students regarding family members' decision-making processes when choosing the most appropriate placement for their loved ones. Each level of care has specific criteria for clients to be accepted. For example, an adult day-care program is not acceptable for an individual who requires complex care.

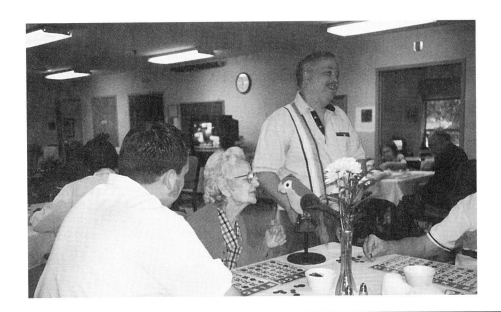

Box 18-1	Student Learning Activity

Teaching the Elderly

Discuss additional accommodations that might be necessary to make when addressing/teaching the elderly.

Consider sensory deficits, educational level, literacy, presence of Alzheimer's, or other mental deficits.

Box 18-2	Student Learning Activity

Care Settings for the Elderly

Identify instances that might require an elderly person who is living independently in the community to move to long-term care.

Can you list conditions that might cause an independent elderly individual to require an acute-care setting, rehabilitation, and then return to independent living in the community?

The directors of each facility confer with the individuals, families, physicians, psychiatrists, and those persons who are able to provide expert opinions regarding appropriate placement for individuals. As individual needs change, the team approach to decision making occurs again. At times, clients need more acute or complex care, and they move along the continuum of care from independent living, to adult day care, to assisted living, to rehabilitation, and eventually long-term care or back to more independent living based on capabilities. Complete Box 18–2 to further discuss care settings for the elderly.

The students were able to become actively involved with families in their quest for assisted living or long-term care placement for their family members. One student developed questions for a daughter to ask at a potential long-term care site for her mother.
- Is there 24-hour registered nurse coverage?
- Can residents bring their own medications or does the agency need to provide them?

- Is there an on-site physician or nurse practitioner available?
- Does the agency have on-site eye care, immunizations, occupational therapy, or physical therapy?
- Are pet visits allowed?
- Are residents encouraged to eat their meals with other residents or do they eat in their rooms?
- Is there a daily exercise program?

We all learned to be sensitive to the needs of the family members who were also the caregivers to the adult day-care participants. Many of these families had children at home, full-time jobs, and one or more parents living in the home. They were not always available for family assessment interviews because of their busy schedules. Again, we honored their wishes, adjusted, and learned to accommodate them. These families were extremely grateful for the resource finding that our students engaged in, especially in finding assistive devices for the home and visiting potential assisted living and long-term care sites.

Box 18–3 contains a client example for you to complete.

Box 18-3	Student Learning Activity

Client Example

Your assignment is to complete a family assessment on a client and his family. You wait by the front door of the center to meet the client and family member. The client does not attend the day-care program that day. What do you do?

You eventually contact the client's daughter. She is very warm and receptive to the idea of meeting with you to complete the family assessment. You suggest that you would be glad to go to the family home for the interview. You are thinking that you would then have the opportunity to assess the home environment for safety. The daughter tells you that she would rather meet at the center on repeated visits than to have you come to the home. What do you do? How can you get the information about the home environment?

Student Feedback

At the George Mason University College of Nursing and Health Science, we value the input of our students regarding our agency selections and their learning experiences. Students have the opportunity to provide this feedback at midterm in formative evaluations and at the end of the semester in summative evaluations. When possible, faculty members are encouraged to modify teaching methods and strategies of achieving course objectives after the formative evaluations are received and realistic suggestions are offered.

One very creative method used by the students to offer feedback regarding this clinical experience was invented by the first group of nursing students to use this combination adult day care/assisted living senior center. They created a video to share how they were able to meet each course objective at this unique site. Still pictures as well as video were taken throughout the semester with the permission of the agency and participants. This video project accomplished two main objectives. First, the students developed a real team spirit in choosing the script for the video and appropriate depictions of their activities. Second, they were able to understand how primary-care services can be delivered in a community-based site. All 10 students collaborated on this project, and their description of how each of the course objectives were met and sample activities follows:

 We have had the opportunity to apply necessary skills, knowledge, and attitudes in a community-based senior center, through interactions with individuals who have physiological, psychological, and social needs.

Adult Day Care is a protective environment geared to serve individuals who, because of mental or physical impairment, cannot remain alone during the day.

The Adult Day Care Center is a stimulating atmosphere aimed at encouraging the individuals to utilize capabilities to their maximum. It is also a place of socialization where effects of isolation can be avoided.

We were given the opportunity to incorporate concepts from pathophysiology, health assessment, and other technologies into the nursing process. [Blood pressures daily, health assessments, medication administration, range of motion exercises, vital signs.]

During the clinical we developed important therapeutic relationships with both the individuals and their families. [Active listening to clients and their families, giving information.] We also collaborated with members of the health-care team, individuals, and family members to determine the health education needs of the participants. [Had access to client admission records to senior center as well.]

We were encouraged to demonstrate caring and sensitive nursing interventions for individuals and their families who are experiencing developmental and situational crises. [Rescheduled assessment sessions, assisted families with emergent issues.]

We also planned and implemented health-promotion and disease-prevention strategies with individuals and small groups. [Sample list of student teaching projects, Table 18–1.]

An important criterion in achieving these objectives was to have fun with this energetic population. [Sang, danced, played Bingo, laughed.]

We assisted with and planned various activities to stimulate the participants creatively, intellectually, and physically. [Teaching projects/activities.]

The staff at the Adult Day Care Center has been very supportive of us in our endeavors to meet our course objectives. We are very grateful for this opportunity to learn.

STUDENTS' EVALUATION OF THE SENIOR CENTER AS A CLINICAL PLACEMENT

Students were asked to evaluate the ease with which course objectives could be met at this site. Varying reactions were received. Some stated that with some effort, the objectives were all obtainable at this senior center, but that the students needed to be creative, imaginative, and collaborative. Student excerpts follow.

- Great opportunity for collaboration with staff, family members, and residents.
- Not all of us were fortunate enough to do a home visit so that assessment was difficult. I found the family that I worked with to be very open to my suggestions [and] help and they helped me with my family assessment.
- [I was able to] apply pathophysiology knowledge to [clients'] situations and look at expected behaviors/outcomes.

- Students have to actively seek out opportunities to meet clinical course objectives, but they are obtainable.
- The site offered a diverse population of elderly. Assisted living and day care provided us opportunities to observe and give out medicines and perform some technologies.
- Because we were the first clinical group to use this agency as a community-based site, there were some initial barriers to overcome. It took time to build a rapport with all interested parties. With the passage of time, meeting course objectives became less challenging.

Strengths and challenges of the clinical site were also assessed. The students listed the following as strengths of the senior center.

- Opportunities for learning are present. Finding enough of them is difficult to fill the full time allotted.
- It is not a nursing home, so we did not feel pressured into doing nursing assistant duties.
- The staff was very supportive and patient with us.
- The residents and participants were very receptive to us and what we had to offer.
- The site allows for a large amount of creativity and independence on behalf of the student—this can present as a challenge if the student is not very driven.
- Plenty of opportunities to learn and grow.
- Faculty is very warm and accepting of nursing students as well as participants and residents.
- Flexibility and openness of staff.
- The availability of the patients and their willingness to participate in student activities.
- This site really presents the elderly in a good light and helps show the student what life over 65 is like.
- [The faculty member] made us find pathophysiology and pharmacology opportunities at the site—some were not obvious.

These comments emphasized the students desire to be accepted and welcomed into the clinical site. The faculty member's role as role model is clearly evident.

The nursing students were also given the opportunity to list the challenges encountered at the Senior Center.

- Developing doable plans of teaching.
- This is a very busy day care with a full daily agenda. It was sometimes hairy to find appropriate times to squeeze in the activities of 10 different students.
- [The day] was much too long.

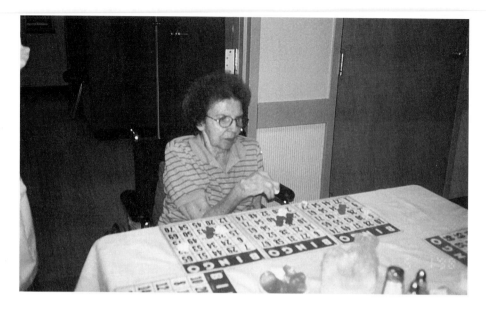

- Adjusting our activities and teaching sessions to fit our audience since our audience had different needs, different interests, and different levels of dementia.
- The only challenge was within myself—I kept myself busy, always looking for an opportunity to learn—self-directed.
- Very difficult to meet "home visit" assignment.
- You really need to work twice as hard to use the "outside" community.
- The biggest challenge . . . was dealing with the dementia and depression of some of the residents.
- You need to look closely to find pathophysiology and pharmacology objectives, but they are there.

Interestingly, the students each had unique needs and challenges at this site. I was not surprised by their list of challenges. It was not easy to develop this site. However, this was a very mature group of students who bonded well and supported each other. Natural leaders emerged and assisted those who needed encouragement. Talents were shared, and the students progressed as a team. Mutual respect was shared among the faculty member, students, staff, and clients. There seemed to be a kind of metamorphosis among the students from the first weeks of the experience to the last days of the clinical. Indeed, tears were shed as we prepared the clients for our departure on our last day. Box 18–4 contains a thought question for you to complete.

Box 18-4	Student Learning Activity

Student Responsibility

Discuss the following question:

Do you think that it is a student responsibility to take initiative in finding activities to meet course objectives? Give the rationale for your response.

Student Perceptions of the Senior Center as Clinical Site

Students had varying perceptions about expectations at this new clinical site. They voiced a great deal of trepidation about the senior center being "just another old folks' home." The transition in their perceptions is illustrated in their descriptions of their experiences.

After my initial experience first semester at the long-term care center, I had a negative opinion of long-term care facilities, and families who would place their loved ones in such a place. I did not want to be at [the senior center]. At [the senior center], I learned that not all long-term care facilities are created equal and how much caring staff makes a difference. It demonstrated how good management and nursing staff could influence a facility. I was able to understand the struggle, both emotional and financial, the family undergoes in their decision to put their family member in long-term care. The interview/home visit with the family was very valuable in demonstrating to me the grieving the family experiences when their family member is unable to function in the role they are accustomed to playing in the family. It was also very valuable to be able to talk to both the resident [in assisted living] and the participants [in adult day care] on their perception of their health and why they were there. After my time at this clinical site, I had a greater understanding of the families, the residents, participants, and the staff and the balance of relationships among them.

Another student shared that he anticipated more correctly the expectations of the clinical agency:

I was expecting a clinical experience at a nursing home, working with the elderly population. I knew that this is what I signed up for and expected to work with the elderly. It added to the experience by spending seven weeks in adult day care and then switching to seven weeks in assisted living.

Working with the elderly population made us understand that their needs are as important as everyone else's. It was an eye-opening experience and gave the group good practice with cultural and age barriers. It provides excellent opportunities to practice technologies such as medication administration, injections, and therapeutic communication. It showed the group the importance of the future of nursing since the population is getting older.

The importance of the students learning to administer medications to the elderly and the students teaching the elderly about their medications cannot be overemphasized. Senior citizens commonly take multiple medications and lack knowledge about proper use and side effects. Seniors often have no access to health professionals to clarify misconceptions about their medications. Frequently, nursing students learn pharmacology in the classroom with no opportunity to apply the knowledge, as it is learned (Wissmann & Wilmoth, 1996).

Our students collected drug histories from the clients in both adult day care and assisted living. Charts were checked from all clients to verify what the clients reported with the documents on record. Following the analysis of the gathered data, our students developed individualized teaching plans for their assigned clients. Many discrepancies were found between the reported drug histories and the clients' current physician orders. The students tailored their teaching for appropriateness after a thorough learning ability assessment and a great deal of critical thinking. The students, in conjunction with the staff, families, and physicians, collaborated frequently. The learning needs of both the clients and the students were met. Wissmann and Wilmoth (1996) used a similar teaching method through a community-based pharmacology experience at a senior center whose clients had drug-knowledge deficits or compliance difficulties.

The students continued to share their impressions of the clinical experience and expressed the value of their presence.

Because we were the first clinical group to use this site, we had a slow start not really knowing our roles. We made a difference and I think the participants, residents, and staff saw and felt the impact we made as a group and were very impressed. As far as I am concerned, I think we made our mark and set the standard for students in this setting.

Yet another student described her experience and first impressions:

I expected to have yet another semester working in a nursing home setting. I immediately thought, "I just had a similar experience, now I have to do 14 more weeks!"

Our [senior center] was not like a nursing home. Working with the participants was such a joy. They were so full of fun and eager to listen to all of our presentations.

The staff was very friendly and extremely supportive, and was happy to assist us in all of our miniprojects. Opportunities were available in this setting to make a difference.

Being "trailblazers" gave us the freedom to try different things and see what worked.

Even though the students freely shared the challenges of the clinical site, some had truly meaningful experiences and wrote about them in their clinical journals. The following student shared his most meaningful experience at the Senior Center:

> *My most meaningful experience at [the Senior Center] was while performing my teaching/learning project. I taught M.S., a resident in the assisted living area, about arthritis. M.S. has had arthritis for about 60 years and knew very little about the disease that has innervated her joints and disfigured her fingers. M.S. voiced interest in the subject during a miniteaching on osteoporosis. During the teaching project, M.S. asked numerous questions and enthusiastically participated in the exercises. Even though M.S. has very limited use of her hands, she has been performing the exercises to help increase flexibility or decrease pain every day since [I presented] the teaching project. The teaching project was interesting and I learned more from the experience than M.S. probably did. I hope that the information that I shared with M.S. stays with her and helps her for years to come.*

It is likely that M.S. benefited greatly from the student's teaching and individual health counseling. A descriptive, exploratory study conducted by Viverais-Dresler, Bakker, and Vance (1995) examined elderly clients' perceptions of individualized health counseling and group wellness sessions. The 36 elderly participants in the study reported that the monitoring of health status, support, and health teaching were valued nursing activities within individualized health counseling. Participants shared that group wellness sessions were an effective means of acquiring general knowledge about aging and lifestyle choices, but that this format could not totally meet all their health-care needs. In this study, blood pressure monitoring was viewed as important to the elderly. The study authors stated that recognition of elderly clients' perceptions was crucial in planning and implementing programs that were appropriate and acceptable for improving the quality of life for this age group.

Additional evidence in a study by Kreidler, Campbell, Lanik, Gray, and Conrad (1994) suggests that health provider actions over time positively influence client readiness to change health behaviors. This suggests that students and faculty members in community-based sites should reinforce lessons taught and be positive role models. Perhaps modeling speaks louder than words.

Not all of the students shared positive remarks concerning this new clinical site. One student was frightened about state boards and worried that she needed more hospital experience. Another bemoaned the fact that some family members preferred to meet with the students at the clinical site instead of the family home. The adult day-care director explained that these were very busy, working families that brought their spouses or parents to day care as a respite. They may have found it easier to spend time with the students while their loved one was engaged in an activity at the senior center. In any case, the students recommended that future students meet their families early in the semester to help the students focus their direction in finding community resources for their families.

Simulated Home Visits/Critical Thinking

Because some of the students were not able to conduct home visits, I compensated by presenting simulated home visit case studies as critical-thinking exercises in postconference each week. Students were given a written scenario and were to write responses in an outline according to the nursing process—assessment, plan, implementation, and evaluation. They were to prioritize problems and actions and state what resources were needed for each individual and family to help the family cope more effectively. Each student shared his or her responses and gave the rationale for the responses. The group constructively critiqued and praised group members. Some of the key concepts discussed through these critical-thinking exercises were community-based primary health care, cultural diversity and sensitivity, community resources, interdisciplinary collaboration, and client advocacy.

Future Directions

As a recommendation for future placement at the senior center, I would like to see additional sites developed in conjunction with the senior center. There are two private elementary schools that border the senior center on each side that may agree to participate. Another interesting site to pursue is an assisted living facility that houses a child-care center. The resident seniors interact with the children in the center. It may be interesting to compare and contrast sites and rotate the students between the two sites. Perhaps the two groups of seniors could develop pen pals and then invite the "sister" group to the adult day-care center for a health fair and picnic to actually meet their pen pals.

Brennan (1992) described the Computer Link project, a specialized computer network designed to support caregivers of persons with Alzheimer's disease (AD). In a randomized field experiment, 102 AD caregivers participated, and 47 caregivers had access to Computer Link for 12 months. During this time, Computer Link was accessed 3,888 times. The researcher stated that these behavioral indicators demonstrate that Computer Link promotes collaboration by providing a means of communication among caregivers and by facilitating their access to information. This type of system could be introduced to AD caregivers at one of the monthly AD meetings at the senior center. Caregivers may feel continuous support as they "link" with other caregivers from their homes if they choose to adopt a system such as Computer Link.

CONCLUSION

One of the 10 students who piloted the use of the senior center as a community-based clinical site made the following statement at the end of the semester:

When the clinical experience in the [Senior Center] was completed, I had a special feeling. It was like a feeling of a job well done; that I knew I did what I could do to help take care of the clients. It gave me a feeling that is hard to describe but I think every nurse would know what I am talking about. Another great experience was the relationship I formed with the group. After spending the semester with the same crew, I saw the teamwork and effort we all put into the Center. Because of this, I was able to see the end result of the positive impact we made on the Center with the clients and the staff.

Although the initiation of this Senior Center as a clinical site required a great deal of effort from both the faculty member's and students' perspective, the experience was worth the effort. The collaboration among all parties—the individuals, families, agency personnel, faculty, students, and community resource persons—enriched the learning. Those students who approached the clinical with a positive attitude toward exploring new challenges developed lifelong skills. Indeed, there was a renewed appreciation for the difference that even novice nurses can make in the application of primary-care skills.

Active Learning Strategies

1. Discuss with your class how you, as nursing students, could create a system (such as a computer modification of the Computer Link) to link caregivers at a senior center through the use of the computer. What other types of communication/collaboration links for family caregivers can you think of?

2. Work with a classmate to make a list of potential teaching projects for clients in a senior center you will visit. Share your list with other groups in your class and prioritize the projects according to which ones appear most important for these clients.

3. Visit a senior center and talk with a client from a culture that is different from yours. Ask the client about how nurses could demonstrate sensitivity to his or her specific cultural needs.

4. What challenges you would encounter if you attempted to teach a client with dementia? With depression? Discuss with a classmate where you would obtain resources to help with this problem.

References

Armentrout, G. (1998). Community based nursing: Foundation for practice. Stamford, CT: Appleton & Lange.

Arrington, D. T. (1997). Retirement communities as creative clinical opportunities. Nursing & Health Care: Perspectives on Community, 18(2), 82–85.

Brennan, P. F. (1992). Computer networks promote caregiving collaboration: The computer link project. Proceedings of the Annual Symposium of Computer Applications in Medical Care, 156–160.

Fries, J. F., Williams, C. A., & Morfeld, D. (1992). Improvement in intergenerational health. American Journal of Public Health, 82, 109–112.

Institute of Medicine. (1978). A manpower policy for primary health care: Report of a study. Washington, DC: National Academy of Press.

Institute of Medicine. (1988). The future of public health. Washington, DC: National Academy Press.

Institute of Medicine. (1994). Defining primary care: An interim report. Washington, DC: National Academy Press.

Kreidler, M. C., Campbell, J., Lanik, G., Gray, V. R., & Conrad, M. A. (1994). Community elderly: A nursing center's use of change theory as a model. Journal of Gerontological Nursing, 1, 25–30.

Magilvy, J. K., Congdon, J. G., & Martinez, R. (1994). Circles of care: Home care and community support for rural older adults. Advances in Nursing Science, 16(3), 22–33.

National Nursing Research Agenda. Developing Knowledge for Practice: Challenges and Opportunities. National Institute of Nursing Research. www.nih.gov/ninr/vol7/chapter1.

U. S. Bureau of the Census. (1990). United States Department of Commerce. www.census.gov.

U. S. Department of Health and Human Services. (1994). Health United States 1993. Washington, DC: U. S. Government Printing Office.

Viverais-Dresler, G. A., Bakker, D. A., & Vance, R. J. (1995). Elderly clients' perceptions: Individual health counseling and group sessions. Canadian Journal of Public Health, 86(4), 234–237.

Wissmann, J. L., & Wilmoth, M. C. (1996). Meeting the learning needs of senior citizens and nursing students through a community-based pharmacology experience. Journal of Community Health Nursing, 13(3), 159–165.

19 Community-based Nursing Practice for Underserved Children in an Elementary School

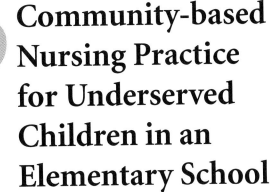

Georgine M. Redmond

Jeanne M. Sorrell

Christine T. Blasser

LEARNING OBJECTIVES

1) Describe the role of the school health nurse.

2) Describe the primary-care skills necessary for nursing practice for underserved children in an elementary school.

3) Describe the unique health-care needs of underserved school-aged children.

4) Discuss health promotion, disease prevention, and risk reduction in a school health setting.

5) Demonstrate cultural competence in working with underserved elementary school students and their families.

While I have enjoyed almost every day working in the clinic in the elementary school this semester, one recent afternoon in particular really touched my heart and made me feel like I made a difference. It had been an average day thus far, with the usual skinned elbows and knees, fevers, nosebleeds, and the ever-pervasive "tummy ache." The clinic was moderately busy at that moment, and the school nurse and I were just finishing up with three or four other students

when a familiar yet hesitant face walked through the door. She is a regular in the clinic, one of many students at the school with asthma. She comes in daily to use her inhaler before recess or PE and also was one of the students the nurse and I chose to participate in my teaching project on asthma management.

There was only an hour or so left in the school day when she arrived, and I thought it was a little late for her to be there for her medicine, so I greeted her quizzically and asked her if she was there to use her inhaler. She quietly replied that she was there for "something else." I immediately had a feeling of what that "something else" might be so I asked her if she would like to wait a few minutes until things were a little quieter (i.e., until the other students had left), to which she eagerly nodded her head. After finishing with the others I guided her into one of the exam rooms and gently asked her what she needed. Her eyes welled up, and through her tears she told me that her period had started. My heart went out to her. I immediately grabbed some tissues and asked her if this was the first time and if she knew what it was all about. She said that yes it was and no she didn't. I asked her if she was scared and she replied yes. As I wiped her tears away I tried to reassure her that this was all natural and perfectly normal and that I would help her to understand the process so that she wouldn't have to be scared.

I knew she must be physically uncomfortable along with emotional distress, so I began by getting her a pad and offering her a fresh pair of underpants. While she was in the bathroom I gathered some materials that I knew the school nurse had from Kotex's "It's a Girl Thing" program and waited for her to return. She and I sat back down in the exam room, closed the door, and together we went over the literature about puberty, female reproductive anatomy, menstruation, and some frequently asked questions. In the end I asked her if she had any questions, and she said no and that she felt much better about it. I gave her the booklet and a little hug and told her that I was glad she felt better and that if she did have any questions at a later time, the school nurse or I would be happy to answer them.

This experience touched my heart on two levels. As a nurse I thought to myself: what a great opportunity to therapeutically communicate and really make a difference for someone in need. It made me feel good that I could teach her about the physical process and, in the process of doing that, quell her fears about it. And on a personal level it has meaning because as a woman I know how scary getting your period for the first time can be even if you are well informed. I was honored to be able to encourage her in this big step in her life.

In today's society, only seriously ill children are likely to be hospitalized. Nurses encounter most children in community-based sites, such as the elementary schools. This creates a need for complex coordination on the part of the school nurse, who may be responsible for as many as 4500 students. Nursing students can gain valuable experience in using elementary schools as clinical learning sites.

Children in some elementary schools can be classified as underserved. These schools have a large number of students from low-income families and diverse ethnic groups. As a nursing student in these elementary schools, you can learn a great deal about planning care for both well and sick children. You may encounter health needs related to chronic illness in the children, preteen and teenage pregnancies, abuse, environmental issues, and a variety of social issues that both children and families face.

A collaborative relationship exists between the College of Nursing and Health Science at George Mason University (GMU), Fairfax County Public Schools, and the Fairfax County Health Department in the education of nursing students in a community-health clinical, which takes place in the spring of the junior year. In particular, nursing students who go to B Elementary School in northern Virginia, have the opportunity to work in a large, language-minority elementary school where schoolchildren learn real-life skills, explore outlets for personal expression, and appreciate differences among many cultures. It is the most culturally, linguistically, and economically diverse elementary school in the county. The nearly 900 children come from 45 countries and speak 20 languages. A focus of the clinical experience has been educating school-age children, families, and small groups, including teachers, in the unique health-care needs of the children. Nursing students and faculty work closely with the school nurse, principal, and teachers to assess, plan, implement, and evaluate a learning experience that is mutually beneficial to all partners.

THE SCHOOL HEALTH NURSE

School health nurses play a critical role in promoting health for underserved children in elementary schools. School nurses often structure their role not only to meet the needs of ill children in the schools, but also around health education, interdisciplinary collaboration, community involvement, and educating others about their role. Also, they communicate positive health practices that are essential to the long-term health and productivity of the nation.

What activities are needed to accomplish this role? The National Association of School Nurses, Inc. (1999) has identified the following strategies to promote student and staff health and safety:

a. Health services—Coordinating the health-services program and providing nursing care

b. Health education—Educating students, staff, and parents about their health needs

c. Healthy environment—Identifying important health and safety concerns to promote a nurturing school environment

d. Nutritional services—Facilitating the implementation of health food services programs

e. Physical education/activity—Promoting appropriate physical activities, including sports policies and practices

f. Counseling/mental health—Assessing and coordinating needed services related to mental health needs for children

g. Parent/community involvement—Promoting parent involvement in school and related community activities

h. Staff wellness—Educating staff about health promotion and healthy environments for children.

Box 19–1 gives you the opportunity to explore the school nurse's role in your community.

Box 19-1	Student Learning Activity

School Nurse Role

Discuss the role of the school nurse in your community.

Identify some of the major activities of the school nurse.

Skills in health promotion are at the roots of the nursing profession. Florence Nightingale exemplified the major concern of nursing as the health of the patient/client and emphasized the need to create an environment conducive to health. At a time when schools are increasingly focused on a broad educational mission, the school nurse helps to articulate the importance of health to learning. Teachers and nurses need to work together as a team to obtain mutual goals (Denehy, 1999).

STUDENT ACTIVITIES IN THE ELEMENTARY SCHOOL CURRICULUM

Although at first you may feel as though you do not know what to do as a nursing student in an elementary school, with help from faculty and others you will see that the children have many needs that you can meet. The learning experiences planned for our junior students are activities that are subsumed under the role of the school nurse. Students are placed in the schools by the local health department. At the beginning of each semester, the health department provides several different orientations for nursing students.

A specific orientation is planned for school health that gives students background on the role of the school nurse as well as orienting them to clinical protocols that guide nursing practice in the schools. Community resources available for school-age children and their families are also discussed. During the next clinical day, students visit the elementary school with their instructor. They meet with school personnel and learn about the demographics of the population of the school, school resources, school philosophy, and the general needs of the students and faculty in the particular school. School personnel also share their perceptions of the health needs of the children in the school, as well as any needs that they have regarding health information or training (e.g., cardiopulmonary resuscitation [CPR] certification).

Over the next few days, students are partnered with a teacher in the classroom, where they can conduct an assessment and engage in "kid watching" to gather data about potential health needs of the children in the classroom. In addition to the classroom, students conduct an assessment of the school, looking at it as a community.

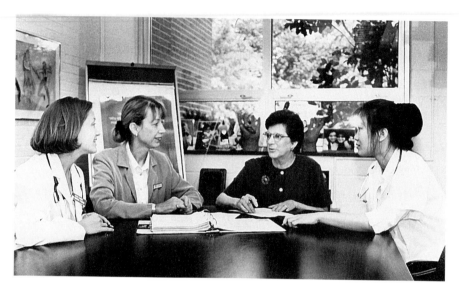

A windshield survey of the surrounding community gives students information regarding the living environment, socioeconomic status, and location of churches, other schools, and health-care facilities. At B Elementary school, 80 percent of the students come from low-income apartments that surround the school. B Elementary also provides trailers adjacent to the elementary school in which Hispanic and Vietnamese liaisons provide services to parents of students in the elementary school. The health needs of the parents who regularly participate in these parental outreach programs are also assessed.

Box 19–2 will help you to think about your classroom assessment.

Within the first two weeks of the semester, nursing students collect a myriad of data, which are later synthesized and analyzed to identify health-care needs of children, parents, and teachers. The county school system uses a health curriculum entitled "Ready, Set, Go For Good Health" (1991). Students use data that they have amassed and compare it with the standard curriculum, which needs to be implemented at each grade level. All levels of prevention—primary, secondary, and tertiary—are addressed in the school experience.

The following are some of the health teaching needs you might need to identify in school-aged children:

a. Dental health
b. Personal hygiene

Box 19-2	Student Learning Activity

Kid Watching

If you were involved in "kid watching" in a classroom, what type of information would you want to gather to prepare for your teaching project? Make a list of information you would want to collect.

---

c. Disease management (e.g., asthma, diabetes)
d. Understanding health-care roles
e. Mental health issues (e.g., self-esteem building and making friends)
f. Smoking prevention and cessation
g. Anatomy and physiology
h. Safety
i. Managing head lice
j. Weight management

An excerpt from one student's journal describes some of the activities she carried out at B Elementary School:

I taught 10 second graders about hand washing. I took three students at a time into the appropriate gender bathroom. I took a dry erase marker and traced two hands on the mirror. I drew a line to separate the hands and wrote "before" and "after" above the respective hand. I asked the kids what germs are and showed them pictures of streptococcus and other bacteria. I asked them why we care about germs (they are everywhere, we can pass the germs on to our friends), what they do to our bodies (they make us sick and we can miss school because of them). I had the kids draw ugly germs on the "before" hand and talked about how we really can't see germs on our hands, but by golly, they are there. Then we talked about what we can do to minimize germs, and they suggested washing our hands. So, we talked about when it is appropriate to wash our hands (after bathroom, before eating, after petting animals, after coughing, after sneezing—showed them a picture of a man sneezing and the expectorate is backlit so the kids could see the huge cloud of "germs"). I showed them how most people wash their hands, a quick wiggle of the fingers under the water. Then I had them scrub up with soap and sing a song—the Pokémon song! As we walked back to class, I reviewed with the kids the steps for appropriate hand washing.

You may also identify health needs of parents, teachers, and staff. These may include breast self-exam, hypertension, stress management, and nutrition. You may want to address these health-care needs through individual teaching projects, class teaching projects, health fairs, or through a closed-circuit television program that reaches the entire school.

Primary-care Skills Used in the Elementary School

Health teaching, communication, health assessment, and family assessment are four important primary-care skills for students to learn in the elementary school.

Health Teaching

Health teaching is the major primary-care skill used by our junior nursing students in the school. Prior to enrollment in the community-based clinical practicum, students are well versed in principles of teaching and learning, in the design of a teaching plan, and in growth and development for school-aged children. As they begin to think about teaching in their classroom, they spend several weeks observing their classroom teacher. They identify the level at which the teacher presents the material to the children and learning activities that engage the children successfully, as well as management of general classroom behavior of the children. Nursing students also explore school resources that will assist with the teaching project (e.g., libraries, audiovisual materials, and teaching supplies). As students prepare to teach either an individual child or a class, they develop the teaching plan, which includes the goal or purpose of the teaching, objectives, teaching/learning activities, and a content outline, as well as a plan for evaluation of the teaching. With the older children, the evaluation may be written in the form of a posttest on what they learned or a written evaluation of the student's performance. Another consideration involved in the teaching plan is whether the teaching materials need to be developed in other languages to meet the needs of the children. Table 19–1 illustrates a teaching plan developed by one of our students on asthma. The teaching plan evolved from a collaborative discussion between the nursing student, classroom teacher, and George Mason University (GMU) faculty.

In determining health-teaching needs it is important to keep the nursing process in perspective at all times, because this is the foundation of health promotion and disease prevention. You will want to begin by doing a needs assessment to devise a teaching project. It is also important to consider the children's experiential knowledge. Even though they are children, many have lived with a chronic illness, such as asthma, for a long time. They may be very knowledgeable about their care and can teach the other children what it is like to live with a chronic illness. It is important to assess not only the children, but also the family and environment in which they live.

Box 19–3 will help you practice your assessment skills.

Table 19-1

Teaching Plan for Asthma
Second-grade Class

Assessment:
Three of my students have asthma; one student has a sibling with asthma. The students are very hyperactive and have a short attention span. They are aware of asthma, that it is treated with an inhaler, and that they can have an asthma attack when they play outside.

Nursing Diagnosis:
Knowledge deficit R/T pathology of asthma.

Theory:
Piaget's child development theory states that children ages 7 to 9 learn concretely and are able to understand spatial concepts.

Purpose:
The purpose of this teaching project is to teach the children about asthma, focusing on the pathology and triggers of asthma.

Objectives:
a. Student will identify the lungs on a model. (Cognitive)
b. Student will list triggers of asthma. (Cognitive)
c. Student will state what a person with asthma does when he or she has an asthma attack. (Cognitive)
d. Student will discuss what happens in the lungs when a person has an asthma attack. (Cognitive)
e. Student will use the trigger or nontrigger cards appropriately by placing the card on the correct section of the poster. (Psychomotor)
f. Student will discuss how it feels to live with asthma. (Affective)

Teaching/Learning Activities:

1. Review anatomy of the lungs and smaller tubes (bronchus, bronchioles).

2. Observe the difference between the bronchioles of a healthy person and those of a person with asthma.

3. List triggers of asthma.
   a. Dust
   b. Cockroaches
   c. Exercise
   d. Cold air
   e. Infections
   f. Mold
   g. Animals
   h. Smoke

4. Review pathology of asthma.
   a. Exposure to a trigger
   b. Tubes tighten and airflow is restricted

5. Demonstrate use of an inhaler.

6. Explain that persons with asthma can live normal, unrestricted lives if they use their medications correctly.

Box 19-3   Student Learning Activity

Assessment of Educational Needs

You have been assigned to prepare a teaching plan related to asthma for fifth graders. What types of assessments would you include in your plan?

An excerpt from a student journal shares the process that one student conducted to accomplish the development of her teaching plan:

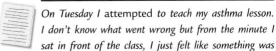

February 15, 2000

Today I did my first official teaching to the kindergarten classes. In preparation I looked in the library for a book about doctors. I found a simple book that I read to the class. We also discussed experiences some of the students had with doctors. After reading a book I asked them to draw a picture of a doctor and write a sentence about what a doctor does. I had made sentence strips with prewritten sentences for them to choose from. After the class I collected the drawings and decided I would keep them for all of the students and we would create a "health book" at the end of the semester.

In between classes I put together a potential teaching plan for the whole semester. I gave a copy to each of the kindergarten teachers and explained that it could change. I included days that I will not be in the classes to go to the outreach trailer and clinic. I also reserved a couple days to work with the asthma booth.

A second journal entry shares a story about the teaching project that was discussed earlier in this chapter, but did not go the way it was planned. The student described it as a "disastrous lesson":

On Tuesday I attempted to teach my asthma lesson. I don't know what went wrong but from the minute I sat in front of the class, I just felt like something was "off." After doing a bit of review from the previous lesson, we started the asthma triggers game. And maybe I didn't explain it well or maybe it was too complex but the kids didn't seem to get it. Granted, my trigger pictures weren't the best, but I thought with some explanation the kids would get the idea, but they didn't. In fact, one of the girls thought that the picture with the cats were actually rats! Same idea I guess but still! I think that while I was designing the game I lost sight of the purpose of the lesson, teaching the kids about asthma triggers, and spent too much time on the game board, pictures, and game pieces. The game was too involved and required too much abstract thinking on the kids' part. Looking back, I could have had a completely different focus and used more visual aids and spent less time on the small details. When I realized the game wasn't working I quickly ended it and shifted gears a little. We ended with the three steps to remember when a friend is having an asthma attack. They all knew the steps and I think at least walked away from the lesson knowing something.

Anyway, I can now look back and laugh, but at the time I was really frustrated with myself. And I realized one of the many great things about kids is that they are completely honest and have no qualms about sharing their feelings. One boy said, "I don't get this game. It's too confusing and it's dumb." I just love kids.

Communication

A second primary-care skill that must be emphasized in the school setting is communication. This includes age-appropriate dialogue with children and communication with staff and parents. Students also complete written documentation of all interventions with children and families for the public health nurse, who is generally in the school only once or twice a week. Nursing students are frequently assigned to children in their classroom who have special health needs, such as diabetes or cystic fibrosis. Nursing students spend time with these children in the classroom, as well as individually, discussing their feelings about the disease, and communicating with them as new health-care needs emerge. In communicating with staff, nursing students must keep their classroom teachers informed of their schedules both orally and in writing. The following story of a nursing student's encounter with a 6-year-old with asthma illustrates how anxiety can impact on students' perception and communication.

> *During my first day at the elementary school for my community clinical, the school nurse was reviewing the children with chronic diseases and their care plans. She ended with a girl in the first grade who she gave the title of "one of the most allergic kids in the country." There on the page sat a picture of an adorable little girl next to a long list of things she was severely allergic to.*
>
> *The nurse went on to tell me about the preparations the school made to bring this girl into the public school system for kindergarten last year. Several meetings went on leading to changes in the classroom ventilation system, carpeting, and products with latex, like the chairs, crayons, and other supplies the children would be using. They had to change the entire room to avoid any reactions this girl may have. The parents and children in this class had to be educated on what not to bring to school and what might happen to this girl if she did have an anaphylactic reaction. For example, products with peanut butter could not be brought into the classroom. Even if another child had peanut butter for breakfast, there was a high chance she could trigger a reaction if her hands were not washed properly.*
>
> *The allergic girl's home environment prior to school was very secluded. The parents explained that they had few visitors, no carpet, and special air filters, and rarely did this little girl go outside. On the occasion that they did take her out she would have reactions requiring EpiPen use and sometimes a call to 911.*
>
> *After explaining the history, the nurse let me know that there have been no severe reactions since the child had been in school. The nurse told me how this little girl knows a lot about her allergies and is very educated on her strict lifestyle. She also stated that the little girl rarely came to the clinic.*
>
> *After lunch that day a familiar face came into the clinic. I immediately felt like my body went into a fight or flight response. I was not sure whether to grab her EpiPen or call 911. I think she sensed this, and she came closer and grabbed my hand and introduced herself. The school nurse told her who I was, and the little girl gave me a big hug. She was only there to get her asthma inhaler. No severe reactions; they were going outside for recess since it was such a nice spring day. She*

> *took her inhaler out of the box and went on to show me how to attach the spacer and she took her two puffs and left giving me another big hug.*

Teachers provide oral feedback regarding individual performance of the students directly to the nursing students as well as to the GMU faculty who are on-site in the schools,. Faculty provide teachers with monthly calendars. It is the student's responsibility to maintain the calendar so that it reflects various activities and times in which they will be present in the individual teacher's classroom. Student nurses are also involved with parents through individual student contacts, home visits, and health fairs. The following journal illustrates how one student prepared materials for Spanish-speaking children and parents:

> *On Tuesday I spent the better part of the day working on "material management." I went through all of my materials and began working on the translation of some materials in preparation for the Asthma Booth for Family Literacy Night at the school. I have been seeking out asthma materials in Spanish and will use those as the primary resources for the booth. But, I feel like I need to really work on my Spanish so that I can use the proper terminology when describing asthma to both kids and their parents. I also met with Pam and Huyen to talk about the booth, and we made up a checklist of things to do and to discuss with the principal of the school. We will meet with her on Tuesday to discuss the details.*

Students also write publicity notices to parents about upcoming educational programs that they have planned, some of which may need to be bilingual. All of these activities teach oral and written communication skills. Table 19–2 is an example of a bilingual letter to parents.

Nursing students complete several process recordings with the children or parents to enhance their therapeutic communication skills. This may often involve a crisis in the classroom when a child comes to school upset. The student may need to take the child aside to talk to him or her individually. The process recording provides the student an opportunity to reflect on the communication

Table 19-2

Bilingual Information Letter

Parents,

At the upcoming Family Literacy Night, to be held March 2, there will be a session about controlling and managing asthma. The session will be lead by George Mason University Nursing students who are working at B Elementary School.

This session will be an opportunity for parents to ask questions, talk with each other, and learn about resources in the community. There will be a video presentation, various handouts, and a discussion.

Please join us on Thursday, March 2 beginning at 6:15 at B Elementary School. If you have any questions, Please contact Ms. R or Ms. L (GMU Nursing Students) at 703 000-0000.

See you on Thursday!

El jueves 2 de marzo tendremos una noche familiar, donde se desarrollaran diferentes actividades como son literatura para niños y habrá una sesión donde se hablará sobre el asma. Será dirigido por estudiantes de enfermería de George Mason University. Usted tendra la oportunidad de preguntar todo lo relacionado acerca del asma.

Reunámonos por favor el jueves 2 de marzo a las 6:15 en la Escuela B Si tienen algunas preguntas, llamen a la Señorita R o la Señorita L (estudiantes de George Mason) al 703 000-0000.

¡Gracias y nos vemos el jueves!

I think I can handle almost anything, but when it comes to kids it seems harder to deal with "bad things." I like these kids so much and want to do my best for them so I've been trying to keep an open mind and open ears when they talk to me. I guess I'm also realizing and seeing that kids can be incredibly resilient.

Health Assessment

Our junior students build on the health assessment course from a previous semester. One of the goals is to expand their knowledge of health assessment, such as providing vision and hearing screening, as well as measuring height and weight. These assessments are normally performed by the public health nurse, who has the responsibility for providing the screenings for all of the elementary school students. Students also incorporate nutritional assessment into the nursing care plans that they complete on the children. A major area of learning in the elementary school is the ability of the nursing student to work with various age groups and complete developmental assessments. These are written up and compared with the norms for various age groups.

Family Assessment

Finally, the ability to work with a family is another primary-care skill that our students develop during their school experience. Students come to this clinical experience process, analyze it, and determine whether it was therapeutic. Table 19-3 provides an example of a process recording by one student. The following narrative is the student's analysis of the process recording in Table 19–3.

Looking back on the conversation, I realize that I was a bit nervous when she said she wanted to talk with me privately. I wasn't sure what to expect, so my mind started racing. I almost felt relieved when she told me what was bothering her. I'm not sure if I was worried that I wouldn't know how to react to something really serious or if I wasn't prepared to deal with a serious issue yet.

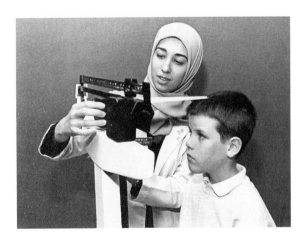

Table 19-3

Process Recording

NURSE—VERBAL	CLIENT—VERBAL	NURSE'S THOUGHTS	ANALYSIS OF INTERACTION
	Can I talk to you a minute?	OK, Wonder what this is about.	
Sure. So, what's up A. C.?	I don't want to talk to you here. Can we go in the back of the room?	Ah, okay. What could this be about? Is she okay? Did something bad happen?	Therapeutic: Trying to be inquisitive while at the same time calm.
Okay, let's go back here. Is this okay?	Okay, but use your quiet voice; I don't want the other kids to hear us.	Oh gosh, this is serious.	Therapeutic: I want A. C. to feel comfortable with me.
So what's on your mind A. C.?	Today, like that girl over there in the purple shirt. She was being really mean to me and said I was fat.	Kids can be brutal sometimes but I didn't expect this.	Therapeutic: Inquiring. Did that hurt your feelings when she said that, A. C.?
Did that hurt your feelings when she said that, A. C.?	Yeah, she's always mean to me.	I'm a little concerned about her having self-esteem issues. I know she is taller and a bit heavier than the other kids.	Nontherapeutic: I should have asked how that made her feel instead of asking a yes/no question.
What did you say to her when she said that?	Nothing, I just told her to shut up.	How did she handle the situation? Did she get upset? Has she heard it before?	Therapeutic: Attempting to find out client's reaction.
It's hard when others hurt our feelings.	Yes, I wanted to cry.	This was painful for her. How can I help her deal with this better the next time?	Therapeutic: Letting client know that I empathize with her.
What do you think you can say to her next time she says something not very nice?	I don't know, it makes me angry.	Maybe we can talk about some ways of dealing with hurt feelings in the future.	Therapeutic: Trying to help client see that she can play an active role in making sure her feelings don't get hurt again.
How about telling her that when she says mean things, it hurts your feelings.	Well, I guess.	I know that telling someone how their actions makes you feel can be tough but, I can at least let her know that it's okay to talk about her feelings.	Therapeutic: Teaching client communication skills to deal with future incidents.
Okay, A. C. Do you feel any better?	Yeah.	Trying to come to some closure with the client.	Nontherapeutic: Could have asked her more to see if she had anything else on her mind.

armed with a general knowledge regarding families, as well as family assessment. Their goal is to work with a family during the semester. This is most often the family of a child in their classroom who has a chronic illness or a special health need. The majority of the students are able to meet with the families in their homes. If this is not possible, arrangements are made to meet before or after school. Faculty visit with the students initially, and later junior students visit in pairs. Students generally meet with the families five to six times during the semester. The first visit is for rapport building. During the second and third visits, students complete their assessment and identify individual and family nursing diagnoses. Students work with the family on the identified problems (for example, teaching interventions or identifying and providing resources for the family) during the fifth and sixth visits. Work with the child on individual needs or problems continues during the school day. Frequently, students must use each other as interpreters or secure an interpreter through the school.

Students enjoy visiting children and families at home, because they get a bigger picture of the children's environments. The following journal entry by a student illustrates this.

> *Today's clinical was amazing. I went on a home visit to see Bobbie. He was home because he is in the P.M. kindergarten. The visit was really interesting. The word "Blood" (gang-related term) was written on their door. The mother, Louanne, had been to the Outreach Trailer several times. She was very nice and receptive to us being there. Chris was great at prompting me to ask the right questions. I got a lot of information about the family. I am going with Bobbie to his clinic appointment on Thursday. He has newly diagnosed asthma. One trigger may very possibly be the black mold that grows along the walls and ceiling of the bedroom. The home was so humid and there was condensation on the windows. Louanne is going to have surgery on the 10th of April and I would love to go with her. It was such an interesting visit.*

Asthma Education in the Elementary School

Health promotion, disease prevention, and risk reduction are all important goals in a school health setting. An example of an important learning focus for GMU students that relates to all three of these areas is a project related to children with asthma (Redmond & Langley, 2000). At George Mason, an asthma education and intervention project is being piloted at two elementary schools, one of which is B Elementary School. Although the metropolitan area of northern Virginia does not meet the definition of a "medically underserved" community, pockets of poverty exist throughout the area, and many groups of people do not have access to adequate and consistent care for chronic illnesses such as pediatric asthma. According to the Fairfax County's "Asthma Coalition Proposal," asthma is the number one chronic illness that is responsible for children missing school. More than three million days of school are missed each year because of asthma in the United States. Pilot schools were selected for both the ethnic and cultural diversity of the student body, as well as for the percentage of students who received free or reduced school lunch as an indication of poverty, using Federal Income Guidelines.

Need for Asthma Education in the Schools

Asthma is the most common chronic illness of children in the United States (Walsh, Kelly, & Morrow, 1999). Asthma mortality is rising, and major efforts are currently directed toward improving the quality of care and patient management skills (Blessing-Moore, 1996). Mortality data are the only surveillance information available at the state and local level, although morbidity data are needed to define high-risk populations and to design and evaluate interventions aimed at preventing the development and exacerbation of the disease. Although several states have added questions about asthma to the Behavioral Risk Factor Surveillance System, those questions are aimed at adults and the Surveillance System has not obtained reliable data for children. Diagnosis of asthma continues to be less reliable among persons under 5 years of age, whereas children continue to be more adversely affected by asthma (Centers for Disease Control [CDC], 1998).

Economically disadvantaged minority children living in the inner cities have experienced disproportionately higher rates of adverse outcomes (Bauer, Lurie, Yeh, & Grant, 1999; Lurie, Straub, Goodman, & Bauer, 1998). According to the "Healthy People 2010 Objectives" (2000), poverty is an important contributing factor to asthma morbidity and mortality. Although medication treatment for chronic asthma has changed over the last 10 years with increased daily use of antiinflammatory medications for moderate to severe asthma, one study of 392 asthmatic children in the inner city concluded that undermedication was common in poor children. Antiinflammatory medications were used less commonly than in the general population, and bronchodilators were used more commonly (Eggleston et al., 1998). A possible explanation for this relates to lack of access to long-term, continuous treatment of the disease. The American Academy of Allergy, Asthma & Immunology (1999) reported that a lack of comprehensive, easily referenced information makes it difficult for primary-care providers to develop adequate pediatric management plans. Many poor children are treated episodically in the emergency room for symptoms. In addition, environmental allergens, as well as exposure to tobacco smoke and other pollutants, hamper long-term management for children with asthma.

The importance of patient asthma education, and in particular children's asthma education, has been recognized since the 1950s. Recent advances in asthma care have improved the understanding of asthma and increased the potential ability to manage asthma effectively. Asthma is now considered a chronic inflammatory disease that requires preventive management, as opposed to an episodic disease requiring intermittent acute treatment (Yamada, 1998).

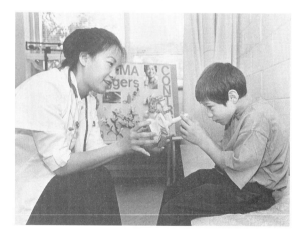

Health education is considered a critical strategy in effective asthma management and prevention (Becker, McGhan, Dolovich, Proudlock, & Mitchell, 1994). Fillmore, Jones, and Blankson (1997) identify the goal of asthma management as achieving normal health and activity, including regular school attendance. High absenteeism is a damaging influence on educational needs and the ability of children to participate in school activities. To address this morbidity, educational authorities must be included in establishing protocols for management of asthmatic children in schools (Speight, Lee, & Hey, 1997). A public program strategy to engage educators in addressing the special requirements of children with asthma can be accomplished by the partnering of health providers and health agencies with community schools (Campbell, Cormier, Daglish, Miles, & Kesten, 1994).

School-based asthma management programs like ours target educators, school nurses, and elementary school children with and without asthma. The development of these programs includes training sessions to educate teachers and nurses on techniques for working with children with asthma. The strategy is to demystify asthma and increase the general awareness of what asthma is and how it should be managed (Campbell et al., 1994). This can be accomplished by a variety of means, including distribution of educational materials to educators, children, and parents; ongoing educational sessions for educators, children, and parents; posters that display suggestions for managing environmental contributors to asthma; and training about specific drug modalities and inhaler use.

Activities for the Project

The educational component of the project for the nursing students builds on their curriculum, including prerequisites and nursing courses. In addition, two training sessions are added in asthma education and management and in cultural competence.

Services provided by the nursing students to children, families, and community include health careers information; community resource guides for all jurisdictions; Internet site information on asthma education, treatment, management, and resources; health education on asthma management for children, families, and teachers; small peer group sessions for children; media (closed-circuit TV, books, games) for all children in schools; and referral as needed to an appropriate primary-care provider (who can develop pediatric asthma treatment plans and provide continuity of care).

Evaluation

The evaluation of intermediate results as well as overall success is built into the fabric of the asthma education program. Ongoing formative evaluation occurs through written systematic evaluations and evaluation meetings with students, faculty, partners, and parents. Two databases are planned: to track all asthma-related activities for each child (e.g., home visits by nursing students, use of resources, and doctors' visits) and to track outcomes. Anticipated outcomes of the project are: (1) hospitalizations for asthma will be decreased by 25 percent, (2) emergency room visits for acute episodes of asthma will be decreased by 25 percent, (3) missed school days because of asthma will decrease by 10 percent, (4) each child will have an appropriate and consistent primary-care provider, (5) an asthma resource book will be available in each of the three Northern Virginia jurisdictions, and (6) an asthma Website will be available for professional and citizen use.

UNIQUE HEALTH-CARE NEEDS OF IMMIGRANT CHILDREN

Underserved children in elementary schools may have unique health-care needs. Many children immigrate from other countries, particularly from Central America; El Salvador is the primary country of origin. They have limited basic resources such as food, shelter, and clothing. Often, they have only one set of clothing (which may not be season appropriate) and no access to a place to regularly bathe and wash their clothing. They may move from one family member or friend's apartment to another. Simple implements of hygiene like a toothbrush and toothpaste may not be available to them.

Poor hygiene presents social problems for these children. Nursing students need to approach these topics sensitively. The school provides a clothes locker where families can secure changes of clothing, and nursing students gather free supplies like soap, toothpaste, mouthwash, toothbrushes, and so on for teaching projects.

The following two journal excerpts illustrate students' interventions with the children concerning hygiene:

April 11

I have been asked in the past by Mrs. C. to teach the class about personal hygiene habits and bathing. I was unsure about how to approach this topic because I did not want to make any of the class members feel bad. I decided to see if there were any books in the library that addressed the topic. I found a great book about a little girl who does not want to take a bath. I took the book with me to class and read it to them. We then talked about why it is important to bathe, how often to bathe, and that they can remind their mothers they need to bathe if their mother is too busy with other things in the house. I taught the bathing topic to two classes during the day.

February 22 and 24

Today was spent planning and working on my projects. I cut out over a dozen little teeth sets for my kids. I got all of my supplies together to teach dental hygiene. I talked with Mrs. D. and I will be teaching dental hygiene on Thursday after I teach in the Outreach trailer. I got free floss from a dentist who goes to my church.

Many of the parents have little education and frequently cannot find jobs. The men often hire out as day laborers in construction or housecleaning. Early in the morning groups of men stand on the street corners waiting to be selected for these jobs. Sometimes parents are here illegally and are afraid to seek health care for their children for fear of being identified.

When the children are ill, their diseases seem more severe because of previous lack of health care in their country of origin and lack of access to health care in this country. The following story reported in a student journal illustrates the lack of access to care for many of these children:

February 24

I also worked in the clinic today. Aside from the usual stomachaches, bloody noses, and runny noses, it was fairly quiet. I returned to the clinic after lunch to make up for the 45 minutes I missed while teaching. A young boy, fifth grade, came in with a serious headache. He didn't have a *temperature, but looked really bad and was teary from the pain. I would venture to guess that the boy had a migraine. Well, we called his mom and she came to pick him up and take him home. The mom . . . spoke only Spanish [and] I learned that the boy had been having the bad headaches for quite some time and she was really worried. She had taken him to a local doctor and he gave her a note saying that she needed to take him to a neurology consult. Well, this woman didn't know what a neurologist was, let alone how to make an appointment or pay for the consultation. I spoke to Sharon [public health nurse] and gave her the background and we made an appointment for the woman to go to the county clinic and fill out the paperwork so that her son could first be seen in the general pediatric clinic and then hopefully somewhere down the line by a neurologist. Unfortunately, the woman has no job besides selling empañadas and tacos in the neighborhood, so it will be difficult for her to qualify for services (because she must provide proof of income) and she knows this, which upsets her. She really, really wants to help her son, but she feels that she has few options. She decided to return to the private doctor and pay the required $40 fee in order to get some kind of medicine for her son so that he can return to school. She said she will go to the appointment at the clinic on March 10 but said she can't wait until then to try and make her son feel better.*

After this exchange, I felt so helpless. Something that seems so easy for me, in this case to call up and make an appointment with a neurologist, seems virtually impossible to this woman. She can barely afford the $40 for a doctor's visit and medication, let alone the costs of seeing a neurologist. The whole experience was both disturbing and enlightening, as I realized that this happens more often than not and there exists a great deal of inequality in health care. I realize that I can't save the world every day, but I can at least try and impact someone's life, however small it may be (in this case of interpreting and lending a listening ear).

Cultural Competence

Working with children in the high-risk elementary schools provides students with many opportunities to develop skills in cultural competence. Children from specific cultures may have health-care practices that differ from the standard in the United States, but may still be appropriate for the specific culture. Some cultural groups, however, may value practices that are not healthful. For example, some cultures may value obesity and may not understand the risks involved with obese children growing up in America. Prevention may not be a common practice for some cultures. Health teaching in these areas must be done with special sensitivity to cultural needs and values. Box 19–4 gives you the opportunity to think of more culturally-determined health care practices.

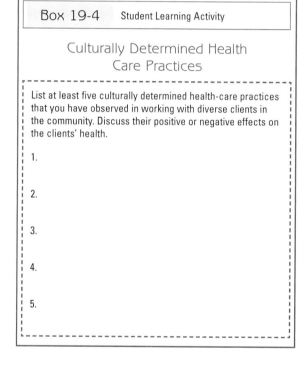

Box 19-4   Student Learning Activity

Culturally Determined Health Care Practices

List at least five culturally determined health-care practices that you have observed in working with diverse clients in the community. Discuss their positive or negative effects on the clients' health.

1.

2.

3.

4.

5.

Language needs are another consideration. Students need to communicate health teaching in a language and style that the children understand and that they can share with their parents. Use of audiovisual materials that the children can take home can help to communicate important concepts to parents.

The following story illustrates how a student was able to sensitively act as a child advocate in the health-care system:

I rushed into the Clinic five minutes late. I expected to walk into a dark, somewhat run-down, possibly smelly, cramped waiting room. Instead, I walked into a bright, well-organized, clean, and uncrowded lobby. I looked for my client, Dan, a 5-year-old obese boy with newly diagnosed asthma. I didn't see Dan or his mother, Lou. I had heard that getting an appointment was a triumph in itself and that if the patient is even a few minutes late, they would move on to the next patient.

I asked the receptionist if Dan had checked in. He had just been called back. Relieved that he made it, I followed a nurse into the examination room. I greeted Dan and Lou in Spanish. I explained to Dan's nurse practitioner (NP) that I was a nursing student doing home visits with this family and I had been asked by Lou to come to the appointment. The NP was also a student and introduced me to her instructor.

I waited with Lou and Dan in the examination room. Lou told me that the doctors are "bad"— they don't listen to her. I saw firsthand what she meant. The NP breezed in and quickly began asking questions. I interpreted and as soon as the NP had the information that she wanted, she turned her back on Lou and began writing her notes. Lou looked at me for help. I suddenly realized that I was the one who had to act as Lou's advocate. I continued to interpret for Lou and we regained the NP's attention.

Dan was given a decongestant for his runny nose, a varicella immunization, and we were finally done. As we waited for the paperwork to go through, Lou showed me Dan's inhaler. It was completely empty. The purpose of the visit was to follow up on Dan's asthma. They hadn't checked his inhaler. Once again, I had to be assertive, and I got Dan a new inhaler with one refill.

We walked to the parking lot, and Lou thanked me for coming. I said goodbye and got in my car. The whole ordeal had taken over two hours. I was so exhausted. I was glad to do what I could for the family, but their situation was overwhelming. Lou was unable to communicate and she was, therefore, pretty much a helpless immigrant mother at the mercy of her health-care providers. I, the little nursing student, had to be the one to speak up to the big nurse practitioner and instructor and act in Lou's interest. I was not used to doing that, and it was a poignant learning experience.

The other day, I walked from my clinical site to my car. An old car drove toward me and as it passed me, the driver honked. I turned around and saw Lou and Dan smiling and waving.

People don't care how much you know until they know how much you care.

In summary, a clinical practicum in an elementary school for underserved children can be a very satisfying learning experience for nursing students. Such experiences can help you to learn the role of the school health nurse, describe the primary-care skills necessary for nursing practice in this setting, and better understand the unique health-care needs of underserved school-aged children. It can also help you to see how the concepts of health promotion, disease prevention, and risk reduction can be integrated into a school health setting while ensuring cultural competence in working with elementary school students and their families.

Active Learning Strategies

1. You are visiting the Rodriguez family in their home. Juan has asthma. You find out that the family is having difficulty paying for Juan's asthma medication. Contact the Lung Association and the pharmaceutical company that manufactures Juan's medication. Do they offer a medication program for low-income families? How would the family access the program? Do a trial run to see if the Rodriguez family will have any difficulty accessing this resource.

2. Plan an age-appropriate health fair for your second-grade class. Consider age and developmental level health needs of this targeted community and topics and activities that fall within the school nurse role.

3. The staff in your school expresses an interest in learning more about chronic diseases in children. Construct a brief survey to identify their specific learning needs.

4. Identify at least three languages that are spoken in your school. Develop a "home safety" guide for children and parents. Work with bilingual classmates or staff to translate the guides.

References

American Academy of Asthma, Allergy & Immunology. (1999). Pediatric Asthma Guide. Washington DC: Authors.

Bauer, E. J., Lurie, N., Yeh, C., & Grant, E. N. (1999). Screening for asthma in an inner-city elementary school in Minneapolis, Minnesota. Journal of School Health, 69(1), 12–16.

Becker, A., McGhan, S., Dolovich, J., Proudlock, M., & Mitchell, I. (1994). Essential ingredients for an ideal education program for children with asthma and their families. Chest, 106(4), 231s–234s.

Blessing-Moore, J. (1996). Does asthma education change behavior? Chest, 109(1), 9–10.

Campbell, M., Cormier, B., Daglish, S., Miles, P., & Kesten, M. (1994). Considerations of public programs and techniques for public/community health education. Chest, 106(4), 274s–278s.

Centers for Disease Control (CDC). (1998, April 24). Surveillance for Asthma—United State s, 1960–1995. Mortality & Morbidity Weekly Reports, 47(SS-1).

Denehy, J. (1999). Health promotion: A golden opportunity for school nurses. Journal of School Nursing, 15(5), 4–5.

Eggleston, P. A., Malveaux, F. J., Butz, A. M., Huss, K., Thompson, L., Kolodner, K., & Rand, C. S. (1998). Medications used by children with asthma living in the inner city. Pediatrics, 103(3), 349–354.

Fillmore, E., Jones, N., & Blankson, J. (1997). Achieving treatment goals for school children with asthma. Archives of Diseases in Childhood, 77, 420–422.

Healthy People 2010 (2000). Understanding and improving health. Washington DC: United States Department of Health and Human Services.

Lurie, N., Straub, M. J., Goodman, N., & Bauer, E. J. (1998). Incorporating asthma education into a traditional school curriculum. American Journal of Public Health, 88(5), 822–823.

National Association of School Nurses. (1999). The role of the school nurse. Scarborough, ME: National Association of School Nurses, Inc.

Ready, Set, Go for Good Health (1991). Fairfax County Public Schools. Fairfax, VA.

Redmond G., & Langley, C. (2000). Asthma education for underserved children. Department of Health and Human Services, HRSA. Rockville, MD. #D11HP00167.

Speight, A., Lee, D., & Hey, E. (1997). Underdiagnosis and undertreatment of asthma in childhood. British Medical Journal, 286, 1253–1256.

Walsh, K. M., Kelly, C. S., & Morrow, A. C. (1999). Head Start: A setting for asthma outreach and prevention. Family & Community Health, 22(1), 28–37.

Yamada, E. (1998). Asthma: The shift from episodic treatment to ongoing prevention, education, and management. Western Journal of Medicine, 169(6), 377.

20 Community-based Nursing Practice on a College Campus

M. Lucille Boland

LEARNING OBJECTIVES

1) Discuss the validity of nursing's role in nontraditional settings.

2) Assess the common health issues of a college campus community.

3) Design at least three interactive methods to deal with selected health problems of a college campus community.

4) Explore the nursing skills that facilitate meeting the health goals of a college campus community.

5) Conduct at least one educational program to address selected health concerns of individuals on a college campus.

6) Evaluate the effectiveness of selected interactive nursing interventions.

When you are a student in a community-based nursing curriculum, you need to be able to think "out of the box." Your role as a nurse may be very different from the image that you currently hold. You need to be able to examine *all* of the skills that you as a nurse possess to understand how you can function in such a nontraditional setting. One of my students shared her initial thoughts regarding our campus clinical with me and, paraphrasing her words, it went something like this:

On our first day of clinical our instructor asked us what we thought we were going to be doing this semester. My hand shot up right away and I said, "Why we'll be taking care of students who come into the student health

center!" I remember being so excited to begin practicing my newly learned skills. Imagine my disappointment and dismay when our instructor said that the student health center would be the last place we would be working! At that point I stopped listening and began to focus on my disappointment. What a waste of my time, I thought. What on earth were we going to do for the next 14 weeks? How were we going to be "real" nurses if we didn't have patients to take care of? Gradually my instructor's voice began to filter back into my consciousness and I remember feeling resignation. There wasn't any thing I could do about things at this point so I decided to try and make the best of a bad situation.

These feelings are common among students when they are exposed to a nontraditional clinical situation. That is when thinking "out of the box" comes in handy. What *are* the skills you need as a nurse when you work in a setting such as a college campus? If you think that nursing skills are just composed of procedures and other "technical"

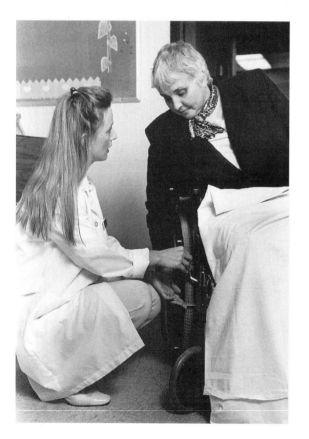

skills, you need to broaden your perspective. I submit that just about anyone can be trained to insert catheters, give injections, or push buttons on a machine. The skills we possess as nurses include not only these technical skills but also the skills of observation, therapeutic communication, analysis, critical thinking, and teaching, to name a few. One area in which nurses have always excelled is that of prevention. To implement prevention programs, the nurse must use all of the skills at his or her command. A college campus is a fertile area in which nurses can have an impact on the health behaviors of a select group of people.

When helping students get started in a community-based clinical setting, I always recommend that they use the nursing process. The nursing process helps the student take many facts and observations and organize them into a meaningful structure. In other words, it is a way of thinking about things. So I tell the students that to decide what nursing interventions they need to implement, they first need to assess their client. In this case, the "client" is the college campus. To assess the campus, you need to know what is out there. An easy way to find out is to walk around and look. Divide the campus up and walk it. Look for the location of health and/or wellness services. Are there any environmental health hazards around? What about safety hazards? Do the buildings conform to the American Disabilities Act (ADA)? Once you have done this, look at your population. Who are your clients? What kinds of people do you find there? Is there cultural diversity? What cultures are represented? What is the general age range of the campus population? Who beside students and faculty make up the campus community? In Box 20–1, list factors that you would like to assess on your campus.

After you have completed your assessment, which is usually a group effort, you need to come together and consolidate your findings. Out of your assessment will come your health needs/concerns list. In addition to your campus assessment, it is important for you to identify the common health problems faced by a college campus population. For this, you must go to the literature. According to the literature, two of the most common problems on a college campus are sexually transmitted diseases (STDs) and eating disorders. List in Box 20–2 at least three additional health concerns to address on your campus.

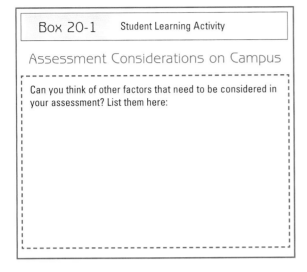

Box 20-1   Student Learning Activity

Assessment Considerations on Campus

Can you think of other factors that need to be considered in your assessment? List them here:

Box 20-2   Student Learning Activity

Campus Health Concerns

Can you identify at least three health concerns for a campus community other than those already given? List them here:

1.

2.

3.

For you to intervene effectively in a wellness/prevention setting, three things need to be present on the part of the client:
1. Interest in the topic
2. Lack of knowledge about the topic
3. Motivation to change the behavior

Even though you might have identified a number of health problems that need to be addressed, your effectiveness will be affected by the presence or absence of these three points. For example, one of my students iden-

tified that our campus had a large international student population. A large number of these students were Muslim. Shortly after the semester began, the month of Ramadan started. In the Muslim religion, Ramadan is a month in which practicing Muslims fast from food and water from sunup to sundown each day. My student noticed that some of her Muslim classmates seemed to be having problems with hypoglycemia during the day. So she approached the Muslim student association on campus and asked if there would be any interest in students learning about what foods they could eat before sunrise and after sunset that would help them maintain a higher blood sugar level during the day when they were fasting. The Muslim student association felt that this information would be very helpful to their group. The nursing student had established that there was interest in the topic, a lack of knowledge about the topic, and motivation to learn, so she proceeded to design a program to meet this perceived need. Another student became aware of a significant group of African-American students on the campus. This student knew that this particular population had potential health risks in several areas outside of the general population. Her search of the literature revealed that African-Americans specifically have a higher risk for developing cardiovascular disease, cerebrovascular disease, hypertension, breast cancer, and sickle cell disease than the general population (Murray & Zentner, 1997; Lewis, Heitkemper, & Dirksen, 2000). In addition, this group consistently delays seeking out health care in a timely manner, compared with the general population (Murray & Zentner, 1997).

The student approached the faculty director of the Black Peer Counseling center on campus to see if there might be interest in developing a series of programs that would focus on health issues specific to this particular group of people. When she received an affirmative answer, she designed a survey with a number of questions focused on assessing the general health of her target group and a list of health topics. She asked students to select the issues of interest to them. Once she correlated the results, she spent a large part of the semester developing a series of presentations that she then implemented with this group of students. These are just are two examples of how students went about developing a single educational program and a series of programs to meet specific health needs of a particular target group of people. In Box 20–3, list target groups to consider on your campus.

Box 20-3   Student Learning Activity

Target Groups on Campus

Who are the specific groups of people on your campus you would like to reach?

What health problems would you like to address?

Ethnic/Cultural Group   Potential Health Problems

List them here:

The preceding information should give you some hints on how to target a specific health need for a specific group of people. Now let's move on to how to influence the college campus as a whole. You have already identified the common health problems associated with a college campus, as previously described. How can you then pique the interest of the individuals you want to reach? My students, working as a group, decided to take a multifaceted approach. The first thing they did was to look at the campus calendar of events. At our university a number of weeks had different themes for events. For example, February was National Heart Month and one week was Eating Disorder Awareness Week. Spring break was in March, and the week before vacation was designated "Have a Safe Spring Break" week. There were other event weeks as well, such as "Drug and Alcohol Awareness Week," "Take Back the Night" (a violence awareness event), and "Exercise Safety Week." As a whole, the clinical group decided to put together a health and fitness

awareness table with materials tied to the various event weeks. They moved the table around the campus on each clinical day. One or two students took responsibility for searching and developing the materials that were used for the table on a weekly or every-other-week basis, and all students took turns staffing the table during clinical time. Some of the places that were used to reach out to the campus community were the student union buildings, the library, and outside on the "quad" (a sort of crossroads on the campus). In Box 20–4, write events on your campus that you might target for teaching projects.

Box 20-4   Student Learning Activity

Scheduled Campus Events

Are there events at your university/school that you could tie into? Identify them here:

Event Week Theme   Health-Related Aspects

Another student had an idea about reaching out to the campus community, and she approached me with her idea as follows:

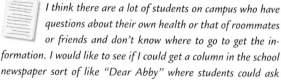 *I think there are a lot of students on campus who have questions about their own health or that of roommates or friends and don't know where to go to get the information. I would like to see if I could get a column in the school newspaper sort of like "Dear Abby" where students could ask questions anonymously and get accurate answers from us. I was thinking of calling it "Ask a Nurse."*

I thought it was a great idea but did think of a few drawbacks. The first drawback was that the school newspaper was a student-produced paper and I as a faculty member had no influence on what the student editors would choose to print. The student herself would have to convince the editors that this was an appropriate and important column for the paper. If she got their approval, we would need to set up a method to obtain the questions anonymously, investigate and write the responses in a condensed format to accommodate space limitations, *and* make it interesting to read. The student not only got the approval of the editors, she got a commitment for a weekly column. To get questions, the student first went to her classmates and got some volunteers to ask appropriate questions. Then came the idea for the "Ask a Nurse" box. The students put together a ballot type box with a sign that read, "Ask your health questions here. See your answers in the *Broadside*" (the school paper).

The box was placed on the health information table on each clinical day so that it was available for anonymous questions. Each student in the clinical then took one or more questions to search and write responses. All responses had to have a documented source. As the instructor, I took the responsibility of editing the student responses for accuracy, style, and approach. We submitted our column each week on floppy disk to the school paper at least 24 hours before the deadline to alleviate anxiety over not having the material when it was needed. The editors were pleased, the students enjoyed getting experience in learning a different form of writing, and the campus community began looking forward to "this week's topic." The project was a great success. After several articles were published in the school newspaper, the campus population began to recognize the "Ask a Nurse" columnists as the Nursenergy group who had the health/wellness table around campus. Students, faculty, staff, and maintenance personnel began to stop by to drop questions into the "Ask a Nurse" box or to look at the health information on display. On more than one occasion, people sought out the students to ask questions about their personal health problems. The students were able to refer them to the appropriate health-care provider who then followed up on the individual's problem.

Another project that the students took on was staffing the campus blood pressure clinic. This clinic had already been established as a program by the health and wellness office on campus. Shortly after the students began to staff the clinic, one of the students came to me with the following concern. She said something like this: " I've been staffing the blood pressure clinic for 2 weeks now and we have had very few participants. I think either people don't

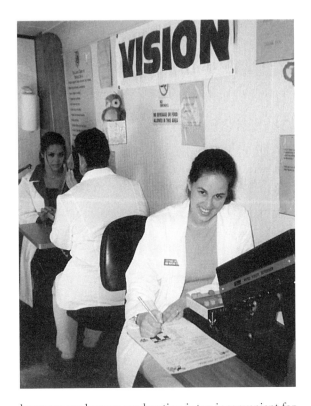

know we are here or our location is too inconvenient for them. I think more people would participate if we were more visible and convenient to them." Out of this observation the "traveling blood pressure clinic" was born. The student organized her classmates and literally took the clinic to the people. The student established a rotation schedule so that each area was visited twice during the semester. Sites included the library, student union buildings, and the physical plant where all the maintenance personnel were located. This was one of our most successful wellness projects. Not only did participation increase, but also a number of people with previously undiagnosed hypertension were identified and referred to appropriate health-care providers. The students not only took blood pressures but also kept records of the results and followed up on any referrals that were made. I, as the instructor, was available by pager if the students had any questions regarding a blood pressure reading or whether or not a referral was necessary.

A third project the students participated in as a group was the campus immunization clinic. In our state, it is mandated that all college students be inoculated for rubella (measles) before the beginning of their second semester. Working in twos, with me as backup, each student participated in at least one immunization clinic during the semester. Not only did the students administer rubella vaccine, but they also got experience with hepatitis B immunizations, tetanus boosters, and the purified protein derivative (PPD) intradermal skin test for tuberculosis. Their participation was more involved than just "giving shots." Not only did they give the injections, they were also responsible for educating the student clients about the particular immunization they were receiving, what side effects to watch for, and when to return to the clinic if necessary. All of the students found this to be a satisfying project because it allowed them to practice their psychomotor technical skills as well as their communication skills.

A final project the entire group took on was participating in a health fair as part of the university's spring campus celebration week. We had several tables located on the quad along with others. As students wandered through the area, the nursing students took blood pressures, performed general vision screening, conducted an "assess your stress" game, and helped students take a computerized alcohol awareness quiz.

As the semester progressed, more and more projects began to be generated by the student clinical group until we needed to acknowledge that there was more to do on the campus than our time and resources would allow. At this point, priorities needed to be identified, and the students began to get some experience in negotiation as they each promoted their own particular project. A priority list was developed by consensus of the group and the list was further divided into recurring and one-time projects. All students were involved in the recurring projects, and individual students took responsibility for one-time projects.

An important activity each week was the clinical conference. Instead of meeting each clinical day for 30 to 45 minutes as is typical in most clinical settings, our group found that meeting once a week for $1\frac{1}{2}$ to 2 hours was the most effective format. Because the students were working on a number of projects at any given time, this longer format allowed each student to share his or her individual activities and ask for help if any was needed. It was also

during these sessions that ongoing or recurring projects were evaluated and adjustments made midcourse, rather than waiting until the end of the rotation to evaluate what did or did not work.

Until now, I have discussed the clinical setting and how the students assessed and identified the health needs on a college campus. Now I would like to discuss how to go about implementing any given student project. Again, I recommend using the nursing process to organize your thoughts and to construct the plan as it lends itself easily to both content and process.

As I have already discussed in depth, the initial step is assessment. Once you have identified the health needs of the campus and prioritized them, you can formulate your nursing diagnosis. In most cases, the diagnosis will involve a lack of knowledge about some health issue (North American Nursing Diagnosis Association [NANDA], 1999/2000). After the nursing diagnoses come the outcomes statements. What do you want to see happen as a result of your intervention? You will want to be sure that your outcomes statements are put in measurable terms. Using "The Taxonomy of Learning Objectives" developed by Bloom (1956), Krathwohl, Bloom, & Masia (1964), and Simpson (1972), you will be able to select the action verbs you need that will make your outcomes measurable. For example, you may want college students to eat a more nutritionally balanced diet. Your outcomes for this might include any or all of the following:

- The client will be able to *verbalize* three sources of calcium-rich foods.
- The client will be able to *identify* three nutritional substitutes for fast-food snacks.
- The client will *report* eating lunch at 3 out of 5 days during the week.

As you can see, each of the outcomes is measurable. This measurability allows for the accurate evaluation of your interventions.

After you have identified your outcomes, you must identify your plan of action. In other words, what information are you going to present? Your information must be geared specifically to the outcome you are trying to achieve. For example, if you are trying to influence the food that students eat on the run, you must identify what they most commonly buy and then substitute equivalent options that are more nutritious. What kind of time will you need? What kind of space? What tools will you need? Table 20–1 presents various resources that should be useful to you when you plan your project.

Once you have identified the content you wish to present, you must look at the methods you will use to present the information. Your methods are your interventions and can include a wide variety of approaches. For example, you might want to form small groups and have each group work on a different piece of information. You might want to design a game for students to play that will increase their awareness of the nutritional pluses or minuses of what they eat. If the game is competitive, all the better. You might want to show a video to get your point across. No matter what methods you decide to use, they need to be geared to a level that your audience can understand. The fact that your target group is on a college campus does not necessarily guarantee a high level of literacy. If, for example, your group is made up of students

---

Table 20-1

Resources

Following is a list of resources you might find helpful in your campus clinical rotation:

National Organizations:
    The American Red Cross
    The American Heart Association
    The American Cancer Society
    The American Diabetes Association
    The Journal of American College Health

Local Service Clubs (e.g., the Lion's Club supports vision screening, used eyeglasses collections, and other activities associated with vision wellness)

Websites:
    www.wnet.org/archive/closetohome/home.html (Moyers on Addiction)
    www.well.com/user/woa/ (Web of Addiction)
    www.nida.nih.gov/ (National Institute on Drug Abuse)
    eatingdisorders.mentalhelp.net/ (All About Eating Disorders—Mental Health Net)
    closetoyou.org/eatingdisorders/ (Eating Disorders Site)
    www.depression.com (Depression Site)
    www.nih.gov/ (National Institutes of Health)
    mentalhelp.net/disorders/sx22.htm (Health Net-Major Depression Symptoms)
    www.cdcnpin.org/ (CDC National Prevention Information Network)
    www.healthlinkusa.com/Sexually_Transmitted_Disease_(STDS).htm (Health Link USA—Sexually Transmitted Diseases (STDs))
    http://www.4contraception.com/ (4 Contraception)
    www.beerboozebooks.com (Resource for Students, Faculty and Administrators on Alcohol Issues on College Campuses)
    www.glness.com/ndhs (Drinking: A Student's Guide)
    www.sada.org/ (Students Against Drugs and Alcohol)
    www.laserbuddy.com/recover/drugs.htm (About.com Substance Abuse: Alcohol)
    www.bloodpressure.com (Hypertension Network)
    www.mayohealth.org/mayo/9905/htm/hyper.htm (Mayo Clinic—Hypertension)
    www.aborcom.com/frame/welcome.htm (Arbor Nutrition Guide)
    cnn.com/HEALTH/diet.fitness/ (CNN.com—Diet and Fitness)
    www.dietitian.com (Ask the Dietitian)
    www.mayohealth.org/mayo/common/htm/dietpage.htm (Mayo Clinic—Nutrition Advice and More)
    www.hquest.com (National Database for Health Professionals)
    www.epa.gov/ (Environmental Protection Agency. Click on "Other Resources")
    www.osha.gov/ (Occupational Safety and Health Administration)

whose primary language in not English, there may be a wide variation in reading comprehension among group members, as well as a wide variety of food preferences. Other learning techniques such as demonstrations or picture boards might be more effective than written materials. If you are working with ancillary service personnel such as maintenance, food service, or groundskeeping, for example, the literacy level may be lower still. Therefore, looking at the level of literacy can become quite important in putting together a meaningful educational program for a group. Doak, Doak, and Root (1996) have a number of helpful ideas for presenting content to people with low literacy skills. These ideas can be valuable as you attempt to have the most positive impact possible on your clients.

Last, you will want to evaluate the effectiveness of your interventions. For this you refer to your outcomes statements. Did you achieve the desired outcome? If not, why not? Were your goals realistic? Were your methods appropriate for your plan? What could you have done differently?

When I think of realistic goals, it always reminds me of a story that happened to me when I was a student:

A middle-aged woman had come into the clinic complaining of polyuria, polyphagia, weight loss, and fatigue. Blood work showed she had developed diabetes mellitus, type II. I was part of an interdisciplinary team involved in planning her care. The team got together and put together a comprehensive approach to her care. The dietitian worked out a food plan, the physician prescribed oral hypoglycemic medication, nursing personnel prepared the finger stick blood sugar routine, and so on. Finally, the "plan" was shared with the client. She looked at it and then looked at us and said, "Who is this for?" You see, none of us had asked the client what her priorities were.

This story illustrates the importance of remembering that when you are establishing outcomes for your clients, whether they are individuals or groups, you need to do it in *collaboration* with your clients. Otherwise, you will more often than not be setting yourself up for failure. Remember, your plans are only as good as your clients perceive them to be relevant to their priorities and within their abilities to accomplish.

The following guidelines may be helpful as you plan various projects:

- Assessment: Be specific. Narrow your focus to one or two health concerns.
- Nursing diagnosis: In a wellness setting, this is usually a lack of knowledge related to (the health concern).
- Outcomes: Some references may call these behavioral objectives. Remember to make them measurable.
- Plan: Includes content to be presented; teaching methods planned; length of time; type of environment needed; teaching tools needed such as posters, videos, charts, and so on; and sometimes rationales for your actions.
- Implementation: What you actually did.
- Evaluation: Were the outcomes established met? If not, why not? What worked in the way of implementation and what didn't? What revisions need to be made if any?

As you progress through the semester, it will be very helpful to both you and your instructor if you keep a daily journal of your activities. The journal is not necessarily graded, so it can be a "safe" place for you to air your concerns, anxieties, and failures as well as your triumphs, client accolades, and feelings of accomplishment. Make it more than a list of activities you engaged in; include your feelings as well. Because your instructor might not be "on-site" with you all the time, the journal gives you an excellent opportunity to communicate to him or her the activities they don't see firsthand, as well as how you feel you are meeting the objectives of the course. This is one important way you can provide feedback to your instructor about your clinical performance. In like manner, your instructor can use your journal to provide written feedback to you about your performance. This approach will not replace face-to-face feedback but rather will complement it. If your instructor uses your journal to provide you with constructive criticism, you can make corrections to your performance in midcourse rather than finding out at the end of the rotation that you did not meet expectations. If there was one thing I did not like as a student, it was not knowing what my instructor was thinking about my performance. The journal approach gives you the opportunity to receive input from your faculty on a weekly basis. In my institution, many instructors use e-mail as a means for students to journal and for them to provide feedback. This system provides a faster response time for the student, cuts down on "paperwork," and can be sent at any time, and allows for entries to be downloaded and saved to help assess an individual student's progress.

Another record you must keep in this type of unstructured clinical is a time log. Some of your clinical time can legitimately be spent searching topic information, preparing audio/visual aids, and collecting handout materials from various sources. It is important that you be able to account for your noncontact time. That is the time you are not directly engaged in working with clients. Your contact and noncontact time should equal the number of hours you are to spend in clinical each week. If you are putting in more hours than your allotted clinical time, your instructor will help you find ways to make your activities more manageable. If you are put-

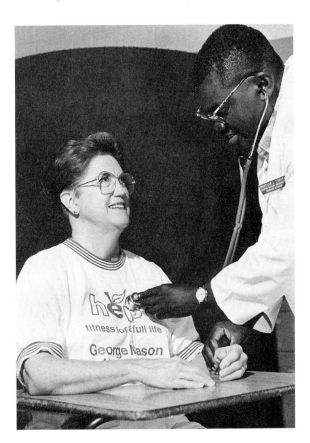

ting in less time, your instructor can help you find ways to be more productive. My students found the time logs to be very helpful. One of them said, "I really didn't have any idea how much time it was taking me to really prepare for my day at the health table. It took more time than I thought."

The last thing you will need to do as a group is to develop a rotation schedule for the semester that includes all the recurring as well as the individual activities in which you will be engaged. You can do this on a monthly basis or for the whole semester. In any case, some kind of schedule is important so that all activities are fully covered and so that you don't double or triple schedule yourself for the same times. This kind of schedule also helps your instructor keep track of who is where on any given day. It is also helpful for the heads of the different offices on campus that you will be interfacing with. Remember, your instructor might not be physically present with you all the time. In this kind of unstructured, wellness-focused clinical, you will most likely be working out of one of the health-related offices on campus, and the people in charge of those offices also need to know who will be working with them and when new students will arrive.

Just a word about the people you will interface with during your clinical. Most, if not all, of them *will not* be nurses. You might find yourself wondering what you as a nursing student can learn from them that relates to your ultimate career plans. I submit that you can learn a lot. On one hand, the people in the various health-related offices have a great deal of knowledge about their particular field. As a nurse, you will constantly find yourself overlapping with other health-related disciplines. Knowing how other disciplines approach common health goals will assist you in complementing their health plans. Also, as a nurse, you can bring a unique perspective to a given situation and can provide nonnurses with ideas they might not have considered. For example, shortly after we began our clinical rotation, Eating Disorder Awareness Week occurred. Because this event happened at the beginning of the semester, much of the planning had already been done the previous semester by the counseling center. My student decided that instead of focusing on the psychological aspects of eating disorders, she would complement the counseling center's information by focusing on the *physiologic repercussions* that result from an eating disorder. Bringing her unique perspective to the event helped to make it more holistic in nature and therefore more complete.

Finally, a few words about confidentiality. Because you will be interfacing with students as well as faculty, staff, and others, keeping the information they share with you confidential is extremely important. As nurses, we are charged to do no harm to those in our care. Sharing information about someone in a casual, social, or public manner not only violates the right to privacy of the person but is also a violation of the Code of Ethics that we as nurses follow (American Nurses Association [ANA], 1991). Be careful with the information that is entrusted to you. You have a professional responsibility to protect the privacy of the clients you see.

The campus clinical can give you an opportunity to develop your teaching and communication skills as well as to refine some of your technical skills. It is an opportunity to make a difference in the lives of a vulnerable group of people. Although it is not what you might think of as a "traditional" nursing role, it is an important role nonetheless. I hope that from reading this chapter you will recognize and value the importance of functioning as a nurse in a nontraditional setting.

And oh, yes, remember the student starting her clinical whose comments I shared with you at the beginning of the chapter? Here's what she had to say at the end of the clinical:

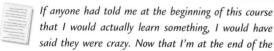

If anyone had told me at the beginning of this course that I would actually learn something, I would have said they were crazy. Now that I'm at the end of the course I'm amazed at how much I have been able to learn. I have been stimulated, challenged, and even had fun. This is the best clinical I've had so far!

Active Learning Strategies

1. Access the Website for "Ask A Nurse" (www.gmu.edu/departments/nursing) and review the archives of columns presented on the site. Do the topics addressed in this column reflect the topics of concern that you found in your review of literature?

2. Talk to three students on your campus who are not in nursing to identify their top three health concerns. Do these differ from those that you found in your literature review?

3. Meet with two other students in your nursing class to identify three potential projects that you could undertake on your college campus. What do you feel is the top-priority project?

4. Talk with a student on your campus from an ethnic group that differs from yours to identify specific health concerns. Does this person have health concerns that are different from those you anticipated?

References

American Nurses Association (ANA). (1991). Ethics and human rights. Washington, DC: ANA.

Bloom, B. S. (Ed.). (1956). Taxonomy of learning objectives, 1. Cognitive domain. New York: Longman.

Doak, C. C., Doak, L. G., & Root, J. H. (1996). Teaching patients with low literacy skills (2nd ed.). Philadelphia: J. B. Lippincott.

Krathwohl, D. R., Bloom, B. S., & Masia, B. B. (1964). Taxonomy of educational objectives. 2. Affective domain. New York: Longman.

Lewis, S. M., Heitkemper, M. M., & Dirksen, S. R. (2000). Medical-surgical nursing: Assessment and management of clinical problems (5th ed.). St. Louis: Mosby.

Murray, R. B., & Zentner, J. P. (1997). Health assessment and promotion strategies: Through the life span (6th ed.). Stamford, CT: Appleton & Lange

North American Nursing Diagnosis Association (NANDA). (1999/2000). Nursing Diagnoses Definitions and Classification. Philadelphia: NANDA.

Simpson, E. (1972). The classification of educational objectives in the psychomotor domain. In Contributions of Behavioral Science to Instructional Technology. Washington, DC: Gryphon.

CHAPTER

21 Community-based Nursing Practice in an HIV/AIDS Network

Loretta Brush Normile

LEARNING OBJECTIVES

1) Discuss the essential components of community-based HIV/AIDS services.

2) Describe the role of the nurse in HIV/AIDS community-based care.

3) Develop a list of HIV/AIDS resources in your community.

4) Describe the skills and competencies used in health promotion and disease prevention of HIV/AIDS.

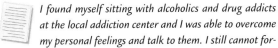

I found myself sitting with alcoholics and drug addicts at the local addiction center and I was able to overcome my personal feelings and talk to them. I still cannot forget the two I became very attached to. I was really moved by one patient whose doctor told him that he had just a few months to live. He believes he is a fighter and will not give up just because someone said he has a few months to live. He thinks nurses are gifted people who can do a lot more than what medication can do—that they help you to help yourself. Another woman I met

was trying to kill herself, but now, after substance abuse treatment, she wants to be a candidate in an HIV treatment research study.

These are the words of a junior nursing student as she reflected back over just one of her clinical experiences in a community-based Human Immunodeficiency Virus/ Acquired Immune Deficiency Syndrome (HIV/AIDS) network. If the HIV epidemic is to be controlled and/or eradicated in our near future, the best hope is through prevention and management of health problems of the individual in his or her community. This chapter teaches you how to deliberately and systematically navigate the community and its resources to prevent HIV disease in the uninfected and to promote health in the HIV infected. Through nursing students' comments and stories from a variety of settings across the life span, you will come to develop an ethic for community-responsive care. You will learn that to be truly effective in that care, it takes a partnership between you and the client and family, interdisciplinary relationships, and community participation.

As the HIV/AIDS epidemic nears the end of its second decade, many changes have come about. The distribution of HIV in populations continues to change over time. We know that HIV surveillance data provide only the minimal estimates of the HIV infected persons in this country. For this reason, the Centers for Disease Control (CDC) surveillance report urges caution in interpretation of its data. We know the CDC estimates nearly 750,000 in the United States are infected with HIV. It is well known that many potentially infected people have not been tested (CDC, 1999). It is estimated that 500,000 of them are not benefiting from treatment and new advances in care. Worldwide, it is believed that 34 million people are living with HIV or AIDS; most of those live in developing countries.

Although the incidence of HIV/AIDS is decreasing in the United States, particularly among homosexuals, selected segments of the population are the exception. The sharp decline in the numbers is not being seen in the African-American and Latino population, especially in women and young adults. We are seeing the numbers of seniors with HIV rise, with the number of adults age 50 and over composing 10 percent of all cases (National Institute on Aging, 1999). Homosexual and heterosexual sexual practices and intravenous drug use remain the three greatest modes of viral transmission.

ESSENTIAL COMPONENTS OF COMMUNITY HIV/AIDS SERVICES

A student nurse reflected on her community-based clinical experience as follows:

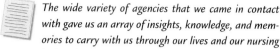

The wide variety of agencies that we came in contact with gave us an array of insights, knowledge, and memories to carry with us through our lives and our nursing career. I had a chance to see HIV clients in schools, hospitals, shelters, clinics, child day care, and of course, their homes. What made this experience so powerful is that I was able to relate to them in their own settings or on their own turf. That gave me special insight into the various needs of individuals with HIV within different settings and also the commonalities, no matter where they are.

You can find clients with HIV or at risk for HIV anywhere in the community. You may choose to explore a network of services and agencies from settings offering highly specialized HIV/AIDS care, such as HIV/AIDS clinics and doctors offices, to care sites providing clinical research protocols and substance abuse centers. Many agencies such as shelters, food banks, jails, schools, local health departments, and voluntary agencies also give access and provide services for HIV-affected clients and families. Other community agencies used to access special population groups include HIV testing and counseling centers, home-health-care agencies, hospices, juvenile detention centers, adolescent and pediatric programs, and of course, the homes of the clients and their families. These settings provide access to vulnerable groups such as intravenous drug abusers, gays and lesbians, and hemophiliacs, as well as those particularly at risk for HIV, such as women of color and their babies and the babies still to be born of HIV-positive mothers and sex trade workers. These diverse populations give contact across the life span from infants to the elderly. Community-based HIV/AIDS care should be carried out in a respectful, compassionate, caring environment that seeks to maintain the dignity of the individual regardless of their gender, age, sexual orientation, race, ethnic background, religious affiliation, or socioeconomic status (Normile, 2000). In Box 21–1, list your ideas for education needs of the older adult.

You will learn about many common problems in the health care of HIV clients. Many of these problems are not idiosyncratic to HIV disease alone. Some of these difficult-to-deal-with issues include access to health care,

```
┌──────────────────────────────────────────┐
│   ┌────────────────────────────────────┐  │
│   │ Box 21-1      Student Learning Activity │  │
│   └────────────────────────────────────┘  │
│                                            │
│        The Older Adult and HIV/AIDS        │
│   - - - - - - - - - - - - - - - - - - - -  │
│   The incidence of HIV/AIDS is increasing in the aging popu- │
│   lation. List three implications of this trend for education of │
│   the elderly in our society.              │
│                                            │
│    1.                                      │
│                                            │
│                                            │
│                                            │
│    2.                                      │
│                                            │
│                                            │
│                                            │
│    3.                                      │
│                                            │
│                                            │
└──────────────────────────────────────────┘
```

Table 21-1

Key Issues and Concerns of HIV-infected Individuals and Their Families

Responding to seroconversion

Disclosing HIV status to others

Coping with disease progression

Coping with HIV as a chronic disease

Adherence to medication regimens

Alteration of body image

Estrangement from relatives and family members

Fear of suffering, dying, and death

Loss of physical capabilities

Loss of mental capacity or emotional stability

Loss of independence

Real or perceived discrimination

Reconciliation of sexual orientation

Treatment considerations and issues (e.g., joining a clinical trial)

Multiple losses and bereavement

Leaving children behind

Loss of control

Loss of personal choices

Loneliness

Approaching death

knowledge deficits, adherence to treatment protocols, and management of a chronic illness. Client problems often seen are similar to those seen with other chronic or terminal diseases—pain management, noncompliance, nutritional deficits, the need for health teaching, and coping with loss, grief, and bereavement.

As you learn to care for HIV/AIDS clients or those at risk for HIV/AIDS, you will discover many unique care issues (Janosik, 1994). Routinely, the individual and family will find it hard to come to terms with a diagnosis of HIV/AIDS. The prolonged uncertainty and complexity of the disease causes the client and family members great difficulty. Family members may rally, cope, and address many of the unique issues of the disease, or the diagnosis may prove to be a catalyst for relationships that have been strained for years. Periods of crisis may be introduced with prolonged uncertainty. The physical and emotional deterioration and frequent intervals of crisis lead to some key issues and concerns (see Table 21–1). These issues often relate to stigma, ethics, sexuality, alternative lifestyles, counseling and support, and multiple losses.

All clients with HIV disease are cared for by a nurse at some point during the course of their illnesses. At this point in the science of care, our emphasis is on maximizing the quality of life, promoting and maintaining health, and ensuring a positive health-care experience for clients' lives. Newly diagnosed clients have special educational needs. List two of these needs in Box 21–2.

The student, the clients, and other health professionals are all equally important and interdependent and should seek out opportunities to support one another. It is essential in these settings to empower each other,

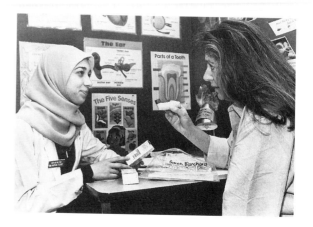

Box 21-2	Student Learning Activity

Educational Needs after HIV-positive Diagnosis

Think about a teenager who has learned she is HIV-positive. List two educational topics you would want to address with her.

1.

2.

welcome new ideas and change, and celebrate life. Allow your tears and the tears of others, and encourage laughter. One student found personal comfort in her assigned clinical experience, as described below.

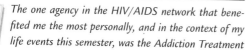

The one agency in the HIV/AIDS network that benefited me the most personally, and in the context of my life events this semester, was the Addiction Treatment Center. Anyone who steps foot through those doors can reap the rewards of listening to and learning from the counselors. You need not be an addict to benefit from their life experiences and their commitment. For me, it had particular impact this semester. My father battled with alcoholism for most of his adult life, and his life ended during this semester. He lost his battle with alcoholism. I truly believe that the memory of my time spent at the Addictions Treatment Center helped alleviate some of my pain and feelings of loss . . . and I am eternally grateful for that.

THE NURSING ROLE IN AN HIV/AIDS COMMUNITY SETTING

A holistic nursing approach is necessary to care for individuals, families, and small groups of clients affected by HIV disease in a community-based setting. You must become familiar with educational strategies so you can protect others from becoming infected. Our messages

on prevention must be specifically tailored and targeted for special groups: socioeconomic, cultural, sexual, and racial- and gender-oriented. We must also possess knowledge of the epidemiology and the demographics of HIV disease, HIV/AIDS treatment modalities and related nursing interventions, mental health concepts, and substance abuse treatment, as well as be capable of providing supportive counseling, advocacy, and, most importantly, connection to services in the community. The demands of this disease require a community-based approach because your clients live and interact as members of a family and a community.

Work with HIV/AIDS poses special challenges: Although the prevalence of HIV/AIDS is increasing, the death rate is declining. People in North America are living longer with HIV/AIDS. The disease is now being managed more like a chronic disease with a primary goal of delaying the occurrence of opportunistic infections and the long-term side effects of therapy. A fatal outcome is always a possibility with a chronic disease, but only a decade ago, many persons with advanced HIV disease spent much of their time in the hospital preparing for death. Who would have thought then that we would have antiretroviral chemotherapy to slow down HIV replication, and that therapy would result in enormously complex personal treatment decisions?

Today, three drug combinations with nucleosides, non-nucleosides, and protease inhibitors are the norm for many, but four- and five-drug combinations are increasingly being prescribed. These highly state-of-the-art aggressive antiretroviral therapies (HAART) can greatly reduce viral load and increase life in both quality and quantity. AIDS clients previously facing death are being returned to a level of health that allows them to reengage in living. This dramatic swing from a high viral load and life-threatening infections to a nondetectable viral load and relative health has been termed the Lazarus Syndrome (in the Bible, Lazarus is returned from the dead). However, maintenance of this health level requires ongoing treatment regimens amid uncertainties about how long this response may last (Gregonis, 1997). Many of these drugs have been approved quickly, and we are asking thousands of people to adhere to a lifelong course of treatment with little data to support its long-term effectiveness and the development of long-term side effects. Many develop resistance, life-threatening reactions to the drugs, and serious drug interactions with other medications used for depression, tuberculosis (TB), and birth control. Pharmaceutical companies are constantly working to develop new, more effective, and less-toxic antiretroviral agents, which will also affect mutant and resistant viral strains. The experimental nature of the drugs can cause concern for clients. List three of these in Box 21–3.

Box 21-3   Student Learning Activity

Experimental Drugs

Your client asks you about the safety of an experimental drug that one of his friends is taking. List three areas of concern you would explore with him.

1.

2.

3.

Perhaps the greatest treatment issues today are when to initiate treatment, long-term management of HIV disease, and adherence to drug regimens. Successful medical treatment centers on closely monitoring viral load, initiating potent combinations of drugs early to drive down the viral load, scrupulous adherence to treatment regimens, and healthy behaviors in all aspects of life (Ungavarski & Flaskerud, 1999).

If you engage yourself in the learning process rather than safeguarding your own feelings, you and the client can both increase understanding of disease and how affected individuals cope. On the other hand, you may approach the details, facts, and data of HIV disease as an intriguing mystery story with you, the student, as the detective. This would be a cold and unfeeling method to apply to clients. Learning about the disease can be appropriately seen as a "sleuthing game," but the human element of suffering of the clients and families experiencing HIV disease cannot be ignored. Open engagement in the learning process helps to develop a strong background from which to practice. Such a perspective also welcomes all messengers with additional news about HIV and is more likely to help distance you from preconceived ideas and beliefs. One junior nursing student expresses herself eloquently in prose to stress how little she really knew about HIV/AIDS and how she grew personally and professionally as she started her experience in the HIV/AIDS Network:

My HIV clinical last spring opened my eyes quite a bit. As a nurse, knowing the wrath of this disease, I had to commit myself to the afflicted, their pain, and their grief far more than I ever encountered in my life, I have to admit.

Reality can be a merciless captor, meeting a HIV patient for the first time as you know death could be approaching at the drop of a dime it's so unfair to witness this misfortune of so many healthy people transforming into the living dead, what a crime.

There is one face and experience that I cannot rid. This HIV-infected heterosexual male who spoke amid the masses of apathetic high school students he told his story, it affected me, I swear it did.

He spoke of his sexual history and his irresponsibility of protecting himself from the things he did while he was in the Navy sleeping with numerous women. Being a man now he was paying for his acts, his stupidity.

I listened and watched, feeling more than empathy in a contrite and reproachful manner as he made his plea to these young kids who feel so superhuman, so free. This could be their destiny, this could actually be me!

He humanized his experience so well and in such depth I felt he was talking to me now, and with each breath I vowed I would make even a small difference as a nurse. If I couldn't save his life, I would try my hardest to prevent another death.

What he taught me that day was that life had to be lived, no matter how hard it was or who you were, there was so much to give by educating others or touching them somehow.

I was his kindred spirit that day, his words channeled through me because now I practice what I preach, and what I teach eagerly is that HIV does not discriminate, it can infect at any moment and it is because of him that I had this epiphany.

Case Management

Case management is an integral part of any community-based experience with HIV/AIDS. It is defined as "a process of identifying needs for and arranging, coordination, monitoring, and evaluating quality, cost-effective health-care services to achieve designated outcomes" (Clark, 2000, p.31). Nursing case management ensures that the client is consistently cared for throughout the illness, from home to hospital to long-term care environments. The case manager can coordinate care to avoid duplication of services and guard against conflicting treatment plans. It is a model for identifying, coordinating, and monitoring the implementation of services needed to achieve desired client outcomes with in a specified period of time (Sullivan & Decker, 1997).

A student reflects on her time with a case manager:

My experience with the case manager was a great way to begin this student rotation. It's so nice to know that nurse clinicians still remember what it was like to be "green" and have empathy for our plight as students. She was wonderful about explaining what she did and why. The client, "K," was wonderful about allowing me to "invade" his personal life. I learned a great deal about prophylaxis, pathophysiology, and human tragedy that day. "K" touched me deeply for many reasons and although I held it together in his presence, I had to cry for a while afterwards in solitude.

Another student's experience with the same nurse case manager was a learning experience about the need for support of the professional caregiver:

The nurse case manager looked stressed to me and the more we talked, the more I realized she has a great deal of responsibility not only at her work, but also personally as a single parent. I realized how important it must be to have a good support system. She was scheduled to see a patient and we examined him for 45 minutes. His CD4 count was 100, and his viral load was 200,000. He had been in the hospital with pneumonia over the holidays. He was doing much better, but when I listened to his lungs, it was clear that his left lung was still affected. He was very nice in letting me be part of the exam. The case manager was very thorough and I would feel very comfortable with her if I were her patient.

You should see the case manager as the human link in a chain of community services. In addition, case managers also serve as excellent mentors for students in a community-based setting. Seeing the case manager "in action" allows you to observe working within interdisciplinary environments and involving clients, family members, and other key support persons.

Working with the case manager is a great opportunity for you to see nursing process and collaboration in action. The HIV/AIDS nurse case manager may have from 10 to 35 clients, often a much higher caseload than a case manager in an acute-care setting. Case managers may or may not provide direct care, and they may follow an HIV client's progress through the system from hospital admission to death. The death of clients continues to be a frequent experience for many HIV/AIDS case managers. Aside from being a knowledgeable clinician caring for clients, the nurse case manager must be highly empathic and caring. In this particular instance, the nurse case manager was able to be empathic to both client and student, and she assumed the roles of a competent clinician and a preceptor.

The HIV/AIDS collaborative practice team is interdisciplinary and may consist of a physician, social worker, nutritionist, substance abuse specialist, clergy, and mental health counselor, in addition to a nurse. All contribute and help to define appropriate intervention. At times, roles may overlap. All depend heavily on collegial support because the risk of becoming emotionally depleted continues to be a prime hazard when working with HIV/AIDS clients. In Box 21–4, list aspects of your role to coordinate with others on the collaborative practice team.

Box 21-4   Student Learning Activity

Interdisciplinary Team

Think about the roles of various members of the HIV/AIDS collaborative practice team. How do you think your role would coordinate with that of:

1. Physician

2. Social worker

3. Nutritionist

4. Clergy

Counseling and Mental Health

HIV/AIDS clients present a great challenge to the nursing student's skills. There are several challenges that face the student:

  b. Developing a comfort level and caregiving skills
  c. Identifying, building, and using support networks
  d. Uncovering personal values and attitudes related to caring for HIV/AIDS clients

Counseling and social support can most simply be defined as effective use of self to help clients and families deal with a set of problems or concerns and includes activities that promote personal competencies. First, you must want to help people from many walks of life and enjoy working with others. Effective communication is a primary skill for the community-based nurse. It is certainly one of the most important aspects of establishing rapport with the client. You need to be honest, be nonjudgmental, and show positive regard for all. These behaviors help to create an atmosphere conducive to open expression of attitudes and feelings. With counseling and support, your task involves helping to recognize feelings and concerns, assisting the client to open up those feelings so they can be explored, and helping to clarify what these feelings may mean for the client. To summarize, you help the person explore, ventilate, understand, and deal with feelings. Your goals for counseling and support may include reduction of anxiety, promotion of successful decision making, and increasing or imparting knowledge.

Because HIV/AIDS presents unique challenges, student nurses are not always comfortable with their skills in counseling and giving support. Many of the people you care for with HIV/AIDS will be young adults. HIV disease is a life-threatening diagnosis with the potential for losses of health, independence, financial security, sexual freedom, and social support, as are other life-threatening diseases. However, HIV disease also carries stigma, blame, the infectiousness and transmissibility of the disease, and the roller-coaster nature of the course of the illness.

You will find the psychosocial issues of HIV disease may be grouped into three constellations. One constellation is loss. A second is stress and includes uncertainty of prognosis and of information, along with rational and irrational fears of rejection and abandonment. The third psychosocial constellation focuses on death and dying (Stine, 1999). Issues vary from person to person and change over the course of the disease. These constellations frequently intersect.

The most essential aspect of your preparation to care for the HIV/AIDS-infected family is an appreciation for this variability and the range of responses you will see. For one client and family, the issue may be disclosure of a diagnosis that has led to estrangement whereas another patient and family may be facing death by planning the funeral. Often, clients need help with immediate needs such as how to disclose HIV status to a lover and the decision of family members to get tested. Later in the disease, as the client becomes sicker, the individual and family may be confronting practical concerns such as dying and issues related to dying and impending death.

Planning for the care of client and family should begin with a comprehensive family assessment, which includes personality characteristics, adherence with treatment, identification of coping skills, realistic awareness of the illness, cultural and religious background, self-esteem, and risk of self-destructive behaviors. As a student, you should be sure to gain a thorough understanding of the key issues for people with HIV disease as identified previously in Table 21–1.

Seeing the client and family regularly requires flexibility and may necessitate home or telephone visits. The focus of your care, however, should always include helping the individual and family reduce stress and obtain as much control over their lives and the disease as possible. Members of special groups living with HIV/AIDS may include intravenous drug users, homeless persons, or women and children; you are in a unique position to advocate for the appropriate services they need. Within the community, you can help these individuals and families develop and build the needed support networks.

Regardless of the client's HIV antibody status, the primary objective of counseling is to provide health information that helps people avoid behaviors that may place them or others at risk for contracting the HIV virus. There are two steps to HIV test counseling; pretest counseling and posttest counseling. Pretest and posttest counseling provide excellent opportunities to educate people who believe they need to be tested. Your role is threefold: (1) provide information, (2) assess sexual behavior and drug history, and (3) counsel concerning what test results mean.

Your experience and personal style will influence the way essential information about the client's situation is collected. Counseling and support of your clients offers them and you opportunities for growth and learning to live life more fully.

Developing a List of HIV/AIDS Community Resources

Information about HIV disease comes from an abundance of sources. For busy students, the temptation to limit information to one reliable source is always present, but that can dramatically narrow your view. Clients will come to you with many things they have heard from sources you are not aware of or may have closed off. It is easier to work with client issues if you are at least somewhat aware of the sources of their information. Questions and statements from clients may run the full range from incredibly inaccurate to highly scientific, from the unreliable to the reliable. If you are prepared, you can talk to them about what you have found reliable. You want to collect a full range of views and facts to let your clients know you are at least aware of the information. Make a list of information sources so you can quickly access the specific information you need (Figure 21–1.).

Fill in contacts, phone numbers, Web sites, and e-mail addresses as you collect the sources you find especially helpful. The list of information sources is enormous and continues to grow (see Table 21–2). Films, plays, journals, news stories, books, and journals written by laypersons as well as professionals, people with HIV and AIDS, celebrity spokespersons, HIV/AIDS treatment newsletters, and official sources such as the Centers for Disease Control (CDC), the World Health Organization, the National Institute of Allergy and Infectious Diseases, and AIDS education and training centers are a few examples. Some of this information may come from questionable sources and some may not be consistent. Some of it is preliminary research. No matter what the source, it is important not to discount the information prematurely.

Now that you have educated yourself about all sources of information, you will want to make a list of referral information sources that you can access quickly when needed. Even the most experienced HIV/AIDS nurse cannot comfortably manage this infectious disease with all of its extraordinary complex pathophysiological, sociological, and psychological aspects without a strong referral network. A referral list can greatly facilitate accessing specific information you may need at any given point in time. As you build your experiences with the resources and continue to add to your referral list, you will find that your expertise in HIV/AIDS care grows. Those resources can include your local community agencies that care for HIV/AIDS clients; the local regional Education and Training Center (sites are listed by the Health Resources and Services Administration Center of the U.S. Public Health Service); HIV/AIDS agencies at the local, county, and state level; a national resource list to include CDC and other national resources such as Project Inform and the Gay Men's Health Crisis Center; your HIV/AIDS medical center and/or clinic; your local

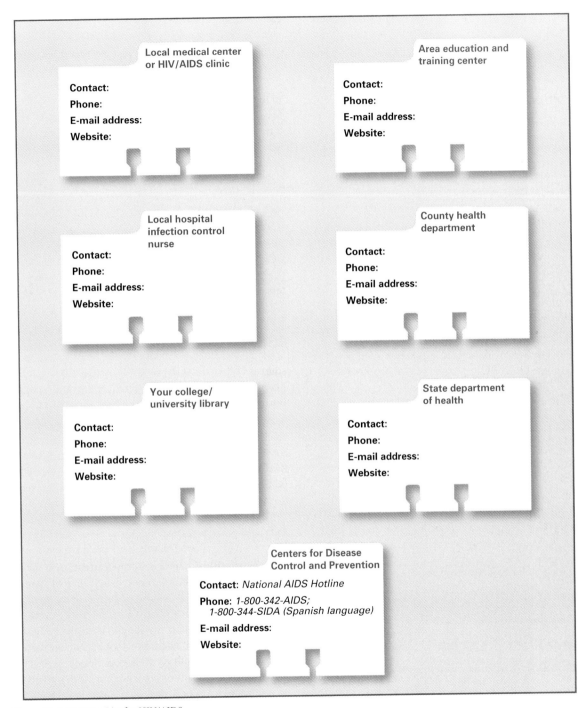

Figure 21–1 Resource List for HIV/AIDS

Table 21-2

Selected HIV/AIDS Internet Resources

AIDS/HIV information

Latest treatment and best news in drug protocol developments and alternative treatment methods. Statistics and facts about HIV/AIDS.

www.geocities.com/HotSprings/6157/AIDS.html

Association of Nurses in AIDS Care (ANAC)

www.anacnet.org/aids/

CDC National Prevention Information Network:

www.cdcnipn.org

e-mail: info@cdcnpin.org

Gay Men's Health Crisis (GMHC)

Provides valuable information on everything from up-to-date treatment to discrimination and employment issues.

www.gmhc.org

HIV Frontline

Add your name to the mailing list for HIV Frontline, a newsletter for professionals who counsel people living with HIV. Provides daily and weekly updates on HIV disease.

www.HIVLine.com

Johns Hopkins AIDS Service Web sites:

hopkins-aids-edu

hopkins-id.edu

The Journal of Test Positively Aware Network:

www.tpan.com

e-mail:tpanet@aol.com

Medscape

Comprehensive summaries by expert authors focusing on clinical implications of HIV/AIDS.

www.medscape.com

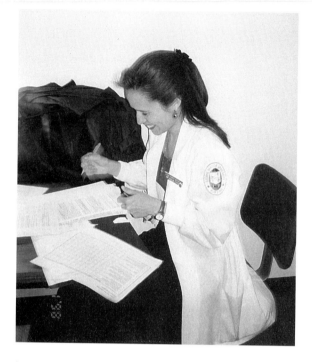

hospital infection control expert; your own support network of colleagues; favorite books on HIV/AIDS; and journals and newsletters. The important thing is to have a good network, a network that is made up of caregivers who are efficient, capable, and caring when dealing with clients and committed to maintaining consistent contact and feedback. By compiling your own resource list you have taken an important step to incorporating HIV disease into your practice of health care.

CONCLUSION

In conclusion, this chapter has drawn attention to the essential components of community-based HIV/AIDS services. You have gained an insight into the role of the nurse in HIV/AIDS community-based care, and the resource list you develop will facilitate meaningful participation in the prevention of HIV/AIDS, care and support of clients, and HIV/AIDS health education of the community. As the HIV epidemic forces its path through human history, your role as a nurse will continue to evolve and connect with the community on a deeper level. I leave you with the words of a lovely poem written about a client by a student nurse.

RENEWAL

We went to the ER as a psych liaison team
to interview a patient who had been deemed
a desperate man that was at the end of his rope
we were there now, two visions of hope.

What we had encountered was such a sad scene
of a body now broken by unfulfilled dreams
a soulless shell with no light in his eyes
he felt there was nothing left but to plan his demise.

As we pursued his history we began to develop
a sense of a man whose life had been enveloped
by the pain of his fate and the weight of his gloom
the air of despair now encompassed the room.

He told us his story like it had been rehearsed
about his addictions, the losses, his curse
of contracting HIV and a life that was battered
banished from the world, he felt nothing mattered.

As momentary silence suspended time and space
tears never fallen now dampened his face
it was then we knew he had to be free
from the darkness that enslaved him, he needed therapy.

He arrived on our unit with only the belief
that the staff would embrace him and provide a relief
safety and comfort were promises we kept
it appeared for the first time he finally had slept.

I talked with him each day and at great length
about self-rediscovery and identifying his strengths
confronting his fears was truly a test
suicide was not the answer, all he needed was a rest.

Because he had HIV, I told him there was a great need
to educate our children, he could plant the seed
he could make a difference with this special giving
and change lives through his new penchant for living.

As the week progressed, the chains of anguish were released
the stage of hopelessness had finally ceased
with the help of the staff his faith had been restored
he forgave himself, resolved issues, his pain was not ignored.

The day of his discharge, the journey began
his growth was evident, he was a new man
with a gleam in his eye, he smiled and waved
and began on the road of new life that I had helped pave.

Active Learning Strategies

1. View the video *The Best Defense* (Intermedia) or *And the Band Played On* (HBO). Following the viewing, discuss the following with a friend: (1) your personal reactions to the video, (2) perceived clinical implications for at-risk groups, and (3) the role of the nurse in reference to the concept/material presented.

2. Select and read four articles concerning HIV/AIDS care in the community. Use nursing journals for this exercise. Use the following guidelines as you select and read your articles.
   A. Select one article from 1985, another from 1990, one from 1995, and one from the current year
   B. Write a summary of your findings to include:
      i. The focus population
      ii. The trends in treatment
      iii. The role of the nurse
   C. Share your summary with your clinical group.

3. Begin a file of articles from journals, newspapers, newsletters, and magazines that discuss HIV disease.

4. Write a short paragraph on how HIV/AIDS disease has changed from a death sentence to a chronic disease.

References

Clark, M. J. (2000). Community health nursing. Stamford, CT: Appleton & Lange.

Centers for Disease Control. (1999). HIV/AIDS Surveillance Report, 11(1), Midyear Edition. Atlanta: Centers for Disease Control.

Gregonis, S. W. (1997). Magic Johnson and Lazarus: The new syndromes. Journal of the Association of Nurses in AIDS Care, 8(5), 75–76.

Janosik, E. H. (1994). Crisis counseling: A contemporary approach (2nd ed.). Boston: Jones and Bartlett.

National Institute on Aging. (1999). HIV, AIDS, and older people. Washington DC: National Institute of Health.

Normile, L. B. (2000). The aging woman and HIV/AIDS: Increasing risk and incidence. Age in Action, 15(3), 1–3.

Stine, G. J. (1999). AIDS update 1999: An annual overview of acquired immune deficiency syndrome. Upper Saddle River, NJ: Prentice Hall.

Sullivan, E., & Decker, P. (1997). Effective leadership and management in nursing. Menlo Park, CA: Addison-Wesley.

Ungavarski, P., & Flaskerud, J. H. (1999). HIV/AIDS: A guide to primary care management (4th ed.). Philadelphia: W. B. Saunders.

CHAPTER

22 Community-based Nursing Practice in a Home-care Setting

Susan W. Durham

LEARNING OBJECTIVES

1) Understand environmental concerns that are unique to the home-care setting.

2) Examine the role differences between the faculty member and the professional nurse as they each encourage the student's autonomous practice in home care.

3) Discuss safety issues related to the home-care setting.

4) Understand the components and sequence of a home visit and apply this to clients with a variety of problems.

5) Understand the concept of case management and allocation of limited resources and services as they relate to the home-care client's health-care needs.

6) Identify some ethical dilemmas specifically related to home care and apply ethical principles to come up with possible solutions.

7) Understand the unique qualities in documentation of a home visit.

8) Identify examples of urgent and emergency situations in the home and what to do when these situations occur.

As the focus of nursing care has moved out of the acute-care setting and into the community, the nurse is faced with the many challenges of providing that care in the client's home rather than in the hospital. As a result, schools of nursing have also been faced with finding settings that prepare their students to meet the changing health-care needs of their clients and to function in a changing practice environment. With this difference in venue, clinical nursing practice has taken on many new dimensions. This chapter will assist you in better preparing to go into the homes and serve your neighbors best.

PREPARING FOR A CLINICAL EXPERIENCE IN HOME CARE

Research suggests that clinical practice is inherently stressful to students, and this stress persists throughout different courses, across curriculums, and without regard to programs (Oermann, 1998). Oermann compared the stresses on students during clinical practice in a variety of different pro-

grams. One of the variables that she found inherent in the stress level was the public nature of the clinical performance. The possibility of many different people and professionals becoming an audience while the student performs a skill is an ever-present reality. This fact leads students to high levels of anxiety, especially if the students perceive the audience as unfair or nonsupportive (Oermann, 1996).

Having to make a home visit and perform clinical skills for the first time in the home environment adds to the nurse's anxiety level because the environment is in the client's control, rather than in the nurse's, as in acute care. In the home, there is an even greater potential for many different kinds of people to become the audience of clinical performance. Some of the people you may encounter on any given visit are a visiting friend, a nonprofessional caregiver, an anxious relative, a home-health aid, a social worker, a physical therapist, or a nurse specialist. Most of the time it is not going to be your choice as to whether they stay during your visit. Usually you must get on with the purpose of your visit in spite of their presence. The pressures of having others watch you perform a clinical technology when it is perhaps only the second or third time you

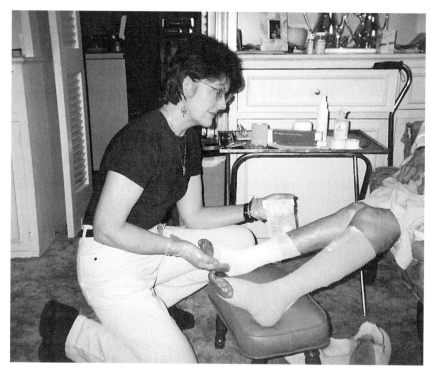

have ever done it can be quite anxiety provoking. However, adequate preparation and planning can lessen the feelings of vulnerability and inadequacy felt when faced with an unexpected audience, as well as offer you experiential learning on which you can make future clinical judgments.

One way nursing schools have found to help students prepare for the uncertainty of the home environment is laboratory simulations. Simulations present students with situations that represent reality without the constraints and pressures of real-life situations. Oermann (1998) suggests that simulations provide a variety of benefits for students, such as problem-solving, decision-making, and critical thinking skills, as well as opportunities for reflective thinking. Therefore, creating a simulated home situation along with practicing with problem-solving scenarios can lesson the "shock factor," improve your ability to make on-the-spot judgments, and increase your confidence level when you enter a home not knowing what or whom you will find.

Creating a realistic laboratory situation that mimics a home environment is pretty easy to do. Most of you are accustomed to performing checklist kinds of clinical procedures on manikins prior to performing them on a client. If you don't have an area of your lab that is set up to simulate a home environment, just choose a bed in your nursing lab and pretend that it is a client's home. Then practice some role-playing scenarios that are characteristic of problems that might be encountered in the home.

Read the following scenario and then answer the questions in Box 22–1.

GAINING CONTROL

You are being sent to the home of a Mrs. C., a 99-year-old lady who has a diagnosis of congestive heart failure and general systems failure. She has been bedridden for about 2 years and lives with her two daughters who are in their late 50s. She has an indwelling, Foley catheter, and you are responsible for doing the bimonthly Foley change. The previous nurse's note states that Mrs. C. has methicillin-resistant Staphylococcus aureus *(MRSA), and precautions must be taken. You are told that the supplies are in the home and there is a nonlicensed caregiver in the home who comes each day at 8 A.M. and stays until 4 P.M. to assist with activities of daily living. You plan to visit during that time so that the caregiver is there to assist you in properly positioning the client. You have reviewed the technique for Foley*

catheter insertion with the nurse and your instructor and you have done the procedure many times successfully on other clients.

When you arrive at the home, the daughters are upset because the regular caregiver has a sick child and could not come. They are both sitting in the living room smoking one cigarette after another. They have been impatiently waiting for you to arrive and are upset about you coming without the nurse even though they told the nurse that it was okay. Fortunately, you have brought along a fellow student to assist you in positioning and holding the client's legs during the Foley change. The nurse said that the client's legs were somewhat contracted and that having another person there would be helpful.

As you are gathering your supplies together in the client's bedroom, you notice that there are no clean gloves left in the glove box and no other clean gloves available in the home. You have only three pairs with you. You begin to count in your head how many glove changes that you will have to make. You know that you will need one pair to remove the old catheter and your student colleague will need one to hold the client's legs, especially because of the MRSA. You will need another pair to clean her up afterward. You should just make it with three pairs of gloves but already you are feeling a little tense. As you prepare and position the client, you realize that her legs are very stiff and will barely open. You need another person to hold the legs. You ask one of the daughters to hold one side. She reluctantly says yes, mumbling something about why the home health agency could not send a real nurse as you hand her the last pair of clean gloves. There is one sterile Foley catheter and one catheter insertion kit. After you set up your sterile field and explain the procedure to the patient, you realize that visibility is minimal at best. You remove the old catheter. Then you ask the other daughter if she would mind holding the light on the perineal area so that you can see. She does so but you still cannot really see. As you begin wiping the urethral opening with Betadine, the client begins yelling and screaming and moving around and pulling her legs together. It is hot in the room and you can feel the sweat running down your back and emerging in little beads on your forehead. You speak calmly to the client about holding still and then the angry daughter explodes. She vents all of her frustrations of the day and tells you to hurry, that you are torturing her mother. You aim for the urethra but do not really see it clearly. You put the catheter in and no urine comes out. You have just contaminated your only sterile Foley. You are forced to tell the daughters that you must get another catheter from the agency. The angry daughter storms from the room and the other one quietly comforts her mother.

Box 22–1	Student Learning Activity

Home Care Scenario

- Make a list of things that were in your control in this scenario and a list of the things that you could not control.

- Look at the list of things that were in your control and decide what decisions could have been made differently that would have increased the likelihood of a successful outcome.

- What must you do at this point to maintain quality care with this patient?

- How will you resolve the conflict that this has caused with the daughters?

- How could using role plays in a lab situation have helped you to better prepare?

- How can the concepts learned in this scenario assist you and other students in preparation for unexpected circumstances in the home?

This situation actually happened. The student called the agency and paged her instructor. The instructor came to the home with clean gloves and two more sterile catheter kits. The daughters were happy to remain in the living room while the instructor inserted the catheter. The instructor decided to do it herself because the student was really flustered and the client's bladder was getting full at that point. With each student holding a leg and a light directed at the perineal area, the instructor successfully reinserted the Foley. The daughters were very happy to have their mother catheterized and comfortable and seemed to have gotten over their frustrations. Both students gave Mrs. P. a bath and changed her bed and left with the instructor. Coming out of the elevator the student in charge of the home visit burst into tears. The instructor and the student went back to the agency and talked about the situation and how it could have been more positive.

They talked about the things that the student could have done differently. The student was in control of when the catheter would be changed. After arriving at the home to find the caregiver absent and a serious lack of supplies, the student could have returned to the agency to secure adequate supplies and to get additional help. The student did the right thing in calling her instructor for help. She knew that the catheter could not be left out longer than five or six hours and the shorter the time better with someone this elderly. The client was never in any danger of permanent harm. The situation was an excellent learning experience for the student, teaching her never to proceed without proper help and supplies. Hopefully, students who have played this out in a lab scenario will take away the same message so that they will be better prepared.

Previsit Preparation

At the home-care agency, your instructor will make your assignments, and you will begin the preparation for your visit. Although you will eventually make independent home visits, for the first few weeks you will be visiting with your nurse or your instructor. Each morning the home-care nurses begin by looking at who they are scheduled to visit for the day. They will most likely know a few days in advance which clients need to be visited. The nurse generally makes a temporary schedule taking into consideration the type of visit and the location. Then she or he calls each client to confirm that they will be home and gives them an approximate time of arrival. The nurse may ask you to telephone the clients that you have already met.

Next comes chart review. Each client will have a permanent chart that stays in the office. It contains all of the admission information, nursing assessments, and a record of each visit made to the home. If you have not read that chart, you need to read it prior to the visit. It will give you up-to-date information about what is going on with your client. In the chart you will see a record of the last visit that lists goals for the next visit. The previous nurse will have made a list of the supplies that have been ordered, and those supplies will be taken to the home on the next visit. In an article on student nurses in the home, one student commented how the home and acute care settings differ and that limited supplies in the home require flexibility and adaptability from the nurse (Cullen, 1998). In the chart you will also find a home environment assessment that will give you some idea about what to expect of the physical home environment. You will also see a list of the present health problems that are being addressed. For Medicare patients, you will see a plan of care based on expected outcomes with the focus on discharge goals. Depending on the agency and type of private pay insurance, clients with health plans funded by private sector insurance will have a projected time line for discharge. This time line may be translated by number of visits or by weeks of service. In the acute-care setting, this may be

written in the form of a Critical Pathway. Critical Pathways are not yet widely used as the basis for reimbursement in home care (Huggins & Phillips, 1998). Because a home-care client requires a skilled procedure to qualify for visits by a professional nurse, the visit schedule and remains skill oriented. As with the use of Critical Pathways in acute care, in home care a treatment plan is used as a case management tool to predict the need for certain interventions that will accomplish projected outcomes.

Finding Your Way in the Community

All patients have been called, all supplies have been secured, and charts have been read in preparation for the day's visits. If you will be driving your own car, it is very important that you know how to get where you are going. If you are unfamiliar with the service area, then it is time to take a brief course in map reading. If you have not had the experience of reading a street map, you must learn to do that prior to leaving the agency. Look at the map and make yourself familiar with the major boundary streets. This will give you a ballpark idea of where you are going and let you know that, when you cross one of those boundaries, you have either just entered or just left your service area. Then find the address of the client you are visiting and attempt to determine the best way to get there from the agency. The chart will contain general directions, but it will not always tell you the best way to get

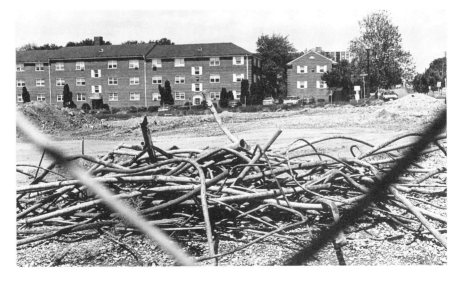

Table 22–1

Pointers for Finding Your Way
in the Community

Table 22–1

Pointers for Finding Your Way
in the Community

- Make yourself familiar with the area that you are visiting.

- Always look up the address and directions before leaving the agency.

- Never leave the office without your map.

- Become familiar with major streets in your visiting area.

- Never read your map while driving.

- Carry a cell phone if you have one.

- Pull over if you get lost and look at your map.

- Stop at an establishment such as a gas station or a place of business to ask directions.

- Do not ask someone on the street for directions (wastes time—may not know the area or could be unsafe).

there. Be prepared for unexpected eventualities in the form of construction, one-way streets, accidents, or heavy traffic. Even if you have mapped out the most direct route, you may still have to find an alternate route because of some of the circumstances just mentioned. Never leave the agency without your map in case you need to find your way if you get lost (see Table 22–1).

THE ROLE OF THE NURSE AND THE INSTRUCTOR IN THE STUDENT'S HOME-CARE EXPERIENCE

Most likely, you will not be assigned exclusively to one nurse or preceptor for your home-care experience. Instead, you will be dealing with whoever is responsible for the client to whom you have been assigned. In home care, each client is assigned a case manager who is the nurse in charge of that client's care. That nurse not only visits the

client, but is responsible for planning, organizing, coordinating, and monitoring services and resources needed to meet the client's health-care needs (Huggins & Phillips, 1998). Your instructor will speak to the case manager to ensure that your assignment is appropriate. This means that the assignment both meets your educational needs and meets the needs of the agency with regard to your client's care. After you have been assigned to a particular client, the case manager is the person who will meet with you to determine the focus of your visit and will most likely be the person who will accompany you on your first encounter with your home-care client. You and your instructor will be receiving constructive feedback from the case manager regarding your clinical performance so that you will have an opportunity to learn and improve.

Building a collaborative relationship with the agency nurse, whether she or he is your preceptor or is just case managing one of your clients, is one of the most important tasks that you can perform. This nurse acts as mentor, an advocate, and a source of valuable feedback regarding your clinical performance. Learning from a practitioner who is in the clinical setting can be one of the most worthwhile experiences of your career. This person can assist in molding you into a nurse with high standards of care. You must be willing to be open-minded, enthusiastic, and self-directed, demonstrating that you are there to learn. This collaborative relationship can also create a supportive environment in which you will receive nongraded feedback on your progress. It will make you realize that your improvement and success is a team effort. A supportive learning environment will make you feel less like you are under a microscope so that you can relax and think clearly. Your instructor is there to assist you in setting logical and realistic goals and to help you process what you have learned so you can begin to put the total client picture together. He or she will be ultimately responsible for grading your clinical performance and certifying your course competence.

THE VALUE OF A CLINICAL JOURNAL

Because the instructor is not on every home visit with you, it is necessary to devise ways, other than by direct observation, for the instructor to evaluate your clinical performance and to assist you in accomplishing your goals for the semester. One excellent way for the instructor to evaluate your critical thinking and clinical judgment is through student journals. The clinical journal can be the instructor's window into your clinical performance. A journal is not just a story or record of a clinical performance; it should contain pertinent information that documents your thought processes, actions, nursing interventions, and emotions. The journal should contain objectives and accurate information describing your actions within the clinical experience. Journals can reflect progression of cognitive development as well as other outcomes (Oermann, 1998). They should be designed to have more than one purpose. They can assist you in articulating the goals that you want to accomplish during your clinical experience; they can help you put your thoughts into a logical sequence so that you are better able to process them; they can help you analyze information demonstrating that you are thinking critically; and they can be an avenue of communication between you and your instructor. Many students use electronic mail to send their journals to the instructor; feedback is more immediate than when the journal is collected and returned. Remember, if you do not dedicate adequate time to writing your journal by following the guidelines and including detailed information, the journal is not going to accurately reflect your clinical accomplishments. A thoroughly written journal will give your instructor in-depth information on which to judge your clinical performance.

Following is an example of a student's journal that details an upsetting experience that she encountered and how she handled it. It also clearly records the clinical day and illustrates how this student met the course objectives.

A CLINICAL JOURNAL

Broad Objective:

Apply the nursing process to provide safe, competent, and therapeutic nursing care, utilizing appropriate technology.

Daily Objectives:

To manage my time effectively.

To perform selected nursing technologies in the clinical setting.

To become confident and competent in giving nursing report.

Thoughts and Feelings:

I had a fantastic week as far as technologies go. I was able to do my first bladder catheterization plus a few more. I also did three in and out caths. When it rains it pours. I also changed the dressing and caps on a triple lumen subclavian catheter and did several Central Venous Line (CVL) dressing changes. Lots of fun stuff!! I was assigned to care for four patients and no one was discharged. I think I'm doing a pretty good job even though sometimes I feel very rushed. I am learning a lot. I am also beginning to relax and enjoy my patients.

One of my patients is a homeless man who I really like a lot. He is quite a character and very demanding, but even so there is something about him that I really like. I've never had an opportunity to know a homeless man before this. I think I was a little scared of homeless people. But he is not so scary and very human. He has a drinking problem—they say in report that he drinks two cases of beer a day. He has also been seen on Route 1 stealing beer. I feel sorry for him because he is a really nice guy. It is such a shame that he has such a wasted life. I understand that he has been living in a friend's shed. If I hadn't already guessed by his drinking history, he is in the hospital with end-stage liver disease. He has a small frame and an enormous belly (ascites). He looks like Humpty Dumpty. The doctor did a paracentesis two days ago and removed 1400 cc of fluid. I'm afraid that he will become hypotensive but so far he is fine. I looked up his liver enzymes and compared them with normal findings. After looking at his blood work I discovered that he had a folic acid deficiency, not uncommon in alcoholics. I told the doctor and they had a nutritionist do a consult on him. He is on fluid restrictions and is always asking for something to drink. I tried to teach him to space his oral fluids throughout the day so that he did not feel too deprived. He must be so used to having a beer in his hands throughout his waking hours. There have been no signs of delirium tremors (DTs). I am sure he has been offered help many times in his life but for whatever reason has been unable to benefit from it. He has been assigned a social worker and he has expressed some interest in getting some clothes. His way of dealing with the hopelessness in his life has taught me a lot but I am not able to articulate it yet.

Problem Solving:

Wow! I had quite a day. Today's experience tested my professionalism, my ability to apply ethical principles to patient care, my caring attitude, and more. I had a patient today who

I cared for yesterday. She was a little difficult but nothing major. She had a way of making a production out of little things. This morning I was also assigned to her roommate who was newly admitted and needed a lot of help. I did my complete care on her roommate but first I made sure she had her things for her morning care. That was my first clue that something was not right. She began yelling in a nasty voice, "I'm in pain over here." I walked over and asked her when she had her last pain medicine. She said that it was two hours ago. I knew that the medication was ordered for every four hours so I knew it wasn't time yet. Then she started saying, "My friends told me not to go to this place." I guess you can pick your nurses but you can't pick your roommates. I thought to myself that she needed some attention so I went over and repositioned her and tried to make her feel more comfortable. It didn't work. While I was there she said, "You've been with her for two hours and have not helped me at all." I said that I was finished with her roommate and I would soon be ready to get her up. "I noticed my roommate's color," she said. I said, "Her color doesn't have anything to do with it." She said, "I'm a Nazi and I don't like Negroes." I'm not even sure what I said. I almost fell over. I just walked to the other side of the room and closed the curtain. Thank goodness her roommate was in the bathroom and didn't hear her. I went out to get my preceptor. By the time the preceptor came back there was all sorts of language flowing. She was using the N word left and right. My preceptor told her not to use that kind of language. The patient said, "You're white, what do you care?" K said she liked to treat everyone with respect. She said, "Well, you should look in the mirror more often." That ended it and K had the lady transferred immediately. Her roommate came out of the bathroom as they were moving her. She had heard the entire conversation. She was thankful that this patient was moving but she did not take it too badly. She just said that it takes all kinds.

It must be hard to live with so much hate inside you. I was proud of myself that I kept my professionalism, yet I let the lady know that what she said was rude and wrong. I also did not let my emotions run away with me. It would have been easy to become rude to her. I was able to control my negative thoughts and feelings even though this lady's attitude repulsed me. I still cared for the Nazi lady, but I only responded to her needs and did not get into any conversations.

Self Evaluation:

The bottom line is my reporting stinks. I keep thinking that I'll get the hang of it. It is time to make it happen. I have to create a system for myself and don't tell any body else about it. I handled the Nazi patient and the homeless patient well and according to their individual needs. I feel that I met my technology objective. I also have begun to integrate the pathophysiology with the total client picture. I did this with my homeless patient. I met the objective on professionalism in dealing with both the Nazi patient and her roommate. I advocated for the roommate by suggesting that we change the other lady's room assignment. I accepted the patient with prejudice with regard to her care and tried not to let my personal views cloud my therapeutic approach.

If the student had just verbally related this experience to the instructor, the emotions of the moment would have probably been expressed clearly, but the opportunity to self-reflect and analyze the client's behavior and her own behavioral response may have been lost. Landeen, Byrne, and Brown (1995) found that journal writing helped students to move beyond feelings of inadequacy. In some instances, the students were able to analyze what had occurred and were able to hypothesize about underlying dynamics. As trust developed throughout the semester and as the students gained increased experience in journal writing, faculty were able to validate students' feelings and at the same time challenge the students to analyze their experiences critically. For the preceding journal entry, having some time to reflect on this incident and to think through what actually happened was very positive. This student was able to gain a perspective on the emotions that the "Nazi patient" provoked in her. Writing this incident down in a journal solidified the learning experience for the student and enabled her to realize that problem solving had taken place while she also worked through her extreme emotions.

SAFETY

Control of your personal safety is a more challenging issue in home care than in a hospital-based clinical because of the unknowns in the environment. Home visiting is very safe, yet there are rules that a wise nurse follows to avoid dangerous situations. Following a few simple rules will assist you in becoming confident and will put you in control while visiting in the community. Use the acronym shown in Table 22–2 to remember a few simple rules about personal safety.

Table 22–2

Safety Tips for Your Home-care Practice

S A F E

S—Stay Alert

Be alert and observant of your surroundings. As you drive up to the client's home, pay attention to who is on the street around or near your client's home. Observe the condition of the neighborhood. Are there abandoned cars? Are the homes in a good state of repair? Are there any thriving businesses in the area or are the streets deserted? Is litter present on the streets or are they clean and well looked after? Pay attention to unusual noises or movement.

A—Announce your arrival in advance

If the client knows you are coming and at approximately what time, he or she will be watching for you. You will be allowed to enter the residence immediately. Home-health nurses are generally viewed as friends of the neighborhood. Neighbors become aware of your schedule and will become protective of you. The informal neighborhood leaders will let you know when something is wrong such as the presence of drug activity or an increase in crime.

F—Follow your "gut"

Intuition is an excellent warning system. Any situations that make you feel uncomfortable should be taken seriously. If you are walking down a street and you see a group of teens that give you a bad feeling, turn around, cross the street, seek shelter in a business; if you are near your car, get in and drive away. If you are in a home and feel threatened by family dynamics or a tense situation, get out. When you are safe, a phone call can be made to do something about the situation.

E—Expect the unexpected

If you expect the unexpected, you will be ready for any eventuality. Being mentally prepared to handle an unsafe situation will help you avoid being caught "off guard." As your confidence level increases, your fear will decrease.

INFECTION CONTROL

As in the hospital, the home environment has the same issues involving the prevention of disease transmission from one person to another (Cecil, 1998). The term used to describe infection precautions is *Standard Precautions* (Twiname & Boyd, 1999). Standard Precautions are aimed at interrupting the chain of infection at the point at which microorganisms leave the body or enter the body. Because the information given to the home-care agency on admission cannot always identify all clients who have a communicable disease, the Centers for Disease Control and Prevention (CDC) recommends certain precautions be taken when handling blood or body fluids for all clients, and these guidelines are also mandated by the Occupational Safety and Health Administration (OSHA). All health-care workers must wear gloves when touching mucous membrane or nonintact skin surfaces of all clients. This means that gloves must be worn while drawing blood, suctioning body fluids, or emptying items containing such fluids. Masks, goggles, and gowns should be worn if aerosolization or splashes are likely to occur (Rice, 1995). Aprons or gowns are required for procedures involving extensive contact with body fluids or with soiled items such as contaminated sheets, heavily soiled dressings, or equipment. Meticulous hand washing is essential. This should be done as soon as you arrive in the home, before beginning care, after removing gloves, after a procedure is complete, and before leaving the home. Soap and paper towels are standard items brought to the home for each visit.

For disposal of contaminated waste or sharps objects such as needles, you should bring a puncture-resistant, leak-proof, hazardous waste container with you into the home. This container should be removed from the home by you and disposed of in the appropriate place in the agency. As in the hospital setting, needles should never be recapped, bent or broken, or removed from disposable syringes (Rice, 1995).

When you are assigned to a home-care clinical, you will be loaned a standard issue agency bag that resembles a multicompartment canvas tote. Every home-care agency has written guidelines for bag use. Table 22–3 provides an example of a Bag Technique Policy.

Table 22–3

Bag Technique

Procedure:

1. The bag is never placed on the floor, on upholstered furniture, or on a bed. It must always be put on a firm, clean surface such as a table, countertop, or a straight-backed chair. Alternatively, it may be hung from the back of a chair (making sure the chair will not tip over) or hung from a doorknob.

2. If there is any doubt as to the cleanliness of the area where the bag is to be placed, a barrier device is to be used. Items appropriate for use as a barrier are (but are not limited to) paper towels, newspapers, large brown grocery bags, or wax paper. The barrier should be discarded at the conclusion of the visit.

3. The interior of the nursing bag is considered clean. It is not to be entered until the hands have been washed

4. Antimicrobial soap, waterless soap, and paper towels provided by the agency are to be carried in an outside pocket of the nursing bag so they are easily accessible. Prior to entering the bag, these items are removed from the pocket for hand washing. In the event that running water is not available or accessible, a waterless cleansing solution is to be used.

5. After the hands have been washed, the nurse may then enter the zippered compartment of the nursing bag. All equipment and supplies needed for the visit are removed from the bag and placed on a clean surface. The bag must not be reentered unless the hands have been washed again.

6. Following the completion of care and after the hands have been washed again, equipment may be returned to the bag. Equipment must be cleaned using a germicidal, disposable cloth prior to its return to the bag.

7. If an item is excessively soiled, it should not be returned to the bag but sealed in a plastic bag and returned to the agency for cleaning and sterilization.

8. In the event that the client's home is excessively dirty or insect infested, the clinician should not take the bag into the home. Essential supplies should be removed from the bag and carried into the home by the nurse.

9. The bag may not be left exposed and unattended in the car, but should be locked in the trunk or other covered compartment.

(Modified from INOVA VNA Home Health Policy Manual, Bag Technique Policy, May 1997)

Box 22–2 presents another problem-solving scenario that can be used to prepare you to handle some of the unusual circumstances that you might find in the home that will challenge your creativity in maintaining infection control standards.

THE HOME VISIT

Going to the home that first time alone can be anxiety provoking and stressful. The environment is really an un-

known. In the hospital setting, students tend to experience anxiety about their inexperience with certain clinical skills and with the rapport-building experience. In the home environment, all those same fears are present but, in addition, the student must accept that many aspects of the environment are out of the provider's control. If a sterile item gets contaminated, you cannot just walk out into the hallway and grab another one. Flexibility, creativity, and adaptability are important traits to possess in the home. Cullen (1998) noted that in the home environment students may

Box 22–2   Student Learning Activity

Problem-Solving Scenario Regarding Infection Control

You walk into the apartment of an 81-year-old man suffering from end-stage chronic obstructive pulmonary disease (COPD) and congestive heart failure (CHF). He has in-home oxygen and is suffering from leg ulcers that are secondary to four-plus pitting edema of his lower extremities. Your goal today is to change his leg dressings.

As you look around you see the most cluttered environment that you have ever encountered. On every surface there are knickknacks, papers, garbage, dust, and spilled liquids. On the one hard-backed chair there is a half-eaten chicken dinner from Kentucky Fried Chicken that appears to be several days old, along with an empty soft drink bottle lying on its side next to a plastic toy necklace. You see at least three roaches climbing on walls and furniture. The client's oxygen tubing is coupled together extending it to a length of several yards. The kitchen is in clear view and the sink is filled with dirty dishes and rotting food. The bathroom is down a dark hallway and has been declared off limits to health-care providers by his caretaker, who is also his 23-year-old-nephew.

Describe how you would accomplish the goals of the visit while maintaining high standards of infection control and caregiver and client safety?

as a partnership in which they have the right to make the ultimate decisions about what type of care is given. Demonstrating your respect for their privacy and property and giving them the opportunity to express their concerns without fear of reprisal go a long way in building a trusting relationship (Clemen-Stone, Eigsti, & McGuire, 1995). There may be some initial embarrassment on the part of the client regarding the condition of his or her home. Unconditional acceptance, tact, and rapport building are essential during that first visit. Clients are more likely to develop a trusting relationship with a provider who is open and honest (Clemen-Stone et al., 1995). For example, it is okay to be empathetic to a client's dilemma but not okay to give advice about the dilemma. That kind of behavior fosters dependency and shows lack of respect for a client's decision-making ability (Clemen-Stone et al., 1995).

After the first home visit, you will begin to realize why certain clients have a difficult time following discharge instructions and remaining compliant with medication regimens. Home visiting has helped students to look beyond the hospital environment and to think about the impact of conditions in the home on the health status of the client (Cullen, 1998). Many students, after visiting a client, have stated that they had no idea that a particular client was dealing with such chaos. That is why an environmental assessment is a crucial part of the plan of care. The nurse and student must be very aware that they are guests in the client's home. Therefore, you are to act as a consultant in assessing shortcomings in the environment and offering suggestions for change (Narayan & Tennant, 1997). The following story illustrates how important it is to consider all aspects of a client's circumstance before judgments are made about willingness to comply with therapy.

DO NOT MAKE ASSUMPTIONS

A student nurse had been seeing Mrs. P. in a clinic setting for her cardiovascular disease and her diabetes. Mrs. P. was in her late 40s and was about 70 pounds overweight. She had serious trouble controlling her blood sugar levels and seemed to be noncompliant with her diet. The student saw her in the clinic a few times and really felt that Mrs. P. was not trying. Mrs. P. had an attack of angina and after a brief hospitalization was sent home. Home care was ordered to attempt to monitor her blood glucose levels and to do some diabetic

find that even a simple dressing change is an adventure. Much of the home-health nurse's job is to observe the environment that he or she has to work with and adapt the goals of each visit to the resources available to the individual client. Explaining the purpose of the visit to the client is essential in case there is an initial lack of understanding about why a nurse must come to the home. You must let clients know that you view their recovery process

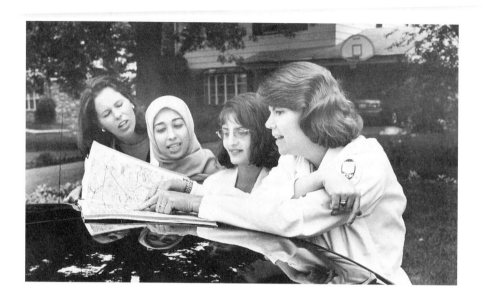

education. The student had the opportunity make a home visit with the home-health nurse. The student could not believe what she saw. Mrs. P. lived in very small dilapidated home. She did not have a car and was unable to get to the pharmacy on a regular basis. To make money, she had agreed to care for a neighbor's 3-year-old daughter who was at her home after her morning preschool, from noon until 6 o'clock. Mrs. P. did not have the energy to properly care for this little girl. In the cluttered living quarters, the little girl sat in front of the TV. Mrs. P. spent her day in the kitchen at the table drinking coffee. She had no transportation to a proper grocery store and managed her meals by buying junk food at a nearby convenience store.

The student saw Mrs. P. in a new light. She no longer passed judgment on her noncompliance but began working to see if there were some available resources for her that would offer her some support. One of the nursing goals was diabetic education but that was not going to work until Mrs. P. received some other assistance. A social worker became involved with her case and began working to get her the help that she needed.

THE ADMISSION VISIT

The admission visit lays the groundwork for the implementation of the plan of care. When you accompany your nurse on an admission visit, be prepared to stay at least two hours to get all of the information necessary for assessment and reimbursement. During this visit you will be building rapport with your client and his or her family members. This is an important time to get to know each other, find out the client's and family members' concerns, allay some of their fears, and obtain important information on which you will base your plan of care. This may include a complete head-to-toe physical assessment, a family assessment, and an environmental assessment. During this time, it is necessary to find out the client's insurance information so that a realistic visit schedule can be established. You will also want to give the client and family information regarding patient's rights and advanced directives.

Generally, the information the home-care agency receives from the hospital regarding the client's health history and problems is very brief and incomplete. Most of the time the actual client situation is much more complex than what is documented on the preadmission forms. The following is a true story about an admission that was much more complex than it seemed on the surface. After you read the story, answer the questions in Box 22–3.

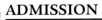

ADMISSION

The nurse receives notification that she will be admitting a new patient today and is given the client's discharge summary from the hospital as follows:

The patient is 77 years old and 5 days posthysterectomy and colon resection. She was discharged from the hospital today. She has a midline, abdominal incision that is healing but requires a daily dressing change. She has a colostomy that requires enterostomal therapy. The patient is married to an 83-year-old man who has a hearing deficit and cataracts. Her 48-year-old daughter will be the primary caregiver and her 40-year-old, mentally disabled son lives at home.

The nurse finds the house on the map and leaves the agency for the home. She drives up to the one-story rambler and sees a woman in her late 40s looking out the door. She introduces herself as Judy, the client's daughter. She is in obvious distress and is chain smoking. She says that her mom is in "bad shape" and she does not know what to do. As the nurse walks into the living room, she notices that the seats of all of the upholstered furniture are covered with 30-gallon trash bags. Judy makes a comment that her younger brother is incontinent, but the nurse has not met him yet. Judy introduces the nurse to her mother, Connie. She appears thin, frail, and scared. She is lying on a sleeper sofa in the living room that has been pulled out and made into a bed. Connie says that she thinks her mother had an accident but she did not know what to do. The nurse cannot help but notice a foul-smelling odor coming from the bed. She asks permission to pull back the covers and discovers that the sheets are dripping with urine. There are no blue moisture pads in place and the urine has soaked through the sheets, saturating the mattress. The colostomy bag has come away from the abdomen and has leaked yellowish-brown, semiformed, soft stool into her partially healed, abdominal wound. Connie says that she needs to urinate again and the nurse begins looking for the bedpan. Under the bed she finds a fracture pan from the hospital that has teeth marks all over it and a few puncture holes. Judy sees the nurse's inquiring eyes and states that the dog had chewed the plastic bedpan when she was not looking. The nurse feels relieved that there is a dog. She asks to use the sink and is shown to a bathroom in the hallway. It is fairly clean and she washes her hands and gets out several pairs of gloves to begin.

Box 22–3   Student Learning Activity

Admission Scenario

- Judy asks the nurse to sit down. Which chair should he or she chose? An upholstered chair covered with a trash bag or a wooden dining-room chair? Why?

- What should the nurse take care of first? Assisting the daughter with the bedpan or beginning the admission interview? Explain your reasoning.

- What additional information does the nurse need to complete the initial assessment and to assist in meeting this client's needs?

- What kinds of things should be ordered that would make Connie more comfortable and would make it easier for the daughter to care for her mother?

- What information will the daughter or caregiver need to know to adequately care for Connie between visits?

- What other family members may need support over the ensuing weeks?

- What wellness issues need to be addressed with this family?

- Name two actual nursing diagnoses and two "at risk" for diagnoses that pertain to this home-care client.

CONTINUITY OF CARE

Students who have spent most of their clinical time in an acute-care settings note crucial differences in the nurse's opportunity to offer continuity of care in the home-care setting. With the changes in the health-care system, many clients stay in the hospital for a very short time. As a result, much of what used to be done in the hospital is now being done in the home by the family members with the support of the home-health nurse. Thus, home-health nurses have the opportunity to see their clients over time and to get to know them and their families in an in-depth way. This has given the home-health nurse a chance to provide clients with continuity of care and to develop "meaningful relationships built on trust and caring" (Cullen, 1998, p. 77). Students find this part of their experience to be very rewarding. They often find it difficult to terminate their relationships with these long-term clients. They spend much of their time in their weekly clinical conferences speaking about the value of the therapeutic relationships that they have developed (Glavinspiehs & Gajdalo, 1997). Many students follow up with the home-health nurses long after their clinical is over with to find out how their clients are progressing.

Managed Care

Necessary attempts at cost containment in health care have caused an explosive increase in the number of home-care clients over the past few years. In the acute-care setting, diagnostic-related groups (DRGs) became the basis for the third-party payment system instead of the historic fee-for-service system. This change has brought on shortened hospital stays and an increased need for home-based care. In addition, the demographic shift toward an aging population has increased the demand for home-care services. With this trend came federal guidelines defining the criteria for financial coverage of the home-care client. They are as follows:
- The client must be homebound.
- The client must require the services of a skilled registered professional nurse or physical therapist on an intermittent basis.
- The services must be ordered by a physician (Rice, 1995).

In home care, there is no billable equivalent to DRGs; however, early in 1999, a new time-intensive and detailed federal requirement called Outcome Assessment Information Set (OASIS) hit the home-care industry. OASIS is a data collection requirement for all home-care clients. Currently, the data must be collected and electronically transmitted to the federal government for Medicare clients only. Eventually this requirement will affect all clients receiving home care. Because of its similarity to DRGs, it is inevitable that this data will eventually be used to mandate guidelines that will equate to a reimbursement standard. As the homebound criteria continue to be defined and redefined, physicians and nurses feel that decisions regarding their clients' welfare no longer rest in their hands. This is a source of extreme stress and frustration for the home-health nurse and has caused many nurses to feel that their standards of care have been compromised (Ellenbecker & Warren, 1998). Has the autonomy that was once such an attractive element of the home-care nurse's job become diluted? With the federal government and the insurance industry calling the shots regarding reimbursement and treatment decisions being made by nonmedical personnel, in many instances, time spent negotiating with third-party payers in an advocacy role for their home-care clients has become an all-consuming task for home-care nurses.

Between 1995 and 1997 the elderly and poor who are covered by Medicare or Medicaid were suddenly given the opportunity, and in some states the mandate, to sign their federal health care benefits over to the private sector (Huggins & Phillips, 1998). Many health maintenance organizations (HMOs) actively recruited the elderly and poor, with their eye on the federal dollars that this move could bring. They often painted a rosy picture of the kinds of coverage that the clients would receive, leaving out the small print regarding such things as preappointment verification and limitation of choice. Most clients did not even realize that they were signing away their federal benefits. When it came time to treat the many chronic illnesses of the elderly and make good on promised services to the poor, some of the HMOs were reluctant to pay. Idealistic students who enter into clinical experiences in home-care agencies are witnesses to these inequities and frustrations and therefore are given a strong dose of reality shock.

As part of the nonbillable first visit, it is necessary for the home-health nurse to speak to the client and the family about the costs of home-care services, insurance coverage, and other financial concerns that the client and family members might have. The type of insurance coverage generally dictates the number of visits with which the agency has to work. Students assigned to a clinical in home health find this one of the most discouraging and disheartening parts of the home-health nurse's job. Although a student would never be required to speak to the client about financial concerns, he or she may be tasked with reaffirming the information discussed with the client during subsequent visits. Many clients and families have very little knowledge regarding the extent or scope of their coverage and depend on their home-health nurse to interpret their insurance coverage for them (Hunt & Zurek, 1997). The number and frequency of visits must be negotiated daily and weekly with many private insurance companies. Medicare remains primarily a fee-for-service system administered by the federal government, so the visit allotment is more reasonable and realistic than for those under managed care (Cochran, 1998). The home-health nurse or an administrative person in the physician's office spends an inordinate amount of time negotiating with private insurance for the care that their clients need.

The following story demonstrates the frustrations felt by a university nursing student assigned to a home-health agency for his clinical preceptorship after seeing the unfair and unrealistic goals set for his client by the client's insurer.

COMMENTARY ON MANAGED CARE

Customer satisfaction is supposed to be a big issue whenever you enter the business world, but I was surprised to see the treatment given to this client by his health insurance company. I find it difficult to believe that these insurance companies have their client's welfare at heart. They do not hesitate to take the premiums but when the time comes for the clients to enjoy their privileges, these same companies begin to "drag their feet." I hate to make generalizations, but after seeing this client's condition, I am tempted to say that most of the insurance companies are only interested in a client's money and not their welfare.

This is a 67-year-old white man. He was admitted to the Visiting Nurses Association (VNA) with a diagnosis of cancer of the mouth, status postsurgical removal of the left jawbone because of a malignant tumor, with implantation of a metal prosthesis where his left mandible used to be. The patient also had radiation therapy and he suffered an infection at the implant site with its subsequent removal. This surgery left him with a deep open wound on the left side of his face healing by tertiary intention. He became dysphagic and a gastrostomy tube was placed in his stomach for nutrition purposes. He had a respiratory arrest, was intubated, and eventually ended up with a tracheostomy. He is alert and oriented but very weak, has an unsteady gait, and ambulates with a cane. What makes this case so interesting are the ethical and moral issues involved. Before my preceptor and I made the first visit to the client's home, she made a series of phone calls in an attempt to gain authorization for the visit. This seemed kind of strange to me so I asked her what was going on. She told me that the client had signed over his Medicare benefits to an HMO and this organization operates under a managed care system. This HMO recommended only a limited number of visits by the home-health nurse. The HMO's goals for this patient were for him to learn to do his own tracheostomy care and dressing changes.

This man lives in a one-bedroom apartment, very congested with books and videotapes, and has no mirror in the apartment except one small circular mirror on the wall of his tiny bathroom. I am not trying to degrade his surroundings but I am just trying to paint the picture clearly so the case can be understood. There was no favorable work area besides the tiny bathroom, which has the only mirror. In order to do the teaching adequately, we all had to be in the bathroom with the client. The client needed to be in front of the mirror to see what he was doing. The task was impossible. First of all the wound was on the left side of his face and he was not able to turn his head to the side so the wound could be viewed in the mirror and see in the mirror at the same time. Obviously, in order to look in the mirror he had to turn his head forward. He was in a very weakened state and had minimal manual dexterity, unable to stand for any length of time without the assistance of his cane. He needed two hands to change both the dressing and the tracheostomy while trying to maintain sterile technique. How can this man be expected to stand for at least one half hour at a time, twice a day to do his dressing changes and tracheostomy care? The wound is about 5 cm by 3 cm in diameter with a depth of 3 cm. It is draining a greenish fluid with a mild odor. The wound is to be irrigated with normal saline and packed with moist, sterile 2-by-2-inch gauze dressings, then covered with dry 4-by-4-inch gauze dressings and then tape is applied. The following is the procedure for the tracheostomy care: Remove the inner cannula of the tracheostomy tube, wash it with hydrogen peroxide, and rinse it with normal saline; clean around the tracheostomy site and outer cannula; change the drainage sponge below the tracheostomy opening, and finally, change the tracheostomy collar and reinsert the inner cannula. Manipulating the tracheostomy tube often causes coughing and expulsion of a large amount of mucous drainage from the tracheostomy site. If not removed immediately, this mucus can obstruct the airway. My client attempted to do this complicated procedure. He stopped after the dressing change and out of anger, frustration, fear, and exhaustion, refused to attempt the tracheostomy care.

This client has fallen on several occasions in his apartment, once in front of my preceptor and me while on his way to the bathroom. I happened to be next to him and broke his fall. He needs physical therapy to build up his strength and endurance. He also needs a home-health aide to assist him with his activities of daily living but unfortunately his HMO does not see the need to provide such services. Because of the federal government's regulations, once he has signed his Medicare benefits over to an HMO the decision is irreversible. He is very dissatisfied but can do nothing about the situation.

The lesson I have learned from this experience is that one should always be cautious when dealing with the insurance industry. I also learned how vulnerable the elderly are to exploitation. This man was clearly taken advantage of because under his original Medicare benefits he would be completely covered. Another thing I learned was about the resiliency of the human spirit. By the end of our visits, his spirits were elevated and he managed to smile. The loving and caring approach used by his home-health nurse was better than any medicine. I hope my experience will help other nursing students to realize the value of patient advocacy and a caring approach in making a difference, in spite of a health-care industry that can be ruthless.

ETHICAL CONSIDERATIONS IN THE HOME

The majority of the ethical issues observed by the home-health nurse are related to autonomy versus safety. Many elderly clients who you will see in the home are hanging on to their independence by a thread. At times, the home-health nurse is the only person who sees the client on a regular basis and is in a position to make a judgment about the safety of the client's home environment. You, too, will be making independent visits and may be asked by the physician or a family member for your perception of your client's ability to safely live alone. Often clients may be in disagreement with family members as to their ability to function on their own. Sometimes the client does not have family or the family is in denial about the client's functional capabilities. These circumstances are truly ethical dilemmas, and there are no right answers. The principles of self-determination (allowing the client to decide what is right for him or herself) and paternalism (the health-care provider deciding something on behalf of the client because of the provider's superior knowledge on the subject, without the client's informed consent) come into play (Burkhardt & Alvita, 1998).

Another ethical principle apparent in home care is that of justice. When clients make unhealthy decisions in spite of recommended treatment, is it just to continue to spend valuable resources on those clients who choose repeatedly not to comply? An example would be continuing with diabetic teaching when a client disregards all diet recommendations and eats a diet full of "empty" carbohydrates.

Ethical issues are complex and multifaceted, and experience gives students the basis on which to make decisions considering all aspects of a client dilemma. Students are taught about nursing's professional code that directs nurses to provide services with respect for the rights and dignity of the patient, regardless of a person's background or the nature of the health concern. Buckhardt and Alvita (1998) state that if nurses find a conflict between responsibilities expected of them in a situation and their own ethical stance, integrity, and accountability, they should remove themselves from the situation after ensuring safety of the clients.

Documentation in the Home

Documentation is one of the most important tasks of the home-care nurse because the home-care client's record has become the basis for third-party payment. The type of documentation necessary in home care is very specific to the specialty. It is based on the illness model that requires documentation to justify reimbursement for specific client care (Hunt & Zurek, 1997). In acute-care facilities, nursing documentation is focused on a problem-oriented format that records client problems and their resolution. In the home, the focus of the documentation is not on which problems have been resolved but on the ones that have not yet been resolved. It must be accurate, specific, clear, concise, and descriptive, but not interpretative. For example, if a nurse has made an attempt to visit a client but was unable to get a response at the door, instead of writing "not at home," which is interpretative and makes an assumption, the nurse should write, " no answer, door locked." The latter statement describes accurately what happened but makes no interpretation or assumption about whether the client was home or not. Another example that illustrates a statement based on the illness model is regarding a patient who has an open wound. In the hospital, after describing the wound you might write that the wound is "healing well," but that is interpretative and evaluative. In home care that same wound would be described as, "wound remains open and draining, with pink epithelial tissue at the edges that gradually becomes light pink in the center." Documentation should also describe the actual size and amount of drainage (Humphrey, 1994). Students have a very difficult time with this documentation at first because it is very different from what they have done in past settings. Preparing a practice note to be reviewed before entering it into the client's permanent record is very helpful and assists students in learning the Medicare language (Loughman, 1997). Many students have commented that this documentation style seems so negative. If you think of your documentation as a form of client advocacy then it makes it easier. What you record about your clients' status will assist them in receiving the home visits that they need for recovery. This is a helpful way to look at the documentation method.

Because of time constraints, many home-care nurses have had to learn to complete their documentation while in the home during the visit. This is difficult for students to accomplish at first. The home-health nurse generally allows students to jot down notes in the home and then record those notes on the actual chart either in the car or back at the agency. Most students eventually learn to complete their charting in the home. Always keep in mind that the chart is a legal document so if a nursing action is not recorded, as far as the courts are concerned it was never done.

Emergency Situations in the Home

When students think of home care, on the bottom of their worry list are emergency situations. Most home-care clients are in stable condition, and the visits are goal oriented but usually not an emergency situation. As hospital stays shorten, the chances of encountering a client who is in acute distress becomes greater and greater. It is not the job of the home-health nurse to respond to emergencies but sometimes there is no choice. If the nurse arrives for the weekly or daily visit and finds a client in acute distress or in an emergency situation, he or she just cannot turn heel and say, "Call 911." He or she must stay with the client until help has arrived or must advise the client regarding the action that should be taken. The same goes for students. If in doubt, the student should always call the nurse or instructor to seek advice or assistance. Sometimes actions must be taken while waiting for the nurse or the rescue squad to arrive. Following is an excerpt from a journal written by a student who was beginning a medical/surgical clinical in the home-care setting and was surprised to find an emergency situation on her very first visit.

A HOME-CARE EMERGENCY

CALL 911! That was the way our first home visit began. The client was breathing rapidly, flushed face with nail beds blue, diminished breath sounds on the left, and no breath sounds on the right. My preceptor quickly explained to the client's wife the need to go to the hospital. The only thing keeping the client from going was the client himself. He refused to go to the hospital without first being guaranteed a private room. My preceptor called the client's doctor and gave the vital signs over the phone and explained the client's wishes. The doctor advised her to call 911, and he would take care of the room arrangements. After conveying this information to the client my preceptor was given permission to call 911 and within minutes the rescue squad was there. They worked quickly, asking a million questions and impressively doing their job. I look back at the case and wonder how I would have reacted if I had gone on that visit by myself. As a visiting nurse coming into the home, you never know what to expect when you knock on the client's door and you are the only hope. Throughout the day, my preceptor introduced me to many other clients and I assisted with their care when appropriate. The day ended very late and I was awestruck at how much we accomplished during the day. My mind kept going back to that first visit, and I decided then that I was going to learn how to respond correctly in the face of an emergency.

Another nursing student who was doing his preceptorship in home health learned that emergencies do not just occur in the hospital. He had to respond to three emergency situations in a 7-week rotation. The first one occurred while with his preceptor. He was nervous because he was planning on doing his first peripheral blood draw that day. His nurse had chosen a nice 95-year-old lady who had good veins. She was a former nurse so she did not mind having students. Just as the student punctured the skin in her right arm, the patient became unconscious. He pulled out the needle and the preceptor checked for a pulse. She could not feel one, and the client had stopped breathing. They laid her on the floor and initiated cardiopulmonary resuscitation (CPR) after calling 911. The little lady came around after a few breaths and a few compressions. She forgot to tell them that she didn't like needles!

A week later, this same student was scheduled to visit an 80-year-old man who was status posttransurethral prostatectomy (TURP) for benign prosthetic hypertrophy. The hospital had sent this man home with his Foley catheter in place because he was unable to void after his procedure. The goals of the visit were to irrigate the Foley catheter and ensure catheter patency. When the student arrived, his client was sitting in a recliner and had been dozing. The lighting in the room was dim and the shades were drawn. The client's wife stated that she had emptied the external urine bag three times during the night but it was full again. She also said that she had cataracts and it was difficult for her to check the color of the urine as was requested in the discharge instructions. When the student looked at the urine bag, the color of the urine appeared to be dark, but it was difficult to see in the present lighting. He asked that the shades be opened and the lights turned up. When he did this he could not believe what he saw. The urine bag was full of dark red blood. He asked to see the catheter insertion site and he found that blood was oozing out around the catheter. He took the client's blood pressure, and it was very low although the client denied any dizziness. The student immediately paged his nurse preceptor. When she did not respond immediately he paged his instructor. His instructor called back very quickly, and he described the

client's symptoms. The instructor told the student to call 911 and to place the client in a supine position. The preceptor walked into the home while the student was talking to the instructor. The patient was rushed to the hospital and did fine after a few pints of blood.

During the second to last week of this student's clinical rotation, he visited a 77-year-old man who had recently been discharged from a rehabilitation hospital, status poststroke. The student had seen this client a few times in the past. The goal of the visit was to do diabetic teaching and insulin administration. The client's wife was going to learn to give the injections. When the student arrived, the client was very agitated and he and his wife had been arguing. The client had right-sided weakness, but he was able to ambulate with a cane. The client told the student that he was planning to kill his wife that night after she went to sleep. He was going to hit her over the head with a brass lamp. The student did not want to agitate the client any further but asked to use the phone in the next room. He paged his preceptor and told her about the conversation. The preceptor said that she was on her way and to stay with the client. When the preceptor arrived at the home the client refused to let her into the house. The student had asked the client's wife to stay in the kitchen, so the preceptor went around to the back door and took the wife outside. The preceptor called 911 and specified that it was a psychiatric emergency. If the client refused to go to the hospital on his own, a court order would have to be obtained. The client would only talk to the student. He refused to allow the rescue squad to enter the house. The nurse began the process of getting a court order to have the client committed to a psychiatric hospital for evaluation. Finally, the student was able to talk the client into going to the psychiatric unit with the rescue squad. The client had developed poststroke psychosis. He was eventually able to go back home on medication.

This student and his classmates learned some very important lessons that semester. Even in home care a student must know how to respond to an emergency by staying calm and using good, safe judgment. Especially in home care, having a solid knowledge base is very important because no second shift is coming along behind you to check your patient. There is no doctor in the hallway that will come and see your client to confirm your assessment. In an emergency situation, you may be the first health professional on the scene. Reviewing your procedures for CPR and first aid and having the courage to use your good judgment in taking immediate action are imperative.

CONCLUSION

No matter where your school of nursing finds itself with regard to a community-based curriculum, you will definitely be confronted with the probability of making home visits at some point in your student career. This chapter looks at the student home-care experience and the benefits and challenges that home care has to offer. Prior to going into a home-care clinical, it is very important to be prepared. This chapter has given you some ideas about how to prepare for and what to expect in the home. The home is a legitimate place to give care, to assist you in accomplishing your educational objectives, and to implement the valuable skills needed for clinical practice.

Active Learning Strategies

1. The home care setting often raises unique challenges in terms of the environment for nursing practice. Working with a classmate, discuss three of the most challenging environmental concerns you have encountered this semester. Share your information with other students in the class. Are there any commonalities among the concerns identified?

2. Although the approaches of managed care and case management are often criticized, it is important that nurses know how to function effectively in this health care environment. Interview a person in the community who is a participant in a managed care health plan and/or who has a case manager. Is the case manager a nurse? How does the person see the role of the nurse in a managed care environment?

3. In your home visits, you may encounter ethical dilemmas for which you feel unprepared. It is important for future students to know potential ethical issues to anticipate. Make a list of ethical dilemmas you have encountered in your home visits and share them as a large group in your class.

4. Discuss with a nurse visiting your client in her or his home some important aspects of documentation that are unique to home visits.

References

Burkhardt, M. A., & Alvita, K. N. (1998). Ethics & issues in contemporary nursing. Albany, NY: Delmar.

Cecil, C. (1998). The spectrum of infection control in home health care, Home Health Care Manage Practice, 10(3), 1–8.

Clemen-Stone, S., Eigsti, D.G., & McGuire, S. L. (1995) Comprehensive community health nursing (4th ed.). St. Louis: Mosby.

Cochran, M. (1998). Managed care: An overview, Home Healthcare Nurse, 16(4), 215–219.

Cullen, J. A. (1998). How student nurses see home health care nurses today. Home Health Nurse, 16, 75–79.

Ellenbecker, C. H., & Warren, K. (1998). Nursing practice and patient care in a changing home healthcare environment. Home Healthcare Nurse, 16(8), 531–539.

Glavinspiehs, C., & Gajdalo, J. (1997). A meaningful clinical experience in home healthcare for associate degree graduate nurses. Nurse Educator, 22(2), 33–37.

Huggins, C. M., & Phillips, C. Y. (1998). Using case management with clinical plans to improve patient outcomes. Home Healthcare Nurse, 16(1), 15–20.

Humphrey, C. J. (1994). Home care nursing handbook (2nd ed.). Gaithersburg, MD: Aspen.

Hunt R., & Zurek, E. (1997). Introduction to community based nursing. Philadelphia: Lippincott.

INOVA VNA Home Health Policy Manual. (1997). Bag technique policy. Falls Church, VA.

Landeen, J., Byrne, C., & Brown, B. (1995). Exploring lived experiences of psychiatric nursing students through self-reflective journals. Journal of Advanced Nursing, 21(5), 878–885.

Loughman K. A. (1997). The essentials for managing home healthcare experiences. Home Healthcare Nurse, 15(3), 189–196.

Narayan, M., & Tennant, J. (1997). Environmental assessment. Home Healthcare Nurse, 15(11), 799–805

Oermann, M. H. (1996). Research on teaching in the clinical setting. In K. R. Stevens (Ed.), Review of research in nursing education, Vol. 7 (pp. 91–126). New York: National League for Nursing.

Oermann, M. H. (1998). Evaluation and testing in nursing education. New York: Springer.

Rice, R. (1995). Handbook of home health nursing procedures. St. Louis: Mosby.

Twiname, G., & Boyd, S. M. (1999). Difficult concepts made easy. Stamford, CT: Appleton & Lange.

CHAPTER **23**

Community-based Nursing Practice in a Faith Community

Margaret M. Moss

LEARNING OBJECTIVES

1) Define nursing in a faith community.

2) Discuss historical and philosophical perspectives of nursing in a faith community.

3) Describe the two key elements that distinguish the faith community nurse model from other models.

4) List the functions of faith community nurses and give examples of application in practice.

5) Describe health-promotion/disease-prevention activities available in a faith community.

A nursing student wrote about her client in a faith community:

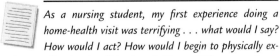

As a nursing student, my first experience doing a home-health visit was terrifying . . . what would I say? How would I act? How would I begin to physically examine my client? What if he doesn't like me? These were just a few of the thoughts racing through my mind as I walked up the pathway and into my client's home.

My home visit training thus far had been reading a few chapters in a community-health nursing textbook, a brief discussion in postconference regarding approaches to home visits, and watching a home video on home-health nursing, of which I remembered almost nothing as I was about to enter my client's house. Partly this was due to my own anxiety. I had been educated enough to know how to do a basic physical exam, and how to converse in a therapeutic manner. I also had enough life experience to appreciate the different ways people cope with life.

But what exactly I would find when I arrived at the door was incredibly anxiety provoking.

My clinical instructor and student nurse partner accompanied me on the first visit. All we knew was that we were going to see an 81-year-old man, who had lost his wife 6 weeks prior to our arrival. William greeted us with enthusiasm, shook our hands, and showed us proudly around his living area. As we gathered our chairs to sit around his minidinette, the first thing William pronounced was, "Well, I don't know that there is anything for you to do here, but I am always happy to help out students." And with that statement, William was off to the races. He talked about his different careers, he talked about his hobbies, he showed us the jewelry he was so proud of making, he told us about his genealogy, and about his son, and grandchildren, and I could not get a word into the conversation. It was difficult to slip in an occasional "um-hum" but briefly, and in a very superficial way, he eventually mentioned that he loved his wife.

When we arrived back at our clinical base, I let my clinical instructor know that I thought William did not need my help as a nurse. He was happy, healthy, and adjusting quite well to his loss. "Please find me another 'sicker' client that I might make an impact on," I said. My instructor firmly stated that it would be more prudent to give this client at least a couple of weeks of my time.

In the 11 visits that followed, William and I played this magnificent game of chess, although there were no board or game pieces involved. William would chat, telling me about his life, and I would hunt for clues and look for ways to attack his incredible defense mechanisms. Some weeks William was more vulnerable than others, and on those visits, we made great connections. Eventually I helped William voice his feelings about the loss of his wife of nearly 55 years. He was able to identify the anxieties he had about his own mortality. He related stories to me that were filled with celebrations of memories. Some were great memories, others were more embarrassing, and still others were filled with poignancy.

In the end, when I terminated with William, I felt that I had been able to be a vehicle for the exploration of his grief. I learned that sometimes as a nurse in a faith community, there is a lot more to healing than just physical assessment.

The decade of the 1990s experienced dramatic changes in the health-care delivery system. Development of innovative models of community-based health care is mandatory to

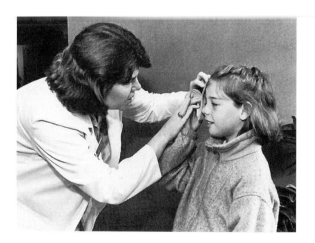

address the myriad changes facing the current health-care delivery system. These changes include rising health-care costs, difficulty accessing primary care, fragmentation of care, and the needs of an expanding elderly population (Baker et al., 1994; Bushnell & Cook, 1995; Weis, Matheus, & Schank, 1997). There is also emerging evidence of relationships between lifestyle behaviors and mortality.

New models for health care must focus on health promotion and disease prevention and emphasize individual responsibility and self-care. They must also incorporate the assumption of health-care reform that health is more than the absence of disease; health is wellness of the whole person. One innovative model that reflects these ideas is Parish Nursing.

Parish Nursing is defined as the practice of "holistic health care" within a faith community, emphasizing the relationship between faith and health (Bergquist & King 1994; Biddix & Brown, 1999). Faith community in this chapter refers to any gathering place where there is an assembly of people whose beliefs about God combine with a common identity, a shared history, a regular worship, and common values (Solari-Twadell & McDermott, 1999). Faith communities have many other titles or names such as church, congregation, temple, parish, synagogue, or mosque, to name a few. Two key elements of the Parish Nurse model that distinguish it from others are a fundamental belief in the relationship between spirituality and health and historical roots in a faith community. According to Donahue (1985), "The history of nursing first becomes continuous with the beginning of Christianity" (p. 93). Nursing has traditionally been concerned with health care to the whole person (Bergquist & King 1994). Florence Nightingale (1886) referred to the human being from physical, psychological, environmental, and spiritual perspectives. Faith communities have been involved in the delivery of health care for more than 2000 years.

HISTORICAL PERSPECTIVE

Faith communities naturally emerge as a place for health care. Throughout history, faith communities have been concerned with the body, mind, spirit, and care of the ill.

Early Egyptian and Babylonian cultures prevailed on priests for the treatment of the sick (Donahue, 1985). Priest–physicians transmitted the principles of good health through religious and mystical teachings in early Eastern cultures (Bergquist & King 1994). Hebrew priests monitored the observance of health rules regarding cleanliness, food, and quarantine. Deacons, deaconesses, monks, and nuns undertook care of the sick and poor in hospitals developed by religious institutions throughout medieval times. The development of hospitals by religious institutions continued until more recent times when modern medicine and nursing emerged. Personal responsibility of faith communities for health care became less prominent; yet members of the congregation—men and women, both religious and lay volunteers—continued to play a major role in the care of the sick. With the recognition of such care as a business and the growing presence of insurance, much of the health ministry role was relinquished to secular agencies (Joel, 1998).

The faith community is a natural support system that enables access to all age, ethnic, and faith groups, in urban and rural sites, and from all socioeconomic levels. Faith communities are natural centers for wellness promotion. Droege (1995) suggests that "everything the congregation does is related to health. . . . Health and healing are the mission of faith communities. . . . Healthy congregations promote solidarity, give meaning and purpose to life, inspire hope, pursue justice, and serve those in need" (pp. 118–119). Faith communities have the capacity to affect physical well-being and illness outcomes as longstanding agents of lifestyle change. The faith community

is a place where support groups can be formed, where ongoing dialogue with respect to struggles can be sustained, where helping relationships have an opportunity to evolve beyond the confines of limited stays or visit allocations, and where informal, nonthreatening environments conducive to learning offer the continued positive reinforcement of caring concern (Rydholm, 1997). According to the Princeton Religion Research Center (1996), 69 percent of all adults claim membership in a faith community. The report also notes that 43 percent of adults indicated they had attended worship services at least once during the past week; this reinforces faith communities as an effective site for community-based health-promotion and disease/illness-prevention programs.

Reverend Granger Westberg (1999), a retired Lutheran minister and hospital chaplain, stated that "the re-emergence of whole person health and faith communities happened quite spontaneously"(p. 35). He and a group of colleagues had been experimenting since the late 1960s with "wholistic" health centers that were family doctors' offices in midwestern churches. The goal was to achieve whole-person health care in a church setting through having spiritually oriented family doctors, nurses, and clergy working together. More than a dozen of these medical clinics were begun in neighborhood churches. The evaluations over a period of 10 years indicated that the quality of care offered when these three professionals worked together under the same roof was measurably more whole-person oriented than the average doctor's office (Westberg, 1999). Westberg reflected, "It was clear that the nurses in each of these centers were the glue that bound these three professionals together in a common appreciation of the healing talents of each" (1999, p. 35). It became apparent that nurses in these clinics could speak two languages: the language of science and the language of religion, thereby acting as translators. As inflation rose, it became more expensive to start new wholistic health centers in churches. One person suggested, "If the nurses in these clinics have proven so valuable, why not try placing a nurse on the staff of a congregation and see what happens?" (Westberg, 1999, p. 36). The decision was made to give it a go!

In 1984, Westberg went to Lutheran General Hospital (LGH), a 608-bed hospital, located in Park Ridge, Illinois.

LGH had long been a leader in pastoral care for its patients, and it showed immediate interest in the idea of partnering with local congregations in a parish nurse project. An administrative team from LGH was organized to plan and implement the first institutionally based program. Six congregations were willing to participate and agreed to a 3-year trial period. In 1985, the first parish nurse network was established with six parish nurses. This initial project was immediately successful, and it became apparent that these six nurses had made extensive inroads into assisting people, many in the early stages of illness, by their presence in the faith community. The members of the faith community saw the nurses as an extension of the church and because the church was already a vital part of their lives, they naturally accepted the parish nurse. It quickly became apparent that a faith community is one organization in our society ideally suited to give leadership to the field of preventive medicine.

Faith communities in America are becoming conscious of their role in keeping people healthy, in addition to the realization that many illnesses are preventable. Our current lifestyle or our way of handling life's many problems may make us ill. If illness is related to our outlook on life or our philosophy of life, then faith communities must be integrated into the health-care system (Westberg, 1999). Parish nurses can step right into this role for faith communities, and nurses have a common bond—both are committed to empowering individuals to achieve their full potential and both believe in the self-care capacity of people (Weis, Matheus, & Schank, 1997). Healing can always occur, even when cure is not possible (Simington, Olson, & Douglas, 1996). Our current health-care system emphasizes individual responsibility for health, making a focus on empowerment extremely important.

Interest in the LGH project grew so rapidly that the National Parish Nurse Resource Center was established in late 1986 to handle the flood of inquiries for information and consultation. The Health Ministries Association was established in 1989. It is a national, nonprofit, interfaith organization whose mission is to promote healing and health ministries in churches. Its membership consists of individual nurses, clergy, and others, as well as organizations. By 1992 there were 1500 nurses in faith communities and more than 50 networks. In 1995, Lutheran General Health System merged with Evangeline Health System to form Advocate Health Care System, which now sponsors the International Parish Nurse Resource Center. In 1998, there were an estimated 3000 nurses in faith communities serving in rural, urban, suburban, and inner-city settings throughout the country. Granger Westberg died in February 1999; he will be remembered as the father of the Parish Nurse concept. His vision has become reality.

PHILOSOPHY OF PARISH NURSING

Now is an excellent time to review your personal philosophy of nursing and to explore where nursing fits in a faith community. Parish nursing is an emerging area of specialized professional nursing practice distinguished by the following characteristics:

- Parish nursing practice holds the spiritual dimension to be central to the practice. It also encompasses the physical, psychological, and social dimensions of nursing practice.
- The parish nurse role balances knowledge and skill; the sciences, theology, and humanities; service and worship; and nursing care with pastoral care functions.
- The focus of practice is the faith community and its ministry. The parish nurse, in collaboration with the pastoral staff and congregational members, participates in the ongoing transformation of the faith community into a source of health and healing. Through partnership with other community health resources, parish nursing fosters new and creative responses to health concerns.
- Parish nursing services are designed to build on and strengthen capacities of individuals, families, and congregations to understand the care of one another in light of their relationship to God, faith traditions, themselves, and the broader society. The practice holds that all persons are sacred and must be treated with respect and dignity.
- The parish nurse understands health to be a dynamic process that embodies the spiritual, psychological, physical, and social dimensions of the person. Spiritual health is central to well-being and influences a person's entire being. Therefore, a sense of well-being and illness may occur simultaneously. Healing may exist in the absence of cure (Solari-Twadell, McDermott, Ryan, & Djupe, 1994).

NURSING MODELS IN A FAITH COMMUNITY

Four different support models for nursing in a faith community have emerged. In the institutional/paid model, the nurse is employed by a hospital, community agency, or long-term care facility that contracts with one or more faith communities and provides salary, benefits, institutional support, and supervision. In this model, the nurse spends 50 percent of his or her time in each facility. In the institutional/volunteer model the nurse volunteers his or her time, but a relationship exists between the faith community and an institution, which may involve the provision of a stipend to the nurse or congregation or education and supervision. The congregation/paid model involves employment of the nurse directly by the congregation with support, benefits, and supervision from the faith community itself. The hours worked by the nurse vary depending on the contractual agreement with the congregation. Nurses in the former model usually form support and resources networks with other faith community nurses in their geographic area. The congregational/volunteer model is similar, except that the nurses volunteer their time (Miskelly, 1995).

Nurses in faith communities have both scheduled and flexible office hours depending on the activities and needs of the congregation. Salaries are based on education, experience, and geographic location (Weis, Matheus, & Schank, 1997).

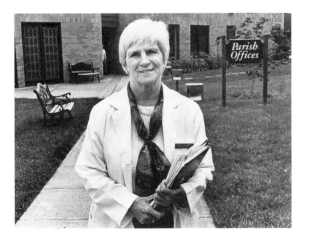

WHAT DO FAITH COMMUNITY NURSES DO?

Nurses working in a faith community assume many different functions depending on their experiences and strengths and the needs of the community they serve. The faith community nurse is sensitive to the relationship between faith and health and the application of spiritual aspects of health care (Westberg, 1999). The faith community nurse is knowledgeable of community-health services and resources, is able to work autonomously, and has good communication skills (McDermott & Burke, 1993). Ideally, the faith community nurse is part of the pastoral team and works with this team to plan and implement health care to the faith community (Bergquist & King, 1994). Faith community nurses interact with clients in a caring manner. The health care they provide is to the body, mind, and spirit.

When asked to reflect on her experiences in a faith community clinical practicum, one student wrote the following:

 The unique mixture of physical, mental, and spiritual care is really caring for the whole person. In this type of nursing a special bond is formed between nurse and client. I experienced this bond visiting home clients as a junior nursing student.

Another student wrote:

 Being a student in a faith community is an ideal setting for the nurse who wishes to combine her professional and spiritual life. In some ways, I believe the sharing of a religious philosophy can enhance the rapport between the nurse and her client. Many clients, especially the elderly, are wary of the seemingly cold and impersonal medical system. They seem to feel more comfortable when the nurse is affiliated with their faith community.

A third student wrote:

 I rejoice as goals of strengthening mind, body, and spirit of both student nurse and client are reached before our eyes.

The International Parish Nurse Resource Center has identified seven functions of the faith community nurse role (Table 23–1). These functions have developed over the past 13 years as the role of nursing in a faith community has evolved. As mentioned previously, not every faith community nurse performs every function.

There are a few functions that nurses in a faith community do not perform. They do not perform any invasive procedures. Less than 2 percent perform hands-on nursing care (McDermott & Burke, 1993). These nurses do not bill for services, do not provide home-health services, and do not duplicate community services. Instead, they collaborate with others to meet unattended needs and enhance the care delivery services to their faith community members. It is the nurse's task to nurture the client, so that even if there is biological disease present, the person can move beyond the circumstances to a feeling of hopefulness and a sense of self-worth and dignity. Box 23–1 will help you expand your understanding of parish nurse functions.

Table 23-1

Functions of a Faith Community Nurse

- *Health Educator* promotes an atmosphere in which individuals of all ages, through a variety of educational activities, explore the relationship between values, attitudes, lifestyle, faith, and health (Solari-Twadell & McDermott, 1999). They are providers of current, accurate information on health and disease (Schank, Weis, & Matheus, 1996).

- *Personal Health Counselor* discusses health issues and problems with individuals; makes home, hospital, and nursing home visits as needed.

- *Referral Agent and Liaison* with congregational and community resources provides referrals to other congregational resources as well as those found in the community at large. A cooperative and collaborative relationship with community agencies is an important aspect of this function (Bergquist & King, 1994).

- *Developer of Support Group* facilitates the development of support groups and self-help groups for members of the faith community and people from the external community. Support groups enhance the healing and caring of faith communities.

- *Facilitator of Volunteers* recruits, coordinates, and resources volunteers within the congregation to serve various health ministries.

- *Integrator of Faith and Health* seeks to promote the understanding of the relationship between faith and health in all activities and contacts.

- *Health Advocate* works with the client, faith community, and primary-health resources to provide what is in the best interest of the client from a whole-person perspective, listening and supporting the clients to do what they can and being their voice when they seem to have none.

Box 23-1   Student Learning Activity

Functions of Parish Nurses

Choose three of the functions listed in Table 23–1. For each function, list two activities that would fulfill that function.

Here is one student's description of her first experience in the role of personal health counselor:

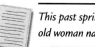

This past spring I was making a home visit to a 96-year-old woman named Ann who had recently had surgery for a recurrence of a mandibular/buccal carcinoma. At first Ann's speech was difficult to interpret but with close attention it quickly became distinguishable. This last surgery was not a major resection. Ann mentioned that she only wished she could go to service on Sunday with her family, but she was concerned about her appearance. She also related that she had not shared these concerns with her daughter and son-in-law with whom she lives. She had not looked in a mirror since the surgery four weeks ago. I spent the next

two weekly visits assisting Ann to verbalize her feelings, concerns, fears, and perceptions of her appearance. The fourth week Ann shared with me that she had the courage to look in the mirror and to her delight the surgery looked rather good. Ann announced that she was planning to attend Easter service with her family the following Sunday. I was able to assist Ann in restoring her self-esteem and dignity. During the next nine weeks further healing took place.

Nursing in a faith community provides endless opportunities for nursing students seeking the challenges of community-based care combined with the spiritual values of promoting health.

DEVELOPMENT OF A PARTNERSHIP FOR HEALTH

A faculty member, who was a member of a faith community with a large multicultural population, initiated the development of a faith community clinical practicum. This particular faith community had a history of a progressive pastoral team who embraced participation in innovative programs. The associate dean for undergraduate nursing education and the nursing program's community liaison met several times with the pastor to define and describe the kinds of services that the nursing students and faculty could provide to the faith community.

George Mason University (GMU) College of Nursing and Health Science in Fairfax, Virginia, adapted a parish nursing model to deliver holistic health care in a faith community. Students are not involved in doing parish nursing as defined in the literature (Solari-Twadell & McDermott, 1999), but they do address the physiological, sociological, and psychological perspectives of health and healing in their work with clients. They refer all spiritual matters to the faith community pastor, priest, or pastoral minister. GMU developed a partnership for HEALTH with Church of the Nativity (referred to as Nativity) in January 1997. The purpose of the partnership is to promote holistic health to the faith community and to prevent disease while facilitating the education of nursing students. The acronym HEALTH (Table 23–2) was selected to denote Health counselor, Educator, Advocate, Liaison to the community, Teacher, and Health promoter. This was the foundation of the Nativity/GMU Partnership for HEALTH.

Table 23-2

Partenership for Health

H—Health Counselor

E—Educator

A—Advocate

L—Liaison to the Community

T—Teacher

H—Health Promoter

Goals and Objectives

The goals for this clinical practicum were: health promotion, disease prevention, therapeutic communications, and health assessments of individuals, families, and small groups. The objectives to meet these goals follow:

- Assess the health-care needs of the faith community.
- Assess health education needs of the faith community.
- Use the nursing process in the delivery of nursing care.
- Develop therapeutic relationships.
- Provide sensitive and caring nursing interventions.
- Provide anticipatory coordination and continuity of care.
- Perform selected technologies in a variety of settings.
- Demonstrate professional behaviors.

Location of Faith Community

Nativity is a faith community located on the outskirts of a major metropolis, with a registered membership of 4000 families from which to draw potential clients and a list of homebound individuals. The church school has a variety of activities including a before- and after-school program, a religious education program involving 1400 students, and an active physical education program, all providing avenues for GMU nursing students to meet their course objectives. One of the classroom teachers mentioned to me, "The GMU nursing students bring youth, enthusiasm, and zest to our school program. Our students seem to be more health conscious when they are here."

PARTNERSHIP IN ACTION

Goals and objectives were in place. The contracts were signed and many planning meetings attended. It was time to get started with this new adventure. Students were excited, anxious, curious, eager, and ready to become active in this fertile environment. Students expressed a number of concerns: What if I'm not a member of this particular faith community, will it matter? What if my home client doesn't like me? What if I don't know the answer to a question? Do I really need to stand in front of a classroom full of students to present a teaching project? What do we wear in this particular clinical setting? All of these questions and others were answered in our first orientation session held at GMU. All the logistics regarding this new clinical site were addressed: introductions to clinical group and instructor; review of syllabus and required assignments; directions to the site; lunch; safekeeping of purses and valuables; appropriate dress, including name tag at all times; lab coat with GMU patch for home visits; clinical hours; phone tree; listing of suggested activities for students to think about for later decisions; and a question-and-answer session.

A daily clinical log was required, which facilitated application of theory and nursing diagnosis to clinical practice. Students were encouraged to express their thoughts and feelings. There were also other questions to ponder related to ideas for teaching, age group of interest, and home-visit preference. Box 23–2 provides an opportunity to answer commonly asked questions.

The first two clinical days were spent in an orientation/exploring mode. Nativity provided a "welcome coffee" and all the significant members of our partnership, (pastor, principal, pastoral ministers, school nurse, and before/after school coordinator) were there to greet and meet the nursing students. Each person presented to the nursing students a short description of his or her particular role within this faith community. A welcome feeling from the onset is valuable for the success of any nursing clinical experience.

A tour of the facility was provided. Much of the morning was spent discussing initial impressions of the facility,

---

Box 23-2   Student Learning Activity

Commonly Asked Questions

These are some common questions that students often ask. Add additional questions that you might want answered.

- What are some of your assumptions about nursing in a faith community?

- What are your expectations of this clinical experience?

- What are your expectations of the clinical faculty?

---

selecting a student partner with whom to work throughout the semester, answering questions, and actively planning activities. Activities suggested by Nativity's partnership members were given first priority. Students had space in the weekly bulletin to present a short column addressing a health fact. All students were eager to participate in this project and immediately signed up. Thus a calendar of events was begun. The column was called Nativity/GMU Partnership for HEALTH.

A second event was an observational visit with the school nurse, who is a registered nurse. All students welcomed this opportunity to examine the role and functions of a school nurse. Students learned that documentation of care is extremely important in this setting.

A third available activity was the before-/after-school program. The program coordinator, who is a registered nurse, was very supportive of nursing students using this population for teaching projects and activities. Students who wanted to participate registered and others knew it was a viable option.

Are you thinking of ideas? GMU students suggested implementation of a blood pressure screening clinic. After brainstorming all possible avenues, it was decided this would be a weekly event held in the vestibule of the church for two hours after a regularly scheduled daily

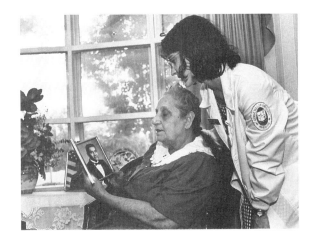

Mass. Two nursing students would participate. The need to advertise was imperative. A poster was constructed and placed in the vestibule and an announcement was written for the weekly bulletin. A request was submitted for permission to add this to the announcements for the upcoming weekend services. The decision to participate was unanimous among the students, and they agreed to begin the following week.

The culminating activity for this orientation day was a windshield survey. As student nurses in a community setting, it is essential to know your surroundings. Students were encouraged to go in pairs to scan the neighborhood surrounding Nativity. They located and recorded the address for the nearest fire and police station, health-care facility, hospital, and library.

Planning continued on the second clinical orientation day. An area of possible involvement for the students, which required some investigation, was the Presidential Physical Fitness Program. This was Nativity school's first year of operation, and the physical education program needed assistance. The principal inquired if the "nurses" could possibly implement this program for the physical education (PE) teacher, who had just terminated. School PE programs have the potential to help children and adolescents establish lifelong, healthy physical activity patterns. It is essential that physical activity be strongly encouraged among young people so that they will continue to engage in physical activity in adulthood and thereby obtain its benefits throughout life (Centers for Disease Control and Prevention

[CDC], 1997). After careful consideration, four students agreed to administer, teach, and evaluate a PE program for grades 2 through 8. A call was immediately placed to national headquarters seeking program requirements. The classes were divided into upper and lower divisions, folders were prepared, a meeting with the PE substitute teacher was arranged, classes were rescheduled to accommodate nursing students' availability, and all students began to practice V-sits and chin pulls. The program was up and running.

Teaching is a core function of the nurse who practices community-based nursing. The more adept you are at teaching, the more you are able to help people help themselves (Armentrout, 1998). Remember that your particular areas of interest and expertise are excellent starting points. At Nativity, teaching projects were completed by all students. The variety of available opportunities, stated needs, and suggested topics were discussed. Grade-school children, teenagers, teachers, staff, parishioners, home clients, and our student group were all receptive to learning. Students considered various modes for accomplishing this task. During the orientation, seeds were planted to bloom further into the semester.

Home visits were an additional bonus of this clinical setting. Many questions immediately rushed to the students' minds. The student story at the beginning of the chapter poignantly articulates these questions: "What would I say? How would I act? How would I begin to physically examine my client?" Another student was concerned that the client might require more assistance than she was prepared to administer. These fears and concerns were addressed through group discussion, role-playing exercises, and a video. I assured the students that I would accompany each of them on their first home visit and shared information about my previous visit with their clients. Decisions were made and a client/student roster was produced.

What would be the equipment required for a home visit? Would it be best to obtain and assemble a nursing bag? What needed to be included in a nursing bag? It was decided that a nursing bag is a necessity and that it should contain pens, pencil, paper, stethoscope, sphygmomanometer, scissors, flashlight, a few pairs of disposable gloves, map, drug book, pocket assessment book, and three file cards. One file card had the client's address, phone number, and directions to his or her home; another card contained the instructor's beeper number; and a third card listed Nativity's main phone number.

One student wrote the following in her clinical log:

Somehow, the prospect of applying what I know (or was supposed to know) in the community presented a whole new set of fears for me. I found myself filling my magazine-size nursing bag to capacity with every pocket-sized nursing reference I owned. After the first few days, I thought the nursing bag might be saying what I didn't want commonly known, "This bag is full of what I don't know." So, I lightened the load . . . a little. By the time I had my last home visit of the semester, I think I had opened one of those books once. I did most of my "looking up" at home, so that I wouldn't have to pull out one of those "I don't know books" during a visit. But I always carried some of them with me, perhaps to unconsciously say, "I may not know the answer to your next question but I do know where to find it in the bag!

Box 23–3 will help you to think through a client situation.

Students decided to plan a Student Health Fair. What a great idea! Health fairs are an excellent venue for impacting large numbers of participants on a variety of health-promotion/disease-prevention topics and activities. Health promotion can and should be integrated into school curricula, programs, and activities. Health promotion encompasses components of environmental health and safety, individual and group preventive health practices, and health education. Each student had the potential to develop a booth for the fair. We reviewed possible booth topics, explored resources, examined the calendar of events for school activities, and analyzed some of the logistics of such an undertaking.

A baby-sitting course was requested on the needs assessment survey. One student volunteered to investigate the available resources for implementing this project. Think of agencies in your community where this could be accomplished.

Another "getting to know the community" activity was to visit a community resource organization for the

---

Box 23-3	Student Learning Activity

Client Example

The client is a 54-year-old male who has become more disoriented, confused, and unable to stay focused or perform activities of daily living. He has recently been diagnosed with early Alzheimer's disease. He lives in a large colonial house in a wooded area with his wife of 25 years and three children ages 15, 20, and 22. His wife notified Nativity that she would like to have a nursing student make a weekly home visit. The student and instructor met with the wife for an hour and a half. The wife had a six-page typed history of her husband's illness.

It was determined that the student and her partner would make a weekly visit to build rapport and assess the client. The student would also explore additional resources for the wife and family. After one visit, when the students opened the front door to leave, the alarm system went off. The client immediately became upset and was pacing about with his hands over his ears. Every time the door was opened the noise was incredible.

- What is the problem?

- Why is it a problem?

- What are the key issues?

- What should the students do first?

- How should the students handle this situation?

- What community resources might be available?

purpose of learning the mission, goals, and objectives of this organization. What are some of the organizations in your community that you might want to explore? Organizations we used were the American Heart Association, the Cancer Society, the Dental Association, the Lung Association, the Alzheimer's Association, the County Center for Aging, the National Osteoporosis Association, the National Dairy Council, the County Center of Children, the National Hospice Foundation, and the American Diabetes Association. All of these were within a 20-mile radius of the clinical setting. Students obtained free samples of available teaching aids and resources (litera-

ture, posters, displays, videos checklists, and equipment), as well as lists of possible speakers and references. They shared their experiences and resources with others in the group. Some helpful community resources are listed in Table 23–3.

What We Did and Its Impact

Activities were organized, calendars filled, resources investigated, clients chosen, and groups defined: Now it was time to carry out the plan of action. The following outlines what we did.

Table 23-3

Resources

Organizations:

The International Nurse Resource Center

205 W. Touhy, Suite 124

Park Ridge, IL 60068

1-800-556-5368

Health Ministries Association

P.O. Box 7853

Huntington Beach, CA 92646

Phone 714-965-0085

Books:

Solari-Twadell, P. A., Djupe, A. M., & McDermott, M. A. (Eds.). (1990). Parish nursing: The developing practice. Park Ridge, IL: National Parish Nurse Resource Center.

Solari-Twadell, P. A., & McDermott, M. A, (1999). Parish nursing. Thousand Oaks, CA: Sage Publishers.

Solari-Twadell, P. A., McDermott, M. A., Ryan, J., & Djupe, M. A. (Eds.). (1994). Assuring viability for the future: Guideline development for parish nurse education programs. Park Ridge, IL: National Parish Nurse Resource Center.

Videos:

The Healing Team: An Introduction to Health Ministry & Parish Nursing. Produced by Bay Area Health Ministries, 415-221-3693/www.bahm.org

The Parish Nurse: A ministry to older adults. Available from the International Parish Nurse Resource Center.

Parish Nurses: Reclaiming their joy. Available from the International Parish Nurse Resource Center.

Yours Are the Hands: Parish Nurse Program, Resurrection Health Care, 773-774-8650.

Articles:

Abbott, B. (1998). Parish nursing. Home Healthcare Nurse, 16(4), 265–267.

Penner, S., & Galloway-Lee, B. (1997). Parish nursing: Opportunities in community health. Home Care Provider, 2(5), 244–249.

Rydholm, L. (1997). Patient-focused care in parish nursing. Holistic Nursing Practice, 11(3), 47–60.

Schank, M. J., Weis, D., & Matheus, R. (1996). Parish nursing: Ministry of healing. Geriatric Nursing, 17(1), 11–13.

Weis, D., Matheus, R., & Schank, M. J. (1997). Health care delivery in faith communities: The parish nurse model. Public Health Nursing, 14(6), 368–372.

Published Health Messages

The column "Nativity/GMU Partnership for HEALTH" appeared in the weekly bulletin for 14 weeks. Every student participated at least once, publishing a health fact. The following are a few examples of published messages:

- Blood Pressure (BP) Screenings will be held Wednesday mornings after the 7:30 A.M. Mass, from 8:00 to 10:00 A.M. This year, in addition to 10 enthusiastic student nurses and our instructor, we have a postgraduate nursing education student joining us. Screenings are free, so stop in, get your BP checked, or just say "Hi!" and spend a few minutes talking with our Nurses/Student Nurses. We look forward to meeting with you!

- Do you know that heart attack is the #1 single cause of death in the U.S.? One simple way to reduce your risk of heart attack is by monitoring your blood pressure. Hypertension (high blood pressure) greatly increases your risk for heart attack, stroke, and kidney failure—and most people with hypertension have no symptoms at all. Remember, free blood pressure screenings are available every Wednesday from 8 to 10 A.M. in the church vestibule. Stop by for more information about preventing heart disease. BE HEART SMART!

- Exercise plays a key role in our overall wellness. It reduces cholesterol, blood pressure, and stress as well as increasing self-esteem, strength, and endurance. We know exercise has multiple positive effects, yet it can be difficult to stick with an exercise program. To ensure compliance with a program, incorporate it into your everyday living and make it a lifestyle change. Here are a few tips to get you started in the right direction.

  1. Keep a log/journal. Recording your activities gives a sense of accountability and is a good record of progress over time.

  2. Set measurable short-term goals and rewards. Set a goal of walking 20 minutes three times a week. At the end of the week, reward yourself by going to a movie you've been wishing to see.

  3. Get an exercise partner. Having a partner allows you to spend time with friends and makes the time go faster as well as have more fun.

  4. Perform activities at the same time on the same days. This helps make exercising a habit.

  5. MAKE IT FUN & SIMPLE!! Try that new sport you have always wanted to do or just go play outside with the children or take the dog for a walk. Once you start experiencing all the wonderful things exercise can do for you, you will wonder how you ever lived without it.

- Did you know that alcohol negatively stresses the body? What starts as an effort at relaxation quickly backfires to cause stress. Alcohol strains the body's detoxification system, the liver, the kidneys, and the pancreas. When alcohol use is frequent, these organs become damaged and do not function as well. Alcohol also affects blood sugar balance and is associated with diabetes and hypoglycemia. Alcohol reduces levels of B and C vitamins and magnesium in the body, which are effective for fighting off the effects of stress. In a worst-case example, what is used as a simple way to relax can become a terrible addiction with serious mental and physical consequences.

Other topics that students addressed included diabetes, the importance of laughter, smoking cessation, dental care, osteoporosis, medication compliance, nutrition, importance of completing antibiotic regimens, and many others. This was a very successful health-promotion initiative.

School Nurse Activities

Spending time with the school nurse was very educational. The role of a nurse in the school setting was experienced first hand. Basic first aid, medication administration, documentation, and techniques for working with a variety of ages of children were observed and explored. The school nurse was available as a consultant and resource for teaching projects. She was an asset to our partnership.

Before-/After-School Programs

The students used the before-school program as an additional experience. It is a "jump start" time, because some students are finishing eating breakfasts, fixing or rearranging their hair, or finishing their homework. Usually, all students needed assistance of some type, and the outcome was positive for all involved. One student took advantage of the after-school program and presented a teaching project on Playground Safety. Prior to his presentation, he spent three hours working with this group of children. He used a multimedia approach to include all students' learning styles and role playing for reinforcement and evaluation of key points. This is an underused opportunity in this clinical setting!

Blood Pressure Screening

Dressed in their white lab coats, each week two students participated in the blood pressure screening clinic. A banner was placed in the church vestibule, a poster was constructed explaining the definition and facts about blood pressure, a handout was designed to record blood pressure, and resource information was made available. This was a very successful health-promotion event, and toward the end of the semester 20 to 25 members were visiting the clinic. Most participants were interested in discussing blood pressure, exercise, or diet implications. If any abnormalities were detected, participants were referred to their primary doctors immediately. One student reported that she was at a loss for words when a middle-aged man replied, " I know my blood pressure is good, I have cancer!" She felt ill prepared and caught off guard. She felt that she didn't respond in a therapeutic manner, for she just replied, "Oh, I'm sorry." She shared this incident with the group, and we discussed techniques to use when these types of situations arise. We all agreed that this client wanted to talk. Box 23–4 allows you to brainstorm responses to a client's communication.

Box 23-4   Student Learning Activity

Communication

Brainstorm how you might have responded if a client stated, "I know my blood pressure is good. I have cancer!" Be prepared to share your ideas with your classmates.

Health Fitness

In warm-up suits, with GMU name tags, equipped with clipboards and whistles, four nursing students welcomed the challenge of implementing the Presidential Physical Fitness Program for the 250 schoolchildren grades 2 through 8. Two students, and the substitute PE teacher on occasion, worked with each class. Every participant had a score sheet that involved accurate record keeping. There are five challenge test items: curl-ups, shuttle run, 1-mile

run, pull-ups, and V-sit reach. Before performing the tests, all students were taught the correct techniques, including proper pacing and running style. The children were then allowed to practice, and when they "felt ready" were tested. There was no limit to the number of tries students could have on each test item, but proper technique had to be maintained throughout the testing phase. The Nativity students were eager to participate and do well. When the program was completed, an awards ceremony was held, and all students were presented with a participant certificate. Students earning National level were also presented with a National Patch and those attaining Presidential level were given special tee shirts, in addition to the Presidential Patch. The first year, 16 students obtained Presidential and 18 obtained National; the second year, 36 earned Presidential and 22 earned National; and the third year, 54 attained Presidential and 45 attained National. The students worked very hard to achieve these awards. Nativity students enthusiastically await this program each spring. One GMU student stated, "Physical activity is great, teaching is fun, you get to be outside, and you wear warm-up suits while having the opportunity to work with children from different age groups and cultures, cheering them on and watching as they succeed. You can't beat it!"

One semester, a Fitness for Life Fair was presented. Some of the booths were "Bike and Helmet Safety," "House and Fire Safety," "Healthy Food Choices," "Fruitful Snacks," and "What Bugs You?" TriEd Fitness, Inc. worked with four students to set up an obstacle course using a new product called Tinix sticks. Every year the fitness programs are different, but all have been well received by the students and staff of Nativity.

Teaching Projects

"Germ Busters," "Stranger Danger," "911," "What Is Depression?" "Hugs not Drugs," and "Importance of Hand Washing" are just a few titles of teaching projects. These were all constructed for various classes at Nativity School. Most can be taught in 20 to 30 minutes. Students selected topics, wrote objectives for the teaching/learning activity, and then approached the classroom teacher for permission to execute their plan, as well as observe the class. The purpose of an observational session was to observe classroom environment, makeup of the class, strategies of teaching, conduct of the teacher, discipline used, and attention span of students. Active learning strategies are incorporated into all teaching/learning projects, as well as use of community resources and handouts to enhance and reinforce learning.

One student elected to develop an educational program specifically aimed toward teachers. She adapted a survey requesting their input on which topics they would like to be presented. Teachers responded to suggested topics with their preferences as follows: first aid (0), recognizing the signs of abuse (1), positive self-esteem building in children (2), healthful snacks for healthy children (2), classroom safety (3), and stress management (5). Stress management was presented in an after-school program for the staff of both the school and church. In a 45-minute session, a stress-reducing environment was created using soft music, low lights, aromatic candles, comfortable chairs, and warm tea. Stress reduction exercises and techniques were discussed and practiced. All participants reported feeling less stressed at the conclusion of the program.

Other students implemented one-on-one client teaching on medications, diabetes, foot care, nutrition, exercise requirements, and alcohol awareness, to mention a few. One student went grocery shopping with her client to teach her how to read and interpret package nutritional labels and make healthy choices. Another student started a weekly caregivers' support group that was structured as a self-help group, which met at the church in the afternoon. It started with four women, and the student served as facilitator; the instructor was also present. Each week there was a suggested topic for discussion, such as caregiver resources. A semiretired parishioner with a degree in social work agreed to continue the group at the end of the semester. Students learned that continuity is extremely important!

Another student planned an international and cultural lesson by presenting "Nursing in Ghana" to his classmates. He went to his embassy for resources and assembled an interesting portrayal not only of nursing, but of the health-care system in this African republic.

Home Visits

Home visits had a significant impact on the clients in this faith community. The weekly visits lasted about an hour, and many clients were seen for 12 to 14 visits, a substantial amount of time to positively impact a client's health care. Basic assessments were completed over the semester,

reviewing medications, nutrition, and exercise and identifying resources for client use. Confidentiality was a top priority. All of the data collected concerning the client were documented in an assessment file and stored at the church.

Visits to clients included a 9-year-old autistic child, who needed help with basic hygiene education and development of a positive relationship with a health professional; a 36-year-old primigravida having twins, requiring bed rest from the fifth month to premature delivery; a 54-year-old man with Alzheimer's disease who spent a great deal of daytime hours alone (safety was a definite issue); a 78-year-old man, poststroke, who needed a great deal of retraining and encouragement; a 34-year-old man who was experiencing alcohol-related seizures; and many others. Each client reflected a unique situation with real health needs and concerns.

Here is a student's description of one home visit experience:

 I had been visiting an elderly couple once a week throughout the semester. On one such weekly visit my elderly gentleman client did not have the usual twinkle in his eye. After just a few questions I discovered he had been suffering from hallucinations, both audio and visual, for several days. Although he had been unable, or unwilling, to share this with his wife, he freely shared it with me. You see, it would have been another burden to lay on his wife as his caretaker. But he knew I was there to help him with just this kind of situation—he trusted me. I referred him to his neurologist—but his wife needed some convincing. My instructor arrived and helped me to help her understand the importance of getting her husband's problem evaluated. The solution was a simple adjustment in medication. This situation is a perfect example of nursing in a faith community—a health-care team working together in partnership with clients through a trusting and a caring relationship.

Another student wrote the following:

Finding a long forgotten faith in the Lord, with the help of a client who knows of its wonder and is a living example herself, students learn too, and I have beautiful memories that will keep me smiling forever.

Home visits provided the opportunity to meet all course objectives and resulted in a vast array of unanticipated learning opportunities. The students were extremely well received by those parishioners who wanted/needed visiting.

Student Health Fair

A student health fair was the culminating activity for this clinical. It was a huge undertaking and took hours of planning and the whole semester to organize. It was a true collaborative effort. The theme of the first fair addressed health issues for children in grades K through 8. The fair took place on a school day, in the school's multiple room. Every participant received a passport for health and goodie bags at registration. Each student constructed a festive, interactive booth and rewarded the participants with a prize for completing the activity. Prizes consisted of healthy snacks, drinks, handouts, and small prizes. The school nurse provided students with a list of children with allergies so that the nursing students could accommodate these needs. Children spent approximately 4 minutes visiting each booth. Some of the themes for booths were "Build a Healthy Pizza," "Fire Safety," "Safety with Animals," "What to Expect When You're in the Hospital," "Car and Bike Safety," "Orthodontics and Dental Care," "Stress Reduction and Importance of Milk and Your Bones," and "What Do Nurses Do?" Points to remember when organizing a health fair include the following: provide extra time for setup and a wide range of activities at each booth for children from 5 years to 13 years of age; arrange enough prizes for all students; develop a carefully planned traffic pattern to eliminate backups; and get a good night's sleep prior to the fair, because you are on all day. Have fun!

The second year, an International Children's Health Fair was presented. The clinical group included nursing students from around the globe. Examples of booths included Italy, "Hugs not Drugs"; Philippines, "Important Foods of the Philippines"; Nigeria, "Water"; Thailand, "Fruits"; Japan, "Relax and Be Happy"; Lebanon, "Sugar"; India, "Ears"; Ireland, "Irish Eyes are Smiling"; Ecuador, "Muscles and Tendons at Work"; and Ghana, "Immunizations." Students dressed in their native costumes, making this a very colorful event, as well as extremely educational. One student nurse responded, " The international health fair was a great idea because it is good for the children to be aware of different cultures. I'm talking about fruit: variety is the spice of life and we need variety in our food, making choices, trying new things."

Baby-Sitting Course

A baby-sitting course was an easy activity to organize and implement. A local hospital system had a nurse on staff that taught just such a course. She agreed to teach the course on a Saturday at Nativity School, for a reasonable fee, to 14 students who were sixth to eighth graders. A letter was drafted and distributed to all eligible students at Nativity. The response was overwhelming. Acceptance letters were sent, the room was reserved, and a school staff member was targeted to open the building. Two courses were implemented that semester and 28 Nativity students were certified. This was a highly successful venture.

CONCLUSION

Nursing in a faith community is emerging as a viable response to the multiple and complex problems that constitute the crisis that we are experiencing in health care. It is also proving to be an excellent clinical site for nursing students whose focus is on health promotion, disease prevention, and holistic care. The challenges and opportunities are endless! GMU student nurses had an immense impact on the health status of this faith community. A student stated, "Parishes are filled with individuals and families who could really benefit from a home visit made by a nurse/student nurse, who takes a genuine interest in her clients." Another student responded, "Faith communities have it all!"

Active Learning Strategies

1. How would you define nursing in a faith community? Compare your definition with a friend's.

2. Write a paragraph on "How spirituality affects health." Share it with your clinical group.

3. What community resources are available in your community to assist clients in a faith community? Select one group (e.g., new mothers) and explore resources available for them in your community. Start a card file of resources with what you find.

References

Armentrout, G. (1998). Community based nursing: Foundations of practice. Stamford, CT: Appleton & Lange.

Baker, J., Bayne, T., Higgs, Z., Jenkin, S., Murphy, D., & Synoground, G. (1994). Community analysis: A collaborative community practice project. Public Health Nursing, 11(2), 113–118.

Bergquist, S., & King, J. (1994). Parish nursing: A conceptual framework. Journal of Holistic Nursing, 12(2), 155–170.

Biddix, V., & Brown, H. (1999). Establishing a parish nursing program. Nursing and Health Care Perspectives, 20(2), 72–75.

Bushnell, F., & Cook, T. (1995). Primary care to the underserved through community empowerment. Nurse Practitioner, 20(8), 21–23.

Centers for Disease Control and Prevention (CDC). (1997). Guidelines for school and community programs to promote life-long physical activity among young people. Journal of School Health, 67(6), 202–220.

Donahue, M. P. (1985). Nursing: The finest art. St. Louis: C.V. Mosby.

Droege, T. (1995). Congregations as communities of health and healing. Interpretation, 49, 117–129.

Joel, L. (1998). Parish nursing: As old as faith communities. American Journal of Nursing, 98(8), 7.

McDermott, M. A., & Burke, J. (1993). When the population is a congregation: The emerging role of the parish nurse. Journal of Community Health Nursing, 1(3), 179–190.

Miskelly, S. (1995). A parish nursing model: Applying the community health nursing process in a church community. Journal of Community Health Nursing, 12(1), 1–14.

Nightingale, F. (1886). Notes on nursing. New York: Dover.

Princeton Religion Research Center. (1996). Religion in America. Princeton: Religious Research Center.

Rydholm, L. (1997). Patient-focused care in parish nursing. Holistic Nursing Practice, 11(3), 47–60.

Schank, M. J., Weis, D., & Matheus, R. (1996). Parish nursing: Ministry of healing. Geriatric Nursing, 17(1), 11–13.

Simington, J., Olson, J., & Douglas, L. (1996). Promoting well-being within a parish. The Canadian Nurse, 92(1), 20–24.

Solari-Twadell, P. A., & McDermott, M. A. (Eds.). (1999). Parish nursing: Promoting whole person health within faith communities. Thousand Oaks, CA: Sage.

Solari-Twadell, P. A., McDermott, M. A., Ryan, J., & Djupe, M. A. (Eds.). (1994). Assuring viability for the future: Guideline development for parish nurse education programs. Park Ridge, IL: National Parish Nurse Resource Center.

Weis, D., Matheus, R., & Schank, M. J. (1997). Health care delivery in faith communities: The parish nurse model. Public Health Nursing, 14(6), 368–372.

Westberg, G. (1999). A personal historical perspective of whole person health and the congregation. In P. A. Solari-Twadell & M. A. Dermott (Eds.), Parish nursing: Promoting whole person health within faith communities (pp. 35–42). Thousand Oaks, CA: Sage.

INDEX

Rights-based theory, 129-130
Risk reduction
    activities, 79-80
    in child-care centers, 334-335
    literature on, 91
RLS. *See* Restless leg syndrome
RN. *See* Registered nurse
Role complementary, 280
Role model, 152
RPh. *See* Registered pharmacist
RRT. *See* Registered Respiratory Therapist
Ruby, Julie Rose, 190-191
Rural Municipality Act, 42

S
Safety
    in home-care setting, 400-401
    shopping for, 86
    strategies to promote, 357
Saint Elizabeth Health Care, 49
Saint Elizabeth Visiting Nurses, 49
Saskatchewan, 42
    Regina, 49
    universal hospital program, 42
Satcher, Dr. David, 216
School Health Policies and Programs Study, 91
School nurse, 153, 356-357
    activities, 424
School programs, 424. *See also* College campus;
    Elementary schools
Scope of practice, 149-150
Search Institute (Minneapolis), 91
Secondary prevention, 81
Seizures, 16
Self-care, 238
Self-determination, 408
    right of, 214-215
Self-disclosure, 255-256
Self evaluation, 400
Senior centers, 90-91
    challenges, 349-350
    critical thinking, 352
    evaluation, 349
    future directions, 352-353
    GMU model, 345-349
    home visits, 352
    nursing practice, 343

primary care concept, 346
    strengths, 349
    student perceptions, 350-353
    student projects, 346
Seniors, 17
    communication with, 262-266
    demographic trends, 344-345
    disabilities, 345
    hearing impaired, 265
    primary-care skills applications, 345-349
    vision and, 265
Setting
    healthcare related, 237
    non-healthcare, 237-238
Sexually transmitted diseases (STDs), 372
Shelters, 89-90
SHMO. *See* Social Health Maintenance Organization
Shortness of breath (SOB), 221, 225
SOB. *See* Shortness of breath
Social Health Maintenance Organization (SHMO), 156
Social isolation, 206
Social justice, 331
Social worker, 154
Sociocultural background, 254-255
Source, 106
Space, 254
    use of, 269
Special populations, 108-118
Speech therapist (ST), 154
Spiritual therapies, 186
ST. *See* Speech therapist
Standard of care, 138
STDs. *See* Sexually transmitted diseases
Stereotyping, 103
St. John's Wort, 179
Stomach cancer, Korean-American rates, 115
Stories
    format, 63
    imagery, 67
    incorporating into practice, 74-76
    never again, 70
    research regarding, 68-69
    rewriting, 72
    writing, 69-74
    writing for publication, 73-74
Storytellers, 66-68
Storytelling
    as art, 60

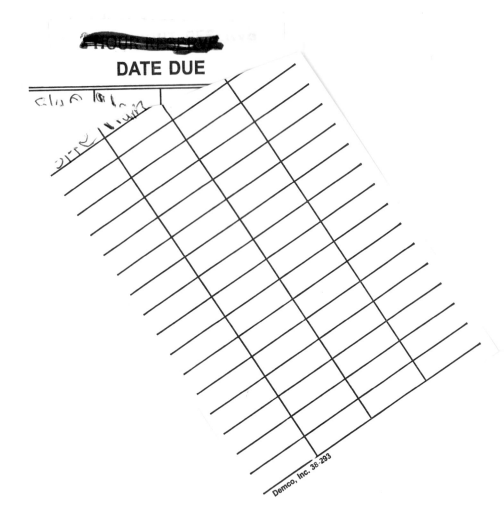

DATE DUE

Demco, Inc. 38-293